Health and Medical Geography

Health and Medical Geography

Edited by Caleb Coleman

hayle medical

New York

Hayle Medical,
750 Third Avenue, 9th Floor,
New York, NY 10017, USA

Visit us on the World Wide Web at:
www.haylemedical.com

ISBN: 978-1-63241-852-4

Cataloging-in-Publication Data

Health and medical geography / edited by Caleb Coleman.
    p. cm.
Includes bibliographical references and index.
ISBN 978-1-63241-852-4
1. Medical geography. 2. Health service areas. 3. Medical climatology.
4. Environmental health. I. Coleman, Caleb.
RA792 .H43 2020
614.42--dc21

Table of Contents

Preface..VII

Chapter 1   **Which environmental factors most strongly influence a street's appeal for bicycle transport among adults? A conjoint study using manipulated photographs**......1
Lieze Mertens, Delfien Van Dyck, Ariane Ghekiere, Ilse De Bourdeaudhuij, Benedicte Deforche, Nico Van de Weghe and Jelle Van Cauwenberg

Chapter 2   **Quantifying multi-dimensional attributes of human activities at various geographic scales based on smartphone tracking**......15
Xiaolu Zhou and Dongying Li

Chapter 3   **The relationship between ethnic composition of the residential environment and self-reported health among Turks and Moroccans**......28
Eleonore M. Veldhuizen, Umar Z. Ikram, Sjoerd de Vos and Anton E. Kunst

Chapter 4   **Using meta-quality to assess the utility of volunteered geographic information for science**......39
Shaun A. Langley, Joseph P. Messina and Nathan Moore

Chapter 5   **Factors related with public open space use among adolescents: a study using GPS and accelerometers**......50
Linde Van Hecke, Hannah Verhoeven, Peter Clarys, Delfien Van Dyck, Nico Van de Weghe, Tim Baert, Benedicte Deforche and Jelle Van Cauwenberg

Chapter 6   **A direct observation method for auditing large urban centers using stratified sampling, mobile GIS technology and virtual environments**......66
Sean J. V. Lafontaine, M. Sawada and Elizabeth Kristjansson

Chapter 7   **Evaluating neighborhood structures for modeling intercity diffusion of large-scale dengue epidemics**......81
Tzai-Hung Wen, Ching-Shun Hsu and Ming-Che Hu

Chapter 8   **Mapping outdoor habitat and abnormally small newborns to develop an ambient health hazard index**......96
Charlene C. Nielsen, Carl G. Amrhein, Alvaro R. Osornio-Vargas and the DoMiNO Team

Chapter 9   **Social and physical environmental correlates of independent mobility in children**......117
Isabel Marzi, Yolanda Demetriou and Anne Kerstin Reimers

Chapter 10   **Estimating the prevalence of 26 health-related indicators at neighbourhood level in the Netherlands using structured additive regression**......134
Jan van de Kassteele, Laurens Zwakhals, Oscar Breugelmans, Caroline Ameling and Carolien van den Brink

Chapter 11   **Determining the spatial heterogeneity underlying racial and ethnic differences in timely mammography screening**..**149**
Joseph Gibbons and Melody K. Schiaffino

Chapter 12   **Evaluation of geoimputation strategies in a large case study**...**161**
Naci Dilekli, Amanda E. Janitz, Janis E. Campbell and Kirsten M. de Beurs

Chapter 13   **Relative risk estimation of dengue disease at small spatial scale**...............................**174**
Daniel Adyro Martínez-Bello, Antonio López-Quílez and Alexander Torres Prieto

Chapter 14   **Influence of Pokémon Go on physical activity levels of university players**...**189**
Fiona Y. Wong

Chapter 15   **Current and future distribution of *Aedes aegypti* and *Aedes albopictus* (Diptera: Culicidae) in WHO Eastern Mediterranean Region**......................**201**
Els Ducheyne, Nhu Nguyen Tran Minh, Nabil Haddad, Ward Bryssinckx, Evans Buliva, Frédéric Simard, Mamunur Rahman Malik, Johannes Charlier, Valérie De Waele, Osama Mahmoud, Muhammad Mukhtar, Ali Bouattour, Abdulhafid Hussain, Guy Hendrickx and David Roiz

Chapter 16   **Where do people purchase food? A novel approach to investigating food purchasing locations** **214**
Lukar E. Thornton, David A. Crawford, Karen E. Lamb and Kylie Ball

Permissions

List of Contributors

Index

Preface

Every book is a source of knowledge and this one is no exception. The idea that led to the conceptualization of this book was the fact that the world is advancing rapidly; which makes it crucial to document the progress in every field. I am aware that a lot of data is already available, yet, there is a lot more to learn. Hence, I accepted the responsibility of editing this book and contributing my knowledge to the community.

The study of health, disease and healthcare approached from a geographical perspective constitutes the field of health and medical geography. The field is focused on the study of the geographies of disease and illness, through descriptive and analytic research. This involves quantifying disease frequencies and distributions as well as the study of the characteristics that make an individual or a population susceptible to disease. An important aspect of health geography is the geography of healthcare, particularly healthcare facility location, utilization and accessibility. All pertinent health risks such as natural disasters, stress, depression, interpersonal violence, etc. are assessed in medical geography. This book aims to shed light on some of the unexplored aspects of health and medical geography and the recent researches in this field. Different approaches, evaluations, methodologies and advanced studies on medical and health geography have been included herein. This book is an essential guide for both academicians and those who wish to pursue this discipline further.

While editing this book, I had multiple visions for it. Then I finally narrowed down to make every chapter a sole standing text explaining a particular topic, so that they can be used independently. However, the umbrella subject sinews them into a common theme. This makes the book a unique platform of knowledge.

I would like to give the major credit of this book to the experts from every corner of the world, who took the time to share their expertise with us. Also, I owe the completion of this book to the never-ending support of my family, who supported me throughout the project.

Editor

Which environmental factors most strongly influence a street's appeal for bicycle transport among adults? A conjoint study using manipulated photographs

Lieze Mertens[1] [iD], Delfien Van Dyck[1,2], Ariane Ghekiere[2,3,4], Ilse De Bourdeaudhuij[1*], Benedicte Deforche[3,4], Nico Van de Weghe[5] and Jelle Van Cauwenberg[2,3,4]

Abstract

Background: Micro-environmental factors (specific features within a streetscape), instead of macro-environmental factors (urban planning features), are more feasible to modify in existing neighborhoods and thus more practical to target for environmental interventions. Because it is often not possible to change the whole micro-environment at once, the current study aims to determine which micro-environmental factors should get the priority to target in physical environmental interventions increasing bicycle transport. Additionally, interaction effects among micro-environmental factors on the street's appeal for bicycle transport will be determined.

Methods: In total, 1950 middle-aged adults completed a web-based questionnaire consisting of a set of 12 randomly assigned choice tasks with manipulated photographs. Seven micro-environmental factors (type of cycle path, speed limit, speed bump, vegetation, evenness of the cycle path surface, general upkeep and traffic density) were manipulated in each photograph. Conjoint analysis was used to analyze the data.

Results: Providing streets with a cycle path separated from motorized traffic seems to be the best strategy to increase the street's appeal for adults' bicycle transport. If this adjustment is not practically feasible, micro-environmental factors related to safety (i.e. speed limit, traffic density) may be more effective in promoting bicycle transport than micro-environmental factors related to comfort (i.e. evenness of the cycle path surface) or aesthetic (i.e. vegetation, general upkeep). On the other hand, when a more separated cycle path is already provided, micro-environmental factors related to comfort or aesthetic appeared to become more prominent.

Conclusions: Findings obtained from this research could provide advice to physical environmental interventions about which environmental factors should get priority to modify in different environmental situations.

Trial registration: The study was approved by the Ethics Committee of the Ghent University Hospital. Trial registration: B670201318588. Registered at 04/10/2013. http://www.ugent.be/ge/nl/faculteit/raden/ec

Keywords: Active transport, Micro-environment, Built environment, Biking, Adulthood, Experiment, Photographs

Background

Although cycling is known as a sustainable form of human transport, it is not yet sufficiently integrated into daily life routines in the global population. In Europe, 50 % of all trips are shorter than 3 km, which is a feasible distance for cycling. However, a large part of these trips is still done by motorized modes of transport [1]. For example in Flanders (Belgium), only 25 % of all trips shorter than 3 km and only 14 % of all trips shorter than 5 km are done actively (i.e. by foot or by bike) among adults between 18 and 65 years old [2]. Several cross-sectional

*Correspondence: Ilse.Debourdeaudhuij@Ugent.be
[1] Department of Movement and Sport Sciences, Faculty of Medicine and Health Sciences, Ghent University, Watersportlaan 2, 9000 Ghent, Belgium
Full list of author information is available at the end of the article

studies among adults indicated that bicycle transport is associated with higher general physical activity levels and lower body weight [3–6]. In addition, bicycle transport also has many other benefits on social (social cohesion), environmental (reduced carbon footprint) and economic (infrastructure costs) level [7–14]. It is therefore in favor of both the individual and the community to create supportive environments that make it easier to engage in bicycle transport [15–18]. Policy development together with relevant sectors such as urban planning, active transport policies, built environment strategies and crime prevention polices should be encouraged at national and subnational level to promote regular bicycle transport by adapting the environment or community [19–24]. By modifying the environment, large populations over long periods of time can be reached. It is therefore important to know which environmental determinants affect bicycle transport among adults.

Built environmental variables can be classified into two broad categories: macro- and micro-scale environmental factors [25, 26]. Macro-environmental factors can be regarded as 'raw' urban planning features; such as walkability, connectivity of the street network, residential density and land use mix diversity. These factors are difficult to change in existing environments because of their large size and complexity, and because they are influenced by different levels of authorities [25, 26]. On the other hand, micro-environmental factors can be defined as relatively small environmental factors such as evenness of the cycle path surface, vegetation and speed limits. These factors are influenced by individuals or local actors and are less complex which makes them more feasible to modify in existing neighborhoods (i.e. lower cost and shorter timeframe) compared to the reconfiguration of the macroscale structural design [25, 26].

In the literature, most research has been conducted on macro-scale environmental factors. Worldwide, consistent strong positive relationships have been found between macro-scale environmental factors and transport-related cycling in adults. Higher levels of walkability, improved access to shops/services/work and higher degree of urbanization were positively related to bicycle transport in adults [27–30]. Unfortunately, research on the micro-environmental factors affecting bicycle transport is scarce and results are inconsistent [31–35]. Previous studies showed inconsistent associations between modifiable micro-environmental factors and bicycle transport [35–38]. For example, some studies found associations of lower road motorized traffic volumes [31] and the presence of traffic calming elements with more cycling for transport [39], while other studies found that higher volumes of motorized traffic were associated with more bicycle transport [36, 38], or found no associations

at all [37, 40, 41]. Mixed evidence was also found for aesthetics. Several studies found a positive association between vegetation and bicycle transport [29, 42–44], while other studies did not find significant associations [5, 40, 45]. Furthermore, although the importance of well separated cycle paths for bicycle transport have already been identified [21, 46], not all research could confirm this positive association [37, 47]. Furthermore, it is still unclear which micro-environmental factors relate most strongly to cycling for transport. Because it is often not possible to change the whole micro-environment at once, it is necessary to explore the individual impact of each parameter and to know which environmental factors should get priority in environmental interventions increasing bicycle transport. Furthermore, since the real environment consists of a combination of several environmental factors simultaneously, it is also crucial to investigate the interaction effects of different micro-environmental factors. For example, a previous pilot study (conducted in a small sample) [48] with manipulated photographs showed that the positive effect of cycle path evenness appeared to increase in an environment with good compared to poorly overall upkeep. Conversely, the street's appeal for bicycle transport decreased when both separations along the cycle path were present (i.e. separation from motorized traffic as well as pedestrians) compared to only a separation with traffic [48]. Furthermore, investigating the relative importance of environmental factors within a particular micro-environmental factor could be interesting for a detailed analysis of these interactions effects. For example, it would be interesting to find out which environmental factors subsequently are important in situations where an even cycle path surface is provided. Unfortunately, this has not frequently been studied in large populations. Therefore, future studies investigating the effect of micro-environmental factors and their interaction effects on the street's appeal for bicycle transport are important.

The main issue with previous studies investigating the effect of micro-environmental factors on bicycle transport is related to the cross-sectional observational study designs [34, 49]. Although usually valid and reliable tools are used (e.g. questionnaires), there are some methodological concerns: participants have to recall features of the physical environment, which involves recall bias [50] and the lack of standardization in neighborhood definitions increases the inconsistency as well [51]. To accommodate these shortcomings, stronger designs are required with improved causal inference [17, 30, 34, 52, 53]. Since natural experiments are complex, time- and cost-consuming to conduct in real environments, an innovative experimental and cost-effective methodology is required.

Therefore, the present study opts for a controlled experiment: it uses experimental manipulations of environmental factors in photographs to examine whether these factors affect the street's appeal for bicycle transport. The validity of color photos in comparison to on-site responses has already been proven in previous studies [54, 55]. Furthermore, respondents who judge photographs do not have to recall features of the physical environment (as is the case when using questionnaires), which improves the reliability of the results. In addition, defining the 'neighborhood' is no longer necessary with this methodology because the assessment of the physical environment happens consistently between participants. Since these photograph experiments control for co-variation (i.e. environmental factors that co-occur), this approach overpowers previous studies by allowing the researcher to differentiate the separate influence of each environmental factor under controlled conditions [55]. This methodology using manipulated photographs results from previous research with non-manipulated photographs [35] and was tested in a recent mixed-method pilot study investigating the effect of a limited number of key micro-environmental factors and the street's appeal for adults' bicycle transport [48]. In this study only five micro-environmental factors were simultaneously manipulated and each factor only had a maximum of two levels. This exploratory study, conducted in a small sample, provided a proof-of-concept to use manipulated photographs to assess a street's appeal for adults in a controlled experiment. From this previous research step, there is a need to carry out a large-scale study in which the effects of all relevant micro-environmental factors are studied. Findings obtained from these controlled experiments might provide guidelines for interventions that use micro-environmental modifications to create more supportive environments for bicycle transport. Only adults in the age range between 45 and 65 years old where included in this study because they assess the physical environment according to their own needs, rather than in perspective of their parental vision (considering their child).

In summary, this study adds to the literature as it is still unclear what type of infrastructure regarding the micro-environment is required to specifically encourage bicycle transport. Furthermore, the experimental design of our study overpowers previously used cross-sectional observational study designs and moreover is a cost-effective methodology compared to natural experiments. Additionally, one of the main novelties compared to existing literature is that the current study creates an order of importance or hierarchy of the different micro-environmental factors and also investigates interaction effects between different micro-environmental factors.

The main aim of the current study was to determine the relative importance of micro-environmental factors for a street's appeal for bicycle transport among middle-aged adults (45–65 years). Second, interaction effects among micro-environmental factors on the street's appeal for bicycle transport were determined to investigate the effect of combinations of micro-environmental factors.

Methods

Protocol and measures

By purposeful convenience sampling, Flemish middle-aged adults between 45 and 65 years were recruited using email, social media, family, friends, clubs, organizations and companies. Additional participants were recruited by snowball sampling. Participants completed a two-part web-based questionnaire, which was developed using Sawtooth Software (SSI Web version 8.3.8.). The online questionnaire was available from the beginning of November 2014 until the end of January 2015 and 1969 middle-aged adults completed the study. Eighteen participants who did not have the proper age (45–65 years old) were excluded from the analysis. Informed consent was automatically obtained from the participants when they voluntarily completed the questionnaire. The study was approved by the Ethics Committee of the Ghent University Hospital.

Photograph development

Prior to data collection, a set of 1945 manipulated panoramic color photographs were developed with Adobe Photoshop© software [56]. The developed photographs were all modified versions of one 'basic' panoramic photograph representing a typical semi-urban (300–600 inhabitants/km²) street in Flanders (Belgium) [57]. The 'basic' photograph was taken from an adult cyclist's eye-level viewpoint under dry weather conditions and depicts a hypothetical cycling route where adults could cycle along. The newly developed photographs differed from each other in at least one micro-environmental manipulation. Seven micro-environmental factors (type of cycle path, speed limit, speed bump, vegetation, evenness of the cycle path surface, general upkeep and traffic density) were manipulated in each photograph and consisted of at least two possible levels. The levels of the environmental factors are presented in Table 1 and the corresponding abbreviations are used throughout the article. These micro-environmental factors and their levels were selected based on existing literature [27, 58] and previous qualitative and quantitative research with (non-)manipulated panoramic photographs [35, 48, 59] studying relationships between the environment and bicycle transport. For example, a previous mixed-methods pilot study with manipulated photographs indicated that it is not inviting for bicycle transport

Table 1 Overview of the manipulated micro-environmental factors and their specific levels

Type of cycle path	C1. No cycle path
	C2. Cycle path, separated from traffic by marked white lines
	C3. Cycle path, separated from traffic with a curb, not separated from walking path by color
	C4. Cycle path separated from traffic with a hedge, not separated from walking path by color
	C5. Cycle path separated from traffic with a curb, separated from walking path by color
	C6. Cycle path separated from traffic with a hedge, separated from walking path by color
Speed limit	S1. 50 km/h
	S2. 30 km/h
Speed bump	B1. Absent
	B2. Present
Vegetation	V1. No trees
	V2. Two trees
	V3. Four trees
Evenness of the cycle path surface	E1. Very uneven surface
	E2. Moderately uneven surface
	E3. Even surface
General upkeep	M1. Bad upkeep (much graffiti and litter)
	M2. Moderate upkeep (a bit of graffiti and litter)
	M3. Good upkeep (no graffiti or litter)
Traffic density	D1. Four cars + truck
	D2. Three cars
	D3. One car

to separate the cycle path and the sidewalk by using bollards [48]. Qualitative data from that study reported that cyclists see these bollards as a disturbing factor that limited their evasive options and also showed that some were afraid to cycle against those bollards. However, from previous research from the Netherlands, Denmark and Germany, we know that it is important to provide a visual and/or physical separation between cyclists and pedestrians for example by grade separation, pavement coloring or surfacing [58]. From this reasoning, we wanted to investigate if a separation by pavement coloration has a more positive effect to separate cyclists from pedestrians instead of bollards as separation. To determine each micro-environmental factor and their levels, a thoughtful reasoning using the literature and previous results was made [27, 35, 48, 58, 59]. An example of the anticipated best and worst street to cycle along are shown in Fig. 1.

The web-based questionnaire

The web-based questionnaire consisted of two parts. First, socio-demographic characteristics were assessed: age, gender, country of birth, marital status, education, and occupational status (see Table 2 for the response categories). Self-reported weight and height were assessed to calculate body mass index (BMI). Additionally, the amount of usual bicycle transport in a week was assessed by using the long form of the International Physical Activity Questionnaire (IPAQ: 'usual week') [60].

In the second part of the questionnaire, a choice based conjoint (CBC) method was used to implement a series

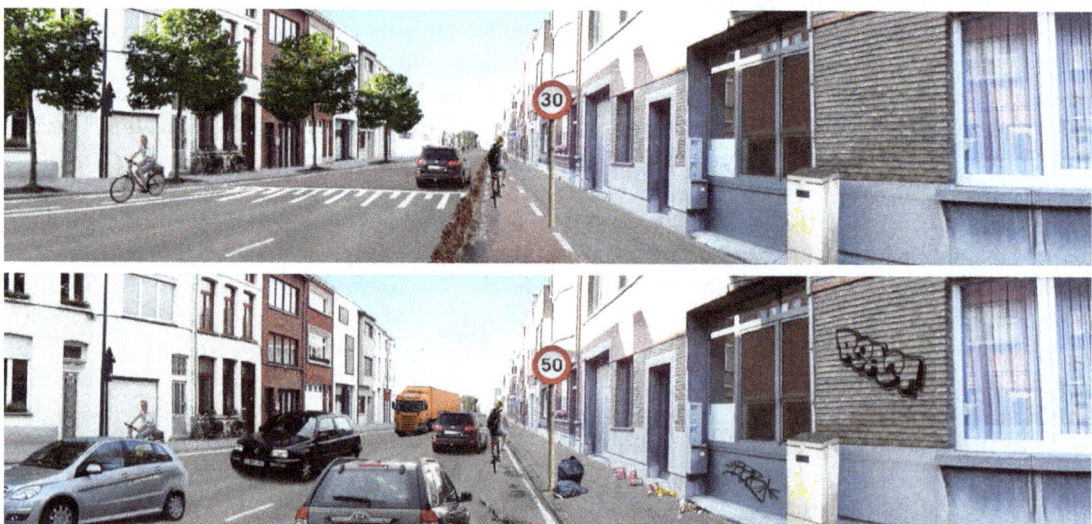

Fig. 1 The anticipated best and worst street to cycle along by manipulating the micro-environmental factors (Table 1). Anticipated best street to cycle along (first photograph): C6, S2, B2, V3, E3, M3, D3. Anticipated worst street to cycle along (second photograph): C1, S1, B1, V1, E1, M1, D1

of choice tasks with manipulated photographs, depicting two possible routes to cycle along. This CBC method is often used in marketing research and aims to identify the relative importance of various components of a product (micro-environmental factors in a street) in the decision process to pursuit the product (cycling for transport in that street) [61]. In this part, the following scenario was presented to the respondents: "Imagine yourself cycling to a friend's home, located at 10 min cycling from your home, during daytime with perfect weather circumstances. For every task you will see two streets, we ask you to choose the street that you find most appealing to cycle along to that friend. Whichever route you choose, the distance to your friend is the same and all cycle paths are one-way. There is no right or wrong solution, we are only interested in which street you would prefer to cycle along." Participants were first shown three examples and afterwards they received a set of 12 randomly assigned and two fixed choice tasks, which is a recommended quantity for such tasks [61, 62]. Figure 2 shows an example of a choice task. Since a full-profile design was used in the choice task, the two photographs in each randomly assigned choice task could differ in one to seven environmental factors [61]. The two fixed choice tasks were identical for all participants and were used to check if participants answered the choice tasks consistently. One respondent was deleted from the analysis as the response to both fixed tasks was not accurate in comparison with the other 1949 participants. We therefore believe that the respondent probably completed the questionnaire without attention.

Table 2 Descriptive characteristics of the participants (n = 1950)

Age (M ± SD) (years)	54.3 ± 5.6	Occupational status (%)	
Women (%)	56.8	Household	5.1
Born in Belgium (%)	96.3	Blue collar	5.3
Marital status (%)		White collar	67.9
Married	68.4	Unemployed	3.2
Widowed	1.6	Retired	17.5
Divorced	13.7	Career interruption	1.0
Single	7.6	Current bicycle transport level	
Cohabiting	8.6	No bicycle transport (%)	21.7
Education (%)		Bicycle transport min/wk (M ± SD)	147 ± 170
Primary	2.2	Living area	
Lower secondary	19.4	Urban (%)	15.4
Higher secondary	13.9	Suburban (%)	74.0
Tertiary	64.6	Rural (%)	10.6
BMI (M ± SD) (kg/m^2)	25.2 ± 4.0		

M mean, *SD* standard deviation, *BMI* body mass index

A priori power analysis (power 0.80 and α = 0.05) was calculated by the following formula: *nta/c > 500* (*n = number of participants; t = 14: number of choice tasks; a = 2: number of alternatives per task; c = 18: the largest product of levels of any two factors*) [61]. This showed that a minimum of 322 subjects was needed when manipulating seven environmental factors in one photograph (with a maximum of six levels) and presenting 14 choice tasks to each participant. It was intended to reach at least three times more this number to allow possibly subgroup analysis.

To assess test–retest reliability of the choice tasks, we conducted a pilot study (n = 28) in which 14 fixed choice tasks were added to the questionnaire. These fixed choice tasks were identical for all participants. The same choice tasks were presented to the participants twice with a 1-week interval. Subsequently, it was examined whether participants chose the same street at both time points. The percentage of agreement for the 14 choice tasks ranged from 72 to 100 % (n = 28). These results indicated that our choice tasks are reliable, since an adequate level of agreement is generally considered to be 70 % [63].

Analyses

Choice-based conjoint analysis (CBC) was used to analyze the data. First, the average relative importance of each environmental factor was calculated from the individual utility data gained from Hierarchical Bayes (HB) estimation using dummy coding. This analysis method has been suggested as the most appropriate method to analyze data gained from choice based conjoint [64]. Average relative importances indicate the influence of an environmental factor on the choice relating to the photograph choice task. These average importances are calculated by the difference in average part-worth utilities between the most and least preferred levels of a factor [61]. Average part-worth utilities represent the degree of preference given to a particular level of an environmental factor and are similar to a beta-value (β) obtained from linear regression analyses [61]. The greater the importance of an environmental factor, the greater the factor has an impact on the choice.

Second, the main effect of each level of each environmental factor on the street's appeal for bicycle transport along the depicted environments was determined using the individual part-worth utilities gained from HB estimation. Average part-worth utilities were calculated and 95 % confidence intervals were determined to compare these part-worth utilities representing the degree of preference for the environmental factor level [61].

Third, interaction effects were also derived from part-worth utilities gained from the HB estimation and were selected using 'CBC interaction search tool'

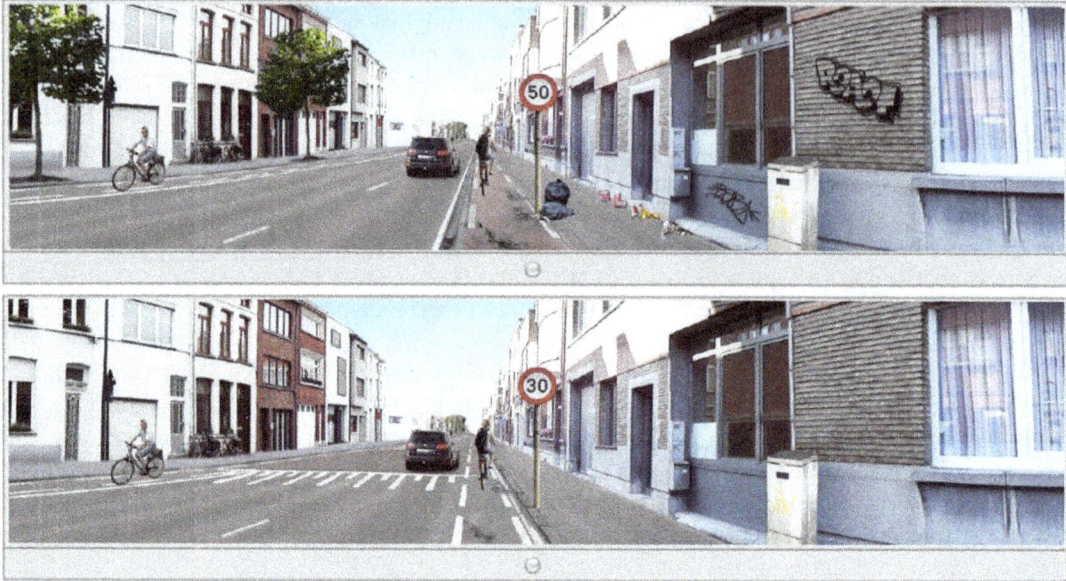

Fig. 2 An example of a randomly assigned choice task used in the questionnaire

of the Sawtooth Software [65]. Separate models were constructed to analyze the interaction effects between different micro-environmental factors. These results were illustrated by graphs and tables in which the total utilities of the different streets were shown. Total utilities were calculated by the sum of the part-worth utilities and representing the degree of preference given to a photograph or for the environmental factors depicted in a street. A 95 % confidence interval was calculated to examine significance.

Last, given that different interaction effects were found with type of cycle path and that this factor is obvious most prominent, the relative importance of all other micro-environmental factors was calculated within each type of cycle path.

Results

Descriptive statistics

The sample consisted of 1950 participants ranging in age from 45 to 65 years: 56.8 % were women, 77.0 % were married or cohabiting, 64.6 % had followed tertiary education (college, university or postgraduate) and 17.5 % was retired (see Table 2). Mean age of the total sample was 54.3 years (SD = 5.6) and mean BMI was 25.2 kg/m^2 (SD = 4.0). Approximately one fifth (21.7 %) of the adults did not cycle for transport in a usual week and the mean

of the entire sample was 147 ± 170 min per week bicycle transport in a usual week.

Relative importance of the micro-environmental factors

'Type of cycle path' (average importance $= 60.14 \pm 14.04$ %; 95 % CI 59.48, 60.81) was by far the most important micro-environmental factor when choosing one out of two streets for bicycle transport (see Fig. 3). The second most important environmental factor was 'speed limit' (average importance $= 8.50 \pm 5.65$ %; 95 % CI 8.25, 8.75) followed by 'evenness of the cycle path surface' (average importance $= 7.76 \pm 5.47$ %; 95 % CI 7.52, 8.00). These factors were chosen over 'traffic density' (average importance $= 7.14 \pm 6.55$ %; 95 % CI 6.85, 7.43), 'general upkeep' (average importance $= 7.11 \pm 5.53$ %; 95 % CI 6.87, 7.36) and 'vegetation' (average importance $= 6.96 \pm 5.17$ %; 95 % CI 6.73, 7.19) which did not significantly differ from each other. The presence of a 'speed bump' (average importance $= 2.38 \pm 1.86$ %; 95 % CI 2.30, 2.47) was significantly less important than any other micro-environmental factor.

Main effects of the environmental factors

Within each micro-environmental factor, all part-worth utilities from the different levels of each environmental factor significantly differed from each other (p < 0.05), with

Relative average importance of micro-evironmental factors

Type of cycle path
Speed limitation
Cycle path evenness
Traffic density
Maintenance
Vegetation
Speed bump

Average importance (%)

Fig. 3 Relative importance of the micro-environmental factors

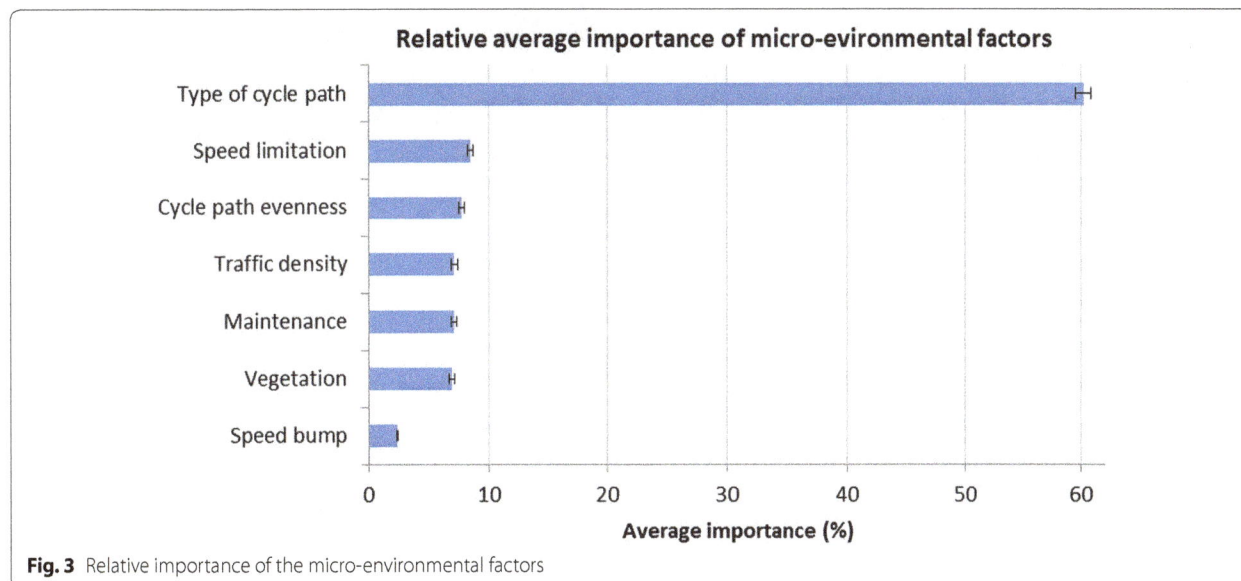

obvious preferences for the anticipated most attractive level over the intermediate and the anticipated unattractive level (see Fig. 4). For example, participants preferred an even cycle path surface (average part-worth utility = 1.90 ± 1.40; 95 % CI 1.84, 1.96) over a slightly uneven (average part-worth utility = 0.47 ± 1.04; 95 % CI 0.43, 0.52) and a very uneven cycle path surface (reference level); and they preferred a slightly uneven cycle path over a very uneven cycle path surface. One notable result was found for 'type of cycle path'. A cycle path separated from traffic with a hedge and not separated from walking path by color was significantly more preferred (C4: average part-worth utility = 16.75 ± 3.64; 95 % CI 16.59, 16.91) than a cycle path separated from traffic with a curb and separated from walking path by color (C5: average part-worth utility = 13.18 ± 5.22; 95 % CI 12.95, 13.42). See Fig. 5 for an illustration of the different types of cycle paths manipulated in this study.

Interaction effects

The combination of all possible interaction effects gave 21 possible interaction effects of which six were significant, namely 'type of cycle path × speed limit', 'type of cycle path × vegetation', 'type of cycle path × evenness of the cycle path surface', 'type of cycle path × traffic density', 'speed bump × traffic density', 'vegetation × general upkeep'. The results of these interaction effects were illustrated by graphs and tables in which the total utilities of the different streets were shown. Total utilities represent the degree of preference and can be found in Additional files 1, 2, 3, 4, 5, 6.

The significant interaction effect between 'type of cycle path' and 'speed limit' (Chi square = 16.87; p = 0.005)

shows that the effect of speed limit has the greatest impact on the street's appeal for bicycle transport when there was no cycle path (C1) (see Fig. 6; Table A.1 in Additional file 1). Adjusting the speed limit from 50 to 30 km/h along all different cycle paths had a significant effect, except for the most preferred cycle path. The effect of speed limit did not provide a significant increase on the street's appeal for bicycle transport when the cycle path was separated from traffic with a hedge and separated from walking path by color (C6).

The significant interaction effect between 'type of cycle path' and 'vegetation' (Chi square = 27.78; p = 0.002) shows that the effect of vegetation was significant in all different types of cycle paths (see Additional file 2). The direction of the effects did not differ, only the magnitude of the effect did. For instance, the greatest effect of vegetation (from zero to four trees) was found when there was no cycle path provided on the street, compared to all types of cycle path.

Similar results were found for the interaction effect between 'type of cycle path' and 'traffic density' (Chi square = 19.01; p < 0.001). The effect of traffic density was significant for all different types of cycle paths in the expected direction, only the strength of the effect differed across the different cycle paths (see Additional file 3). The greatest effect of traffic density on the street's appeal for bicycle transport was found when there was no cycle path.

The significant interaction effect between 'type of cycle path' and 'evenness of the cycle path surface' (Chi square = 44.94; p = 0.040) showed that the greatest effect of evenness of the cycle path surface (from very uneven or moderately uneven to an even cycle path surface) was

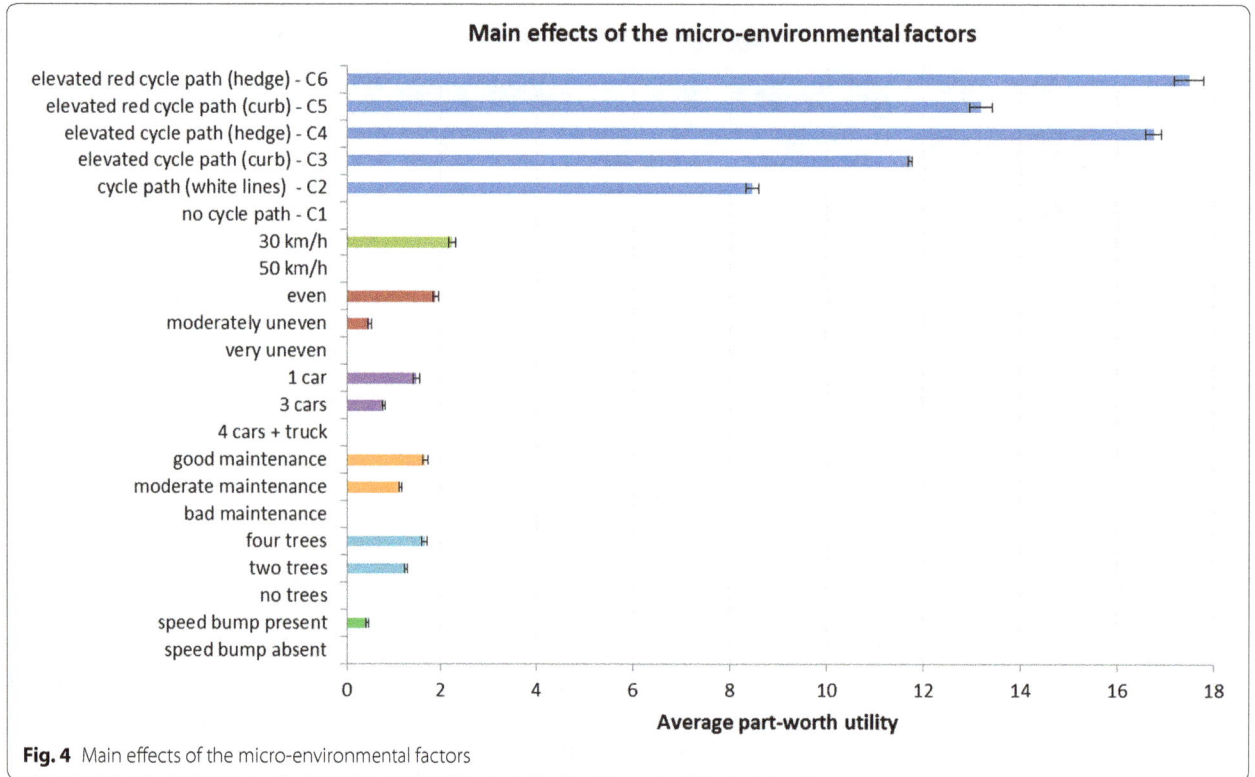

Fig. 4 Main effects of the micro-environmental factors

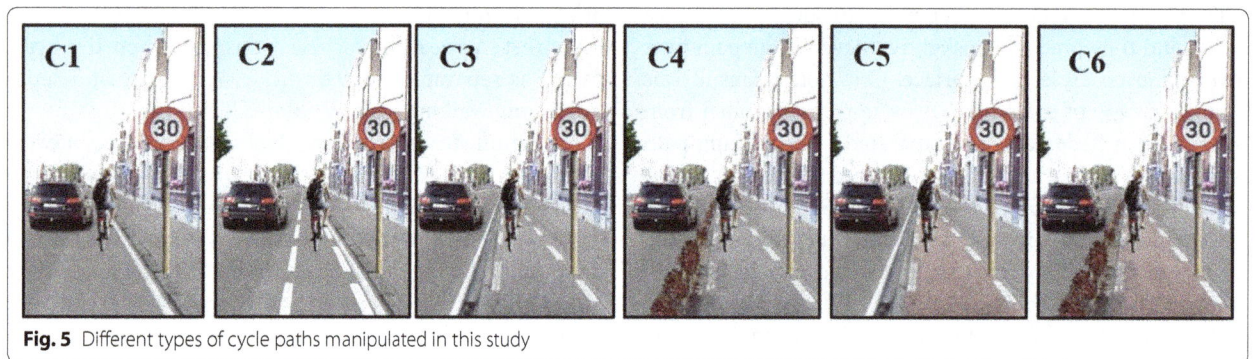

Fig. 5 Different types of cycle paths manipulated in this study

found with cycle paths where a separation with motorized traffic by a curb is provided (see Additional file 4). The greatest effects from a very uneven to an even cycle path surface on the street's appeal for bicycle transport was found with a cycle path separated from traffic with a curb and separated from walking path by color (C5). Additionally, the greatest effect of evenness from a moderately uneven to an even cycle path surface on the street's appeal was found with a cycle path separated from traffic with a curb and not separated from walking path by color (C3).

There was also a significant interaction effect between 'speed bump' and 'traffic density' (Chi square = 9.71;

$p = 0.008$). The effect of a speed bump (installing a speed bump on the street) on the street's appeal for bicycle transport, was greater when the traffic density was lower (reducing the number of cars to the intermediate or lowest level) (see Additional file 5).

Finally, the significant interaction effect between 'vegetation' and 'general upkeep' (Chi square = 10.19; $p = 0.040$) showed that depending on the number of trees another effect of general upkeep was found (see Additional file 6). The effect of general upkeep from moderate to good upkeep was greater if there were no trees present in the environment. The effect of general upkeep from bad to good upkeep was greater in an environment

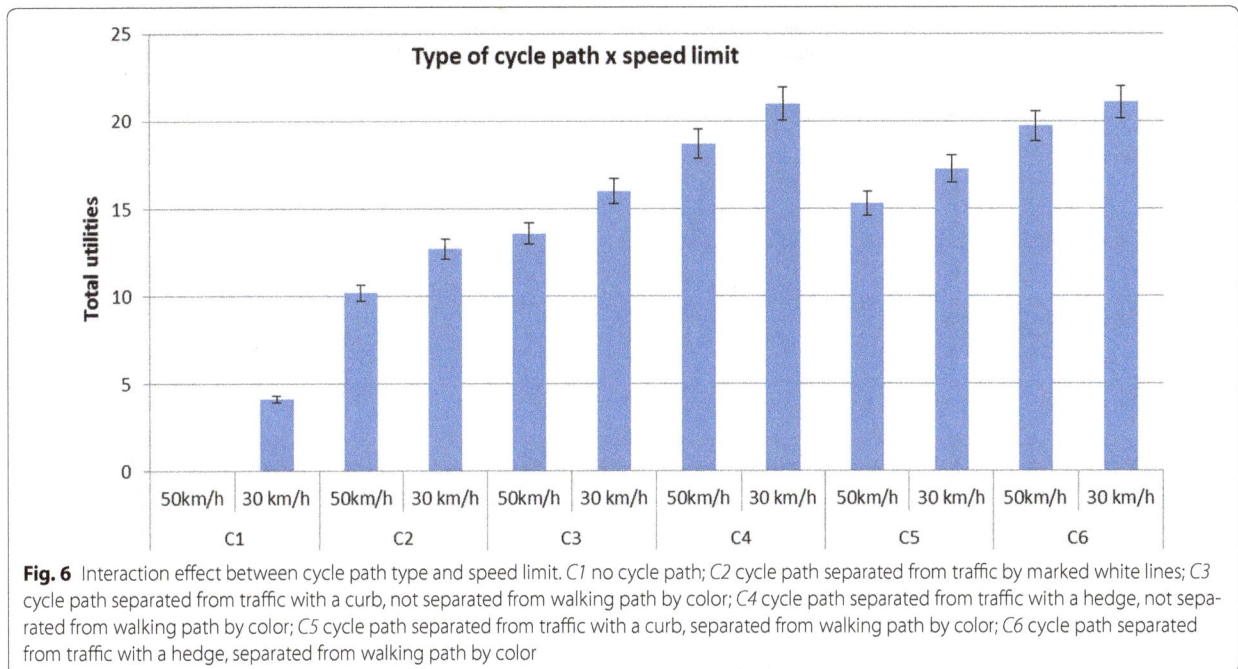

Fig. 6 Interaction effect between cycle path type and speed limit. *C1* no cycle path; *C2* cycle path separated from traffic by marked white lines; *C3* cycle path separated from traffic with a curb, not separated from walking path by color; *C4* cycle path separated from traffic with a hedge, not separated from walking path by color; *C5* cycle path separated from traffic with a curb, separated from walking path by color; *C6* cycle path separated from traffic with a hedge, separated from walking path by color

with two trees and the effect between bad and moderate upkeep was greater in an environment with four trees.

Relative importance of the micro-environmental factors within different cycle paths

Given that several interaction effects were found with 'cycle path type' and it appeared to be by far the most important micro-environmental factor in making choices among different street alternatives, the relative importance of all other environmental factors within each type of cycle path was defined. It is useful to determine which priority must be given in adapting the environment if a community does not have the ability to build a desired cycle path.

In Fig. 7, the relative importance of the remaining six environmental factors is presented for each type of cycle path. The results showed that modifying the speed limit was the most important environmental factor in situations where there was no cycle path (C1), no elevated cycle path (C2) or no cycle path with separations at both sides (C3 and C4). When there was no cycle path present in the environment (C1), the effect of speed limit (average part-worth utility = 23.97 ± 10.96 %; 95 % CI 23.48, 24.45) and traffic density (average part-worth utility = 21.46 ± 9.75 %; 95 % CI 21.03, 21.89) created the largest impact on the street's appeal for bicycle transport. Furthermore, with increasing separation (going from C1 to C6), speed limit appeared to become less important. In situations where the most preferred type of cycle path was already present (C6: elevated cycle

path, separated from motorized traffic with a hedge and separated from the walking path by color), the first three micro-environmental factors did not significantly differ from each other: traffic density (average part-worth utility = 20.87 ± 9.93 %; 95 % CI 20.43, 21.31), evenness of the cycle path surface (average part-worth utility = 20.61 ± 9.98 %; 95 % CI 20.17, 21.05) and general upkeep (average part-worth utility = 20.01 ± 9.77 %; 95 % CI 19.58, 20.44). Moreover, the effect of speed limit was significantly lower when the most preferred cycle path was present (C6) compared to situations when less preferred cycle paths were present.

Discussion

We identified the micro-environmental factors that should get priority when adapting the micro-environment to increase the street's appeal for middle-aged adults' bicycle transport. In addition, we investigated the interaction effects between different micro-environmental factors. The current study proved that the 'type of the cycle path' appeared to be the most important micro-environmental factor affecting the street's appeal for adults' bicycle transport under optimal conditions in terms of trip length and trip objective. A cycle path separated from traffic with a hedge was significantly more preferred than a cycle path separated from traffic with a curb, regardless of the separation from walking path by color. Previous research already showed a positive outcome of having a good separation between cyclists and motorized traffic on bicycle transport but did not focus

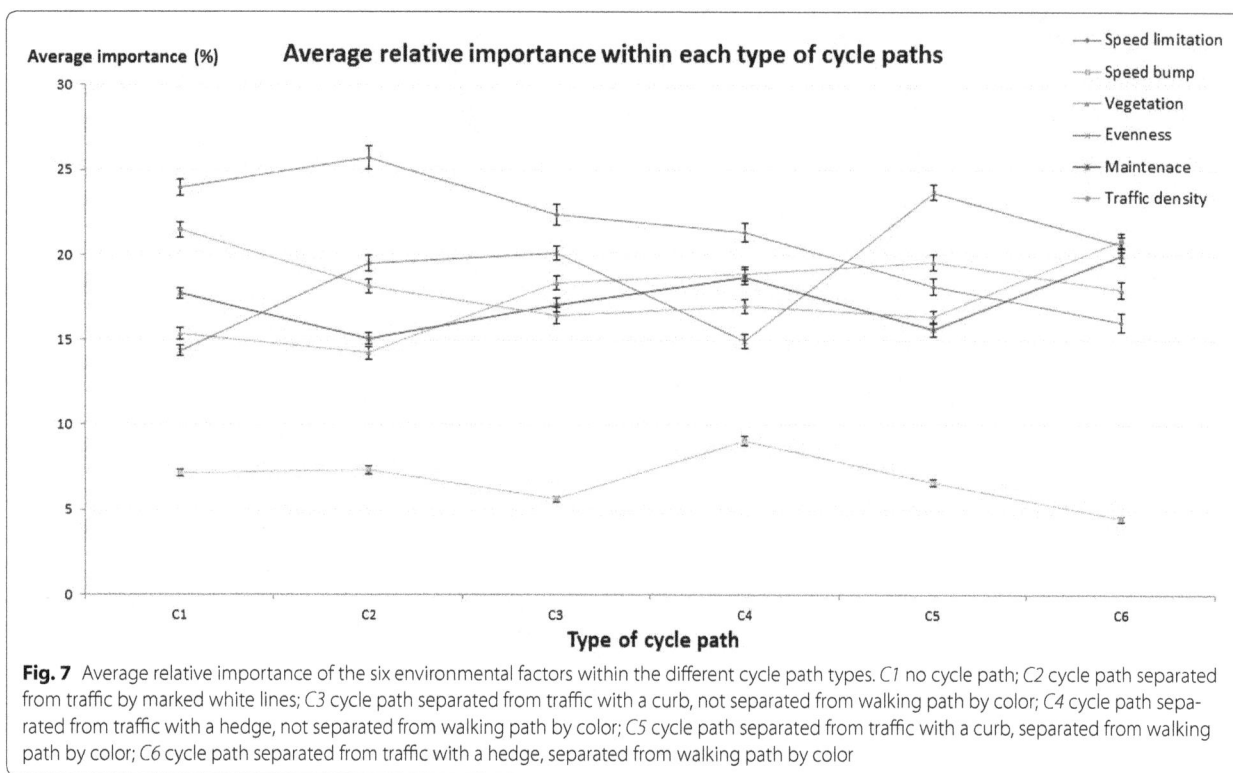

Fig. 7 Average relative importance of the six environmental factors within the different cycle path types. *C1* no cycle path; *C2* cycle path separated from traffic by marked white lines; *C3* cycle path separated from traffic with a curb, not separated from walking path by color; *C4* cycle path separated from traffic with a hedge, not separated from walking path by color; *C5* cycle path separated from traffic with a curb, separated from walking path by color; *C6* cycle path separated from traffic with a hedge, separated from walking path by color

on the relative importance of different types of 'separations' [49, 66, 67]. One of these studies indicated that research should also focus on the different designs to separate cyclists from cars [67]. The present study presented an initial possibility to investigate different gradation levels for possible separation between motorized traffic and cycle path (i.e. marked white lines—curb—hedge). A remarkable result in the present study was the large effect on the street's appeal of the most preferred type of separation, a small hedge. As a small hedge will not provide complete protection for cyclists from cars, it will merely be the perception of a separation that apparently makes them feel safer. Increased traffic safety or only the perception of it will be of great importance. This corresponds to recent findings, indicating that implementing measures to improve cyclists' safety from cars could increase cycling [66]. The current study showed that adapting the cycle path should get priority over other micro-environmental factors, such as speed limit, speed bump, vegetation, evenness of the cycle path surface and general upkeep. Even when it is not possible to actually separate cyclists from motorized traffic with a hedge, the presence of a curb or an indication by marked white lines may stimulate bicycle transport. An additional separation between cycle path and walking path by color will increase the street's appeal even more, but much less

pronounced in comparison with the benefit obtained by a suitable separation with motorized traffic.

Changing the type of cycle path might not be possible in all situations (e.g. financial or space constraints). Therefore, we also investigated the relative importance of the environmental factors within each type of cycle path which has not been studied previously. When there are no possibilities to provide a separation between cycle path and motorized traffic, adjusting the speed of the traffic from 50 km/h to 30 km/h may ensure an increase in the street's appeal for bicycle transport. Furthermore, traffic density was found to be the second most important environmental factor to adapt when there is no cycle path in the street. Similar results were found for the interaction effects; decreasing the traffic speed or traffic density has a larger effect on the street's appeal for bicycle transport when there is no cycle path provided in the street compared to situations where other cycle paths are present. On the other hand, modifying the speed limit from 50 to 30 km/h has no additional effect on the street's appeal when the most preferred cycle path is present. These results indicate that in situations where there is no cycle path provided, micro-environmental factors associated to traffic-related safety appear to be most prominent. These findings should be communicated to policies at national and subnational level encouraging bicycle transport. The first priority when executing environmental interventions is the provision of a cycle path. If this adjustment is not practically feasible, micro-environmental factors related to safety (i.e., speed limit, traffic density) may be more effective in promoting bicycle transport than micro-environmental factors related to comfort (i.e. evenness of the cycle path surface) or aesthetic (i.e. vegetation, general upkeep). The importance of traffic safety regarding bicycle transport has also been mentioned in the literature [10, 49, 67]. The study of Fraser and Lock [49] noticed that when we want to create safe environments, we need to improve our research on the built environment prioritizing the needs of cyclists, including the evaluation of both rates of physical activity and road injury [49].

Furthermore, when a more separated cycle path (going from C1 to C6) is provided, micro-environmental factors related to comfort (i.e. evenness of the cycle path surface) or aesthetic (i.e. vegetation, general upkeep) appeared to become more important. For example, the effect of evenness obtained from the interaction analysis showed that increasing the evenness of the cycle path surface has the greatest effect on the street's appeal when a cycle path is separated from traffic with a curb. Improving the evenness of the cycle path surface could increase the street's appeal for bicycle transport even more when there is already a separation by means of a curb present. Moreover, when the most preferred cycle path is present (separated from traffic with a hedge and separated from walking path by color), the relative importance of the other environmental factors became more similar. In this situation, it does not matter which of the three micro-environmental factors ('traffic density', 'evenness of the cycle path surface' or 'general upkeep') will be modified first. They may achieve the same effect on bicycle transport because these factors did not significantly differ in importance from each other.

The effect of vegetation (from the lowest or intermediate to the anticipated most attractive level) on the street's appeal for bicycle transport was the greatest when there was no cycle path provided in the street. But on the other hand, we also know that when there is no cycle path provided, other micro-environmental factors turn out to be more important than vegetation. Nevertheless, the presence of vegetation may contribute to the street's appeal as second important factor in situations with a cycle path separated from traffic with a hedge (C4) or a cycle path separated from traffic with a curb and separated from walking path by color (C5).

Although, speed bump is the least preferred micro-environmental factor of all seven, the effect of the presence of a speed bump can be enhanced by reducing traffic density. Providing the street of a speed bump should not get priority over the other environmental factors, but a recommendation

to the transport policies could be that adapting both factors together (speed bump and traffic density) is better than just focusing on installing a speed bump. A possible explanation for this effect could be found with the help of qualitative data from a recent mixed-method study [48], in which participants argued that the presence of a speed bump indirectly shows that many cars drive in the street.

The main strength of the current study was the used methodology (i.e. the choice based conjoint method using manipulated photographs) to answer the research questions. In real life, when people choose a route to cycle along to go to a place, they have to choose between combinations of factors. For example, people could make a decision by considering multiple factors such as limited speed of the cars, an even cycle path, some green along the route. Therefore, it is important to identify which factors are more important than others in such complex decisional contexts in order to understand how to create more encouraging cycling environments. The CBC method using manipulated photographs could identify the relative importance of micro-environmental factors in a street's appeal to cycle for transport [61]. This methodology allows studying the effects of environmental changes (manipulations) under controlled conditions, i.e. controlling the variation within and between the manipulated micro-environmental factors. The controlled manipulations of micro-environmental factors in the photographs are a cost-effective approach and could be used to experimentally find out which factors affect a street's appeal for bicycle transport under optimal conditions in terms of trip length and trip objective. Findings obtained from this study could provide practical guidelines for environmental interventions focusing on adapting micro-environmental factors to create more supportive environments for bicycle transport. From a previous study we know that these findings are not only valid for the street context depicted in the photographs of current study (i.e. a typical street environment in a semi-urban (300–600 inhabitants/km^2) Belgian municipality [57]), but most likely also for other street contexts (i.e. an environment with low building density and single land use or an environment with high building density and mixed land use) [59]. To our knowledge, this is the first study that creates an order of importance or hierarchy of the different micro-environmental factors. Furthermore, also interaction effects between different environmental factors were examined. Finally, by disseminating the research through the web, a very large sample was reached. However, this method also involved some disadvantages. Participants with a tertiary education (64.6 %) and a white collar occupation status (67.9 %) were over-represented in our study compared with the statistics of the Flemish population [68]; where 28.1 %

has a tertiary degree and the majority of the adults has a blue collar occupation. With our research, we have reached mainly highly educated people. Future research needs to establish whether these findings can be generalized to the entire Flemish population of mid-aged adults. Another limitation of current study is the two-dimensional character or the lack of movement/noise in the photograph environments. This can be overcome by using three-dimensional methods like manipulating computer-generated virtual walkthrough environments [69]. Nevertheless, using such methods is very expensive and only small samples can be reached. Finally, the most important weakness is that the current study did not assess effects on actual cycling behavior, but only on the street's appeal for bicycle transport. Consequently, these findings need to be confirmed by on-site research.

Some suggestions for future research can be made. A first suggestion is to compare our findings with results of other age groups. In the current study, only middle-aged adults between 45 and 65 years old were included to assess the viewpoint of the adult population. Besides this, also the viewpoint of younger adults assessing the environment in the perspective of their child is an important contributor as well as the viewpoint of older adults. Since, interventions targeting the built environment to encourage active transport, can reach a large proportion of the population [15], it is important to determine whether the same micro-environmental factors are important for different age-groups. Secondly, the current study fixed both trip objective and trip length. It would be interesting for future research to investigate the role of these environmental factors in relation to the preferred cycling route. Thirdly, integrating the role of socio-environmental factors (e.g. neighborhood safety) might enrich future studies' inputs and results. Finally, future research should also investigate the moderating effects of socio-demographics, psychosocial correlates and bicycle use on the relationship between the micro-environment and bicycle transport.

Conclusions

To our knowledge, this is the first study that creates an order of importance or hierarchy of relevant micro-environmental factors. Furthermore, also interaction effects between different environmental factors were examined as well as the relative importance of environmental factors within a particular micro-environmental factor. Providing streets with a cycle path separated from motorized traffic seems to be the best strategy to increase the street's appeal for adults' bicycle transport. A cycle path marked by white lines can already contribute to this, but a separation between cycle path and motorized traffic by means of a curb or a hedge appeared to be preferred. An additional separation with the walking path by color would

increase the street's appeal for bicycle transport even more. If this adjustment is not practically feasible, micro-environmental factors related to safety (i.e., speed limit, traffic density) may be more effective in promoting bicycle transport than micro-environmental factors related to comfort (i.e. evenness of the cycle path surface) or aesthetic (i.e. vegetation, general upkeep). Furthermore, when a more separated cycle path is provided, micro-environmental factors related to comfort (i.e. evenness of the cycle path surface) or aesthetic (i.e. vegetation, general upkeep) appeared to increase in importance. Findings obtained from this research could provide advice to physical environmental interventions about which environmental factors should get priority to modify in different environmental situations.

Additional files

Additional file 1. Interaction effect between cycle path type and speed limit.

Additional file 2. Interaction effect between cycle path type and vegetation.

Additional file 3. Interaction effect between cycle path type and traffic density.

Additional file 4. Interaction effect between cycle path type and evenness.

Additional file 5. Interaction effect between speed bump and traffic density.

Additional file 6. Interaction effect between vegetation and general upkeep.

Abbreviations
C1: no cycle path; C2: cycle path, separated from traffic by marked white lines; C3: cycle path, separated from traffic with a curb, not separated from walking path by color; C4: cycle path separated from traffic with a hedge, not separated from walking path by color; C5: cycle path separated from traffic with a curb, separated from walking path by color; C6: cycle path separated from traffic with a hedge, separated from walking path by color.

Authors' contributions
LM, AG and JVC developed the photograph material and research protocol, in correspondence with NVdW, DVD, BD and IDB. LM, AG and JVC conducted the data collection. LM performed the data analysis and drafted the manuscript, supervised by DVD and JVC. All other co-authors critically reviewed and revised versions of the manuscript. All authors read and approved the final manuscript.

Author details
[1] Department of Movement and Sport Sciences, Faculty of Medicine and Health Sciences, Ghent University, Watersportlaan 2, 9000 Ghent, Belgium. [2] Research Foundation Flanders (FWO), Egmontstraat 5, 1000 Brussels, Belgium. [3] Department of Public Health, Faculty of Medicine and Health Sciences,

Ghent University, De Pintelaan 185, 4k3, 9000 Ghent, Belgium.   Department of Human Biometry and Biomechanics, Faculty of Physical Education and Physical Therapy, Vrije Universiteit Brussel, Pleinlaan 2, 1050 Brussels, Belgium. [5] Department of Geography, Faculty of Sciences, Ghent University, Krijgslaan 281, S8, 9000 Ghent, Belgium.

Acknowledgements
The authors would like to thank Daphne Reinehr for developing the photographs.

Competing interests
The authors declare that they have no competing interests.

Funding
AG (Grant Number: GA11111N), JVC (Grant Number: 11NO313N), and DVD (Grant Number: FWO12/PDO/158) are supported by a Grant from the Fund for Scientific Research Flanders (FWO).

References
1. Rudinger G, Donaghy K, Poppelreuter S. Societal trends, mobility behaviour and sustainable transport in Europe and North America. Eur J Transp Infrastruct Res. 2006;6(1):61–76.
2. Vlaamse overheid Departement Mobiliteit en Openbare Werken. Onderzoek Verplaatsingsgedrag Vlaanderen 4. Brussel.
3. Wanner M, Götschi T, Martin-Diener E, Kahlmeier S, Martin BW. Active transport, physical activity, and body weight in adults: a systematic review. Am J Prev Med. 2012;42:493–502.
4. World Health Organization. Global Recommendations on Physical Activity for Health. 2010. p. 1–60. http://apps.who.int/iris/bitstream/10665/44399/1/9789241599979_eng.pdf. Accessed 25 Aug 2016.
5. Oja P, Titze S, Bauman A, de Geus B, Krenn P, Reger-Nash B, Kohlberger T. Health benefits of cycling: a systematic review. Scand J Med Sci Sports. 2011;21:496–509.
6. Kelly P, Kahlmeier S, Götschi T, Orsini N, Richards J, Roberts N, Scarborough P, Foster C. Systematic review and meta-analysis of reduction in all-cause mortality from walking and cycling and shape of dose response relationship. Int J Behav Nutr Phys Act. 2014;11:132.
7. Rissel CE. Active travel: a climate change mitigation strategy with co-benefits for health. N S W Public Health Bull. 2009;20:10–3.
8. Woodcock J, Edwards P, Tonne C, Armstrong BG, Ashiru O, Banister D, Beevers S, Chalabi Z, Chowdhury Z, Cohen A, Franco OH, Haines A, Hickman R, Lindsay G, Mittal I, Mohan D, Tiwari G, Woodward A, Roberts I. Public health benefits of strategies to reduce greenhouse-gas emissions: urban land transport. Lancet. 2009;374:1930–43.
9. Departement of Health, Physical Activity. Health improvement and prevention: at least five a week. 2004. p. 1–128. http://www.bhfactive.org.uk/sites/Exercise-Referral-Toolkit/downloads/resources/cmos-report-at-least-five-a-week.pdf. Accessed 25 Aug 2016.
10. Pucher J, Buehler R, Bassett DR, Dannenberg AL. Walking and cycling to health: a comparative analysis of city, state, and international data. Am J Public Health. 2010;100:1986–92.
11. Rabl A, de Nazelle A. Benefits of shift from car to active transport. Transp Policy. 2012;19:121–31.
12. Active Transport. https://secure.ausport.gov.au/clearinghouse/knowledge_base/organised_sport/sport_and_government_policy_objectives/active_transport.
13. de Hartog JJ, Boogaard H, Nijland H, Hoek G. Do the health benefits of cycling outweigh the risks? Environ Health Perspect. 2010;118:1109–16.
14. Rojas-Rueda D, de Nazelle A, Tainio M, Nieuwenhuijsen MJ. The health risks and benefits of cycling in urban environments compared with car use: health impact assessment study. BMJ. 2011;343:d4521.
15. World Health Organization. Interventions on diet and physical activity: what works (summary report). 2009. p. 1–48. http://www.who.int/diet-physicalactivity/summary-report-09.pdf. Accessed 25 Aug 2016.
16. Vandenbulcke G, Thomas I, de Geus B, Degraeuwe B, Torfs R, Meeusen R, Panis LI. Mapping bicycle use and the risk of accidents for commuters who cycle to work in Belgium. Transp Policy. 2009;16:77–87.
17. Jongeneel-Grimen B, Busschers W, Droomers M, van Oers HA, Stronks K, Kunst AE. Change in neighborhood traffic safety: does it matter in terms of physical activity? PLoS ONE. 2013;8:e62525.
18. Sallis JF, Cervero RB, Ascher W, Henderson KA, Kraft MK, Kerr J. An ecological approach to creating active living communities. Annu Rev Public Health. 2006;27:297–322.
19. Gaffron P. The implementation of walking and cycling policies in British local authorities. Transp Policy. 2003;10:235–44.
20. Pucher J, Dill J, Handy S. Infrastructure, programs, and policies to increase bicycling: an international review. Prev Med. 2010;50(Suppl 1):S106–25.
21. Buehler R, Pucher J. Walking and cycling in Western Europe and the United States. TR NEWS (280) 2012.
22. Commission of the European Communities. GREEN PAPER towards a new culture for urban mobility. Commission of the European Communities: Brussels; 2007.
23. World Health Organization. Global Status report on noncommunicable diseases. 2014. p. 1–302. http://apps.who.int/iris/bitstream/10665/148114/1/9789241564854_eng.pdf. Accessed 25 Aug 2016.
24. Pucher J, Buehler R. Cycling for everyone: lessons from Europe. J Transp Res Board. 2007;2074:58–65.
25. Swinburn B, Egger G, Raza F. Dissecting obesogenic environments: the development and application of a framework for identifying and prioritizing environmental interventions for obesity. Prev Med. 1999;29(6):563–70.
26. Cain KL, Millstein RA, Sallis JF, Conway TL, Gavand KA, Frank LD, Saelens BE, Geremia CM, Chapman J, Adams MA, Glanz K, King AC. Contribution of streetscape audits to explanation of physical activity in four age groups based on the Microscale Audit of Pedestrian Streetscapes (MAPS). Soc Sci Med (1982). 2014;116:82–92.
27. Van Holle V, Deforche B, Van Cauwenberg J, Goubert L, Maes L, Van de Weghe N, De Bourdeaudhuij I. Relationship between the physical environment and different domains of physical activity in European adults: a systematic review. BMC Public Health. 2012;12:807.
28. Saelens BE, Sallis JF, Frank LD. Environmental correlates of walking and cycling: findings from the transportation, urban design, and planning literatures. Ann Behav Med. 2003;25:80–91.
29. Van Dyck D, Cerin E, Conway TL, De Bourdeaudhuij I, Owen N, Kerr J, Cardon G, Frank LD, Saelens BE, Sallis JF. Perceived neighborhood environmental attributes associated with adults' transport-related walking and cycling: findings from the USA, Australia and Belgium. Int J Behav Nutr Phys Act. 2012;9:70.
30. McCormack GR, Shiell A. In search of causality: a systematic review of the relationship between the built environment and physical activity among adults. Int J Behav Nutr Phys Act. 2011;8:125.
31. Foster CE, Panter JR, Wareham NJ. Assessing the impact of road traffic on cycling for leisure and cycling to work. Int J Behav Nutr Phys Act. 2011;8:61.
32. Wendel-Vos W, Droomers M, Kremers S, Brug J, van Lenthe F. Potential environmental determinants of physical activity in adults: a systematic review. Obes Rev. 2007;8:425–40.
33. McCormack G, Giles-Corti B, Lange A, Smith T, Martin K, Pikora TJ. An update of recent evidence of the relationship between objective and self-report measures of the physical environment and physical activity behaviours. J Sci Med Sport. 2004;7(1 Suppl):81–92.
34. Bauman AE, Reis RS, Sallis JF, Wells JC, Loos RJF, Martin BW. Correlates of physical activity: why are some people physically active and others not? Lancet. 2012;380:258–71.
35. Van Holle V, Van Cauwenberg J, Deforche B, Goubert L, Maes L, Nasar J, Van de Weghe N, Salmon J, De Bourdeaudhuij I. Environmental invitingness for transport-related cycling in middle-aged adults: a proof of concept study using photographs. Transp Res Part A Policy Pract. 2014;69:432–46.
36. Vandenbulcke G, Dujardin C, Thomas I, De Geus B, Degraeuwe B, Meeusen R, Panis LI. Cycle commuting in Belgium: spatial determinants and "re-cycling" strategies. Transp Res Part A Policy Pract. 2011;45:118–37.
37. de Geus B, De Bourdeaudhuij I, Jannes C, Meeusen R. Psychosocial and environmental factors associated with cycling for transport among a working population. Health Educ Res. 2008;23:697–708.

38. Titze S, Stronegger WJ, Janschitz S, Oja P. Environmental, social, and personal correlates of cycling for transportation in a student population. J Phys Act Health. 2007;4(1):66–79.

39. Titze S, Giles-Corti B, Knuiman MW, Pikora TJ, Timperio A, Bull FC, Van Niel K. Associations between intrapersonal and neighborhood environmental characteristics and cycling for transport and recreation in adults: baseline results from the RESIDE study. J Phys Act Health. 2010;7:423–31.

40. Van Dyck D, Cardon G, Deforche B, Giles-Corti B, Sallis JF, Owen N, De Bourdeaudhuij I. Environmental and psychosocial correlates of accelerometer-assessed and self-reported physical activity in Belgian adults. Int J Behav Med. 2011;18:235–45.

41. Parkin J, Wardman M, Page M. Estimation of the determinants of bicycle mode share for the journey to work using census data. Transportation. 2008;35:93–109.

42. Lee C, Moudon AV. Neighbourhood design and physical activity. Build Res Inf. 2008;36(5):395–411.

43. Zlot AI, Schmid TL. Relationships among community characteristics and walking and bicycling for transportation or recreation. Am J Health Promot. 2005;19:314–7.

44. Wendel-vos W, Schuit J, De Niet R, Boshuizen HC, Saris WHM, Kromhout D. Factors of the physical environment associated with walking and bicycling. Med Sci Sports Exerc. 2004;36(4):725–30.

45. Kondo K, Su ÆJ, Kiyoshi LÆ, Yusuke KÆ, Takagi H, Sunagawa ÆH, Akabayashi ÆA. Association between daily physical activity and neighborhood environments. Environ Health Prev Med. 2009;14(3):196–206. doi:10.1007/s12199-009-0081-1.

46. Caulfield B, Brick E, Thérèse O. Determining bicycle infrastructure preferences—a case study of Dublin. Transp Res Part D. 2012;17:413–7.

47. Evenson KR, Herring AH, Huston SL. Evaluating change in physical activity with the building of a multi-use trail. Am J Prev Med. 2005;28:177–85.

48. Mertens L, Van Holle V, De Bourdeaudhuij I, Deforche B, Salmon J, Nasar J, Van de Weghe N, Van Dyck D, Van Cauwenberg J. The effect of changing micro-scale physical environmental factors on an environment's invitingness for transportation cycling in adults: an exploratory study using manipulated photographs. Int J Behav Nutr Phys Act. 2014;11:88.

49. Fraser SDS, Lock K. Cycling for transport and public health: a systematic review of the effect of the environment on cycling. Eur J Public Health. 2010;21:738–43.

50. Carpiano RM. Come take a walk with me: the "go-along" interview as a novel method for studying the implications of place for health and well-being. Health Place. 2009;15:263–72.

51. Spittaels H, Foster C, Oppert J-M, Rutter H, Oja P, Sjöström M, De Bourdeaudhuij I. Assessment of environmental correlates of physical activity: development of a European questionnaire. Int J Behav Nutr Phys Act. 2009;6:39.

52. Sallis JF, Bowles HR, Bauman A, Ainsworth BE, Bull FC, Craig CL, Sjöström M, De Bourdeaudhuij I, Lefevre J, Matsudo V, Matsudo S, Macfarlane DJ, Gomez LF, Inoue S, Murase N, Volbekiene V, McLean G, Carr H, Heggebo LK, Tomten H, Bergman P. Neighborhood environments and physical activity among adults in 11 countries. Am J Prev Med. 2009;36:484–90.

53. Ferdinand AO, Sen B, Rahurkar S, Engler S, Menachemi N. The relationship between built environments and physical activity: a systematic review. Am J Public Health. 2012;102(10):e7–13.

54. Nasar JL. Assessing perceptions of environments for active living. Am J Prev Med. 2008;34:357–63.

55. Wells NM, Ashdown SP, Davies EHS, Cowett FD, Yang Y. Environment, design, and obesity: opportunities for interdisciplinary collaborative research. Environ Behav. 2007;39:6–33.

56. Adobe Systems Incorporated: Adobe Photoshop CC. 2013. p. 1–87. http://wwwimages.adobe.com/content/dam/Adobe/en/devnet/photoshop/pdfs/photoshop-cc-scripting-guide.pdf. Accessed 25 Aug 2016.

57. Lenders S, Lauwers L, Vervloet D, Kerselaers E. Afbakening van het Vlaamse platteland, een statistische analyse. 2006. p. 1–63. http://www2.vlaanderen.be/landbouw/downloads/volt/38.pdf. Accessed 25 Aug 2016.

58. Pucher J, Buehler R. Making cycling irresistible: lessons from the Netherlands, Denmark and Germany. Transp Rev. 2008;28:495–528.

59. Mertens L, Van Cauwenberg J, Ghekiere A, Van Holle V, De Bourdeaudhuij I, Deforche B, Nasar J, Van de Weghe N, Van Dyck D. Does the effect of micro-environmental factors on a street's appeal for adults' bicycle transport vary across different macro-environments? An experimental study. PLoS One 2015;10:1–17.

60. Craig CL, Marshall AL, Sjöström M, Bauman AE, Booth ML, Ainsworth BE, Pratt M, Ekelund U, Yngve A, Sallis JF, Oja P. International physical activity questionnaire: 12-country reliability and validity. Med Sci Sports Exerc. 2003;35:1381–95.

61. Orme BK. Getting started with conjoint analysis: strategies for product design and pricing research. Madison: Resarch Publishers; 2009.

62. Sawtooth Software Inc. The CBC system for choice-based conjoint analysis. 2013. p. 1–27. https://sawtoothsoftware.com/download/techpap/cbctech.pdf. Accessed 25 Aug 2016.

63. Multon KD. Interrater reliability. In: Salkind NJ, editor. Encyclopedia research design. Thousand Oaks, CA: Sage; 2012. p. 627–629. doi:10.4135/9781412961288.n194. http://methods.sagepub.com/reference/encyc-of-research-design/n194.xml. Accessed 25 Aug 2016.

64. Allenby GM, Arora N, Ginter JL. On the heterogeneity of demand. J Mark Res. 1998;35:384–9.

65. Interaction Search Tool. https://www.sawtoothsoftware.com/help/issues/ssiweb/online_help/index.html?interaction_search_tool.htm.

66. Sallis JF, Conway TL, Dillon LI, Frank LD, Adams MA, Cain KL, Saelens BE. Environmental and demographic correlates of bicycling. Prev Med. 2013;57:456–60.

67. Winters M, Davidson G, Kao D, Teschke K. Motivators and deterrents of bicycling: comparing influences on decisions to ride. Transportation. 2010;38:153–68.

68. Statistics Belgium. http://statbel.fgov.be/.

69. Cubukcu E, Nasar JL. Influence of physical characteristics of routes on distance cognition in virtual environments. Environ Plan. 2005;32:777–85.

Quantifying multi-dimensional attributes of human activities at various geographic scales based on smartphone tracking

Xiaolu Zhou[1,2*] and Dongying Li[3]

Abstract

Background: Advancement in location-aware technologies, and information and communication technology in the past decades has furthered our knowledge of the interaction between human activities and the built environment. An increasing number of studies have collected data regarding individual activities to better understand how the environment shapes human behavior. Despite this growing interest, some challenges exist in collecting and processing individual's activity data, e.g., capturing people's precise environmental contexts and analyzing data at multiple spatial scales.

Methods: In this study, we propose and implement an innovative system that integrates smartphone-based step tracking with an app and the sequential tile scan techniques to collect and process activity data. We apply the OpenStreetMap tile system to aggregate positioning points at various scales. We also propose duration, step and probability surfaces to quantify the multi-dimensional attributes of activities.

Results: Results show that, by running the app in the background, smartphones can measure multi-dimensional attributes of human activities, including space, duration, step, and location uncertainty at various spatial scales. By coordinating Global Positioning System (GPS) sensor with accelerometer sensor, this app can save battery which otherwise would be drained by GPS sensor quickly. Based on a test dataset, we were able to detect the recreational center and sports center as the space where the user was most active, among other places visited.

Conclusion: The methods provide techniques to address key issues in analyzing human activity data. The system can support future studies on behavioral and health consequences related to individual's environmental exposure.

Keywords: Individual activity tracking, Location-based step, Smartphone, Tile systems, Geographic information systems

Background

The interaction between human activities and the environment has been an important topic in many disciplines, such as transportation research, urban planning, and public health [4, 15, 29–31]. An increasing number of studies over the past decades have aimed to achieve better understandings of the environmental and health consequences related to travel behavior. Among these studies, tasks such as collecting and processing data related to human activities are mostly laborious and time-consuming. Several challenges exist in collecting and processing human dynamic data.

Regarding data collection, technology advancements have spurred new ways of recording activity data. Many studies have used wearable devices such as global positioning system (GPS) receivers and accelerometers to measure people's activity space and physical activities [22, 26, 27]. Although activity-tracking devices are

*Correspondence: xzhou@georgiasouthern.edu
[1] Department of Geology and Geography, Georgia Southern University, 68 Georgia Ave, Herty Bldg 0201, Statesboro, GA 30460, USA
Full list of author information is available at the end of the article

becoming more affordable, logistical challenges still exist in carrying out experiments, especially when large sample sizes are needed. Wearing additional devices such as an accelerometer or GPS is cumbersome for participants. In recent years, with rapid growth in smartphone ownership [21], studies have explored using smartphones as sensors to measure travel behavior [19, 31]. However, most studies have focused on total steps averaged across a day based on the daily step counting apps. There is much less discussion on location-based steps, i.e., registering steps to different locations. Issues such as battery consumption and positioning accuracy in covered areas are considered challenging when using smartphone as a tool to track movements [1, 11].

Even for the studies that have considered location-activity interaction, point locations and point density are usually the only information captured as the characteristics of the activities or the individuals' activity space. Data that are critical to understanding the activity, such as the intensity and duration of the activity that occurred in different locations are usually missing. Another missing piece of information in the empirical studies using smartphone-tracked activity is how accurate the point locations are at various locations. This piece of information is vital because positioning can be less precise in covered areas or urban canyons, resulting in finding that may be less reliable.

Second, in studies analyzing activities, data regarding environmental features are often examined as correlates. Conventional approaches rely on official and commercial datasets, which demonstrate issues of data availability, hierarchy and subjectivity. Nowadays, crowdsourcing geographic data, such as OpenStreetMap (OSM) are increasingly detailed and accessible. As approaches to collectively produce knowledge, OSM offers new ways in unfolding the fine-scale phenomena that are usually neglected by official datasets. If smartphone-based tracking can be integrated and analyzed with OSM data easily, researchers could gain greater access to rich data regarding a broad range of place of interests (POIs). In addition, OSM uses hierarchical tile systems (i.e. a grid system that controls the level of detail a map should display) to store and display geographic information. The strength in the tile system is that data are extracted and prepared at different scales, boosting the computational efficiency. In order for the human activity research community to take advantage of the rich OSM dataset, new approaches that can process activity data and link them with OSM data become critical.

To fill these gaps, we proposed and implemented an innovative system that integrated smartphone-based step tracking and the sequential tile scan techniques to collect and process activity data at various spatial scales.

For data collection, the system involved using smartphones as mobile sensors to collect location-based steps. We used a smart sensor coordination approach to track users' locations and steps. Such an approach can improve the previously reported limitations in using smartphone as an activity tracker. For data processing, we proposed the sequential tile scan technique to calculate the activity routes and the associated attributes (i.e. probability, step, and duration surfaces). We applied OSM tile system to aggregate the positioning points at variable scales. The duration surface represents the duration of activity in every tile. The step surface measured the spatial distribution of steps and displayed the tiles that were associated with more steps. The probability surface estimated how accurate the location logs were in every tile. With this approach, researchers can readily link a multifold of activity data, e.g., steps during physical activity, duration of stay in a certain area, with OSM information at various scales. In the following sections, we introduce related studies, explain the system in detail, and present an example application of the approach.

Related studies
Monitoring individual's environmental exposure in behavioral research

Prolonged inactivity poses a critical, life-long health risk. A growing body of evidence indicates that built environment characteristics influence lifestyles. For example, people who live in neighborhoods that are close to stores, recreational places, green spaces, playgrounds, walkways, and bike paths participate in more active travel and have a lower body weight [6, 12, 29].

Previous studies point out that one challenge for healthy behavior research is to contextualize people's spatial behavior and activities [16]. Many studies used predefined boundaries such as census blocks [17, 23], or various sized buffer areas around points of interest, such as home location [13] to represent activity spaces. However, neither boundaries nor buffer areas around a point of interest capture the actual environment where physical activity takes place. In fact, most people's physical activities happen in a broader range of space beyond their residential neighborhood. The environmental features where physical activity takes place may also differ from those in the residential neighborhoods [27, 29]. A review found that 90% of the studies in the area of physical activity and environment measured environmental characteristics of participants' residential neighborhoods and that only 4% of studies examined nonresidential locations [18]. To identify the environmental characteristics that promote active behaviors, it is critical to overcome this limitation by using actual location-based data.

The limitation exists in studies analyzing people's dietary environment. Many studies have computed dietary environment based on pre-defined areal units or buffer areas around individuals' home addresses [7]. However, the measured environment may be very different from where individuals choose to eat. For example, when one drives along the highway, the neighborhoods close by are not easy to access despite the proximity. The uncertainty of contextual influences that individuals experience calls for a detailed activity data and multi-facet business information to ensure the rigor of the measured environment [10].

Smartphone-based tracking

Issues related to GPS devices and accelerometers in activity tracking involve the cumbersomeness in wearing two sets of devices, technical difficulties, and time commitment [30, 31]. In comparison, smartphone tracking demonstrated fewer participant dropouts and greater capabilities in incorporating acceleration values [16]. As a result, smartphones have been used as "urban sensing" devices and are used in studies examining travel and activity patterns [24].

Despite its advantages, smartphone tracking is not without limitations [9]. Recording accuracy, especially with signal losses in indoor areas and areas with dense foliage or buildings, has been a challenge for all types of GPS tracking [3]. In addition, step counting has become common in different smartphone operating systems. Most modern smartphones are equipped with motion sensors. For Android, since API level 19 (KITKAT), most Android phones provide step counter that tracks the number of steps taken by users. For iOS, since iPhone 5 s, similar sensors have been used to record daily steps. Experiments have reported that smartphone-based step detectors perform as accurately as most wearable devices [8]. However, beyond the summary number of total step count, applications to record steps along with the location information on a continuous base have been lacking.

Shifting scales and the OSM tiles systems

In the past two decades, the environmental health research community has more attention on disaggregated and individual scales. Regarding GIS-based analysis, the traditional uneven access to data and tools between experts and local citizens poses important hurdles. Public participation geographic information systems (PPGIS) initiatives were proposed to combat such unevenness [14, 25]. As an innovative type of PPGIS, the OpenStreetMap takes inputs and edits from certified users, who usually are locals with knowledge about their environments. The data collected for OSM are at the most disaggregated, individual scale and can support inquiries at a variety of levels. To assist flexible data output, the tile system is used so that data can be presented based on the zoom level specified by the user.

This approach has huge potentials in analyzing and visualizing individual travel behavior. These strengths call for a platform that could integrate activity location collection, storage, visualization, and analysis using the OSM tile systems. Based on the tile system, data and analysis can be dynamic and flexible.

Methods

Location-based steps

In this study, we used the Android platform to implement the location-based steps. Both motion sensors and position sensors were applied in our program. For position sensors, devices used GPS or network (cellular tower or WiFi access points) to determine the locations. Table 1 shows the strengths and limitations of of the three types of the positioning sensors [28], based on which we developed our system using a hybrid-positioning scheme to detect location-based steps.

We used several techniques to reduce the battery cost, such as sensor rotation and activity controlled switch [32]. Generally, sensor rotation aims to rotate network-based and GPS-based positioning. The activity controlled switch turns on location sensor when people start moving while turns off the location sensor when people become still. In this study, we developed two modules to control the sensors, i.e., control module and sensor module. Location and step information from the sensor module is sent to the control module every 30 s. The control module determines the sensor statuses and sends commands back to the sensor module. We set the frequency of location updates to be 10 s and 10 m in minimum displacement between location updates if positioning sensor is switched on. Outputs of the program included movement trajectories and steps in continuous space and time dimensions.

Table 1 The strengths and limitations for each of these sensors [28]

Techniques	Spatial accuracy (m)	Battery Consumption	Limitations
GPS (A-GPS)	8	High	Indoors or high rise areas
WiFi	74	Low	Areas without access points
Cell-Id	600	Very low	Regions without cell signals

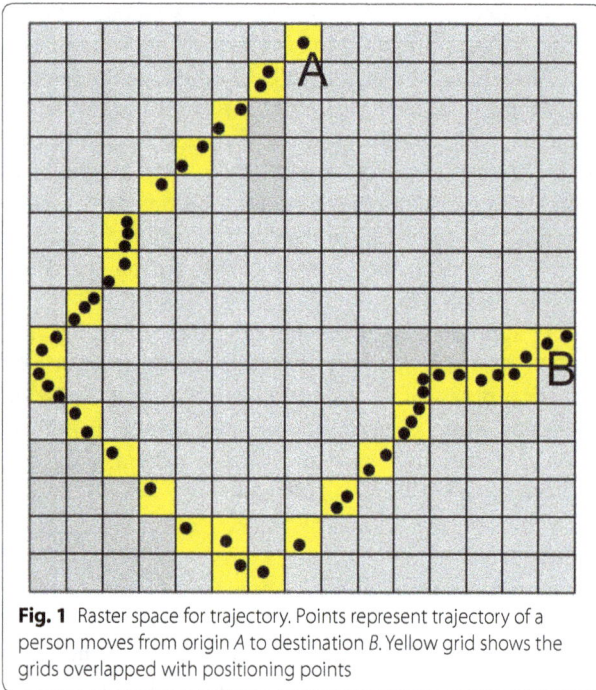

Fig. 1 Raster space for trajectory. Points represent trajectory of a person moves from origin A to destination B. Yellow grid shows the grids overlapped with positioning points

OSM tile system

Once the steps and movement data were collected, the next step was to construct the activity space and associate activities with the environment. Currently, OSM and some other mapping service providers, such as Google Maps, offer rich geographic information. It would be ideal to link location-based steps with their tile systems directly. One approach would be directly converting

The OSM tiles that are associated with different zoom levels are predefined for the entire earth. Therefore, we set up the positioning points with the tiles at different zoom level directly. There are three advantages to set up the activity data display and analysis system in such a way. First, instead of creating a grid of tiles within the rectangular extent defined by all the positioning points, we only needed to identify the tiles that intersected with the positioning points. This process largely addressed the storage redundancy problem. Second, because the tile systems were associated with multiple zoom levels, it was fast and easy to switch research granularity at different spatial scales. For instance, for the same dataset, higher zoom levels (e.g., zoom 22) could be selected when the research question was at the scale of urban streets, while lower zoom level (e.g. zoom 18) could be used when there was a need to aggregate the data to a larger area. Third, tiles from the OSM offered rich geographic information (e.g., stores, parks, and road networks). Such geographic information can be directly tied to the activity data to analyze the association between human behavior and the environmental context.

The OSM use a Spherical Mercator Projection coordinate system. The tile system includes tiles in a hierarchical structure based on zoom levels. For instance, at zoom level 0, the world is represented by 1 tile while at zoom level 2, the world is divided into 16 tiles. Tile number is determined by $N = 2^n \times 2^n$, where n is the zoom level [20].

To convert positioning points to tile IDs, the following equations were applied to the latitude and longitude pairs [20].

$$L = 2^n$$

$$IDx = Math.floor\left(L * \left(\frac{(lon + 180)}{360}\right)\right)$$

$$IDy = Math.floor\left(L * \frac{1 - \frac{Math.\log\left(Math.\tan\left(Math.toRadians(lat)\right) + \frac{1}{Math.\cos\left(Math.toRadians(lat)\right)}\right)}{Math.PI}}{2}\right)$$

positioning points into grids. Tools such as Points to Grid are available in most GIS programs to achieve such a conversion. However, it would be redundant to store every grid when no activity falls in the grid (grey grids in Fig. 1). The storage redundancy is especially significant if the raster covers a wide area with high resolution but the actual activities happen sparsely. The following sections introduce our proposed method.

In our system, we used a tile system that modeled activity data using a system similar to the OSM tile system.

where *lat, lon* are the coordinates, *toRadians* converts angle degrees to radians.

Mapping positioning points to the tile system

Once we converted points into the tile system, we need to determine the path that connected adjacent positioning points to form activity routes. In computer graphics, the Bresenham's line algorithm [5] provides an efficient way to form a close approximation of straight-line grids between two given points. In this project, we extended Bresenham's line to construct the activity routes.

Algorithm 1 (Bresenham, 1977)

```
Function line(x, y, x2, y2)
    w <- x2 - x
    h <- y2 - y
    dx1, dy1, dx2, dy2 <- 0
    if w<0 then dx1 <- -1  else if w>0 dx1 <- 1
    if h<0 then dy1 <- -1  else if h>0 dy1 <- 1
    if w<0 then dx2 <- -1  else if w>0 dx2 <- 1
    lg <- abs(w)
    st <- abs(h)
    if lg <= st then
        lg <- abs(h)
        st <- abs(w)
        if h < 0 then dy2 <- -1 else if h > 0 then dy2 <- 1
        dx2 <- 0
    numerator <- lg >> 1
    i<-0
    while
        if i>lg then end while
        SelectTile(x,y)
        numerator <- numerator+st
        if numerator >= lg then
            numerator <- numerator-lg
            x <- x+dx1
            y <- y+dy1
        else
            x <- x+dx2
            y <- y+dy2
        i<- i+1
    end while
end Function
```

Suppose we used LINE1 to link two adjacent positioning points and we aimed to find the tiles intersect with such line. If we scanned tiles horizontally, when $|\Delta x| \geq |\Delta y|$ (LINE1), the y-axis increment associated with one unit x-axis increase would be less than one. This process would produce continuous tiles. However, when $|\Delta y| \geq |\Delta x|$ (LINE2), the above-mentioned equation would generate disconnected tiles (Fig. 2). Hence, we considered conditions in different octants. In addition, when calculating the slope, using floating-point data type and considering infinitely large slope would decrease the efficiency. Therefore, we used the Bresenham's line algorithm to simplify the line tile intersection problem by only using integer variables and removing the costly division operation for slope calculation (Algorithm 1). This process was efficient in generating straight-line grids between two given points.

Step and duration surfaces

After mapping points to the tile system and connecting tiles with straight-line grids, we computed the number of steps and activity duration within each tile. We assumed uniform motion between two adjacent points, which was reasonable with a short sampling interval. Hence, we divided the steps and duration by the tile numbers between the adjacent positioning points. The results were assigned to each tile. Because the sum of the probabilities of all the tiles along each perpendicular scan equaled to one, the total numbers of steps (or duration) was calculated as $S_{total} = \sum_i^{range} \sum_j^{seq} p_i \times s_j$, where *range* is the width of the possible tiles on the perpendicular direction, *seq* is the total number of tiles between the two points, and p and s are the probability score and step number allocated to each tile.

Probability surface

We also estimated the activity probability surface. The accuracy of the positioning points could vary from meters to thousand meters. Therefore, quantifying the probability of a point locating in a certain tile was important. The app reported both the locations and the estimated accuracy range. The red points on Fig. 3 were the measured positioning points, and the dashed circles were the accuracy ranges. When the accuracy range was smaller than the tile resolution, the person was very likely located inside the tile. When we increased the zoom level, the certainty of person in a particular tile decreased. In addition, the tiles along the route that connected two adjacent points became more uncertain. In this study, we assumed that people were more likely to move in a straight line between two adjacent points. The assumption was especially safe with short intervals (e.g. 30 s). It was also reasonable to assume that the probabilities decreased when the distance increases away from the central straight line. For instance, at Zoom Level III in Fig. 3, tiles intersected with the straight line between two points had the highest present probability. The probabilities gradually fell as the tiles moved away from the central straight line.

To calculate the probability surface, one way is to find the bounding polygons for the possible activity space (the yellow polygons on Fig. 3) and intersect with the tile system. However, it is computationally expensive to calculate bounding intersection. In this study, we used sequential tile scan technique to calculate the probability surface. This technique involved four steps. We first calculated the possible tile range for the two consecutive positioning points based on the tile resolution and the accuracies of the positioning points. This step helped to determine the numbers of tiles to be considered surrounding the positioning points. Second, we computed the tile sequence connecting the positioning points using Bresenham's line algorithm. Third, we scanned through all tiles sequentially to create perpendicular tiles. The widths of the perpendicular tiles were determined by the tile range of the current center tile. Fourth, an inverse proportional function was applied to each perpendicular tile to calculate the present probability scores for each tile. This step guaranteed that probability scores decreased when tiles were away from the central straight lines and the sum of the probabilities of all tile along the perpendicular line equaled one (Fig. 4).

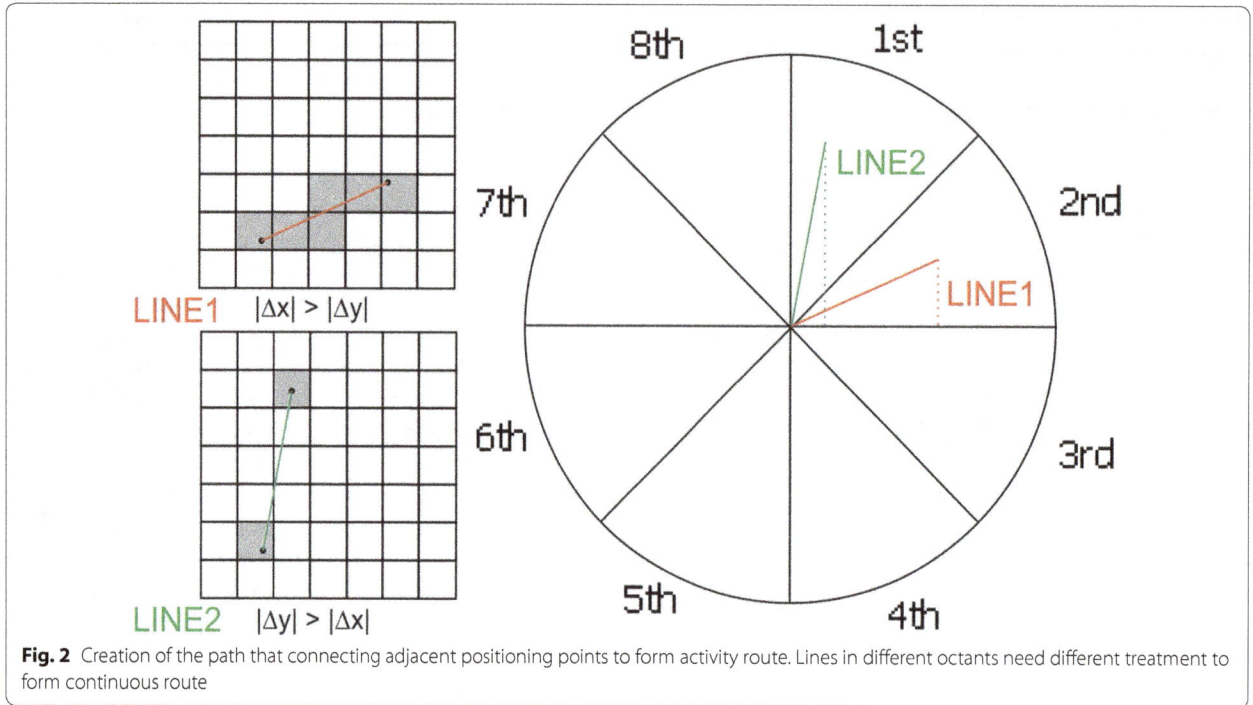

Fig. 2 Creation of the path that connecting adjacent positioning points to form activity route. Lines in different octants need different treatment to form continuous route

Algorithm 2

```
Function ProbSurf(x0,y0,x1,y1,acc1,acc2,res)
    tRange1 <- floor(acc1/res)
    tRange2 <- floor(acc2/res)
    centerL <- line(x0, y0, x1, y1)
    interpolateRange(centerL,tRange1,tRange2)
    for t in centerL
      tRan<- getTileRange(t)
      while itte < tRan
          newTile <- movePerpen(t)
          newProb <- computeKernel(newTile,
          "Linear")
          itte++
      end while
    end for
end Function
```

Extracting place of interest from OSM

After detecting when and where people were active at multiple geographic scales, we needed to extract environmental associates of human activities from OSM. OSM provides rich and free geographic data available across the world. The tags along with geographic data also bring additional information, such as names, addresses, and land use type to complement activity information. We first extracted POIs from all OSM tags. The POI set was based on OSM Map Feature List (https://wiki.openstreetmap.org/wiki/Map_Features). We applied OsmPoisPbf (https://github.com/MorbZ/OsmPoisPbf) to filter geographic features and stored them in Post-GIS database. The tags in key-value pairs were stored as hstore data type. Second, we conducted spatial queries in PostGIS to select geographic features that overlap with activity tiles and appended the tag information from OSM to the end of corresponding activity tiles.

Application of the system in public health

There is a growing interest in developing new ways to measure personal activity and determine the environmental features that are relevant to the behavioral patterns and health consequences. Dietary environment is one of the topics.To demonstrate the effectiveness of our system within the context of human's dietary environment, we tested the application for 5 days, aiming to capture information about physical activity and dietary space. In the result section, we present the performance of the application in capturing and integrating information such as steps, activity duration, locations, and patterns generated by examining the smartphone and OSM datasets.

Results
App interface

Figure 5 shows the main functionalities of the application. The interface is easy-to-follow and self-explanatory. We focused on the main functions and techniques that coordinated location and motion sensors rather than interface design in this project. Screen (a) shows the login

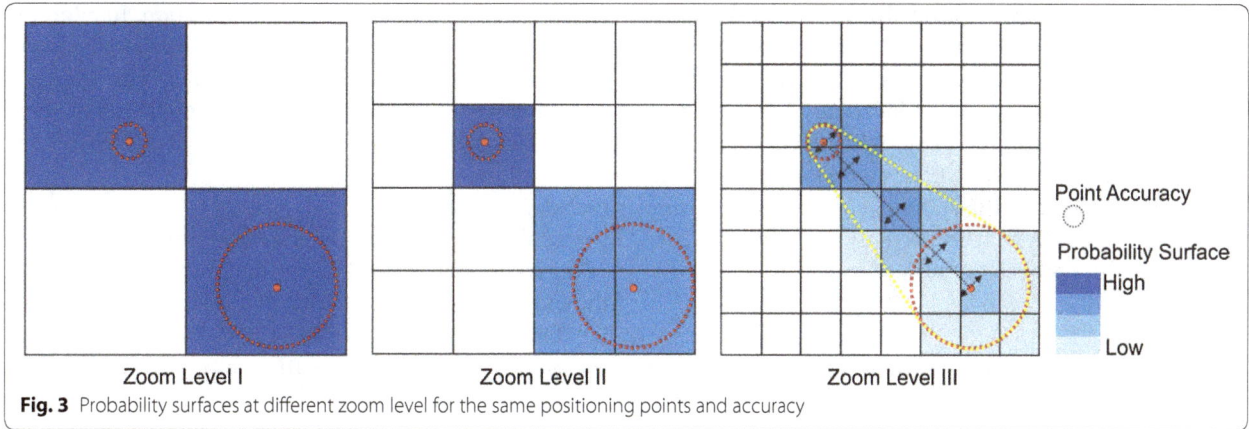

Fig. 3 Probability surfaces at different zoom level for the same positioning points and accuracy

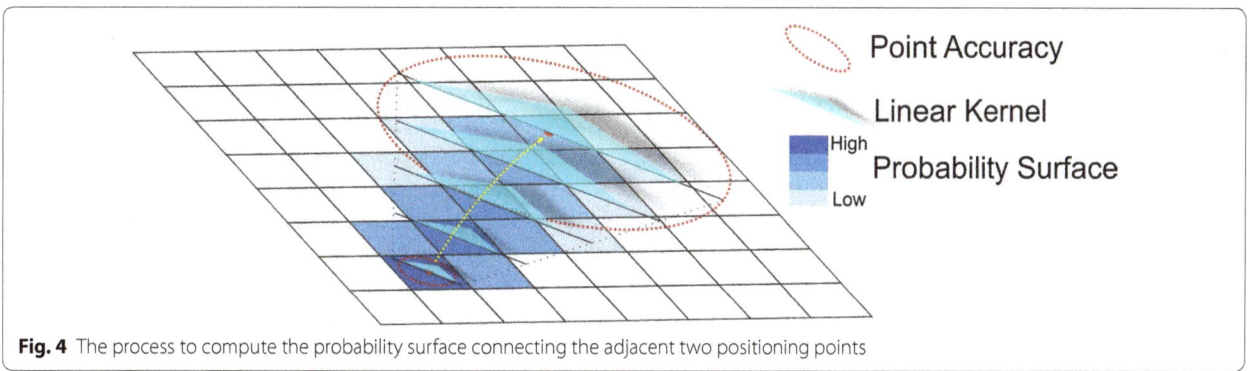

Fig. 4 The process to compute the probability surface connecting the adjacent two positioning points

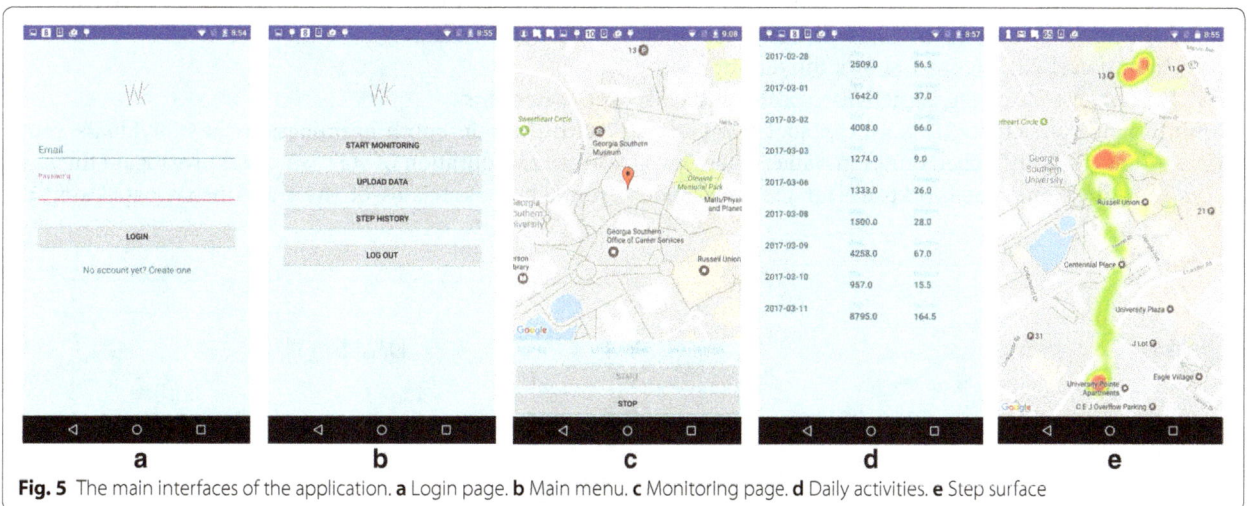

Fig. 5 The main interfaces of the application. **a** Login page. **b** Main menu. **c** Monitoring page. **d** Daily activities. **e** Step surface

page. Screen (b) shows the main menu. It allows users to start or stop monitoring, upload data, and look up previous location-based steps. Screen (c) is the monitoring page; the instantaneous steps and locations are updated on the map and the information section at the bottom of the page. Screen (d) shows a list of recorded steps and activity durations for each day. Once a record is selected, Screen (e) will display the step surface.

Multi-dimensional attributes of travel behaviors
To demonstrate the effectiveness of the application in capturing multi-dimensional attributes of travel

behaviors, one researcher used the app for 5 days and analyzed the trajectories and relevant information. The resulting test data include a sum of 43.11 h of information. We collected 2245 point locations, translating to 1053 tiles at level 19. The positioning accuracy ranged from 3 meters to 2900 m, with a median accuracy of 12 meters. In our project, the system generated three layers to represent the activity space: activity step surface, duration surface, and probability surface.

Step surface

The step surface demonstrated the locations where the user actually walked. People's activity space may cover a broad area, but the places where people actually walked can be very limited. For the step surface, the value associated with each tile is the actual steps accumulated in the corresponding tile. Figure 6 shows the distribution of moving trajectories at zoom level 19. The colors in the map represent the number of steps: the green end of the color ramp representing fewer steps and the red end of the color ramp representing more steps. Numbers at the bottom present the daily step counts. From this surface, we could identify the locations where steps concentrated.

Duration surface

In addition to the step surface, we also produced the duration surface to map where and how long people stay in each area in their daily life. By doing so, we could find anchor points (e.g. home or workspace) for users' daily activities. To better illustrate the duration surface, we plotted the travel behavior on Day 5 at a higher zoom level (Zoom Level 22). Figure 7 shows the duration surface. The longest duration of activity within a tile is 47 min. Among all activity tiles, we can spot two places (Spots A and B) with higher duration value. These two places were the home and workplace for the user. Spot

C also emerged as an important destination. In addition, the tile system at level 22 displays very detailed ground information about the locations visited. For example, Fig. 7d, e show the buildings where the individual spent most of his/her time.

Probability surface

Probability surface was generated to show the accuracy of the locations. Figure 8 shows the probability surface of the individual's daily activities. We used two zoom levels (i.e. Level 18 and 22) to reflect the probability surface on Day 5. At Level 18, the resolution for each tile was about 128 meters in this area. Most tiles at this zoom level had a probability of 100%, which suggested that we were very positive that the individual had their footprints on these tiles. At level 22, the resolution for each tile was about 8 meters in the study area. This level provided detailed movement information. In addition, when the positioning accuracy was high, we could acquire very certain estimation about the actual movement path (such as route A). On the other hand, when the positioning accuracy was relatively low (lower than the resolution level), we still could map out the possible path and the associated probability scores (such as area B). Figure 8c shows the contrast between outdoor and indoor activities. GPS provided high positioning accuracy outdoors, so the certainty of tiles was very high (Area C). When using network positioning inside the building, although the overall accuracy was lower, we could still map out the most possible activity space (Spot D) in the building by using the probability surface.

POI detections

With these in-depth examinations of individual's route, steps, and duration of stay, we could investigate the environmental associates of the travel behaviors. Using the

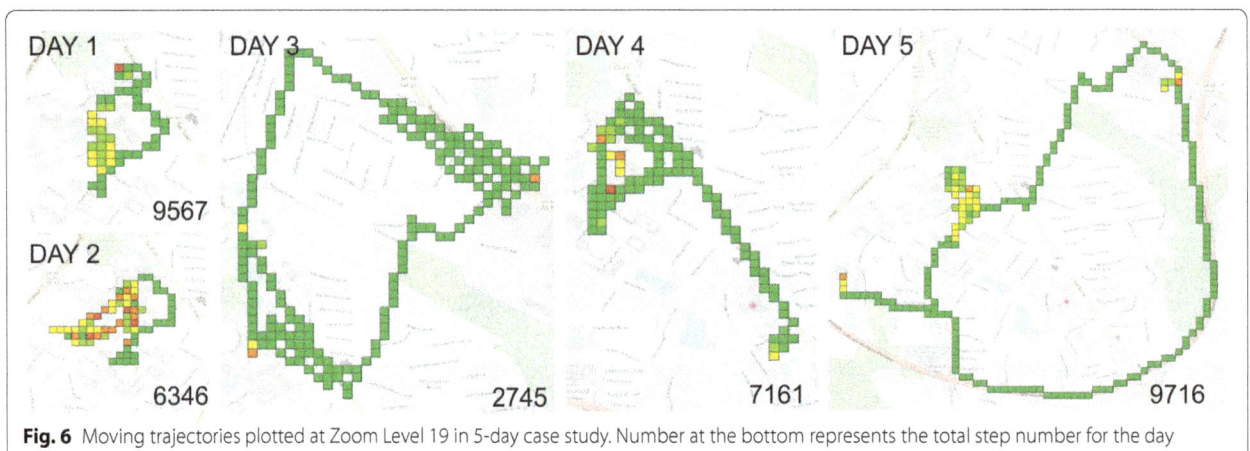

Fig. 6 Moving trajectories plotted at Zoom Level 19 in 5-day case study. Number at the bottom represents the total step number for the day

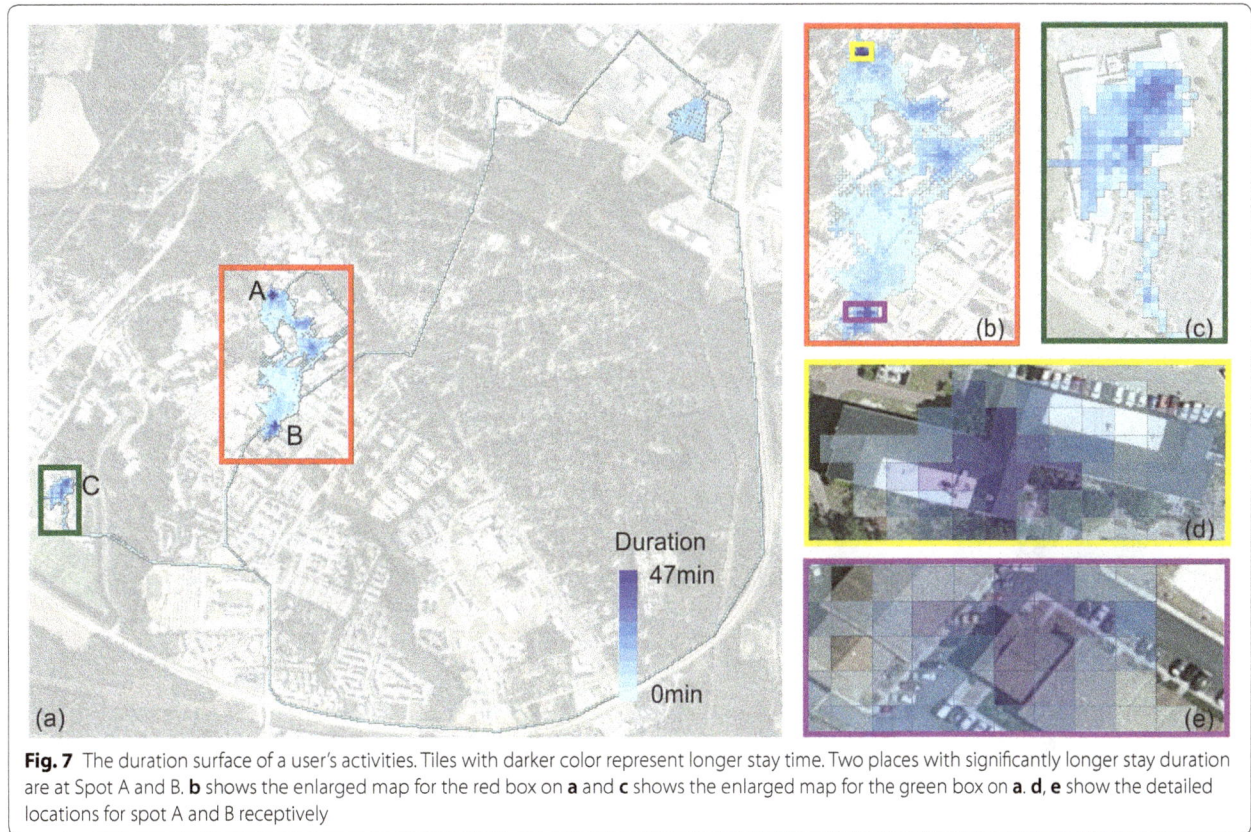

Fig. 7 The duration surface of a user's activities. Tiles with darker color represent longer stay time. Two places with significantly longer stay duration are at Spot A and B. **b** shows the enlarged map for the red box on **a** and **c** shows the enlarged map for the green box on **a**. **d**, **e** show the detailed locations for spot A and B receptively

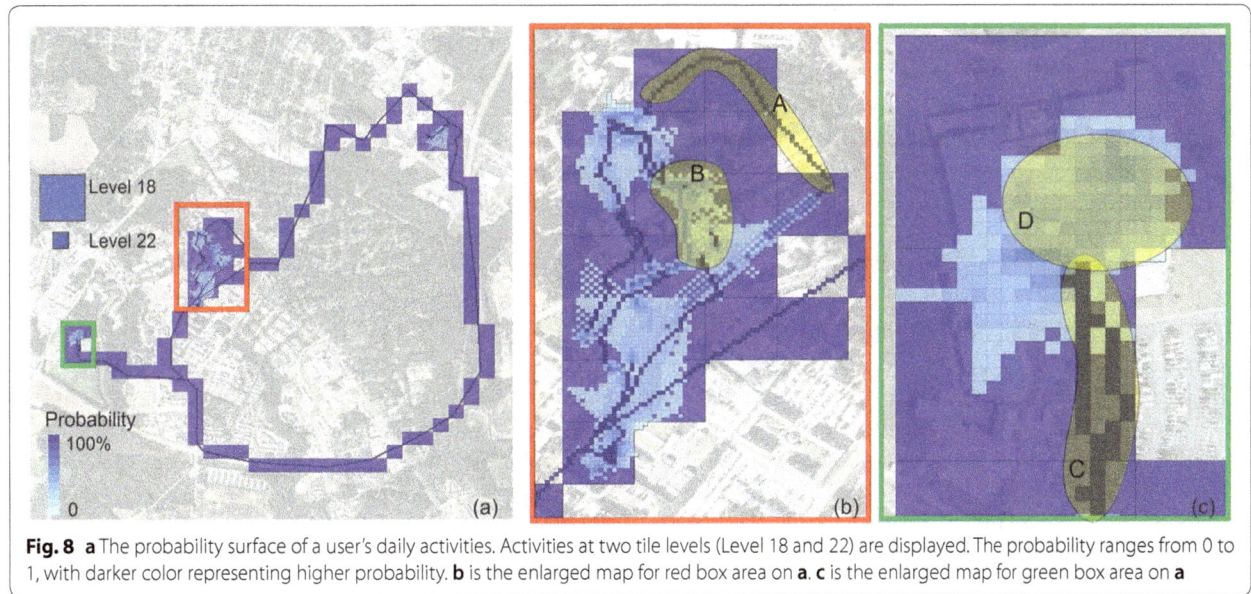

Fig. 8 **a** The probability surface of a user's daily activities. Activities at two tile levels (Level 18 and 22) are displayed. The probability ranges from 0 to 1, with darker color representing higher probability. **b** is the enlarged map for red box area on **a**. **c** is the enlarged map for green box area on **a**

OSM tile system, travel behavior were directly linked with points of interests (POIs) provided by OSM data. This feature supported visual assessment and further spatial statistical analyses in examining the correlation between characteristics of destinations and physical activity. To show the corresponding POIs where high number of steps concentrated, we queried the OSM database to detect POIs. Figure 9 shows the most active

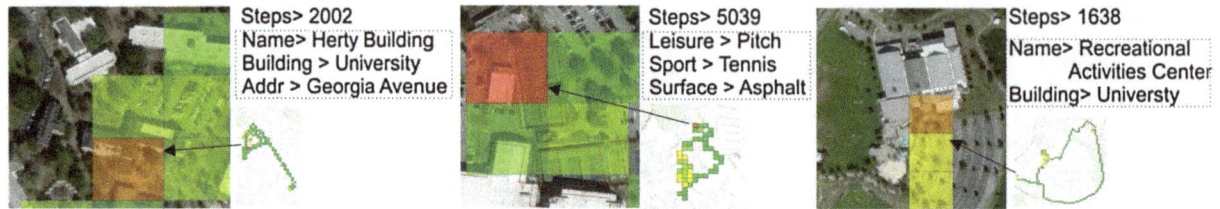

Fig. 9 POIs, corresponding tags, and steps numbers at the most active places in the 5-day moving trajectory. Information in the dashed boxes is derived from OSM tags

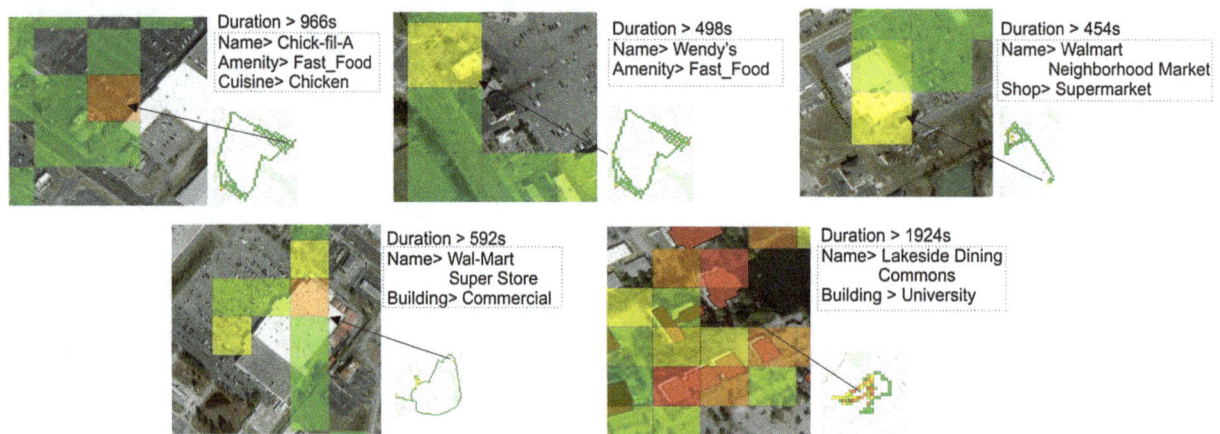

Fig. 10 POIs, corresponding tags, and durations for the dining and grocery activities in the 5-day case study

places and their POI information. We identified that the user was most active in the recreational activities center, tennis courts, and the Herty Building. The corresponding steps at these places were also displayed.

Activities happen in restaurants or grocery stores are important indicators in analyzing people's dietary behaviors. We integrated the trajectory data with OSM data to detect dining or grocery shopping activities. POIs in tiles related to food and grocery were selected if trajectories intersected with those tiles for more than 5 min. Figure 10 shows the POIs related to dining and grocery places the user visited in the 5-day case study. From the POIs, we found that the user visited at least two fast food venues (Chick-fil-A and Wendy's) and two grocery stores.

Change between spatial scales

Flexible and agile methods to process activity data across multiple scales help facilitate activity data analysis. In order to evaluate the performance of our methods to process activity data across multiple scales, we collected a larger scale dataset with GPS positions to test the algorithm. Figure 11 shows the user continuously drove for 164.3 miles on the highway while using the app. Each black dot on the figure represents one positioning point.

We collected 1003 points along this route. Using this dataset, we compared the computation time, resolution, and tile numbers generated for multiple zoom levels. Figure 11b shows an enlarged road segment, which shows the tiles at zoom levels from 17 to 23. The higher the zoom level, the better the tiles fit the actual route. When the zoom level is greater than 21, the generated tiles can mostly represent the actual route.

Table 2 shows the process time in milliseconds, tile resolutions in meters, and the generated tile numbers associated with each zoom level. At zoom level 22, the system generated 42,562 tiles in 3.4 s on a computer with 16 GB memory and Intel i7-4770 at 3.4 GHz processor. A resolution of 8 meters was high enough for most applications and it was very fast to generate these tiles.

To summarize the results, the sequential tile scan technique can estimate the step, duration and probability surfaces efficiently, which is very useful in quantifying multi-dimensional attributes of the activity spaces. We applied OSM tile system to aggregate the positioning points at various scales. Activity spaces were compatible with OSM tile systems, which facilitated geographic data collection and examination along with the human activity data.

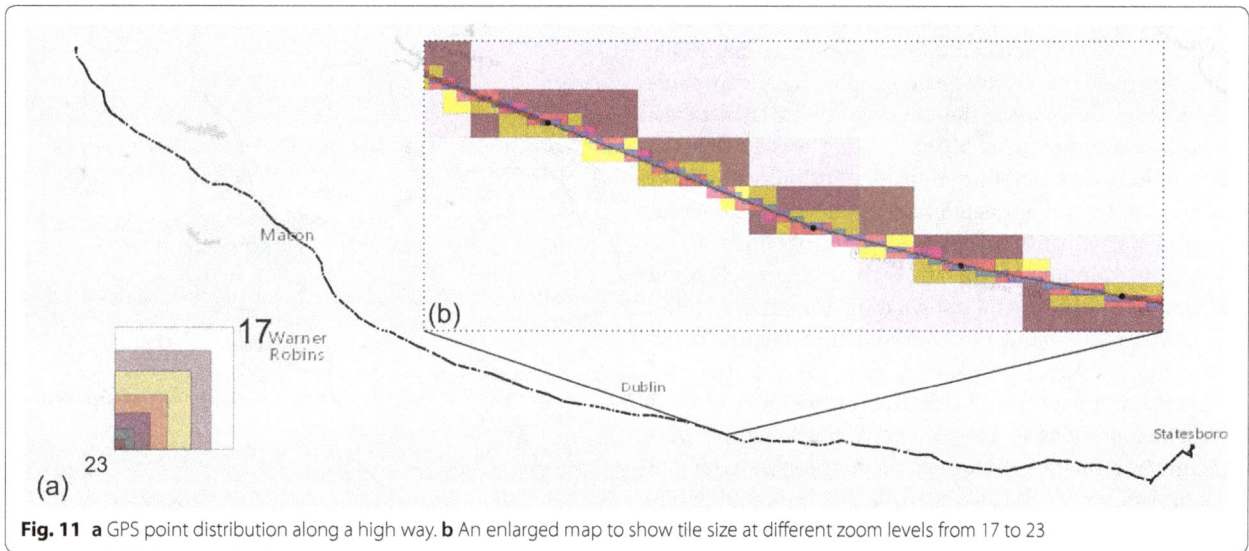

Fig. 11 a GPS point distribution along a high way. **b** An enlarged map to show tile size at different zoom levels from 17 to 23

Table 2 Process time, resolution, and tile numbers that corresponding to different zoom level

Zoom level	Process time (MS)	Resolution (m)	Tile number
17	1190	256.42	1954
18	1229	128.21	2880
19	1338	64.105	4722
20	1561	32.05	8497
21	1998	16.03	16,751
22	3408	8.01	42,562
23	15,230	4.00	178,946

Discussion

Conceptually, this study offers a new way of examining and aggregating individual GPS trajectories. First, this platform supports research that examines individual's travel trajectories. By focusing on daily activity places instead of the arbitrary residential neighborhood, this approach represents improvements in capturing the environmental exposure associated with behavioral and health outcomes. Moreover, based on the collected positioning points, we computed a continuous probability surface to quantify the likelihood of individuals being at certain locations.

Another methodological contribution of this study is to tie multi-dimensional attributes, e.g. the step and duration surfaces with travel patterns. In human–environment research, methods have been proposed to delineate the contextual areas to which individuals expose based on GPS points, but limited attention has been paid to identifying walking behavior and recording the duration of activities in specific environmental context. As a result, the entire activity space is usually given equal consideration when analyzing the environmental associates of behavior. However, as we know from previous research, the health and behavioral outcomes vary based on type of activity, intensity, and duration [2]. Our approach provides data regarding steps and duration of activity in the different tiles that could be examined in relation to different environmental characteristics.

Also, the aggregation process helps safeguard the privacy issue associated with personal location data. Researchers and individual users can select to release data at the level where private information cannot be traced, which is particularly useful in generating visualizations to show the spatial patterns of travel behavior.

Finally, this proposed platform combines a number of GPS data collection, visualization and analysis functionalities for research and everyday use. The technical issues regarding transforming and converting data across platforms present challenge for researchers and limits the use of GPS tracking in a variety of research. Our platform, however, supports processes that involves the collection of individual data, aggregation based on specific research goals and analytical needs.

There are several limitations in this study. First, because the possible tiles that connect origin and destination were interpolated based on the consecutive location points, locations where the signal is weak or the participant is sedentary were not recorded. Therefore, the data has to be cleaned and incorrect trajectory records needed to be removed. In future studies, we will incorporate the road network data and map matching methods to address such situations. Second, the comprehensiveness of OSM data varies in different cities. When analyzing the

activities along with OSM data, the richness of the findings rely heavily on detailed information regarding POIs.
In the future, we can combine geographic data from multiple sources to increase the coverage of POIs in cities.
Third, because our focus of this project was to develop
the functionality to capture multi-dimensional attributes
of activities, we did not deploy our application to a larger
group of participants. Instead, we only obtained a test
dataset by running the app for 5 days. The application
was able to capture useful information at multiple scales.
We also demonstrated the captured information could
be used in projects in measuring physical activities and
environmental exposure. In the future, we plan to conduct a comprehensive assessment. We will recruit participants and invite them to use the app for an extended
period. Along with the app, we will also use pedometers
and accelerometers and self-reported activity diaries to
validate the app-based step and duration measures. We
also plan to apply the proposed system in empirical studies investigating issues regarding the human–environment interaction, such as crime risk modeling and food
exposure analysis.

Conclusion
To conclude, in this study, we proposed and implemented
a system that integrates smartphone-based step tracking and the sequential tile scan techniques to collect and
process activity data at various scales. Such a system
can be applied to a number of human dynamics studies
to achieve better understandings of the behavioral and
health consequences related to individual's environmental exposure.

Authors' contributions
XZ developed the concept of the multiple attributes of human travel. XZ
implemented the concept, XZ and DL jointly collected and analyzed the data,
as well as prepared the manuscript. Both authors read and approved the final
manuscript.

Author details
[1] Department of Geology and Geography, Georgia Southern University, 68
Georgia Ave, Herty Bldg 0201, Statesboro, GA 30460, USA. [2] Yunnan University
of Finance and Economics, Longquan Road 237, Kunming 650221, Yunnan,
China. [3] Department of Landscape Architecture and Urban Planning, Texas
A&M University, College Station, TX 77843, USA.

Acknowledgements
The authors are very grateful to the editor and reviewers' comments and suggestions to the manuscript.

Competing interests
The authors declare that they have no competing interests.

Funding
Not applicable.

References
1. Abdulazim T, Abdelgawad H, Habib K, Abdulhai B. Using smartphones
   and sensor technologies to automate collection of travel data. Transp Res
   Rec: J Transp Res Board. 2013;2383:44–52.
2. Barton J, Pretty J. What is the best dose of nature and green exercise for
   improving mental health? A multi-study analysis. Environ Sci Technol.
   2010;44(10):3947–55.
3. Bellad V, Petovello MG, Lachapelle G. Intermittent tracking in weak signal
   environments. Paper presented at the Indoor Positioning and Indoor
   Navigation (IPIN), 2015 International Conference on (2015).
4. Boarnet M, Crane R. The influence of land use on travel behavior:
   specification and estimation strategies. Transp Res Part A: Policy Pract.
   2001;35(9):823–45.
5. Bresenham J. A linear algorithm for incremental digital display of circular
   arcs. Commun ACM. 1977;20(2):100–6.
6. Carroll-Scott A, Gilstad-Hayden K, Rosenthal L, Peters SM, McCaslin C,
   Joyce R, Ickovics JR. Disentangling neighborhood contextual associations
   with child body mass index, diet, and physical activity: the role of built,
   socioeconomic, and social environments. Soc Sci Med. 2013;95:106–14.
7. Caspi CE, Sorensen G, Subramanian SV, Kawachi I. The local food environment and diet: a systematic review. Health Place. 2012;18(5):1172–87.
8. Case MA, Burwick HA, Volpp KG, Patel MS. Accuracy of smartphone applications and wearable devices for tracking physical activity data. JAMA.
   2015;313(6):625–6.
9. Chen R. Introduction to smart phone positioning. Ubiquitous positioning and mobile location-based services in smart phones. Hershey, PA: IGI
   Global, 1–31; 2012.
10. Chen X, Kwan MP. Contextual uncertainties, human mobility, and per-
    ceived food environment: the uncertain geographic context problem in
    food access research. Am J Pub Health. 2015;105(9):1734–7.
11. Cottrill C, Pereira F, Zhao F, Dias I, Lim H, Ben-Akiva M, Zegras P. Future
    mobility survey: experience in developing a smartphone-based travel
    survey in Singapore. Transp Res Rec: J Transp Res Board. 2013;2354:59–67.
12. Duncan MJ, Winkler E, Sugiyama T, Cerin E, Leslie E, Owen N. Relationships
    of land use mix with walking for transport: do land uses and geographi-
    cal scale matter? J Urban Health. 2010;87(5):782–95.
13. Feng J, Glass TA, Curriero FC, Stewart WF, Schwartz BS. The built environ-
    ment and obesity: a systematic review of the epidemiologic evidence.
    Health Place. 2010;16(2):175–90.
14. Haklay M. Citizen science and volunteered geographic information:
    overview and typology of participation. In: Crowdsourcing geographic
    knowledge. Dordrecht: Springer; 2013. p. 105–22.
15. Handy S. Methodologies for exploring the link between urban form and
    travel behavior. Transp Res Part D: Transp Environ. 1996;1(2):151–65.
16. Kerr J, Duncan S, Schipperjin J. Using global positioning systems in health
    research: a practical approach to data collection and processing. Am J
    Prev Med. 2011;41(5):532–40.
17. Koohsari MJ, Badland H, Giles-Corti B. (Re)Designing the built environ-
    ment to support physical activity: bringing public health back into urban
    design and planning. Cities. 2013;35:294–8.
18. Leal C, Chaix B. The influence of geographic life environments on cardio-
    metabolic risk factors: a systematic review, a methodological assessment
    and a research agenda. Obes Rev. 2011;12(3):217–30.
19. Nitsche P, Widhalm P, Breuss S, Brändle N, Maurer P. Supporting large-
    scale travel surveys with smartphones: a practical approach. Transp Res
    Part C: Emerg Technol. 2014;43:212–21.
20. OSM. (n.d.). Slippy Map Tilenames. from http://wiki.openstreetmap.org/
    wiki/Slippy_map_tilenames.
21. PRC. (2015). Mobile Fact Sheet. from http://www.pewinternet.org/fact-
    sheet/mobile/.
22. Quigg R, Gray A, Reeder AI, Holt A, Waters DL. Using accelerometers and
    GPS units to identify the proportion of daily physical activity located in parks
    with playgrounds in New Zealand children. Prev Med. 2010;50(5):235–40.

23. Riva M, Gauvin L, Barnett TA. Toward the next generation of research into small area effects on health: a synthesis of multilevel investigations published since July 1998. J Epidemiol Community Health. 2007;61(10):853–61.

24. Shin D, Aliaga D, Tunçer B, Arisona SM, Kim S, Zünd D, Schmitt G. Urban sensing: using smartphones for transportation mode classification. Comput Environ Urban Syst. 2015;53:76–86.

25. Sieber R. Public participation geographic information systems: a literature review and framework. Ann Assoc Am Geogr. 2006;96(3):491–507.

26. Stewart OT, Moudon AV, Fesinmeyer MD, Zhou C, Saelens BE. The association between park visitation and physical activity measured with accelerometer, GPS, and travel diary. Health Place. 2016;38:82–8.

27. Troped PJ, Wilson JS, Matthews CE, Cromley EK, Melly SJ. The built environment and location-based physical activity. Am J Prev Med. 2010;38(4):429–38.

28. Zandbergen PA. Accuracy of iPhone locations: a comparison of assisted GPS, WiFi and cellular positioning. Trans GIS. 2009;13(s1):5–25.

29. Zenk SN, Schulz AJ, Matthews SA, Odoms-Young A, Wilbur J, Wegrzyn L, Stokes C. Activity space environment and dietary and physical activity behaviors: a pilot study. Health Place. 2011;17(5):1150–61.

30. Zhou X, Li D, Larsen L. Using web-based participatory mapping to investigate children's perceptions and the spatial distribution of outdoor play places. Environ Behav. 2016;48(7):859–84.

31. Zhou X, Yu W, Sullivan WC. Making pervasive sensing possible: effective travel mode sensing based on smartphones. Comput Environ Urban Syst. 2016;58:52–9.

32. Zhuang Z, Kim K-H, Singh JP. Improving energy efficiency of location sensing on smartphones. Paper presented at the Proceedings of the 8th international conference on Mobile systems, applications, and services; 2010.

The relationship between ethnic composition of the residential environment and self-reported health among Turks and Moroccans in Amsterdam

Eleonore M. Veldhuizen[1*], Umar Z. Ikram[2], Sjoerd de Vos[1] and Anton E. Kunst[2]

Abstract

Background: Previous studies from the US and UK suggest that neighbourhood ethnic composition is associated with health, positive or negative, depending on the health outcome and ethnic group. We examined the association between neighbourhood ethnic composition and self-reported health in these groups in Amsterdam, and we aimed to explore whether there is spatial variation in this association.

Methods: We used micro-scale data to describe the ethnic composition in buffers around the home location of 2701 Turks and 2661 Moroccans. Multilevel regression analysis was used to assess the association between three measures of ethnic composition (% co-ethnics, % other ethnic group, Herfindahl index) and three measures of self-reported health: self-rated health, Physical and Mental Component Score (PCS, MCS). We adjusted for socioeconomic position at individual and area level. We used geographically weighted regression and spatially stratified regression analyses to explore whether associations differed within Amsterdam.

Results: Ethnic heterogeneity and own ethnic density were not related to self-rated health for both ethnic groups. Higher density of Turks was associated with better self-rated health among Moroccans at all buffer sizes, with the most significant relations for small buffers. Higher heterogeneity was associated with lower scores on PCS and MCS among Turks (suggesting worse health). We found spatial variation in the association of the density of the other ethnic group with self-rated health of Moroccans and Turks. We found a positive association for both groups, spatially concentrated in the sub-district Geuzenveld.

Conclusions: Our study showed that the association of ethnic composition with self-reported health among Turks and Moroccans in Amsterdam differed between the groups and reveals mainly at small spatial scales. Among both groups, an association of higher density of the other group with better self-rated health was found in a particular part of Amsterdam, which might be explained by the presence of a relatively strong sense of community between the two groups in that area. The study suggests that it is important to pay attention to other-group density, to use area measurements at small spatial scales and to examine the spatial variation in these associations. This may help to identify neighbourhood characteristics contributing to these type of area effects on urban minority health.

Keywords: Neighbourhood ethnic composition, Ethnic density, Ethnic heterogeneity, Self-reported health, Spatial scale, Geographically weighted regression

*Correspondence: e.m.veldhuizen@uva.nl
[1] Department of Human Geography, Planning and International Development Studies, Faculty of Social and Behavioural Sciences, University of Amsterdam, Nieuwe Achtergracht 166, 1018 WV Amsterdam, The Netherlands
Full list of author information is available at the end of the article

Background

European societies have become increasingly ethnically diverse over the last decades, and this demographic shift is likely to continue given the relatively high influx of immigrants [1, 2]. Evidence indicates that ethnic minority groups overall tend to have worse self-rated health than the ethnic majority group in European countries [3]. This has been attributed to low individual socioeconomic status (SES) and psychosocial factors (e.g., discrimination, acculturation, social network) [4–7], amongst other factors.

Contextual factors such as characteristics of the residential environment may also shape the health of ethnic minority groups. One such characteristic is ethnic composition, which is conceptualized as ethnic diversity or as own-group density (i.e., the presence of the same-ethnic group in the residential environment) [8]. The association between ethnic composition of the residential environment and health presumably operates through social capital and exposure to discrimination [9]. However, evidence from the United States (US) and Europe is equivocal, in that the strength and direction (both negative and positive) of the association vary by ethnic minority group, spatial scale, and outcome measure [8–12].

Furthermore, the existing literature on this topic has three potential limitations. First, most epidemiological studies have focused on own-group density or ethnic diversity, while relatively few studies have assessed other-group density (i.e., co-presence of a specific other ethnic group). This might be particularly relevant for some cities in which two or more (large-sized) ethnic minority groups reside. Other-group density might affect health through material and psychosocial processes. The association could be either positive or negative, largely depending on the inter-relationship the groups have (e.g. mutual trust, discrimination, sharing job information) [13–15].

Second, previous studies have used large spatial scales (e.g., census tracts, electoral wards), making it potentially difficult to assess the associations with health outcomes accurately [16]. Most inter-ethnic interaction and the underlying material and psychosocial processes are likely to occur at smaller spatial scales in the direct environment. Hence using smaller spatial scales could possibly better capture the associations between ethnic composition of residential environment and health [16].

Third, most studies have presented the aggregated effects of ethnic composition on health at city-level [8–11]. This may possibly obscure the spatial variation within a city. Different parts of a city may differ in the opportunities they provide for social interaction between groups. These opportunities might be different due to differences in physical environments (e.g., built environment) and social environments (e.g., social cohesion,

local institutions) [16]. So far, it is unknown whether the association between ethnic composition of residential environment and health differs within a city.

In the present study, we aimed to fill these gaps in the literature. First, we aimed to investigate the association between other-group density of the residential environment and self-reported health outcomes in two ethnic minority groups. We further considered other measures of ethnic composition of residential environment: ethnic heterogeneity and own-group density. Second, we assessed the associations at different spatial scales (both small and large). Third, we explored spatial variation, by assessing whether the associations differed within the city.

We focused on Turkish and Moroccan adults residing in Amsterdam, the Netherlands. These two groups are considered the largest ethnic minority groups in Europe, and tend to co-exist in many different cities (e.g. Paris, Berlin). Our study extended previous studies on this topic conducted in Amsterdam. A 2014 study found own-group density was not associated with psychological distress in Turkish and Moroccan adults living in the four largest Dutch cities (including Amsterdam) [12]. A more recent study from Amsterdam suggested that a high density of Moroccan residents was associated with poor self-rated health among Turkish residents, but not vice versa [13]. In the present study, we delve into these findings by using a much larger dataset, more health outcomes and different spatial scales, as well as by assessing variation within the city.

Study population and methods

Study population

The data were obtained from the HELIUS (Healthy Life in an Urban Setting) study. The aims and design of the HELIUS study have been described elsewhere [17]. Briefly, HELIUS is a large-scale cohort study on health and healthcare among different ethnic groups living in Amsterdam. It included individuals aged 18–70 years from the six largest ethnic groups living in Amsterdam, i.e. those of Dutch, South-Asian Surinamese, African Surinamese, Ghanaian, Moroccan and Turkish origin. Participants were randomly sampled from the municipal registers, stratified by ethnicity. Data were collected by questionnaire and a physical examination. At the end of 2014, response rates were estimated between 20 and 40% with some variations across ethnic groups.

For the current study, baseline data collected from January 2011 until December 2014 were used, including 2962 Turkish and 3000 Moroccan participants. Individuals with missing data on self-reported health, individual characteristics, area ethnic composition or area socioeconomic position, and individuals living at locations with

<25 inhabitants within a buffer of 50 m were excluded from the analysis (n = 600). Our final sample comprised 5362 participants: 2701 Turks and 2661 Moroccans.

Individual level measurements

Participant's ethnicity was defined according to the country of birth of the participant as well as that of his/her parents. Specifically, a participant is considered of Turkish/Moroccan origin if: (1) he or she was born in Turkey/Morocco and has at least one parent born in Turkey/Morocco; or (2) he or she was born in the Netherlands but both his/her parents born in Turkey/Morocco [18].

Three measures of self-reported health are used: self-rated health and generic physical and mental health (PCS and MCS). Self-rated health was measured by the response to the question, 'In general, would you say your health is excellent, very good, good, fair or poor?' The answers were classified into two categories: excellent/very good/good and fair/poor. In the remainder of the paper we refer to the first category as better self-rated health. Generic mental and physical health were assessed using the component summary measures of physical (PCS) and mental health (MCS) from the Medical Outcomes Study Short Form 12 (SF-12) [19]. Scores range from 0 to 100 with higher scores reflecting better health.

From the same survey, we obtained data on characteristics of the participants that were used as control variables at the individual level. These include age, sex, marital status, household composition, educational level, length of residence in the country and a measure of general wealth (whether the participant experienced difficulties living on his or her current household income). See Table 1 for a description of these variables.

Area-level measurements

For area-level measurements we used integral demographic and socio-economic registries at the level of full 6-digit postcodes maintained by the Department of Research and Statistics of the Municipality of Amsterdam. Data on the spatial level of 6-digit postcode area is the most detailed data available. On average, these units are sized 50 × 50 m and include 10–20 households.

To describe the ethnic composition for each participant, we constructed three variables: *own-group density* (i.e., percentage of co-ethnics), *other-group density* (i.e., percentage of the other ethnic group—Turks or Moroccans) and *ethnic heterogeneity* described by the Herfindahl-index. This index yields the probability of two randomly selected individuals from the same neighbourhood being of different ethnic origin. The theoretical range of the index runs from 0 to 1, with 0 representing an area in which every individual is from the same ethnic group and 1 representing an area in which every individual is from a different ethnic group. To calculate this index, we sum the squared proportion of each ethnic group (Surinamese, Antilleans, Ghanaians, Turks, Moroccan, other non-western migrants, other western migrants and Dutch) and subtract this total from one.

When studying the association between ethnic composition and health, it is not enough to control for individual characteristics only. Veldhuizen et al. [13] showed that it is necessary to control for the socio-economic environment as well, because this variable can act as a confounder. To describe the socio-economic environment we constructed two socio-economic variables: the percentage of residents living on a minimum income and the average property value of houses.

In general, the multicollinearity between the independent variables is not very high. Most correlations are 0.5 at most. Only the correlations between percentage Turks/percentage Moroccans/heterogeneity (Herfindahl index) and percentage of minimum income households are high for the larger buffers (0.7). However, because socioeconomic environment is an important determinant of self-rated health we cannot remove the variable from our model.

Within a Geographical Information System (ArcGIS) we created buffers of varying sizes, with radiuses ranging from 50 to 1000 m, around the central point location of each participant's 6-digit postcode area. The ethnic composition and socioeconomic characteristics of each of these buffers were estimated by aggregating the postcode data to the buffers. For a more detailed description of the procedure see Veldhuizen et al. [20].

Statistical analysis

The associations between ethnic composition of the residential environment and self-rated health were assessed using multilevel logistic regression analysis, with better self-rated health as the dependent variable and 6-digit postcode as the variable indicating the higher level (participants living in the same postcode area have identical buffers). We adjusted for the individual characteristics age, sex, marital status, household composition, education, length of residence in the country and wealth and for socio-economic environment measured by the percentage of households living on minimum income and average property value.

To enable comparison of the results of these analyses between different predictors and the different buffer sizes, we present standardised odds ratios of the three measures of ethnic composition. These odds ratios can be interpreted as the change in the odds of better self-rated health if a predictor variable increases with one standard deviation. The odds ratios take into account the

Table 1 Characteristics of participants and their socio-economic environment, per ethnic group

Ethnic group	Moroccan	Turkish
N	2661	2701
Self-rated health (%)		
Excellent	4.7	4.0
Very good	9.7	10.8
Good	48.1	49.6
Fair	30.5	26.4
Poor	7.1	9.3
Physical Component Score		
Mean	46.0	45.3
Standard dev	10.2	10.7
Mental Component Score		
Mean	46.1	44.8
Standard dev	10.9	11.3
Length of residence in the country (years)		
Mean	28.6	28.2
Standard dev	8.7	8.2
Age (%)		
18–29	28.3	25.0
30–39	22.3	21.1
40–49	22.4	29.5
50–64	24.4	22.7
≥65	2.6	1.7
Sex (%)		
Male	36.6	46.3
Marital status (%)		
Married couple	57.6	62.6
Unmarried couple	2.3	3.4
Never been married	28.4	21.5
Divorced	10.1	10.2
Widow/widower	1.7	2.3
Household composition (%)		
Single	7.2	9.2
Couple without children	7.3	10.3
Family	49.2	52.1
Other (living with parents, parents in law, institution)	36.3	28.4
Education (%)		
No/elementary	33.1	33.3
Lower secondary	18.0	25.5
Intermediate/higher secondary	33.1	27.5
Higher	15.9	13.6
Living on household income (%)		
No problems at all	22.3	16.8
No problems, but I have to watch what I spend	35.6	25.4
Some problems	26.3	31.3
Lots of problems	15.7	26.5
Property value of houses at postcode of residence (€)		

Table 1 continued

Ethnic group	Moroccan	Turkish
Mean	198,216	193,880
Standard dev	55,915	53,692
% Households living on a minimum income at postcode of residence		
Mean	28.4	25.9
Standard dev	14.4	15.5

differences in standard deviation according to predictor and buffer size (Table 2).

The associations between neighbourhood ethnic composition and PCS and MCS were assessed using multilevel linear regression analysis, adjusting for the same individual and environmental variables as mentioned above. We present standardised regression coefficients. These coefficients can be interpreted as the change in the standardised dependent variable in case the predictor variable increases with one standard deviation.

In total, 2251 postcode areas were included in the analysis; 1507 for the Turks and 1572 for the Moroccans. We applied random effects (intercept) estimators using STATA's melogit and mixed commands. Random effects appeared to be significant in all empty models and in approximately half of the models with variables. Because a significant number of postcode areas include only one or a limited number of participants, it was not possible to accurately measure both variations between and within the areas. As a result, likelihood ratio tests indicated that our random intercept models were not statistically significant in several models, implying limited meaning of random effects models compared to models without random effects. We present the parameters of the multilevel models because these models generated greater standard errors for our variables of interest than models without random effects.

The dependent variables show substantial variation over Amsterdam. For instance, across 22 administratively defined areas, for Turks the percentage of participants with good self-rated health varies between 44 and 77, for Moroccans between 50 and 73.

Geographical analysis

Additionally, we used logistic geographically weighted regression (GWR) within the software GWR4 to explore whether the most important association we found from the multilevel regression analyses spatially differed within Amsterdam. GWR enables us to explore if the association varies within the city, without a priori assumptions with respect to the geographic scale at which these variations would occur. GWR is a local form

Table 2 Characteristics of the participant's neighbourhood ethnic composition per ethnic group and spatial scale

Ethnic group	Moroccan		Turkish	
	Mean	SD	Mean	SD
Own ethnic density (%)				
Buffer50	26.6	16.5	17.2	10.5
100	23.5	14.9	15.0	8.6
150	22.2	14.1	14.3	7.9
300	19.7	11.7	12.9	6.8
500	18.3	10.3	12.2	6.3
750	17.2	9.0	11.7	6.0
1000	16.3	8.3	11.3	5.9
Other ethnic density (%) (Turks resp. Moroccans)				
50	12.6	9.9	22.9	15.3
100	12.3	8.6	22.6	13.4
150	12.0	8.1	22.2	12.6
300	11.1	7.1	20.7	10.5
500	10.5	6.5	19.7	9.0
750	10.0	6.1	18.7	8.0
1000	9.6	5.9	18.0	7.5
Ethnic heterogeneity (range 0–1)				
50	0.711	0.085	0.722	0.083
100	0.721	0.079	0.735	0.072
150	0.723	0.079	0.738	0.070
300	0.728	0.078	0.744	0.066
500	0.729	0.077	0.747	0.064
750	0.728	0.075	0.745	0.063
1000	0.725	0.073	0.742	0.062

of (in this case logistic) regression to model spatially varying relationships. It constructs a separate equation for every participant incorporating the dependent and explanatory variables of all participants living within a specific distance around the target participant. We used a bandwidth (Gaussian Kernel) of a fixed distance of 500 m which means that a 500 m kernel is used over the whole study area. The alternative for a fixed spatial kernel, an adaptive kernel, varies the size of kernel according to the spatial distribution of observation. This would mean that in areas with relatively few participants the kernel would become large which would obscure local relationships. We considered 500 m as a reasonable compromise between two conflicting demands: (1) to include a reasonable number of participants in the analyses, and (2) to allow for the exploration of sufficient spatial variation. We mapped the resulting odds ratios to visually explore spatial patterns.

Based on the observation that the spatial pattern of the OR values more of less coincides with sub-districts of Amsterdam, we decided to perform an additional stratified multilevel analysis by sub-district. This allows us to assess the associations more accurately than within GWR because of the limited number of observations in the local regressions. We restricted the stratified analysis to Nieuw-West where most participants reside.

Results

Table 1 describes the characteristics of the study population in both ethnic groups. In general, no substantial differences in poor self-rated health, PCS and MCS were observed between Turkish and Moroccan participants. The two groups also had similar scores on most other characteristics although more Turkish participants were lower educated and had a little more difficulties in making ends meet.

Table 2 shows the average levels and standard deviations of own-group density, other-group density and ethnic heterogeneity by spatial scale for the two ethnic groups. Compared to Turkish participants, the residential environment of Moroccan participants was characterized by a higher share of co-ethnics. Levels and standard deviations of own-group density decreased with increasing buffer size, especially among Moroccans. Turkish participants had a higher percentage of Moroccans in their residential environment than vice versa. The difference between Turkish and Moroccan participants on the measures was approximately 10% points at all buffer distances. Levels and standard deviations of other-group density decrease with increasing buffer size, especially among Turkish participants. The level of ethnic heterogeneity of the residential environment of Moroccan and Turkish participants is comparable. Ethnic heterogeneity increases for buffers up to 500 m.

Table 3 shows the association of own-group density, other-group density and ethnic heterogeneity with self-rated health per ethnic group. Overall, own-group density and ethnic heterogeneity were not significantly related to self-rated health in both groups. For other-group density, a higher percentage of Turks in the neighbourhood was associated with higher odds of reporting better self-rated health among Moroccans. These results were consistent with more significant relations found for smaller buffers. Self-rated health of Turks was not significantly associated with higher density of Moroccans in the neighbourhood.

Table 4 shows the associations of own-group density, other-group density and ethnic heterogeneity with PCS and MCS per ethnic group. Among Moroccans a higher density of Turks within a 50 m buffer was significantly associated with a healthier PCS. Among Turks, higher ethnic heterogeneity was significantly associated with worse PCS at buffer sizes up to 300 m and with worse MCS from 150 to 500 m buffers.

Table 3 Association of density of Moroccans, density of Turks and ethnic heterogeneity with better self-rated health, per ethnic group and spatial scale

Ethnic group	Moroccan	Turkish
	Standardised OR[a] (CI[b])	Standardised OR[a] (CI[b])
Density of Moroccans (%)		
Buffer50	1.01 (0.89; 1.14)	1.05 (0.94; 1.19)
100	1.08 (0.95; 1.23)	1.08 (0.95; 1.23)
150	1.10 (0.96; 1.26)	1.05 (0.92; 1.20)
300	1.09 (0.95; 1.25)	1.05 (0.92; 1.20)
500	1.09 (0.96; 1.24)	1.04 (0.92; 1.19)
750	1.11 (0.98; 1.26)	1.08 (0.96; 1.23)
1000	1.15 (1.02; 1.30)*	1.08 (0.96; 1.23)
Density of Turks (%)		
50	1.19 (1.07; 1.33)**	1.10 (1.00; 1.22)
100	1.16 (1.04; 1.30)**	1.06 (0.95; 1.18)
150	1.17 (1.04; 1.31)**	1.07 (0.96; 1.19)
300	1.15 (1.03; 1.30)*	1.05 (0.94; 1.17)
500	1.14 (1.01; 1.28)*	1.08 (0.97; 1.21)
750	1.14 (1.01; 1.28)*	1.09 (0.97; 1.22)
1000	1.16 (1.02; 1.31)*	1.07 (0.95; 1.21)
Ethnic heterogeneity		
50	0.98 (0.89; 1.09)	0.98 (0.89; 1.08)
100	1.03 (0.93; 1.15)	0.97 (0.88; 1.08)
150	1.03 (0.92; 1.15)	0.99 (0.89; 1.10)
300	1.10 (0.97; 1.24)	0.97 (0.86; 1.08)
500	1.15 (1.01; 1.31)*	1.03 (0.92; 1.16)
750	1.11 (0.97; 1.26)	1.06 (0.94; 1.20)
1000	1.14 (0.99; 1.31)	1.09 (0.96; 1.24)

* Significant at the 0.05 level

** Significant at the 0.01 level

[a] OR represents the standardised Odds Ratio (i.e. change in odds of having better self-rated health with one standard deviation increase in the predictor variable)

[b] CI represents 95% confidence interval

Based on the results of Table 3, we performed additional GWR-analyses to explore the spatial variation in the association of the density of Turks within 50 m buffers with self-rated health of Moroccans. The map in Fig. 1 shows some degree of spatial variation in this association, although most OR values were not significantly different from 1. In the district Nieuw-West, for example, the association of the density of Turks with self-rated health of Moroccans is more positive in the northern part of the district than in the southern part. In the district West mainly positive associations cluster and in East positive as well as negative associations were observed.

Table 5 assesses associations per sub-district in Nieuw-West. We stratified the additional MLR analyses by sub-district because the results of the GWR suggested variations at the level of sub-districts. We restricted the stratified analysis to Nieuw-West where most participants reside. Positive significant associations of density of Turks with self-rated health of Moroccans were found in the district Nieuw-West and mainly in the sub-district Geuzenveld. The density of Moroccans was significantly positively associated with self-rated health of Turks in Geuzenveld as well. For both groups, no significant association of own-group density with self-rated health was found in any district.

Discussion

In this study, we assessed associations between ethnic composition of the residential environment and self-reported health among people of Turkish and Moroccan origin living in Amsterdam. At the city-scale of Amsterdam, own-group density and ethnic heterogeneity were not associated with self-rated health for either Moroccan or Turkish participants. For Turks significant associations between ethnic heterogeneity and PCS and MCS were found, suggesting more negative health outcomes with increasing heterogeneity. With regard to other-group density, for Moroccans, greater density of Turks was significantly associated with higher odds of reporting better self-rated health and higher scores on PCS. Such associations were not found for Turks.

Additional geographical analyses suggest that the relationship between the density of the other group and self-rated health varies within Amsterdam. Associations were particularly observed in the sub-district Geuzenveld within the district Nieuw-West. In this specific area, other-group density is positively associated with self-rated health for both groups.

Evaluation of data and methodology

A major strength of our study is that the HELIUS data provides a large number of participants from different ethnic groups and detailed health measurements and socio-demographic data. We further derived precise data about place of residence using the 6-digit postcode of the home addresses of the participants, and we accessed detailed socio-economic and demographic data from registries at the level of 6-digit postcodes. On average, 6-digit postcode areas in Amsterdam include no more than 10–20 households and are sized 50 by 50 m. The large number of participants and information on their precise place of residence enabled us to use advanced geographic techniques to explore varying associations within the city. The importance of using environmental variables at small spatial scales derives from the fact that most of the significant associations were found at small spatial scales. It suggests that no associations could have been demonstrated if the environmental characteristics

Table 4 Association of density of Moroccans, density of Turks and ethnic heterogeneity with Physical and Mental Component Score per ethnic group and spatial scale

Ethnic group	Moroccan		Turkish	
	Standardised b[a] (CI[b])		Standardised b[a] (CI[b])	
	PCS	MCS	PCS	MCS
Density of Moroccans (%)				
Buffer50	0.01 (−0.04; 0.05)	0.03 (−0.02; 0.07)	0.01 (−0.04; 0.05)	−0.01 (−0.06; 0.04)
100	0.02 (−0.03; 0.07)	0.00 (−0.05; 0.06)	0.01 (−0.04; 0.06)	−0.02 (−0.07; 0.04)
150	0.01 (−0.04; 0.06)	0.00 (−0.05; 0.06)	0.01 (−0.04; 0.06)	−0.04 (−0.10; 0.01)
300	0.00 (−0.05; 0.05)	0.01 (−0.04; 0.07)	−0.01 (−0.06; 0.04)	−0.01 (−0.07; 0.04)
500	−0.00 (−0.05; 0.05)	0.01 (−0.04; 0.06)	−0.00 (−0.05; 0.05)	−0.03 (−0.08; 0.02)
750	0.01 (−0.04; 0.05)	0.00 (−0.05; 0.05)	0.01 (−0.03; 0.06)	−0.02 (−0.07; 0.03)
1000	0.01 (−0.04; 0.06)	0.00 (−0.05; 0.05)	0.02 (−0.02; 0.07)	−0.02 (−0.07; 0.04)
Density of Turks (%)				
50	0.04 (0.00; 0.08)*	0.01 (−0.03; 0.06)	0.01 (−0.03; 0.05)	−0.01 (−0.05; 0.03)
100	0.04 (−0.00; 0.08)	0.01 (−0.03; 0.06)	0.01 (−0.03; 0.05)	−0.01 (−0.06; 0.03)
150	0.04 (−0.00; 0.08)	0.01 (−0.04; 0.05)	0.01 (−0.03; 0.05)	−0.02 (−0.06; 0.03)
300	0.03 (−0.02; 0.07)	0.01 (−0.04; 0.05)	0.01 (−0.03; 0.05)	−0.02 (−0.07; 0.02)
500	0.01 (−0.03; 0.05)	0.01 (−0.04; 0.05)	0.02 (−0.02; 0.06)	−0.01 (−0.06; 0.03)
750	0.01 (−0.03; 0.05)	−0.01 (−0.05; 0.04)	0.02 (−0.02; 0.06)	−0.01 (−0.06; 0.04)
1000	0.01 (−0.04; 0.05)	−0.01 (−0.06; 0.04)	0.03 (−0.01; 0.08)	−0.02 (−0.07; 0.03)
Ethnic heterogeneity				
50	−0.02 (−0.05; 0.02)	−0.02 (−0.06; 0.02)	−0.06 (−0.09; −0.02)**	−0.01 (−0.05; 0.03)
100	0.00 (−0.04; 0.04)	−0.01 (−0.05; 0.03)	−0.05 (−0.09; −0.01)**	−0.02 (−0.06; 0.02)
150	0.00 (−0.04; 0.04)	−0.02 (−0.07; 0.02)	−0.04 (−0.08; −0.00)*	−0.05 (−0.09; −0.01)*
300	0.04 (−0.01; 0.09)	−0.01 (−0.06; 0.03)	−0.06 (−0.10; −0.02)**	−0.07 (−0.11; −0.02)**
500	0.05 (−0.00; 0.09)	0.00 (−0.05; 0.05)	−0.02 (−0.06; 0.03)	−0.06 (−0.10; −0.01)*
750	0.03 (−0.02; 0.08)	−0.02 (−0.07; 0.04)	−0.02 (−0.07; 0.02)	−0.05 (−0.10; 0.00)
1000	0.03 (−0.02; 0.08)	−0.01 (−0.06; 0.05)	−0.00 (−0.05; 0.04)	−0.03 (−0.08; 0.02)

* Significant at the 0.05 level

** Significant at the 0.01 level

[a] b represents the standardised regression coefficient (i.e. change in the dependent variable with one standard deviation increase in the predictor variable)

[b] CI represents 95% confidence interval

of administrative areas were used because these areas may be too large to detect any health effects.

This study has some limitations as well. First, because buffers partly overlap, observations are not entirely independent. This results in a slight overestimation of significance levels. However, this problem of partial overlap applies particularly to larger buffers and less to smaller buffers, for which we found the most significant associations. Second, because our data are cross-sectional, our interpretations ought to refer to associations rather than to causal relationships. Nevertheless, we might interpret these associations as evidence for environmental influences on health. Reverse causality should refer to selective migration, which in our study would imply that healthy Moroccans would move to places with a lot of Turks or unhealthy Moroccans would leave such areas, which is not very plausible. Third, since we focused on

two specific ethnic minority groups living in Amsterdam, our findings could possibly not be generalized to other populations or areas. Nonetheless, numerous large European cities have large migrant populations from Turkey and Morocco, so our findings might have relevance for these cities as well. Finally, PCS and MCS have not been validated among Turkish and Moroccan participants. However, these instruments have been positively validated across other cultures and countries [21, 22].

Our conceptualization of the residential environment, buffers, can be associated with two discussions in the research field, referred to as the 'local trap' [23] and the 'residential trap' [24]. The local trap refers to the question whether the local scale is the best scale for analysis and the residential trap refers to the neglect of other environmental context besides the residential context. Because we use different buffer sizes in our study, we

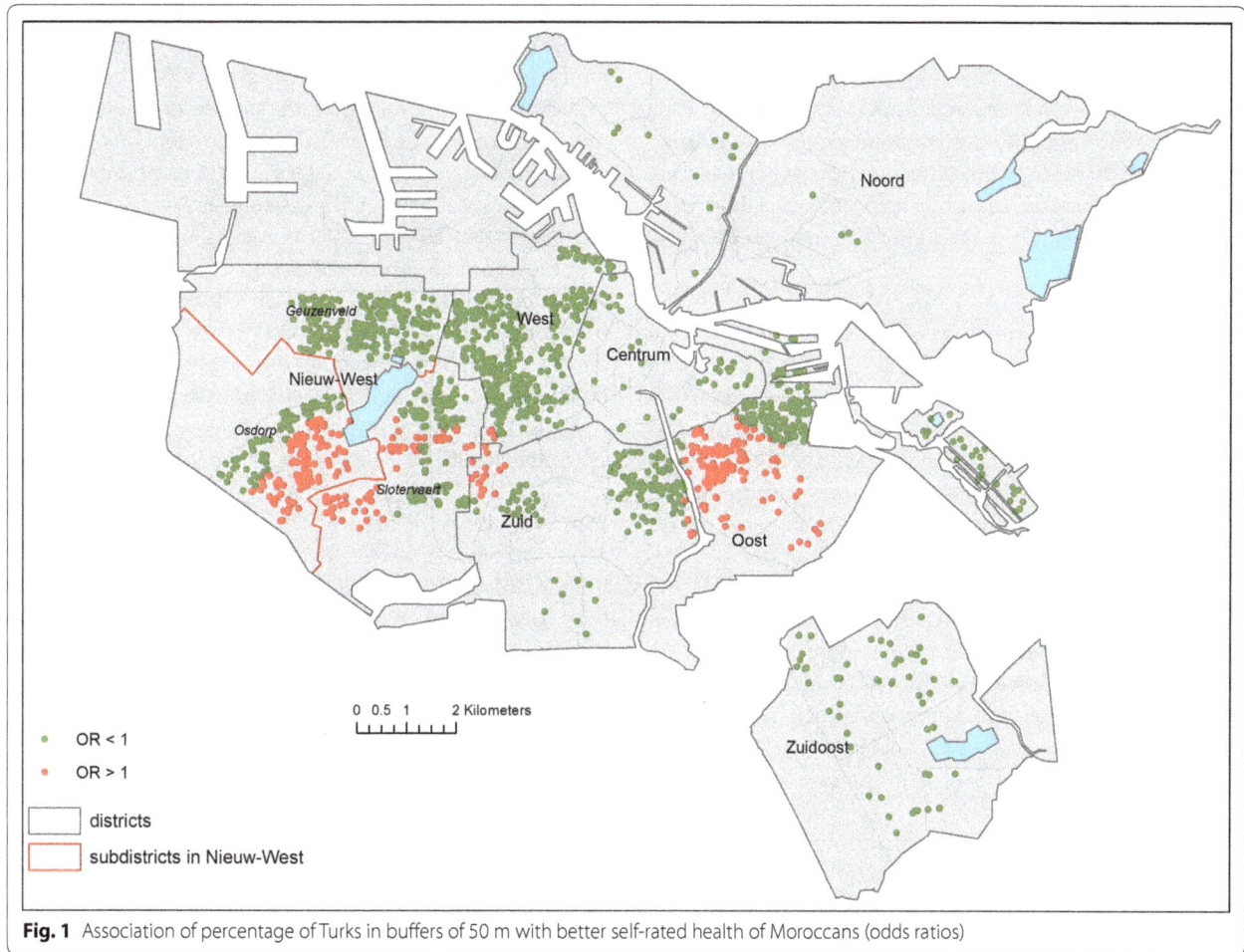

Fig. 1 Association of percentage of Turks in buffers of 50 m with better self-rated health of Moroccans (odds ratios)

Table 5 Association of other- and own-group density within 50 m buffer with better self-rated health, per ethnic group and sub-district

Ethnic group			Moroccan		Turkish	
			Standardised OR[a] (CI[b])		Standardised OR[a] (CI[b])	
Density of			Turks (%)	Moroccans (%)	Moroccans (%)	Turks (%)
(Sub-)district	N Mor	N Tur				
Nieuw-West	1238	1365	1.16 (1.00;1.35)*	0.93 (0.76;1.12)	1.03 (0.86;1.23)	1.10 (0.96;1.26)
Geuzenveld	433	626	1.39 (1.04;1.86)*	0.86 (0.62;1.20)	1.32 (1.02;1.71)*	1.05 (0.86;1.29)
Osdorp	388	383	1.11 (0.85;1.45)	0.97 (0.67;1.40)	0.87 (0.59;1.28)	0.99 (0.74;1.32)
Slotervaart	416	356	1.02 (0.76;1.37)	1.01 (0.70;1.45)	0.81 (0.53;1.25)	0.98 (0.72;1.33)

* Significant at the 0.05 level

[a] OR represents the standardised odds ratio (i.e. change in odds with one standard deviation increase in the predictor variable)

[b] CI represents 95% confidence interval

could evaluate the local trap problem. In fact, the results imply that this problem is not so relevant on our cases, as the strongest associations were observed in the smaller buffers.

With regard to the residential trap, we admit that other environmental contexts are also important in determining people's exposure to the own and other ethnic groups. To improve our understanding of the influence of other contexts, future research could try to combine different environmental contexts based on activity spaces. Activity spaces can be separated into domains such as a residential, transportation and work domain and for each domain the exposure to a certain environmental characteristic, for instance ethnic diversity, can be measured. Finally, the effects of the three exposure variables on a health outcome, such as mental health, can be assessed. This may yield new insights.

Interpretation and comparison with previous studies

For Turks and Moroccans in Amsterdam we did not find associations of own-group density with self-rated health, PCS or MCS. These findings are not in line with 'classic' ethnic density theory which suggests better health if a high proportion of the own ethnic group lives in the neighbourhood. This positive influence on health is presumably due to increased social support and less discrimination if your own group lives around [25–28]. Several studies in the US and UK found effects of own-group density on health, sometimes positive [9, 29, 30], but sometimes negative [31–33]. However, similar to our results, Schrier et al. [12] found no association between own-group density and psychological distress for Surinamese, Turks, and Moroccans in the four largest Dutch cities (including Amsterdam).

The absence of an ethnic own-group density effect especially among Turks is surprising considering that the Turks are known as a group with a strong orientation towards their co-ethnics. It might be explained by segmentation within the Turkish community. Turks are a heterogeneous group, divided along often crosscutting lines associated with political, ethnic, religious and geographical differences [34]. Our measure for own-group density, which is based on the country of birth of the participants or their parents, may fail to comprehensively capture the own-group effects. If the subgroups would have lived entirely segregated, an own-group density effect for the Turkish participants might be expected. However, probably the subgroups live mixed because most of the Turks and Moroccans depend on social housing which means little room for own choice regarding place to live [35]. Unfortunately we miss the essential accurate information about the home location of subgroups for further examination.

The negative influence of ethnic heterogeneity on PCS and MCS among Turks accords with conclusions of Putnam's study in the US [36] which suggested worse health conditions in heterogeneous neighbourhoods because of lower social capital in these neighbourhoods. For the Netherlands, Lancee and Dronkers [37] also found that more heterogeneous neighbourhoods are characterized by less social capital. However, our study did not find

a negative effect of heterogeneity among Moroccans. Recently, it has been suggested that Putnam's theory may not be generalizable to all ethnic groups [38], but depend on ethnic group identities and specific inter-group relations. In Amsterdam, for Turks a heterogeneous environment might be experienced as negative, because Turks are known as a group with a strong orientation towards (some of) their co-ethnics. Moroccans are known to have lower levels of co-ethnic cohesion [39]. Hence it could be suggested that Turks rely more on 'bonding' social capital (relations within the own group), while Moroccans may find it easier to link with other ethnic groups and thus rely on 'bridging' social capital (relations with other groups).

We found a positive influence of density of Turks on self-rated health of Moroccans. A previous study, based on a smaller survey among six ethnic groups in Amsterdam [13], found a negative influence of the density of Moroccans on self-rated health of Turks. Although the findings of the two studies are not identical, both imply that co-residence with Turks has no negative effect on self-rated health of Moroccans, and the Moroccans have no positive effect on Turks. This asymmetric relation might be explained by a lesser positive opinion of Turks towards Moroccans, partly because Moroccans are more stigmatized in Dutch politics and media than Turks [39, 40]. In such a context it is less favourable for Turks to be associated with Moroccans living in the same neighbourhood than vice versa. Another reason might be that Turks seems more oriented on the own group unlike Moroccans as already mentioned in the previous paragraph.

The positive influence of other-group density in the direct residential environment on self-rated health of both groups in Geuzenveld might be related to specific conditions in this area. Geuzenveld is an area with a relatively strong sense of community among Turkish and Moroccan inhabitants. Compared to other administratively defined areas in Amsterdam, Geuzenveld is smaller in size and the ethnic composition is dominated by only a few groups. Turks and Moroccans together comprise almost 50% of the population. This implies a relatively high degree of dependency and interaction between the two groups, with possibly stronger social support systems between these groups. This is reinforced by a low number of relocations and outmigration among ethnic groups in ethnic concentration areas such as Geuzenveld [41]. Moreover, the two groups may have forged stronger alliances with each other, given the context of strong tensions between ethnic minorities and those of Dutch origin in Geuzenveld [42], and relatively low socio economic position of Geuzenveld residents as compared to most other parts of Amsterdam [43].

Our findings may give some direction to policy aimed to improve urban health. The health effects of residential ethnic composition we found in this study reveal generally at small spatial scales and varied within the city. This suggests that to improve urban minority (self-rated) health, area-based local interventions are more appropriate than global city-wide interventions; health benefits will be larger if interventions are adjusted to specific problem locations. For instance, in areas with negative associations between other group density or heterogeneity and health, policy interventions could aim to increase interactions and social cohesion at the very local level.

Conclusion

Our study suggests that in studies on the influence of neighbourhood ethnic composition on health three aspects are important. First, other-group density, the density of a specific ethnic group, deserves attention aside from common measures such as own-group density and ethnic heterogeneity. Additionally, it is important to use area measurements at small spatial scales. Finally, to improve our understanding of the underlying mechanisms, it might help to examine the spatial variation in the relationship within urban areas. The relationship between ethnic composition and health may depend on specific local factors influencing relations and ties between ethnic groups.

Abbreviations

GIS: geographic information systems; MCS: Mental Component Score; PCS: Physical Component Score.

Authors' contributions

EV, UI and AK conceptualized this paper and determined the research plan. EV completed the statistical analyses with support of SV. EV, UI and AK wrote the majority of the paper with input of the other author. All authors read and approved the final manuscript.

Author details

[1] Department of Human Geography, Planning and International Development Studies, Faculty of Social and Behavioural Sciences, University of Amsterdam, Nieuwe Achtergracht 166, 1018 WV Amsterdam, The Netherlands. [2] Department of Public Health, Academic Medical Centre, University of Amsterdam, Meibergdreef 9, 1105 AZ Amsterdam, The Netherlands.

Acknowledgements

The authors gratefully acknowledge the Department of Research and Statistics of the Municipality of Amsterdam for providing the environmental data and Mr Mohamed Bensellam, district- manager of Nieuw-West, for being an important key informant.

Competing interests

The authors declare that they have no competing interests.

Funding

Not applicable (time for research was fully covered by the University of Amsterdam).

References

1. Lee JJH, Guadagno L. World Migration Report 2015. Migrants and cities: new partnerships to manage mobility. Geneva: International Organization for Migration; 2015.
2. StatLine. Bevolking; generatie, geslacht, leeftijd en herkomstgroepering, 1 Januari 2015. http://statline.cbs.nl/. Accessed 20 Novembre 2015.
3. Nielsen SS, Krasnik A. Poorer self-perceived health among migrants and ethnic minorities versus the majority population in Europe: a systematic review. Int J Pub Health. 2010;55:357–71.
4. Finch BK, Vega WA. Acculturation stress, social support, and self-rated health among Latinos in California. J Immigr Health. 2003;5:109–17.
5. Harris R, Tobias M, Jeffreys M, Waldegrave K, Karlsen S, Nazroo J. Effects of self-reported racial discrimination and deprivation on Māori health and inequalities in New Zealand: cross-sectional study. Lancet. 2006;367:2005–9. doi:10.1016/s0140-6736(06)68890-9.
6. Lindström M, Sundquist J, Östergren PO. Ethnic differences in self reported health in Malmö in southern Sweden. J Epidemiol Community Health. 2001;55:97–103.
7. Reijneveld SA. Reported health, lifestyles, and use of health care of first generation immigrants in The Netherlands: do socioeconomic factors explain their adverse position? J Epidemiol Community Health. 1998;52:298–304.
   Mair C, Diez Roux AV, Galea S. Are neighbourhood characteristics associated with depressive symptoms? A review of evidence. J Epidemiol Community Health. 2008;62:940–6, 948 p following 946. doi:10.1136/
8. jech.2007.066605.
   Pickett KE, Wilkinson RG. People like us: ethnic group density effects on health. Ethn Health. 2008;13:321–34. doi:10.1080/13557850701882928.
10. Bécares L, Shaw R, Nazroo J, Stafford M, Albor C, Atkin K, et al. Ethnic
9. density effects on physical morbidity, mortality, and health behaviors: a systematic review of the literature. Am J Public Health. 2012;102:e33–66.
11. Shaw RJ, Atkin K, Bécares L, Albor CB, Stafford M, Kiernan KE, et al. Impact of ethnic density on adult mental disorders: narrative review. Br J Psychiatry. 2012;201:11–9.
12. Schrier AC, Peen J, de Wit MA, van Ameijden EJC, Erdem O, Verhoeff AP, et al. Ethnic density is not associated with psychological distress in Turkish-Dutch, Moroccan-Dutch and Surinamese-Dutch ethnic minorities in the Netherlands. Soc Psychiatry Psychiatr Epidemiol. 2014;49:1557–67. doi:10.1007/s00127-014-0852-x.
13. Veldhuizen EM, Musterd S, Dijkshoorn H, Kunst AE. Association between self-rated health and the ethnic composition of the residential environment of six ethnic groups in Amsterdam. Int J Environ Res Public Health. 2015;12:14382–99. doi:10.3390/ijerph121114382.
14. Damm AP. Ethnic enclaves and immigrant labor market outcomes: quasi-experimental evidence. J Labor Econ. 2009;27:281–314.
15. Damm AP. Neighborhood quality and labor market outcomes: evidence from quasi-random neighborhood assignment of immigrants. J Urban Econ. 2014;79:139–66.
16. Diez Roux AV, Mair C. Neighborhoods and health. Ann N Y Acad Sci. 2010;1186:125–45. doi:10.1111/j.1749-6632.2009.05333.x.
17. Stronks K, Snijder MB, Peters RJG, Prins M, Schene AH, Zwinderman AH. Unravelling the impact of ethnicity of health in Europe: the HELIUS Study. BMC Public Health. 2013; doi:10.1186/1471-2458-13-402.
18. Stronks K, Kulu-Glasgow I, Agyemang C. The utility of 'country of birth' for the classification of ethnic groups in health research: the Dutch experience. Ethn Health. 2009;14:1–14.
19. Ware JE, Kosinski MMA, Keller SD. A 12-Item Short-Form Health Survey: construction of scales and preliminary tests of reliability and validity. Med Care. 1996;34:220–33.
20. Veldhuizen EM, Stronks K, Kunst AE. Assessing associations between between socio-economic environment and self-reported health in Amsterdam using bespoke environments. PLoS ONE. 2013;. doi:10.1371/journal.pone.0068790.

21. Jenkinson C, Chandola T, Coulter A, Bruster S. An assessment of the construct validity of the SF-12 summary scores across ethnic groups. J Public Health Med. 2001;23:187–94.

22. Gandek B, Ware JE, Aaronson NK, Apolone G, Bjorner JB, Brazier JE, Bullinger M, Kaasa S, Leplege A, Prieto L, Sullivan M. Cross-validation of item selection and scoring for the SF-12 Health Survey in nine countries: results from the IQOLA Project. J Clin Epidemiol. 1998;51:1171–8.

23. Cummins S. Commentary: investigating neighbourhood effects on health-avoiding the 'local trap'. Int J Epidemiol. 2007;36:355–7.

24. Chaix B, Merlo J, Evans D, Leal C, Havard S. Neighborhoods in eco-epidemiologic research: delimiting personal exposure areas. A response to Riva, Gauvin, Apparico, and Brodeur. Soc Sci Med. 2009;69:1306–10.

25. Smaje C. Ethnic residential concentration and health: evidence for a positive effect? Policy Polit. 1995;23:251–69.

26. Halpern D. Minorities and mental health. Soc Sci Med. 1993;36:597–607.

27. Hunt MO, Wise LR, Jiguep MC, Cozier YC, Rosenberg L. Neighbourhood racial composition and perceptions of racial discrimination: evidence from the black women's health study. Soc Psychol Q. 2007;70:272–89.

28. Bécares L. The ethnic density effect on the health of ethnic minority people in the United Kingdom: a study of hypothesised pathways. Doctoral dissertation. London: University College London; 2009.

29. Veling MD, Susser E, van Os J, Mackenbach MD, Selten JP, Hoek HW. Ethnic density of neighborhoods and incidence of psychotic disorders among immigrants. Am J Psychiatry. 2007; doi:10.1176/appi/ajp.2007.07030423.

30. Das-Munshi J, Becares L, Dewey ME, Stansfeld SA, Prince MJ. Understanding the effect of ethnic density on mental health: multi-level investigation of survey data from England. BMJ. 2010; doi:10.1136/bmj.c5367.

31. LeClere F, Rogers R, Peters K. Ethnicity and mortality in the United States: individual and community correlates. Soc Forces. 1997;76:169–98. doi:10.1093/sf/76.1.169.

32. White K, Borrell LN. Racial/ethnic neighborhood concentration and self-reported health in New York City. Ethn Dis. 2006;16:900–8.

33. Grady SC. Racial disparities in low birthweight and the contribution of residential segregation: a multilevel analysis. Soc Sci Med. 2006;63:3013–29.

34. Inglis C, Akgonul S, De Tapia S. Turks abroad: settlers, citizens, transnationals—introduction. IJMS. 2009;11:104–18.

35. Van Praag C, Schoorl J. Housing and Segregation. In: Crul M, Heering L, editors. The position of the Turkish and Moroccan second-generation in Amsterdam and Rotterdam. Amsterdam: Amsterdam University Press; 2008. p. 49–62.

36. Putnam R. E pluribus unum: diversity and community in the twenty-first century the 2006 Johan Skytte Prize Lecture. Scan Polit Stud. 2007;30:137–74.

37. Lancee B, Dronkers J. Ethnic diversity in neighborhoods and individual trust of immigrants and natives: A replication of Putnam (2007) in a West-European country. In: Hooghe M, editor. Social cohesion. Contemporary theoretical perspectives on the study of social cohesion and social capital. Brussels: Royal Academy of Belgium; 2010. p. 77–103.

38. Abascal M, Baldassarri D. Love thy neighbour? Ethnoracial diversity and trust re-examined. Am J Sociol. 2015;121:722–82.

39. Slootman M, Duyvendak JW. Feeling Dutch: the culturalization and emotionalization of citizenship and second-generation belonging in the Netherlands. In: Foner N, Simon P, editors. Fear, anxiety, and national identity: immigration and belonging in North America and Western Europe. New York: Russell Sage Foundation; 2015. p. 147–68.

40. Identities Groenewold G, Relations Intercultural. In: Crul M, Heering L, editors. The position of the Turkish and Moroccan second-generation in Amsterdam and Rotterdam. Amsterdam: Amsterdam University Press; 2008. p. 105–29.

41. Musterd S, de Vos S. Residential dynamics in ethnic concentrations. Hous Stud. 2007;22:333–53.

42. Boers J, van Marissing E, Slot J, Boutellier H. Samenleven met verschillen: Signalering van spanningen en versterken van vertrouwen in Amsterdamse buurten. Amsterdam: Gemeente Amsterdam Bureau Onderzoek en Statistiek en Verwey-Jonker Instituut; 2012.

43. Municipality of Amsterdam. Gebiedsanalyse 2015. Retrieved from: http://www.ois.amsterdam.nl/pdf/2015_gebiedsanalyses_overkoepelende%20analyse.pdf.

Using meta-quality to assess the utility of volunteered geographic information for science

Shaun A. Langley[1], Joseph P. Messina[2] and Nathan Moore[2*] (iD)

Abstract

Background: Volunteered geographic information (VGI) has strong potential to be increasingly valuable to scientists in collaboration with non-scientists. The abundance of mobile phones and other wireless forms of communication open up significant opportunities for the public to get involved in scientific research. As these devices and activities become more abundant, questions of uncertainty and error in volunteer data are emerging as critical components for using volunteer-sourced spatial data.

Methods: Here we present a methodology for using VGI and assessing its sensitivity to three types of error. More specifically, this study evaluates the reliability of data from volunteers based on their historical patterns. The specific context is a case study in surveillance of tsetse flies, a health concern for being the primary vector of African Trypanosomiasis.

Results: Reliability, as measured by a reputation score, determines the threshold for accepting the volunteered data for inclusion in a tsetse presence/absence model. Higher reputation scores are successful in identifying areas of higher modeled tsetse prevalence. A dynamic threshold is needed but the quality of VGI will improve as more data are collected and the errors in identifying reliable participants will decrease.

Conclusions: This system allows for two-way communication between researchers and the public, and a way to evaluate the reliability of VGI. Boosting the public's ability to participate in such work can improve disease surveillance and promote citizen science. In the absence of active surveillance, VGI can provide valuable spatial information given that the data are reliable.

Background

We are standing on the apex of a scientific transition as technological and communications barriers are toppled [1, 2], and the distinction between amateur and professional scientist is eroded. Neogeography characterizes the "blurring of the distinctions between producer, communicator, and consumer of geographic information"; the separation of scientist and layperson, expert and novice, is obscured as citizens engage in the generation of new knowledge [3]. As citizens engage in Science, we need to reconsider our traditional notions of authority, expertise, and purpose.

Neogeography, a type of citizen science, is the democratization of geographic tools and methods for non-traditional mapmaking. It has garnered a great deal of attention in the literature as we struggle to conceptualize the nature of "geographic expertise"; however, the involvement of citizens in science has long been established [3, 4]. Participatory science has sought to involve citizens directly in academic research and related exploits [5–7] on the premise that citizens are more informed actors with respect to their local environment than researchers operating externally. Citizens are perceived to hold authority through experience and status, and are

*Correspondence: moorena@msu.edu
[2] Center for Global Change and Department of Geography, Environment, and Spatial Sciences, Michigan State University, East Lansing, MI, USA
Full list of author information is available at the end of the article

acknowledged for their capacity to convey unique understanding, or indigenous knowledge [1, 5].

With the advent of Web 2.0 [8, 9] and the widespread availability of new technologies [6, 10], citizens are increasingly exposed to geographical information. Citizens also increasingly volunteer spatially explicit (geographical) information that is of relevance or interest to them, often integrating this information with existing datasets, or mashups, utilizing it for their own gain [4, 11]. Boulos [12, 13] first introduced this concept of collaboratively developed spatial information as the "Wikification of GIS by the masses". Goodchild coined the term "volunteered geographic information" (VGI) to refer to spatial data that is contributed by ordinary citizens, irrespective of their training in scientific methods [14]. The notion of VGI grew out of recognition of the limitations of traditional methodologies for adequately mapping and assembling spatial information around the world that provided both good coverage and fine temporal resolution [15–17]. As a framework, VGI encompasses citizen participation from a range of social classes and computing practices with the express purpose of harnessing the collective intelligence [5, 18]; it builds on the notion that data can be shaped by social and political processes and an individual's expertise, context, and spatial awareness [15, 19–21]. Local knowledge is crucial to an accurate geographic description of communities and social groups, involving the citizen in the process of data collection.

VGI in practice is now commonplace, e.g. Google Maps. Arguably one of the most successful, if not the most widely cited, outlet for VGI has been Wikimapia [14, 16]. Here individuals contribute knowledge of the physical, built environment around them in order to create as accurate a representation as possible. Recent events have also demonstrated the potential for VGI to assist in disaster response [22].

However, the utility of VGI remains limited. In the context of the broader GIS literature, data quality has always been a concern [16, 23]. In the case of VGI, this concern is exacerbated due to the lack of expertise, or credibility, of the individual [23]. Given that VGI is user-generated information by non-experts, there is no quality assurance of the data [24]. Others have raised concerns over the motivations of the individual, whether data is volunteered with intent to inform or mislead, an act of digital vandalism [25].

Many approaches have been taken to assess the quality and reliability of VGI [e.g. 10, 20, 23, 26], but mainly conceptual. The most common of these methods involves social trust networks and reputation models [10, 27]. Under this approach, data quality is checked by other project participants for errors and inconsistencies. In this model, no single expert is tasked with reviewing each

volunteered report. Another approach recommended has been to use existing data sets (collected using more authoritative methods) to check for inconsistencies in data. However, quality is not absolute; a datasets fitness-for-use is contextual and may have varying degrees of suitability for different users [28]. No single metric can be used to determine whether a data set is suitable across all ranges of potential uses. Thus, the context of a user's participation and interaction with VGI must be taken into account when considering accuracy/quality of VGI.

Given the concerns raised over the uncertainty of data quality in VGI, there is significant debate as to the utility of VGI for science. Elwood et al. [16] inventoried 99 projects utilizing VGI and found only 3% to have academic affiliations. One of the most prominent examples of VGI in science is the Audubon Society's Christmas Bird Count. This project has amassed a significant volume of volunteered data; however despite attempts to train volunteers in data collection, lingering questions of data quality, of reliability, have limited any analytical value and integration potential with authoritative datasets [29].

The credibility (or believability) of VGI can be described objectively by traditional measures of data quality—the degree to which the information can be considered accurate, or as the subjective perception on the part of the consumer [23]. However, for VGI to be useful for science, it is the traditional, objective "credibility-as-accuracy" measure demanded [23]. To fully quantify error in data, it is necessary to have a measure or to make assumptions as to the nature of the population being measured, to compare the distribution of data against the population as a whole. It is in this way we measure attribute accuracy, completeness, thematic resolution, and variability, to name only a few. Other measurements rely on feedback from measurement equipment, such as positional accuracy, temporal accuracy, spatial and temporal resolution, among others. Participatory science and VGI Science (VGIS) often involve datasets for which the nature of the population is not immediately known. Therefore, a direct quantification of the error of VGI is only possible in a post hoc analysis. However, it is the immediate benefit VGI can provide us that is of interest here and so we must develop a mechanism to evaluate the merits of VGI in real time (as it is contributed). In the absence of an ability to directly measure error and uncertainty parameters of volunteered data, we can use a surrogate measure, *meta-quality*, a measurement of the collective quality of the data [30].

The objective of our work here is to improve the perceived value of VGI for science by demonstrating a methodology for VGI data quality assessment. We accomplish this through a mechanism to explicitly assess the reliability of reporters based upon their respective VGI contributions.

To better illustrate our approach, we apply the methodology to a case study in disease ecology where we model the distribution of the tsetse fly, the principle vector of African Trypanosomiasis in sub-Saharan Africa. The "Tsetse Ecological Distribution model" or TED is based on an assessment of environmental characteristics critical for the persistence of the fly [31]. The model is a conservative estimation of the population distribution specifically minimizing errors of commission; therefore, the TED model is an estimation of the minimum extent of tsetse at each point in time. However, the model is reliant on a static land cover classification and makes no adjustment for error intrinsic to the model [31]. The TED model produces estimates of the spatial distribution as binary outputs indicating presence/absence of the fly for each time period.

Potentially the most important contribution to incorporating VGI into a species distribution model of the kind here is the fact that we can explicitly address one component of model error (omission) without contributing additional error. TED was developed as a conservative model of the minimum expected distribution of tsetse. By incorporating VGI into the model results, we can effectively facilitate the population expanding over gaps of unsuitable habitat, either due to actual conditions or poor input data. It is known that microclimates provide refuge for tsetse in areas where the habitat would be otherwise unsuitable [32, 33]. The spatial resolution of the underlying MODIS data misses these microsites and therefore omits these cells in the estimated distribution. Allowing the distribution to be updated based on the VGI would allow us to more accurately reflect conditions as they exist reflecting sub-pixel dynamic that otherwise would not be possible. Incorporating VGI into the model results to expand the distribution can therefore reduce errors of omission without contributing additionally to errors of commission, thereby reducing total error, and thus improving data quality. Incorporating VGI into TED requires two distinct steps: (1) determine the reliability of the reporter to assess whether the VGI meets the threshold for acceptance, and (2) update the tsetse distributions by changing the binary tsetse presence/absence value for the cell (in which the datum is located) to 1—indicating presence of the fly. In cases where VGI reflects the predicted distribution, no change is made.

Methods

Here we undertake a series of experiments to illustrate the integration of VGI into a traditional analytical model. First, we explore the characteristics of VGI and its impact on model results. Second, we evaluate the sensitivity of the model to three types of error common to crowdsourced data. Finally, we explore the importance of reliability, as measured by a reputation score [26, 27, 34]

in determining the threshold for accepting the data for inclusion in the model, under both static (a pre-defined score) or dynamic (a varying score) conditions.

To simulate the generation of VGI, we first consider the different kinds of reporters and the characteristics of the data they might contribute (Table 1). We identify four basic types of reporters: (1) "always right", (2) "always, intentionally wrong", (3) "random", and (4) "normal". The "always right" reporter represents individuals who are judged, post hoc, to be highly reliable and the data they contribute are of high quality, often promoted to the role of moderator in online forums [27]; there is no (or minimal) spatial or temporal error component to the data they contribute. The "always, intentionally wrong" reporter represents individuals who consistently, and/or intentionally provide erroneous data [35, 36]; these reporters are unreliable and the data they contribute should always be rejected. The "random" reporter represents individuals who generate data, falling on a random distribution, reporting tsetse fly presence, for example, at apparently random locations across the landscape (whether or not they are actually present) ignorant of underlying habitat conditions [37, 38]; due to the random nature of the reports, the data are therefore unreliable. Finally, the "normal" reporter represents the typical individual who volunteers information; the individuals have a high degree of credibility and the data are usually high quality [23], but there is a spatial and temporal error component to the data they contribute. It is this type of reporter that we are most interested in evaluating reliability.

In the context of our case study, the simulated data for each reporter are based on habitat suitability criteria. In a real scenario, it is not possible to assess the accuracy of any report by itself; rather we can only assess the fitness-for-use of the data by placing it in application context and asking whether it is plausible [39, 40]. We simulate this by evaluating the data based on the likelihood of the data being correct given the underlying habitat conditions. To simulate the data, we identify a set of conditions that would be consistent with reports made for each reporter type, and use these conditions to identify points that can be used in our sample data set. Table 1 fully describes

Table 1 Reporter types and the criteria used to simulate their behavior

Reporter	Type	Model criteria
1	Always right	Tsetse predicted
2	Always, intentionally wrong	Tsetse not predicted, habitat unsuitable
3	Random	Spatially random
4	Normal	Suitable habitat + one occupied neighbor

the types of reporters and the set of conditions used to simulate data. For completeness, we explore the impact on the predicted occurrence of tsetse by simulating data, not only from the four reporter types but also from data generated from all combinations of habitat suitability criteria. It is based, in part, on these simulations that we identified the specific combination of criteria that would be used to render simulated VGI (Table 2).

The simulated data are based on the underlying conditions present at each time step in the model, but not necessarily on the predicted occurrence for that simulation. For each set of criteria and combination thereof, we ran 100 simulations, identifying 100 points in each time step to serve as mock reports. Pooling these data points together results in 10,000 potential locations (some locations are represented more than once in the pool due to random selection in the simulations) for reports for each time step from which we randomly draw from when simulating reporters. This allows us to incorporate a minimum amount of stochasticity that would exist with reporters in a real-world scenario.

The basic TED model was implemented in GRASS based on the methods outlined by DeVisser et al. [31]. Building on our implementation of the TED model, we model the predicted distribution of tsetse, incorporating VGI, and evaluate the magnitude of the difference. Each model was written in BASH, a UNIX shell-scripting language. The models were run on the High Performance Computing Center (HPCC) cluster at Michigan State University for a total of 9321 simulations representing an estimated 13,981 h of computing time.

The normal reporter is defined as an individual who usually provides credible data, but has the potential to submit erroneous data. Incorporating these inaccuracies into the data stream produces some degree of error in the model output. In reality, it is not possible determine the truthfulness of the data; therefore we must be able to determine the influence of error on the model output.

The standard "normal" reporter is assigned an error rate of 10% (an arbitrary assignment); we measure the effects of this error by evaluating the impact on the resulting distribution when the "normal" reporter is assigned an error rate of 50%. The arbitrary choice would likely have an impact on the results because higher error rates would require more trials to identify credible reporters. However, since this presents a proof-of-concept just to see if the process works, we did not perform a sensitivity analysis on these error rates yet. As the data are constructed based on the combination of habitat suitability criteria, we evaluate introducing error into the model in different ways. Erroneous data are simulated by selecting points in areas of unsuitable habitat by shifting the location of the point (simulating positional error), or by holding the data until the following time step (simulating temporal error). A z-score is computed comparing each set of criteria against a simulation where points are selected at random, as well as a test of significance against the output from the TED model alone (no VGI data incorporated).

An assessment of the reliability of the VGI requires us to first generate a dynamic history for each reporter that reflects the plausibility of the data as determined by habitat suitability criteria. Each reporter is assigned a score, a measurement of their reputation, which is a product of these criteria (slightly modified from Langley and Messina 2013 [26] to allow for negative changes in reputation). The index returns an ordinal measurement of reliability; it is not constraint to a particular range, rather is structured such that positive scores convey reliability. It is computed as:

$$Reliability = \theta + \rho + \frac{\kappa}{4} + \gamma \tag{1}$$

θ = reporter's score, ρ = the number of times a cell was previously occupied (-1 if 0), κ = the number of occupied cells in 4-cell neighborhood (-1 if 0), γ = the number of supporting reports (-1 if 0).

Table 2 Simulation results for simulated conditions

Sim	Criteria	% Gain				Variance			
		Overall	2004	2005	2006	Overall	2004	2005	2005
1	Random	9.81	4.23	13.66	11.85	144.02	76.83	105.73	106.62
2	Suitable habitat	14.06	7.22	17.94	17.58	108.26	73.41	80.88	77.11
3	One neighbor	0.29	0.17	0.39	0.32	93.37	27.62	66.28	65.48
4	Suitable habitat + one neighbor	0.03	0.02	0.04	0.05	19.65	10.86	16.52	13.97
5	Tsetse present	0	0	0	0	0.01	0.01	0.01	0.01
6	Tsetse not present	10.59	4.78	14.57	12.71	128.16	75.51	97.03	91.45
7	Habitat unsuitable	8.23	3.46	11.75	9.66	138.43	79.15	112.02	109.58

Values represent percent increase over the base TED model

We arbitrarily selected threshold scores of 5 and 8 for incorporation of the VGI into the TED model results. This arbitrary choice would affect results when exercised in a real-world case; however, for our purposes, we merely needed threshold scores of any value to see whether or not the process actually worked. Higher or lower threshold scores would just require fewer or more trials to assess correctness. A paired t test is used to measure the significance of adjusting the threshold and the potential importance the specific selection has on the resulting predicted occurrence. An alternative approach to the arbitrary assignment of scores is to determine the threshold at which reporter types can be distinguished from each other. We subject the history of reporter scores to a k-means test; this analysis tries to iteratively place each reporter into one of two clusters (we define these clusters to mean reporters of "plausible" or "erroneous" data). Cluster centers were defined at random from the set of scores for each test. As reporter scores increase over time, we expect it will take a certain number of model time steps before they will group properly. The average reporter score (for the plausible group) from 100 iterations can be interpreted as a reasonable threshold score under a static model.

Over time, the scores for reporters quickly exceed the small thresholds we set (reaching values > 100 at the end of the simulation), which results in unqualified acceptance of the VGI into the model. As such, we cannot detect or respond (within a reasonable time) to changing behavior among reporters, reflecting the inability of arbitrary, static thresholds to capture potential declining reliability and reputation of reporters over time. In the final set of simulations, we explore the possibility of using a dynamic score model, where the threshold for acceptance is drawn from the distribution of all reporter scores at each time step. For each simulation, we set a threshold equal to the 1st quartile score, mean, or 3rd quartile score from the distribution of all reporters' scores at that time. This allows us to include only the most reliable reporters from our total pool of participants, and the longer the model operates over time, the more reliable our output becomes. The net benefit to the model should thus improve over time. Sets of paired t-tests are used to measure the significance of the difference in predictions from the three threshold models.

In our case, the likelihood that tsetse are present in an area (the subject of the VGI in question) is correlated with the habitat suitability as measured by land cover, land-surface temperature, and NDVI (Normalized Difference Vegetation Index). A reporter's score is a measurement of their reputation, akin to eBay's ratings system, which quantifies the history of the individual to perform in a manner that is perceived positively by their peers [27]. We assume that if a reliable reporter contributes information that confirms another's data, the likelihood that datum being accurate is improved. However, this method of confirmation by peers necessitates a set of reporters who have attained a data history. Until a reporter attains a certain reputation, we do not have enough information to assess data quality; however, we have seen that different reporters themselves quickly separate from each other, allowing us to partition out individuals who are either reporting randomly (and thus frequently inaccurately) or are simply providing erroneous data intentionally. Partitioning out these two types of reporters alone immediately improves the quality of the contributed data.

Results

Varying the criteria for spatially locating VGI greatly influences the overall impact on the predicted occurrence of tsetse, however the impact varies markedly from year to year due to environmental conditions and shifts in the habitat suitability. Randomly locating points results in an overall 9.81% (4.23–13.66% for individual model years) increase in the number of cells in which tsetse are predicted to occupy over the time period in the model (recall that incorporating VGI into the TED model can only increase the prevalence of tsetse). However targeting specific locations where habitat is suitable and at least one neighbor is predicted to be occupied (the criteria we assign to our normal reporter), yields an overall 0.03% (0.02–0.05%) increase in occupied cells. Notably, selecting suitable habitat alone as our criteria influenced the results the most, with an overall 14.06% (7.22–17.94%) increase in predicted occurrence. Likely this speaks to the design goal of the TED model to minimize errors of commission. Predictably, constraining report locations to only those cells in which tsetse are predicted to occur (the condition for our "always right" reporter) yields no increase in the predicted occurrence of tsetse over the base model. Selecting locations in which tsetse are not predicted to occur or where habitat is unsuitable (conditions for the "wrong" reporter or a component of error in the normal reporter, respectively) yields an overall 10.59% and 8.23% increase in the predicted occurrence. All criteria tested yielded significantly different results over the random model ($p < 0.001$ in each case).

In the static threshold score model, there was no significant difference in the overall predicted occurrence of tsetse ($p > 0.4$). However, utilizing a dynamic threshold score model resulted in significant differences between all three models (1st quartile, mean, and 3rd quartile) with p values < 0.001 in each case. The overall increase in predicted occurrence was 0.8, 0.43, and 0.12% respectively; however, the results varied widely from year to year for both static and dynamic threshold models (see Table 3).

Table 3 The percentage increase in the prevalence of tsetse over the base TED model for simulations 8–12

Sim	Score	% Gain				Variance			
		Overall	2004	2005	2006	Overall	2004	2005	2006
8	5	1.28	0.27	1.94	1.68	139.56	46.8	113.56	100.52
9	8	1.22	0.23	1.88	1.6	138.6	44.09	112.57	99.1
10	1st quartile	0.8	0.13	1.15	1.2	120.62	37.76	92.9	95.07
11	Mean	0.43	0.05	0.6	0.68	109.46	28.92	83.06	83.27
12	3rd quartile	0.12	0	0.14	0.24	77.36	10.47	55.49	66.11

Table 4 The percentage increase in the prevalence of tsetse over the base TED model for simulations 13–20

Sim	Error type	% Gain				Variance			
		Overall	2004	2005	2006	Overall	2004	2005	2006
13	10%	1.38	0.39	2.07	1.74	139.44	48.86	116.26	95.18
14	50%	5.23	1.88	7.94	5.95	144.9	70.59	124.32	99.84
15	Spatial shift 5%	1.39	0.39	2.13	1.7	137.33	49.43	112.58	92.83
16	Spatial shift 10%	1.39	0.44	2.22	1.52	142.05	54.59	118.36	97.97
17	Spatial shift 25%	1.41	0.44	2.18	1.65	131.66	50.61	108.22	95.31
18	Temporal shift 5%	1.46	0.43	2.21	1.79	135.71	50.68	112.63	97.89
19	Temporal shift 10%	1.54	0.45	2.4	1.81	149.88	52.54	124.28	97.73
20	Temporal shift 25%	1.61	0.5	2.47	1.9	148.95	55.65	119.68	97.55

[Note: simulations 8 through 12 in the table consider the cases for only normal reporters].

The four types of reporters cluster into two groups—see simulations 13 and 14 (Table 4) for the cases where all reporter types are considered. The four reporters are not fully distinguishable from each other at any time in our models (k-means with four clusters). Figure 1 presents the distribution curve (for all 100 replications) for the time step, at which point the reporters can be distinguished using a k-means clustering approach. For simulation 13, where a threshold score of 5 is used, the reporters can be separated, on average, in the 5th time step (mean = 4.93, median = 5). The average reputation score in the 5th time step is 10.87 for the "plausible" group. Reporters in simulation 14 (50% error rate) do not consistently cluster together into two groups.

The arbitrary 10% error threshold

Considering the dynamic score models, there were no significant differences in the time needed for reporters to group together. For the 1st quartile threshold score (simulation 10), reporters clustered into two groups, on average, in the 5th time step (mean = 4.61, median = 5). The average score for the "correct" reporters in the 5th time step was 18.87 (Fig. 2). In the mean threshold score models (simulation 11), reporters clustered together in the 4th time step (mean = 4.32, median = 4). The average reputation score for reporters in this time step was

15.06 (Fig. 3). Finally, for the 3rd quartile threshold score model, reporters clustered together in the 4th time step (mean = 4.21, median = 4) with an average reputation of 15.14 (Fig. 4).

The nature of error (positional vs. temporal) introduced into our models through incorporating VGI did not appear to change the magnitude of the impact on predicted occurrence. This was also true when varying the magnitude of the error, at least for the range tested (5–25%). We did observe a significant increase in the predicted occurrence of tsetse when the magnitude of the error introduced was 50% (where each reporter had a 50% chance of contributing erroneous data); introducing error of any type, though, results in a significant

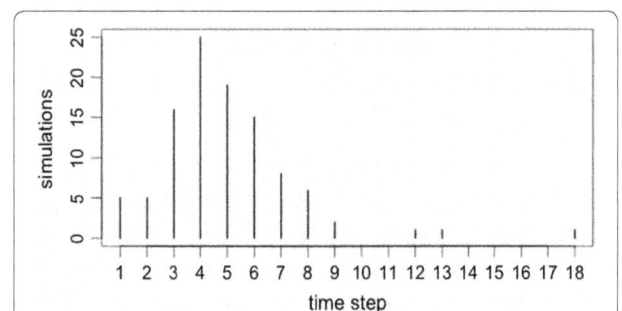

Fig. 1 A frequency plot representing the time-step in which reporters cluster into two groups, for 100 replications of simulation 13

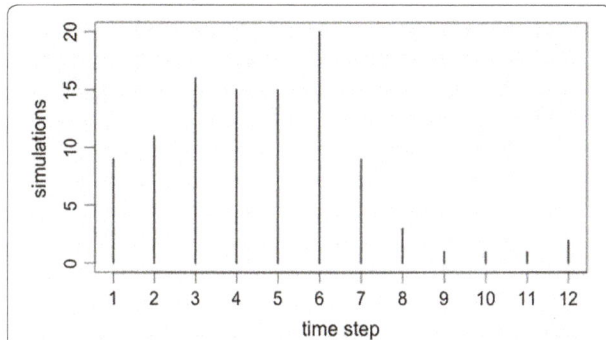

Fig. 2 A frequency plot representing the time-step in which reporters cluster into two groups, for 100 replications of simulation 10

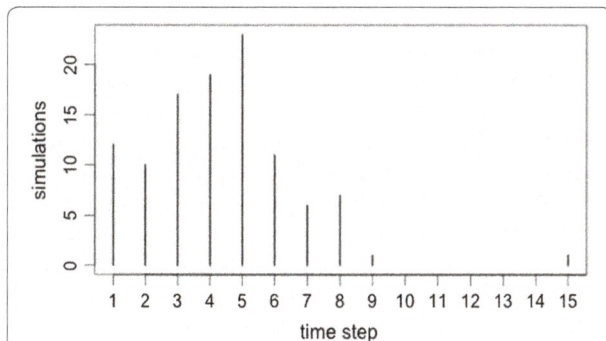

Fig. 3 A frequency plot representing the time-step in which reporters cluster into two groups, for 100 replications of simulation 11

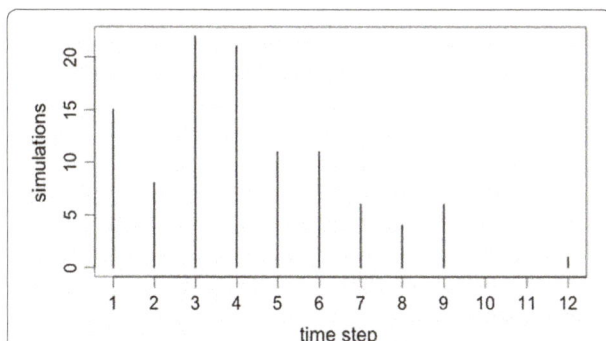

Fig. 4 A frequency plot representing the time-step in which reporters cluster into two groups, for 100 replications of simulation 12

While the analysis reveals significant differences in the predicted tsetse occurrence from incorporating VGI into the TED model, global metrics are difficult to interpret given the importance of spatial structure in the dataset. To this extent, visualizing the structure of tsetse distribution patterns can lead to novel interpretations of the influence of VGI. Figures 5, 6 and 7 present the predicted distribution of tsetse over our study area (for simulations 10, 11, and 12 respectively); cell values indicate the proportion of time steps in the model (every 16 days between 2004 and 2006) where tsetse are predicted to occur, averaged across 100 replications. The distributions incorporating VGI closely mirror the base TED model with marked differences between core tsetse areas. These maps illustrate specific areas where VGI is particularly influential, likely due to the ability of tsetse populations to "jump" patches of unsuitable habitat.

Time is a significant factor to consider when evaluating the results of our models. In describing the output of

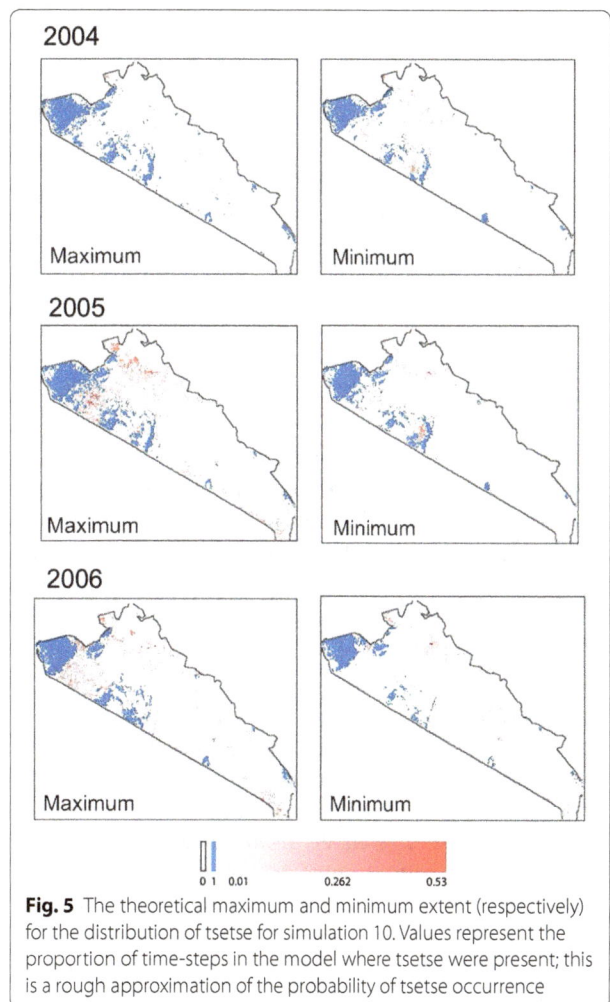

Fig. 5 The theoretical maximum and minimum extent (respectively) for the distribution of tsetse for simulation 10. Values represent the proportion of time-steps in the model where tsetse were present; this is a rough approximation of the probability of tsetse occurrence

increase in the predicted occurrence compared to the case where no error is considered (simulation 4). Therefore, at least in our case study, the error introduced from VGI is not expected to a statistically significant effect on the prevalence of tsetse. This suggests that our models are resilient to the introduction of some erroneous data. Adaptations of our model to different studies will nevertheless necessitate an exploration of the role of introduced error from VGI to assess the resiliency of scientific models.

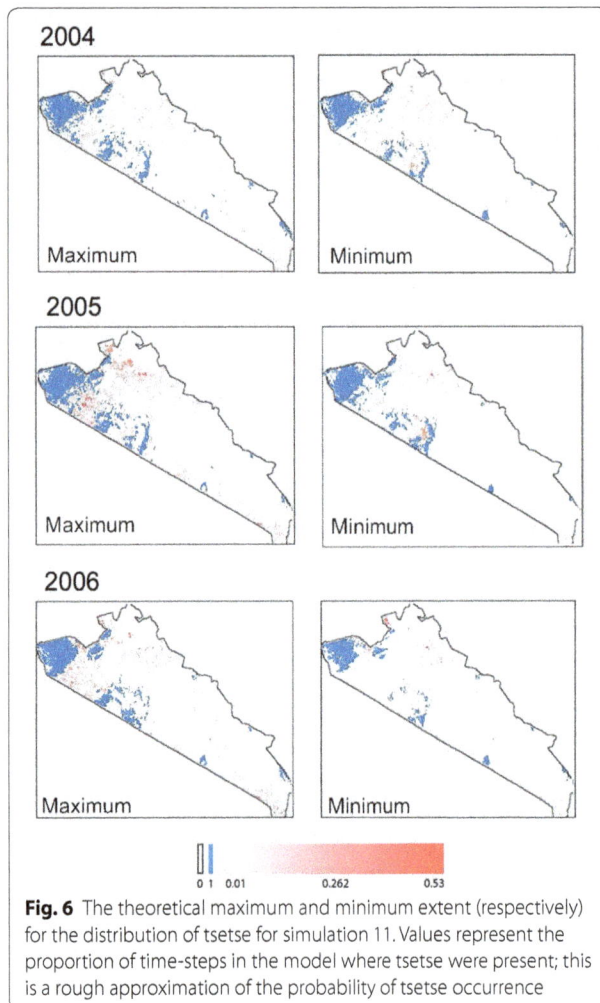

Fig. 6 The theoretical maximum and minimum extent (respectively) for the distribution of tsetse for simulation 11. Values represent the proportion of time-steps in the model where tsetse were present; this is a rough approximation of the probability of tsetse occurrence

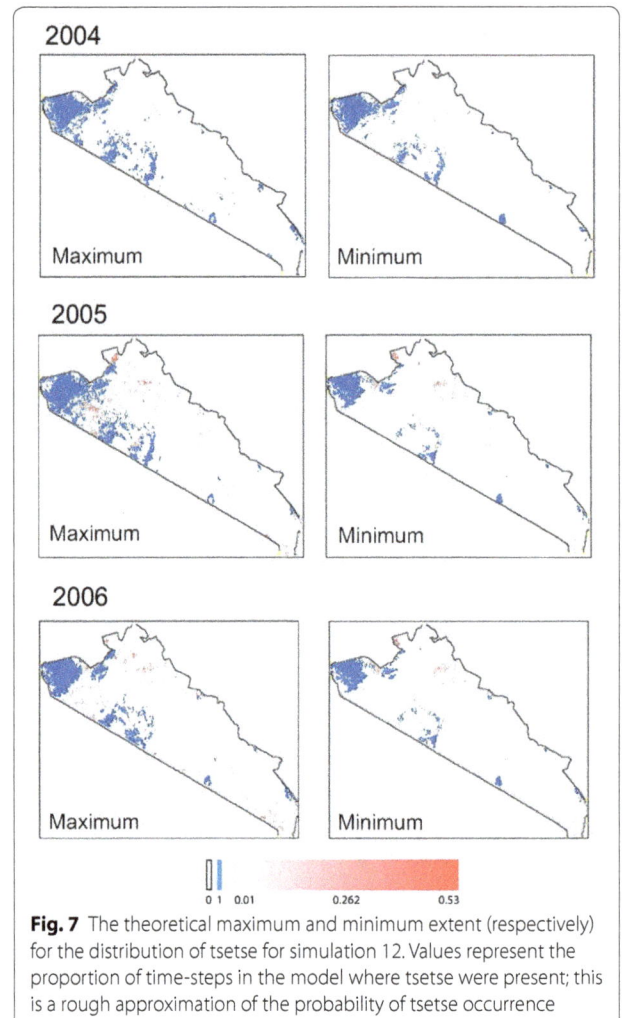

Fig. 7 The theoretical maximum and minimum extent (respectively) for the distribution of tsetse for simulation 12. Values represent the proportion of time-steps in the model where tsetse were present; this is a rough approximation of the probability of tsetse occurrence

TED model predictions, DeVisser et al. [31] noted that tsetse populations tended to reach their maximum extent at the end of the long rains (ending the beginning of June). Populations tended to reach their minimum extent at the end of the cool dry season (mid- to late-October). This interpretation of tsetse population distributions comports with what is observed in my simulations, and is grounded in an ecological understanding of tsetse population dynamics.

Conclusions

Volunteered geographic information can make valuable contributions to science, enhancing datasets from more authoritative sources. However, integrating VGI data necessitates assessing the error and uncertainty of those data. Direct quantification of data quality in this context is difficult; the traditional components (e.g. accuracy, precision, and variance) typically cannot be ascertained for VGI. It is critical for us to at least be able to qualify data quality, as it serves as the foundation from which we

assess fitness-for-use. We have proposed using reputation or reliability (of the reporter) as a surrogate measure of meta-quality. As an initial assessment, meta-quality allows us to begin to break through the cloud of uncertainty inherent with VGI.

We build on the power of the reliability/reputation assessment by considering a dynamic threshold-scoring model. While we considered three different criteria for establishing a threshold (defined as the 1st quartile, mean, and 3rd quartile values in the distribution of reporter scores in each time step), we did not find a significant difference between them—as measured by an overall increase in the prevalence of tsetse in our models. In considering only those individuals whose reliability exceeds the mean score for all reporters, we only incorporate VGI from a subset of reporters we deem the most reliable. As scores improve for all individuals (regardless whether we have incorporated their data into our models), the threshold for acceptance/inclusion in our models also increases (approximately linearly in our models—Fig. 8 shows the trend for one simulation). Over time, the quality of VGI data that we incorporate will improve, and the impact of any erroneous data we have included should decrease. Most importantly, a dynamic threshold model facilitates detection of declining performance (of a reporter) and a rapid response to limit the acceptance of poor quality data. Figure 8 illustrates that over time, random or erroneous reporters get consistently lower scores, with accurate reporters get consistently higher scores. This shows that this approach produces strong and clear divergence separating out erroneous reporting.

The potential value of a means to assess data quality of VGI is immense. The strongest hurdle to fully utilizing VGI has been our inability to measure data quality and uncertainty. In demonstrating a valuation system for VGI (based on the reputation of reporters themselves), we have, in part, overcome this hurdle. To date, the utilization of VGI for science has been reserved for those cases only where the performance of reporters is controlled through training and guidance while closely monitoring the entire process from data collection to communication [7, 20, 29]. But this runs contrary to many of the perceived strengths of VGI, the dissolution of traditional roles [1, 3, 6, 41] and the establishment of a two-way communication model for geographical information [14]. Projects that have tried to embrace VGI have done

so under the old model of participatory science, and thus are subject to all the perceived and actual limitations [5, 11]. Many factors influencing quality remain difficult to measure, including rates of participation and motivation to participate; the value of VGI cannot be fully appreciated until we can reliably assess these factors and the role they play in determining data quality.

It is our position that incorporating VGI into standard scientific models, particularly those where available data are sparse, can significantly improve the performance of the models and the predictive or explanatory power of the results. Consider the case of "Digital Earth"; first conceived by then US Vice-President Al Gore, it represented a push to represent the planet in high-resolution, multi-dimensional space for the primary purpose of improving our predictive capabilities of Earth's ecosystems [24, 42]. Twelve years later, significant gaps still exist, particularly in terms of our capacity to collect certain types of data of sufficient quality and resolution [42]. Harnessing the collective power of earth's citizens, the aggregate power of "six billion sensors", we can make significant strides to improving the predictive capacity of our models through incorporating new types of information [14]. Therefore, it is critical we continue to explore ways to assess the credibility of VGI, to embrace the new geographical traditions, while respecting the scientific paradigms of the past.

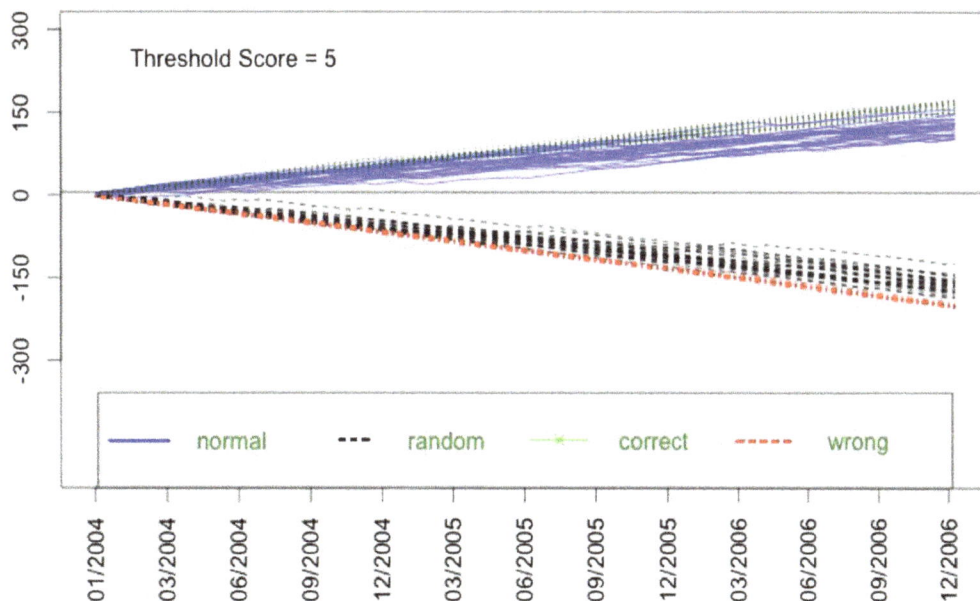

Fig. 8 This figure overlays the scores of 100 reporters for simulation 8

Authors' contributions

SAL developed the model design. SAL and JPM conducted the data analysis. JPM and NJM provided input on spatial analysis. SAL, JPM and NJM wrote the manuscript. All authors read and approved the final manuscript.

Author details

[1] Urban GIS, 1143 W Rundell Pl Suite 301, Chicago, IL, USA. [2] Center for Global Change and Department of Geography, Environment, and Spatial Sciences, Michigan State University, East Lansing, MI, USA.

Acknowledgements

We thank Dr. Joseph Maitima at Ecodym (http://ecodymafrica.co.ke), Nairobi, Kenya, for providing local tsetse distribution data. The opinions expressed herein are those of the authors and do not necessarily reflect the views of the NIH, NIGMS, NIFA, USAID, or the US government.

Competing interests

The authors declare that they have no competing interests.

Funding

This research was supported in part by the National Institutes of Health Office of the Director (Roadmap Initiative). It was also supported by NIGMS (Award No. RGM084704A), NIFA, and the USAID-supported Global Center for Food Systems Innovation (GCFSI).

References

1. Elwood SA, Goodchild MF, Sui D. Prospects for VGI research and the emerging fourth paradigm. In: Sui D, Elwood SA, Goodchild MF, editors. Crowdsourcing geographic knowledge. Dordrecht: Springer; 2013. p. 361–75.
2. Gray J, Szalay A. eScience: the next decade will be exciting. Lecture presented at ETH, Zurich. 2006; Retrieved from: http://research.microsoft.com/en-us/um/people/gray/talks/ETH_E_Science.ppt.
3. Goodchild MF. NeoGeography and the nature of geographic expertise. J Locat Based Serv. 2009;3(2):82–96. 10.1080/17489720902950374.
4. Turner A. Introduction to neogeography. Sebastopol: O'Reilly; 2006.
5. Elwood SA. Negotiating knowledge production: the everyday inclusions, exclusions, and contradictions of participatory GIS research. Prof Geogr. 2006;58(2):197–208. https://doi.org/10.1111/j.1467-9272.2006.00526.x.
6. Haklay MM, Singleton A, Parker C. Web mapping 2.0: the neogeography of the GeoWeb. Geogr Compass. 2008;2(6):2011–39. https://doi.org/10.1111/j.1749-8198.2008.00167.x.
7. Tulloch DL. Is VGI participation? From vernal pools to video games. GeoJournal. 2008;72(3–4):161–71. https://doi.org/10.1007/s10708-008-9185-1.
8. O'Reilly T. What is web 2.0? 2005; September 30. Retrieved June 30, 2013, from http://oreilly.com/web2/archive/what-is-web-20.html.
9. O'Reilly T. Web 2.0 Compact definition: trying again. 2006; December 10. Retrieved June 30, 2013, from http://radar.oreilly.com/2006/12/web-20-compact-definition-tryi.html.
10. Corbett J. "I Don't Come from Anywhere": exploring the role of the geoweb and volunteered geographic information in rediscovering a sense of place in a dispersed aboriginal community. Dordrecht: Springer; 2012. p. 223–41.
11. Miller CC. A beast in the field: the Google maps mashup as GIS/2. Cartogr Int J Geog Inf Geovis. 2006;41(3):187–99. https://doi.org/10.3138/J0L0-5301-2262-N779.
12. Boulos MNK. Web GIS in practice III: creating a simple interactive map of England's strategic Health Authorities using Google Maps API, Google Earth KML, and MSN Virtual Earth Map Control. Int J Health Geogr. 2005;4(1):22.
13. Boulos MNK, Resch B, Crowley DN, Breslin JG, Sohn G, Burtner R, Chuang KYS. Crowdsourcing, citizen sensing and sensor web technologies for public and environmental health surveillance and crisis management: trends, OGC standards and application examples. Int J Health Geogr. 2011;10(1):67.
14. Goodchild MF. Citizens as sensors: the world of volunteered geography. GeoJournal. 2007;69(4):211–21.
15. Elwood SA. Volunteered geographic information: key questions, concepts and methods to guide emerging research and practice. GeoJournal. 2008;72(3–4):133–5. https://doi.org/10.1007/s10708-008-9187-z.
16. Elwood SA, Goodchild MF, Sui DZ. Researching volunteered geographic information: spatial data, geographic research, and new social practice. Ann Assoc Am Geogr. 2011;102(3):110809092640007. https://doi.org/10.1080/00045608.2011.595657.
17. Goodchild MF. Commentary: whither VGI? GeoJournal. 2008;72(3):239–44.
18. Connors JP, Lei S, Kelly M. Citizen science in the age of neogeography: utilizing volunteered geographic information for environmental monitoring. Ann Assoc Am Geogr. 2012;102(6):1267–89. https://doi.org/10.1080/00045608.2011.627058.
19. Elwood SA. Volunteered geographic information: future research directions motivated by critical, participatory, and feminist GIS. GeoJournal. 2008;72(3–4):173–83. https://doi.org/10.1007/s10708-008-9186-0.
20. Elwood SA, Leitner H. GIS and community-based planning: exploring the diversity of neighborhood perspectives and needs. Cartogr Geogr Inf Syst. 2012;25(2):77.
21. Harvey F. To Volunteer or to contribute locational information? Towards truth in labeling for crowdsourced geographic information. Dordrecht: Springer; 2012. p. 31–42.
22. Goodchild MF. Crowdsourcing geographic information for disaster response: a research frontier. Int J Digit Earth. 2010;3(3):231–41. https://doi.org/10.1080/17538941003759255.
23. Flanagin AJ, Metzger MJ. The credibility of volunteered geographic information. GeoJournal. 2008;72(3–4):137–48. https://doi.org/10.1007/s10708-008-9188-y.
24. Craglia M. Volunteered geographic information and spatial data infrastructures: when do parallel lines converge. Position paper for the VGI Specialist Meeting, Santa Barbara 13–14 December 2007.
25. Tulloch DL. Many, many maps: empowerment and online participatory mapping. First Monday. 2007;12(2). Retrieved from http://www.firstmonday.dk/ojs/index.php/fm/article/view/1620/1535.
26. Langley SA, Messina JP. Utilizing volunteered information for infectious disease surveillance. Int J Appl Geospat Res. 2013;4(2):54–70.
27. Maué P. Reputation as tool to ensure validity of VGI. Position paper for specialist meeting on VGI. Santa Barbara, CA. 2007; Retrieved from http://www.ncgia.ucsb.edu/projects/vgi/docs/position/Maue_paper.pdf.
28. Goodchild MF. Assertion and authority: the science of user-generated geographic content. In: Proceedings of the proceedings of the colloquium for Andrew U Frank's 60th Birthday, Department of Geoinformation and Cartography, Vienna University of Technology, Vienna. 2008.
29. Wiersma YF. Birding 2.0: citizen science and effective monitoring in the web 2.0 world. Avian Cons and Ecol. 2010; 5(2):13–21.
30. van Oort P. Spatial data quality: from description to application. (PhD), Wageningen University. 2005; Retrieved: http://edepot.wur.nl/38987.
31. DeVisser M, Messina JP, Moore NJ, Lusch D. A dynamic species distribution model of Glossina subgenus Morsitans: the identification of tsetse reservoirs and refugia. Eco Soc Am. 2010;1(1):1–21.
32. Ford J. The role of the trypanosomiases in African ecology. A study of the tsetse fly problem. Oxford: Clarendon Press; 1971.
33. Moore NJ, Messina JP. A landscape and climate data logistic model of tsetse distribution in Kenya. PLoS ONE. 2010;5(7):e11809. https://doi.org/10.1371/journal.pone.0011809.
34. Frew J. Provenance and volunteered geographic information. In: Workshop on volunteered geographic information. 2007; Retrieved

June 30, 2013. http://www.ncgia.ucsb.edu/projects/vgi/docs/position/Frew_paper.pdf.

35. Bishr M, Kuhn W. Geospatial information bottom-up: a matter of trust and semantics. In: Fabrikant SI, Wachowicz M, editors. The European Information Society: leading the way with geo-information. Berlin: Springer; 2007. p. 365–87.

36. van den Berg H, Coetzee S, Cooper AK. Analysing commons to improve the design of volunteered geographic information repositories. In: Proceedings of the AfricaGEO 2011, Cape Town, South Africa. 2011; May 31–June 2.

37. Chow TE. "We know who you are and we know where you live": a research agenda for web demographics. Dordrecht: Springer; 2012. p. 265–85.

38. Coleman D, Sabone B. Volunteering geographic information to authoritative databases: linking contributor motivations to program characteristics. Geomatica. 2010;64(1):27–40.

39. Grira J, Bédard Y, Roche S. Spatial data uncertainty in the VGI world: going from consumer to producer. Geomatica. 2009;64(1):61–71.

40. Groot RTA d. Evaluation of a volunteered geographical information trust measure in the case of OpenStreetMap. (MS), University of Münster, Germany. 2012; Retrieved http://run.unl.pt/handle/10362/8301.

41. Goodchild MF. Citizens as voluntary sensors: spatial data infrastructure in the world of web 2.0. Int J Spat Data Infrastruct Res. 2007;2:24–32.

42. Craglia M, de Bie K, Jackson D, Pesaresi M, Remetey-Fülöpp G, Wang C, Woodgate P. Digital Earth 2020: towards the vision for the next decade. Intl J Digital Earth. 2012;5(1):4–21. https://doi.org/10.1080/17538947.2011.638500.

Factors related with public open space use among adolescents: a study using GPS and accelerometers

Linde Van Hecke[1,2,3] ⓘ, Hannah Verhoeven[1,2,3], Peter Clarys[2], Delfien Van Dyck[3,4], Nico Van de Weghe[5], Tim Baert[3,5], Benedicte Deforche[1,2] and Jelle Van Cauwenberg[1,3]*

Abstract

Background: Low physical activity levels and high levels of sedentary time among adolescents call for population wide interventions. Public open spaces can be important locations for adolescents' physical activity. This study aimed to describe the prevalence, frequency and context of public open space visitation and to gain insight into the individual, social and physical environmental factors associated with public open space use among 12- to 16-year-old Flemish (Belgian) adolescents.

Methods: Global positioning system devices, accelerometers and one-on-one interviews were used to measure location-specific activity levels, time spent at, reasons for using and accompaniment at public open spaces among 173 adolescents. Multilevel hurdle and gamma models were used to estimate the associations between the independent variables (age, gender, ethnicity, education, sport club membership and accompaniment) and the amount of time, sedentary time, light-, moderate- to vigorous- and vigorous-intensity physical activity at public open spaces.

Results: Three out of four participants had visited a public open space (for recreational purposes) and participants were most often accompanied by friends/classmates. Mainly public transportation stops/stations were used, and subsequently the most reported reason for public open space use was "to wait for something or someone". Furthermore, boys, younger adolescents, non-western-European adolescents and lower educated adolescents were more likely to use public open spaces. Additionally, boys and younger adolescents were more likely to accumulate physical activity at public open spaces. The only social environmental variable associated with time spent at public open spaces was accompaniment by siblings: adolescents spent more time at public open spaces when accompanied by their siblings.

Conclusions: Public open spaces may be effective areas to promote physical activity among groups at risk for physical inactivity (i.e. low educated and non-western-European adolescents). Additionally, girls and older adolescents were less likely to visit and be physically active at public open spaces. Therefore, urban planners should consider adding attractive features, in order to encourage physical activity among girls and older adolescents at public open spaces. Furthermore, creating public open spaces that are attractive for youth of all ages could contribute to adolescents visiting public open spaces accompanied by siblings.

Keywords: Global positioning device, Physical activity, Sedentary time, Youth, Leisure time, Public spaces

Background

The World Health Organisation (WHO) recommends adolescents to engage in 60 min of moderate- to vigorous-intensity physical activity (MVPA) daily [1] in order to obtain health benefits such as lower risk for overweight and obesity, diabetes type 2, high blood pressure and depressive symptoms [2–5]. In addition, adolescents engaging in extended periods of sedentary time (i.e. time spent sitting or lying down at low energy expenditure [6]) are at higher risk for higher Body Mass Index

*Correspondence: Jelle.VanCauwenberg@ugent.be
[3] Fund for Scientific Research Flanders (FWO), Brussels, Belgium
Full list of author information is available at the end of the article

(BMI), decreased fitness and lower psychosocial health [7, 8]. However, during the transition from childhood to adolescence a steep decline in physical activity (physical activity) levels [9–11] and an increase in sedentary time occurs [10, 11]. Subsequently, more than half of the adolescent population worldwide does not meet the physical activity recommendations [12–14] whilst European adolescents' sedentary time rises to 4–8 h per day on average [15]. Furthermore, healthy behaviours concerning physical activity and sedentary time developed in adolescence are known to track into adulthood, so being sufficiently active and having low levels of sedentary time during adolescence are of high importance [16–18].

Consequently, there is a need for population wide interventions to increase adolescent physical activity levels and decrease sedentary time. In the past, mostly individually-oriented models were used for intervention development [19]. During the last decade however, a shift has been made to socio-ecological models, which emphasize the interactions between individuals and their physical and socio-cultural environment [19, 20]. The different layers of the socio-ecological model are build up around four active living domains where adolescents can be active: at home, at school, during active transportation, and during leisure time [20]. Leisure time, physical activity can occur in an organized setting such as sport clubs or in non-organized settings such as at home, in streets, parks and playgrounds. Little is known about the locations where adolescents' non-organized leisure time physical activity (away from home) takes place and the need for more information on location-specific physical activity levels has been emphasized previously [21].

Studies in the US have shown that public open spaces (POS) are used for physical activity and recreational activities among children, adolescents and adults [22–24]. They are suitable for non-organized physical activity as they are public spaces that are freely accessible to all people, without entrance fee and present in most communities [24–26]. POS can have different appearances such as parks, playgrounds and squares, but also streets, vacant lots and parking lots. POS may be especially important for adolescents under the age of sixteen because they do not have the possibility to drive a car or moped and are, therefore, still limited in their ability to visit places located at greater distance from their residence and have to rely more on public transportation. Moreover, qualitative research has indicated that adolescents attach great importance to POS as a place where they can spend time without parental supervision or to be away from the bustle at home or school [27, 28].

On the one hand, a POS can be a suitable location for physical activity (and thereby directly increase overall physical activity levels), but on the other hand, a POS can also be a destination that adolescents can visit using active transportation (and thereby increase overall physical activity levels through active transportation) [7, 8]. This implicates that when only physical activity in POS would be considered in research (and thus not including physical activity during trips to and from POS), an underestimation of the physical activity related to POS visitation would be made. Therefore, physical activity accumulated during trips to and from POS should be included in research concerning POS use among adolescents, as these can contribute to overall activity levels even if adolescents do not accumulate physical activity in POS.

Research on POS use among adolescents is limited, but some studies have emerged recently. An Australian survey study reported almost 40% of 13-year old adolescents to have used a park at least once a week during the past 3 months. Additionally, only 12% of the adolescents reported not to have visited a park in the past 3 months [29]. Furthermore, a US study among 11- to 14-year-old adolescents using accelerometers and global positioning system (GPS) devices reported that an average of 45 min was spent daily on streets and sidewalks, 25 min at playgrounds and 17 min in parks [30]. A Danish study among 11–16-year olds with similar methodology reported lower levels of POS use, with a median of only 11.7 min/day spent at school grounds (during leisure time), 5.2 min/day in urban green space, 0.0 min/day at playgrounds and 0.0 min/day at sport facilities [31]. However, the differences in POS use between the two studies can be attributed to the fact that active transport to POS and in POS was included to calculate time spent in POS in the US study, while this was not the case in the Danish study.

However, research on the prevalence and frequency of POS visitation, the activity levels in POS, types of POS used and reasons for POS visitation among adolescents remains scarce, especially in Europe. Therefore, additional research is needed to gain insight into the prevalence and frequency of POS visitation and the activity levels in POS. Furthermore, the types of POS that are used and reasons for POS visitation should be explored in order to better understand the different aspects of (active) POS use.

As mentioned above, socio-ecological models emphasize the importance of individual-, physical- and social environmental factors to explain physical activity behaviours and sedentary time. Currently, information is lacking about factors associated with time and physical activity in POS whilst (to our knowledge) no studies have investigated the factors associated with sedentary time in POS. Because sedentary time is independently related to health problems [12, 13], identifying factors associated with sedentary time in POS is especially important. Identifying the physical and social environmental factors that could induce sedentary behaviour in POS enables to define the necessary strategies to reduce sedentary time at public open spaces. Additionally, this allows to target specific population groups at risk for sedentary time in POS.

Two Danish studies using GPS and accelerometers showed that older adolescents (mean age 14.2) spent less time [31] and less MVPA [32] at school grounds during leisure-time and more time and MVPA at sport facilities and shopping centres compared to younger adolescents (mean age 12.4) [31]. Furthermore, boys aged 11- to 16-year-old spent more time at sport facilities, accumulated more MVPA at school grounds during leisure time [31, 32] and less MVPA at playgrounds and urban green space compared to girls [32]. Furthermore, a Canadian study using GPS and accelerometers indicated that adolescents living in suburban areas performed more MVPA in POS locations such as green spaces or shopping malls compared to adolescents living in urban and rural areas, whilst no differences were found in MVPA at different POS locations according to adolescents' Socio-Economic Status (SES) [33]. These studies indicate that individual factors such as gender and age could possibly be associated with time spent and physical activity in POS whereas, no previous research has looked into the individual factors associated with sedentary time in POS. Furthermore, it is possible that the social environment (e.g., accompaniment in POS) is associated with adolescents' time, sedentary time and physical activity in POS, however, no studies have investigated this matter. Additionally, some physical environmental factors associated with physical activity in POS, have been identified, whereas no research has studied the associations for environmental factors with sedentary time in POS. Recent observational research has indicated that different park areas such as playgrounds, open fields or sport fields were associated with different activity levels across all age groups [34–37]. This evidence suggests associations of individual, social- and physical environmental factors with time and physical activity in POS among adolescents. However, European research is limited and additional insight is needed into the factors associated with sedentary time in POS among adolescents.

Many of the studies investigating the association between POS availability, POS use and physical activity levels have used questionnaires, geographical information systems (GIS) or audits of POS in the participants' neighbourhood [23, 38–41], assuming that these are the locations that are most frequently used. However, adolescents may use other POS than those closest to home and, therefore, it is important to use methods such as diaries or GPS-measures that allow to investigate the locations that are actually used by the adolescents. GPS devices have been identified as more accurate compared to activity diaries [42–44]. Furthermore, when GPS devices are combined with accelerometers, it is possible to objectively measure location-specific physical activity [45].

Summarized, evidence on adolescents' POS use and its associated individual, physical and social environmental factors is limited, with most studies originating from North-America and Australia. Only two studies originate from Europe. Most of the existing studies included measures of POS use, some included measures of physical activity in POS, whilst none included measures of sedentary time in POS. Furthermore, many studies have used methods that cannot capture the specific POS that is used. POS can be suitable locations for physical activity among adolescents. However, in order to develop interventions to promote physical activity and reduce sedentary time in POS, insight is needed into the use of POS, physical activity and sedentary time in POS and into the factors associated with POS use, physical activity and sedentary time in POS. Therefore, this study used GPS devices and accelerometers in order to (1) describe the prevalence, frequency and context (i.e. company, locations and reason) of POS visitation and (2) gain insight into the individual, social and physical environmental factors associated with time, sedentary time and physical activity in POS among 12- to 16-year-old Flemish (Belgian) adolescents.

Methods
Study area
The study took place in Ghent, the capital city of the province of East Flanders (Belgium). Belgium is ranked 22th in the Human Development index developed by the United Nations, with a value of 0.90 (maximum score = 1) [46]. Ghent comprises an area of 156.18 km^2 and has 253,266 inhabitants (population density: 1622 inh/km^2) [47, 48]. Ghent is a modern city that was founded in the eighth century at the confluence of two rivers and has a densely built historical inner city surrounded with nineteenth and twentieth century workers districts. The north of the city comprises an international harbour, whilst the south is characterised by the new train station [49].

In Ghent, the unemployment rate is 12.5, 2.0% of the population is entitled to a living wage and 18.8% is part of an ethnic-cultural minority whilst the remaining 81.2% is predominantly white [50–52]. In total, 37.0% of the inhabitants of Ghent have access to public green space (< 1 ha) within 150 m of their home and 41.9% has access to public green space (> 1 ha) within 400 m from their home [50]. Additionally, 1.8 km^2 of the city is designated to playgrounds, woods or parks where people are allowed to play [50].

Four of the participating schools were located in the city centre whilst two were located in the outskirts of the city (Fig. 1).

Participant and school recruitment

Participants (12- to 16-year-old) were recruited through schools. Before recruitment, the study design and purpose were presented in a meeting with all principals of the governmental schools located in Ghent (Flanders, Belgium). Six out of twelve schools were willing to participate. In each school at least two classes in the first to fourth grade (12- to 16-year-old) were selected by the principal or a staff member and all students from these classes were invited to participate (total of 18 classes: Additional file 1: Table S1). Participation in the study was voluntary and participants received a movie ticket as an incentive after measurements were finished.

Study protocol

Data were collected from September to December 2015 (mean daily rainfall = 0.4 mm/day, mean daily hours of sunshine: 4.1 h/day, mean maximum temperature: 15.1 °C/day). Participating schools were visited three times by the research team. Before school visits took place, all schools were asked to distribute a parental information and consent form to all parents of students in participating classes. Parents who did not give permission for their children to participate, had to sign the parental consent form and their children could hand in these parental consent forms to the researchers at the first school visit. During the first school visit, participants were asked to read and sign a participant consent form. This approach was used because adolescents had to fill in a questionnaire on a non-sensitive topic [53, 54]. This consent procedure and the research protocol for minors were approved by the medical ethics committee of the University Hospital of Ghent University (2015/0317) referring to the privacy act of December 8th, 2012 on the protection of privacy in relation to the processing of personal data [55]. Participants received a personal ID number they could use to anonymously complete a questionnaire concerning demographics. Every participant received an accelerometer, GPS device and charger for the GPS device. The participants were given verbal

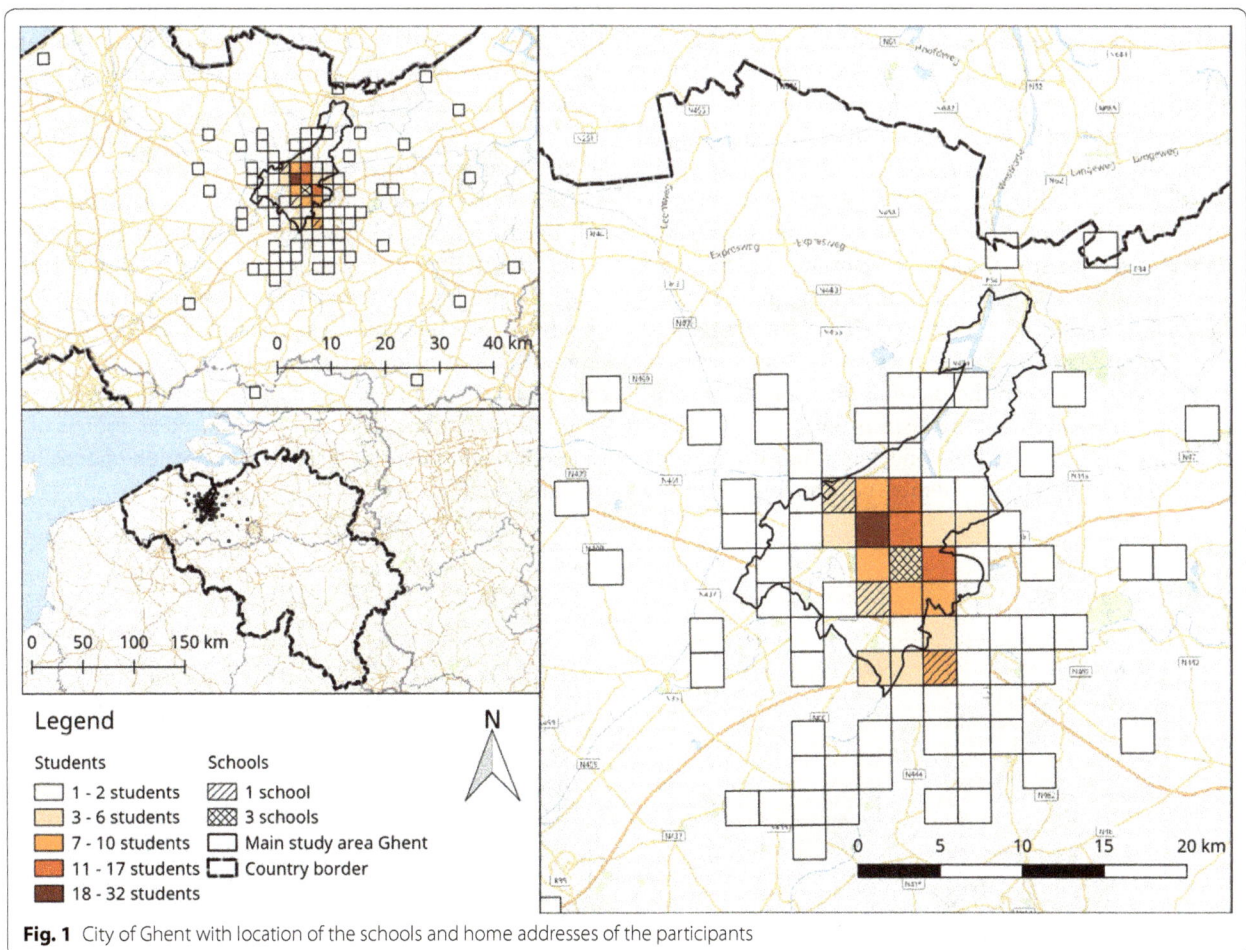

Fig. 1 City of Ghent with location of the schools and home addresses of the participants

and written instructions on how and when to wear the devices and how to charge the GPS overnight. All participants were asked for their phone number and those willing to give their number (n = 140; 49.5%), received two text messages daily: every morning to remind them to wear the devices and every evening to remind them to charge the GPS device.

After 4–5 days the devices were collected during the second school visit and the GPS and accelerometer data were downloaded from the devices. A web application was created to visualize the data from each participant on a map for each day the devices were worn.

The third school visit comprised a one-on-one interview of 10–20 min during which the personal maps were used. During this interview, participants were asked about the reasons, activities and company in POS locations that were used. An overview of the data collection process is presented in Fig. 2.

Measurements
Questionnaire
All participants were asked to complete a questionnaire that included the following questions on demographics: date of birth, place of birth, sex, address (address was used to define area of residence: rural < 300 inh/km^2, suburban: 300–600 inh/km^2, urban > 600 inh/km^2 [56]), education (general, technical, vocational or arts), school grade (first to fourth year), nationality of parents, highest education of the parents (primary education, secondary education, higher education-non university, higher education-university, I don't know [57]) and sport club membership (yes/no). Based on parental educational level, low SES was defined as: none of the parents possessed a higher education diploma whereas high SES was defined as: at least one parent possessed a higher education diploma. Based on the place of birth of the participant and the parents, a non-western-European ethnicity was defined as having at least one parent born outside of the EU15 as defined by the Flemish government [58].

Physical activity measurement
Physical activity was measured with ActiGraph GTX-3 devices which were worn during waking hours for 4–5 consecutive days on a belt on the right hip. The Actigraph GTX-3 is a reliable and valid instrument to measure physical activity in youth and adults [59–61]. The Actigraph accelerometer uses a piezoelectric acceleration sensor, that, when it undergoes an acceleration, produces a voltage signal that is expressed as 'counts' [62]. These counts were averaged in periods (called epochs) of 15 s, as recommended [63]. The counts were stored onto the accelerometer device and later on downloaded using Actilife software version 6. For each 15 s epoch, the activity level [sedentary time (e.g., watching TV while sitting down), light-intensity physical activity (LPA) (e.g., walking slowly), moderate-intensity physical activity (MPA) (e.g., walking at 7.2 km/h) and vigorous-intensity physical activity (VPA) (e.g., running) [64–66]) was determined using Evenson cutpoints (sedentary time ≤ 100; LPA > 100, < 2296; 2296 ≥ MPA < 4012, VPA ≥ 4012) [67]. Continuous periods of 60 min of zero values were classified as non-wear time and removed from the data. Only participants with at least 1 day with at least 9 h of valid data were included in the analysis [32, 68]. Thus, when GPS devices were turned off for a substantial amount of time, this could have led to that day being excluded from analysis.

Spatial measurements: locations
A GPS device (Qstarz BT-Q1000XT) was worn on a belt on the left hip to track the locations of the participants. The devices were configured and data downloaded using the program Q-travel. Data were logged every 30 s. Epochs of 30 s have been used successfully for GPS data processing in previous studies with adolescents [69, 70]. Additionally, Schipperijn et al. [71] showed that limited differences exist between GPS data stored at epochs of 5, 15 and 30 s and that the three data collection epochs had the same median error.

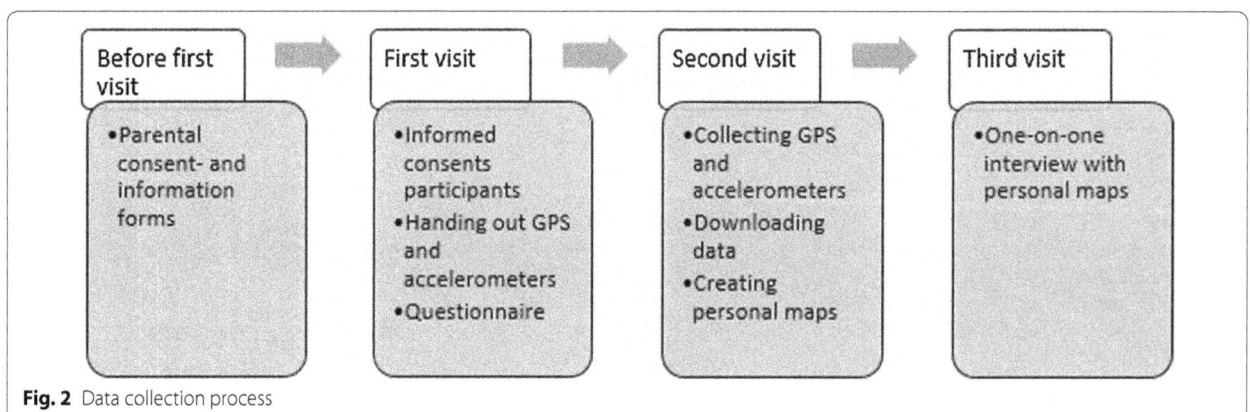

Fig. 2 Data collection process

One-on-one interview with personal maps

The data from the GPS devices were stored in a Post-greSQL database with PostGIS in order to visualize the visited locations of each participant in the self-made web application. The personal ID was used to log each participant in a self-made web application, where an individual map was available for each day the participant wore the devices (Fig. 3). On this individual web based map, the trip of the participant was visualized by placing a dot on the map every 30 s. Additionally, a light to dark colour scheme was used, to give an indication of the time during the day. The exact time of a point could be seen by clicking on a point. It was possible to zoom in on the map, which gave a clear overview of the locations that were visited. By using OpenStreetMap as a background layer, contextual information on the visited places of the participant could be gathered. The first week- and weekend day with complete data were selected (excluding the day the devices were handed out) and discussed with the participants. When no weekdays with complete data were available, two weekend days were selected and vice versa. For participants with only 1 day with complete data, this day was selected. For these selected days, the participants had to indicate the type of each location (e.g., school, home, a park, train station) they visited. For the locations that were classified as outdoor POS (street, shopping street/mall, square, park, outdoor sports ground/playground, parking lot, vacant lot and public transportation stop/station) three additional questions were asked: "who accompanied you here?"; "which activities did you engage in?"; "why did you choose this place?".

The colours of the dots represent the time course of the day: every 30 s a dot was placed on the map (Temporal resolution: 30 s). Lighter colours represent the start of the day, darker colours represent the end of the day. The green arrow represents the first data point registered by the GPS and the "finish flag" represents the last registered data point by the GPS.

Data processing

An overview of the data processing can be found in Fig. 4. First, all GPS and accelerometer data were created as CSV (comma separated value) files and imported into the Personal Activity and Location Measurement System (PALMS©) which was developed by the Centre for Wireless and Population Health Systems, University of California, San Diego.

Secondly, PALMS was used to merge all corresponding GPS and accelerometer data points (i.e. all data points-in epochs of 30 s-were matched according to the timestamp). PALMS identified speeds above 130 km/h, changes in distance higher than 1 km and elevations higher than 100 m between two data points (that are 30 s apart) as invalid data. In PALMS every data point (i.e. corresponding with an epoch of 30 s) was categorized into either an event or a transport related data point according to the acceleration measured. The transport related data points were further categorized into pedestrian ($\geq$ 1 km/h < 10 km/h), bicycle ($\geq$ 10 km/h, < 25 km/h) or motorized transport ($\geq$ 25 km/h) [72] (data not reported). All data points that were not identified as transport, were categorized as an event. Additionally, all

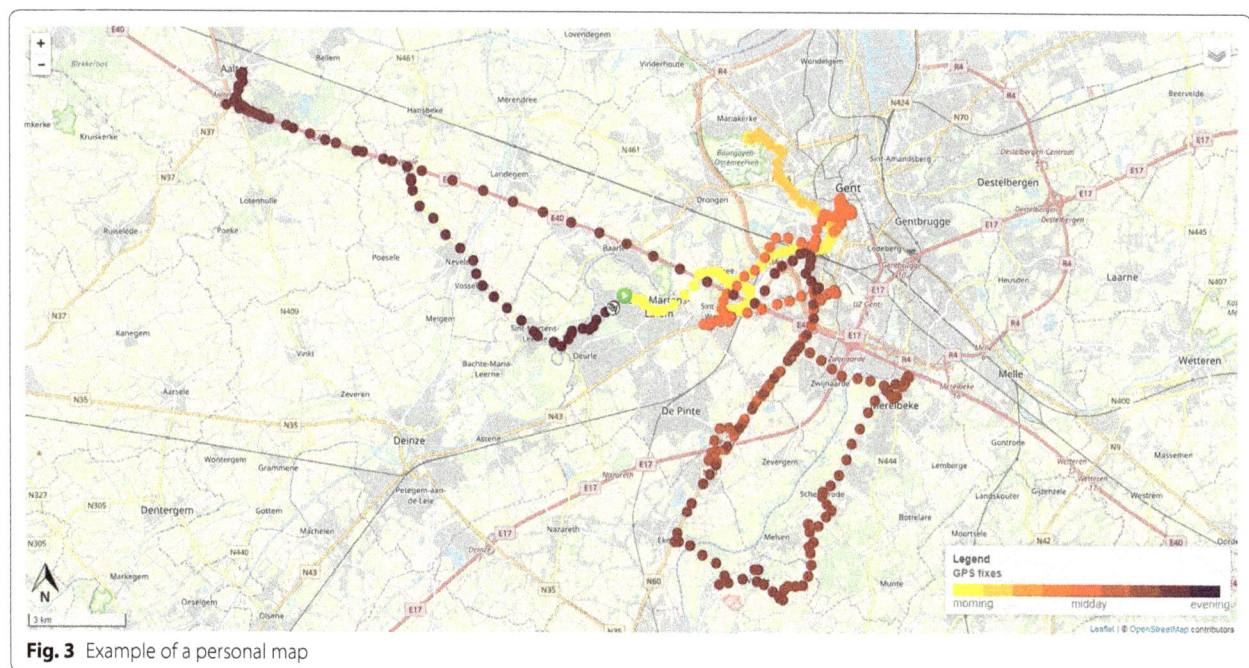

Fig. 3 Example of a personal map

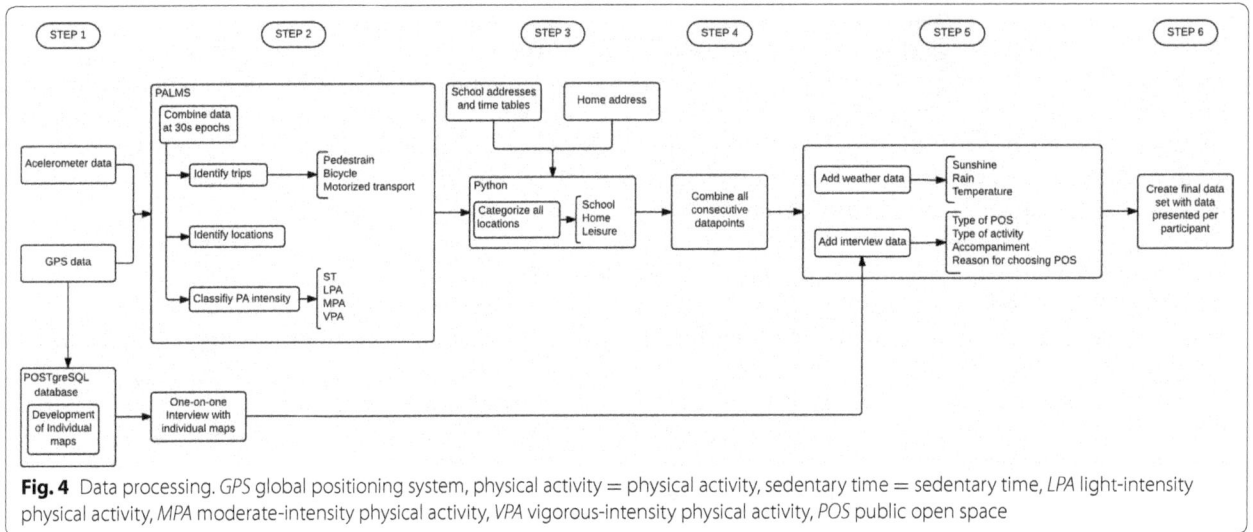

Fig. 4 Data processing. *GPS* global positioning system, physical activity = physical activity, sedentary time = sedentary time, *LPA* light-intensity physical activity, *MPA* moderate-intensity physical activity, *VPA* vigorous-intensity physical activity, *POS* public open space

epochs were classified according to the physical activity intensity using Evenson cutpoints [67].

Thirdly, the PALMS dataset was combined with information on the home and school addresses and school time tables in Python. All data points that were identified as an event (i.e. not a trip) were categorized into three domains: school, home or leisure. The data were categorized in the domain school during school hours, when the participant was located at school (100 m buffer). Within the domain school, a distinction was made between physical education classes, other classes and recess based on the time tables of the participating classes. The home domain was defined as being at the home address with a 100 m buffer around the home. All other data were categorized in the leisure domain. A similar approach was used in previous Danish research [68].

Fourth, all consecutive data points allocated to the same domain were combined, resulting in a database with data per trip and event.

In the fifth step, all data from the individual interviews (i.e. for each POS location, the accompaniment, reason why they chose that POS and activities performed) and weather data (mean min sun/day, mean mm rain/day and average temperature/day) were added to the database. All trips or locations misclassified by PALMS were corrected using the interview data (e.g., when a participant indicated that a certain trip was done by bus, however, due to traffic congestion the speed was rather low (< 25 km/h) and this trip was falsely allocated to the bicycle category by PALMS, this was picked up during the interviews and corrected).

In order to perform the analyses, the data had to be presented per participant (instead of per event, as was the case after step five). Therefore, in the final data

processing step, data were extracted from the data file created in step five, in order to create a new data file with data per participant. New variables were created with following information: mean wear time; mean number of POS visits accompanied by friends/classmates, siblings/cousins, parents/grandparents, organisation or alone; average sedentary time/day, in LPA/day, MVPA/day and VPA/day in total, located in POS (inclusive LPA, MVPA and VPA accumulated during trips to and from POS).

In this study, only time spent in the "leisure" category in POS and transportation to and from a POS was included. In other words, when a participant went to a park by bike, the time on the bike and the time spent in the park was included in the analyses. However, when a participant went to school by bike and cycled through a park, this trip was not included as this was categorized as a trip to school (and not POS) using active transportation.

Data analysis

Descriptive statistics were calculated using IBM SPSS statistics 22 software. Chi^2 tests and independent sample t tests were performed in SPSS to calculate differences between included and excluded participants (based on valid data).

Associations of individual factors (i.e. age, gender, ethnicity, education and sport club membership) and social environmental factors (accompaniment in POS with friends/classmates, siblings/cousins, parents/grandparents, organisation or alone) with the outcome measures (time, sedentary time, LPA, MVPA and VPA in POS, inclusive trips to and from POS) were examined using Multilevel Hurdle models and Gamma models (level 1 = subject, level 2 = school) using the package lme4 [73] in R version 3.4.1.

Different statistical models were used for the different outcomes as data were distributed differently. The outcome 'time spent in POS', was positively skewed and contained a high number of zeros (i.e. when a participant did not use a POS) demanding a multilevel hurdle model. A hurdle model includes two parts, first associations between the independent variables and the odds of having visited a POS were estimated by means of logistic regression analysis (binomial variance and logit link function) among all participants (n = 173). Second, a multilevel regression model with gamma variance and log link function was used to estimate the associations between the independent variables and the amount of time that was spent in POS among the participants who had used a POS (n = 130). The exponentiated regression coefficients represent the proportional difference in min spent in POS with a one-unit difference in the independent variables.

For the outcomes sedentary time, LPA, MVPA and VPA in POS, only the participants who had used a POS during data collection (n = 130) were included. This was done because participants who did not use a POS, logically also did not engage in any sedentary time, LPA, MVPA or VPA in POS. The outcomes 'sedentary time in POS', 'LPA in POS' and 'MVPA in POS', were skewed but did not contain many zeros and, therefore, multilevel regression models with gamma variance and log link function (selected based on Akaike's Information Criterion) were fitted. These models estimate the association between the independent variables and the amount of time spent in sedentary time, LPA and MVPA in POS among the participants who had used a POS for sedentary time, LPA and MVPA. For the outcome VPA, a multilevel hurdle model was selected as data were skewed and contained a high number of zeros.

A stepwise procedure was used to build the models. First, all potential covariates (residence-urban, suburban or rural-, mean wear time, mean POS visits/day, number of days with valid data, rain, sun, temperature, total time in POS, mean min sedentary time/day for outcome sedentary time in POS, mean min LPA/day for outcome LPA in POS, mean min MVPA/day for outcome MVPA in POS and mean min VPA/day for outcome VPA in POS) were entered simultaneously into a model to identify those that were significantly related to the outcomes. Based on this, residence, temperature, mean wear time, mean POS visits/day, and number of days with data were included as covariates in all subsequent analyses. Mean min LPA/day, MVPA/day and VPA/day were included as covariates in the analyses with the outcome variables LPA, MVPA and VPA in POS, respectively, and total time in POS was included as a covariate in the analyses with the outcome variables sedentary time, LPA, MVPA

and VPA in POS. Second, all individual factors (i.e. age, gender, ethnicity, education and sport club membership) were entered separately into a model adjusted for the appropriate covariates (see above).

Third, all individual factors that were significantly related to the outcome in the previous step were entered together into one model, again adjusting for the relevant covariates.

In a fourth step, each social environmental variable was entered separately into a model adjusting for the significant individual factors identified in step 2 and the relevant covariates. These four steps were performed separately for each outcome variable.

POS visitation in the company of an organisation was not included in the analyses, as only 2.5% of all POS visits were done in the company of an organisation. It was not possible to analyse associations between the environmental factors (i.e. location: street, shopping street/mall, square, park, outdoor sports ground/playground, parking lot, vacant lot and public transportation station/stop) and the outcome variables (SB, LPA, MVPA, VPA), because more than 70% of all POS visits were located at a public transportation stop/station. Level of significance was set at α = 0.05.

Results
Descriptive statistics
In total, 283 adolescents were invited to participate in the study of which ten had no consent from their parents or were not willing to participate themselves. Of the remaining 273 participants, 100 were excluded from the analyses. Reasons for exclusion were: absence when handing out material or during interview (n = 49), no days with valid data for at least 9 h (n = 22), being older than 16 years (n = 12), forgot to wear material (n = 7), no longer enrolled at this school/class (n = 4), material forgotten at home (n = 3) or the GPS did not work properly (n = 3). Eventually, 173 participants aged 12–16 years were willing to participate, had parental consent and valid data for at least 1 day (Fig. 5).

No differences were found for gender, SES and ethnicity between the participants who were included for analysis (n = 173) and those who were excluded (n = 100) ($p > 0.05$). The excluded participants were significantly older than the included participants (15.6 vs. 14.2; $p < 0.05$) because participants older than 16 years were excluded from analyses.

The sample had a mean age of 14.2 ± 1.1 years, consisted of 54.4% girls and 93.1% was living in an urban or suburban environment. Most participants were enrolled in general education (68.8%), 28.3% had a non-western-European ethnicity and 22.5% had a lower SES based on parental educational level. Almost 60% of

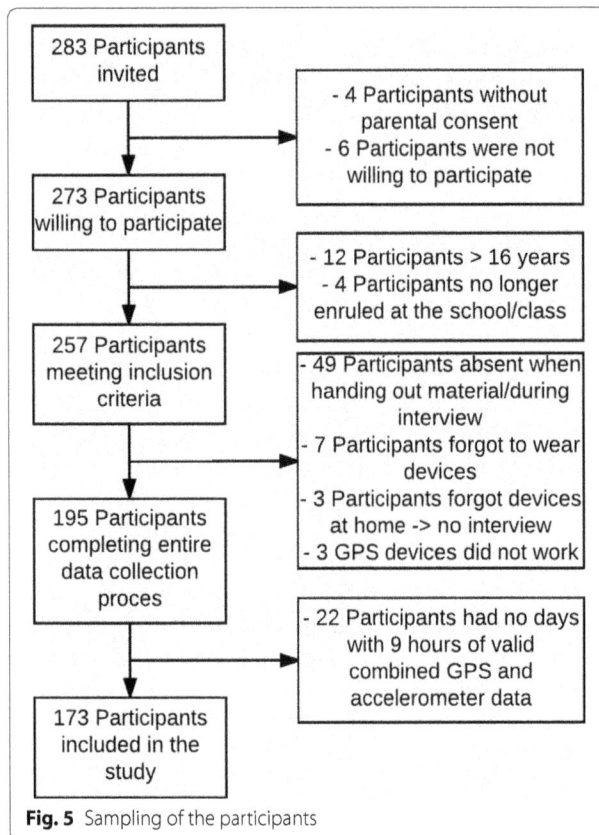

Fig. 5 Sampling of the participants

The flowchart contains:

- 283 Participants invited
  - 4 Participants without parental consent
  - 6 Participants were not willing to participate
- 273 Participants willing to participate
  - 12 Participants > 16 years
  - 4 Participants no longer enruled at the school/class
- 257 Participants meeting inclusion criteria
  - 49 Participants absent when handing out material/during interview
  - 7 Participants forgot to wear devices
  - 3 Participants forgot devices at home -> no interview
  - 3 GPS devices did not work
- 195 Participants completing entire data collection proces
  - 22 Participants had no days with 9 hours of valid combined GPS and accelerometer data
- 173 Participants included in the study

Table 1 Descriptive characteristics of the sample (n = 173)

Age (mean ± SD)	14.2 ± 1.1
Gender (% girls)	54.4
Living environment (%)	
Rural	6.9
Sub-urban	16.8
Urban	76.3
Education (%)	
General	68.8
Vocational	22.0
Technical	9.2
Other ethnicity (%)	28.3
Lower SES (%)	22.5
Sport club membership (%)	58.0
Sedentary time (mean h/day ± SD)	8.8 ± 1.6
LPA (mean h/day ± SD	3.3 ± 1.0
MVPA (median min/day; Q1, Q3)	36.5; 22.9, 51.4
% of participants who used a POS	75.1
Mean number of POS visits among participants who used a POS	1.83 ± 1.2

Skewed data were reported as median and interquartile range

SD standard deviation, *SES* socio-economic status, *MVPA* moderate- to vigorous-intensity physical activity, *Q1* 25th percentile, *Q3* 75th percentile, *min* minutes, *POS* public open space

the participants were member of a sport club and the median min of MVPA/day was 36.5. Among the participants who used a POS (75.1% of the participants), the mean number of POS visits per day was 1.8 ± 1.2 (Table 1).

All participants with one (n = 63) or 2 days (n = 110) of complete GPS and accelerometer data for 9 h minimum/day were included in the study. During the 283 included days 373 events took place at an outdoor POS. Participants reported that more than half of the POS visits were done in the company of a friend/classmate (59.8%) and most POS visits were located at a public transportation stop/station (71.0%). The most frequently mentioned reasons to visit a specific POS were: to wait for something/someone here (e.g., train) (30.3%), because friends/classmates/siblings/cousins wanted to go to that POS (17.4%), for 'other reasons' (e.g., for shopping purposes, easy to meet up) (17.4%) or because the POS was close to school or their home (13.8%). Standing was most frequently reported by the participants as the main activity in POS during a POS visit (43.1%), followed by walking (38.5%) and sitting or lying down (13.8%). The one-on-one interviews revealed that participants often indicated to 'just hang around' in POS while talking to friends (Table 2).

Associations of individual factors and company with time spent in pos

The logistic regression model shows that the odds for having used a POS were 2.20 times higher for participants with a non-western-European ethnicity compared to participants with a western-European ethnicity and 8.09 times higher for participants enrolled in technical education compared to participants enrolled in general education (both trends towards significance, see Table 3). In the multivariate model (data not shown in table), education became significant (OR: 8.68; 95% CI 1.03–72.75) while ethnicity remained borderline significant (OR: 2.33; 95% CI 0.93–5.86). For the participants who had visited a POS at least once during the days that were measured, results showed that with each additional visit accompanied by siblings, on average 60% more time was spent in POS per day (Exp. B: 1.60; 95% CI 1.26–2.04; data not shown in table). In other words, the higher the number of POS visits with siblings, the higher the total time spent in POS daily.

Associations of individual factors and company with sedentary time and physical activity in pos

None of the individual and social environmental factors was significantly associated with sedentary time and LPA in POS (see Table 4). The analyses for the outcome

Table 2 Descriptive characteristics of POS visits (n = 373)

Company (% of POS visits; multiple answers possible)	% (n = 373)
Friends/classmates	59.8
Siblings/cousins	16.4
Parents/grandparents	16.4
Alone	15.6
Organisation	2.5
Location (% of POS visits)	
Public transportation stop/station	71.0
Street	9.4
Parking lot	5.4
Square	3.5
Shopping street	3.2
Sport field/playground	2.9
Park	2.9
Shopping mall	1.3
Vacant lot	0.3
Reasons for POS visit (% of POS visits; multiple answers possible)	
I had to wait for something/someone here (e.g., train)	30.3
My friends/classmates/siblings/cousins wanted go there	17.4
Other (e.g., for shopping purposes, easy to meet up)	17.4
This POS is close to my home/school	13.8
I was going somewhere else and decided to stay there	10.1
It is a habit to go there	8.3
There is a nice atmosphere	4.6
My parent want me to go there/I am not allowed to go anywhere else	4.6
There is sport infrastructure available	4.6
This POS is easy accessible	3.7
I know this place for a long time and I am familiar with this POS	1.8
Activity in POS (self-reported; multiple answers possible)	
Standing	43.1
Walking	38.5
Sitting/lying down	13.8
Ball sports	6.4
Biking	2.8
Other	1.8
Skateboarding/BMX/roller-skating	0.9
Active games	0.9
Jogging	0.9

POS public open space

Table 3 Associations between individual factors and time spent in POS

Individual factors	Logistic regression[a]		Gamma model[b]	
	OR	95% CI	Exp. B	95% CI
Gender (ref = male)	1.82	0.88–3.79	0.98	0.69–1.38
Education (ref = general)				
Vocational	1.09	0.41–2.88	1.42	0.65–3.11
Technical	8.09°	0.97–67.62	1.15	0.61–2.15
Age	1.00	0.70–1.43	1.05	0.88–1.26
Ethnicity (ref = Belgium)	2.20°	1.88–5.49	1.25	0.84–1.86
Sport club membership (ref = yes)	1.80	0.85–3.85	1.21	0.87–1.68

OR odds ratio, *CI* confidence interval, *Exp. B* exponent of B, *POS* public open space, *ref* reference category, *min* minutes, ° $\alpha < 0.1$ = trend towards significance

[a] The logistic regression model estimated the association of the independent factors with the odds of having visited a POS

[b] The Gamma models (Exp. B) estimated the proportional difference in min spent in POS associated with a one-unit difference in the independent variables for adolescents that had visited a POS. Analyses were controlled for mean temperature, residence, POS visits/day, total wear time (mean min/day), and amount of days. All Gamma models were fitted using the log link function

MVPA in POS revealed that among the participants who had used a POS, girls engaged on average in 43% less min of MVPA/day in POS compared to boys. None of the other individual or social environmental factors were significantly associated with MVPA in POS.

The logistic regression model for the outcome VPA in POS shows that girls had a 79% lower odds of having used a POS for VPA compared to boys and an increase in age with 1 year was associated with a 40% lower odds of having engaged in VPA in POS (trend towards significance for age, see Table 5). When gender (OR: 0.16; 95% CI 0.05–0.52) and age (OR: 0.52; 95% CI 0.30–0.93) were entered simultaneously into a model, both were significant (data not shown in table). Among those who had used a POS for VPA, girls engaged on average in 40% less min of VPA in POS/day compared to boys and participants enrolled in vocational education spent on average 41% less min in VPA in POS/day compared to participants enrolled in general education (trend towards significance for education). When gender and education were entered in the multivariable gamma model, only gender remained significant (Exp B: 0.63; 95% CI 0.41–0.98).

Discussion

In this study, a socio-ecological approach was used to gain insight into the prevalence, frequency and context (i.e. company, locations and reason) of POS visitation and the factors associated with time, sedentary time and physical activity in POS among adolescents. Our study revealed that 75% of the participants used a POS and during most POS visits, participants were accompanied by friends/classmates. Mainly public transportation stops/stations were used, and subsequently the most reported reason for POS visitation was "to wait for something/someone (e.g., bus)". Furthermore, ethnicity, education, gender and age were the individual factors associated with at least one outcome. The only social environmental

Table 4 Associations between individual and social environmental factors with sedentary time, LPA and MVPA spent in POS

Individual factors	Gamma model sedentary time		Gamma model LPA		Gamma model MVPA	
	Exp. B	95% CI	Exp. B	95% CI	Exp. B	95% CI
Gender (ref = male)	0.89	0.63–1.27	0.73	0.53–1.00	0.57**	0.41–0.80
Education (ref = general)						
Vocational	1.43	0.85–2.40	0.71	0.42–1.19	0.74	0.44–1.24
Technical	1.11	0.62–2.00	0.93	0.51–1.67	0.72	0.40–1.29
Age	1.08	0.91–1.29	0.98	0.82–1.16	0.96	0.80–1.15
Ethnicity (ref = Belgium)	1.12	0.78–1.61	1.09	0.74–1.60	0.96	0.64–1.42
Sport club membership (ref = yes)	0.94	0.66–1.36	0.75	0.52–1.09	0.83	0.57–1.19

The Gamma models (Exp. B) estimated the proportional difference in sedentary time, LPA and MVPA in POS associated with a one-unit difference in the independent variables for adolescents that had used a POS. Analyses were controlled for mean temperature, residence, POS visits/day, total wear time (mean min/day), total time in POS and amount of days. All Gamma models were fitted using the log link function

LPA light-intensity physical activity, *MVPA* moderate- to vigorous-intensity physical activity, *OR* odds ratio, *CI* confidence interval, *Exp. B* exponent of B, *POS* public open space, *ref* reference category, *min* minutes, ° = α < 0.1 = trend towards significance

**α < 0.01

Table 5 Associations between individual and social environmental factors with VPA in POS

Individual factors	Logistic regression[a]		Gamma model[b]	
	OR	95% CI	Exp. B	95% CI
Gender (ref = male)	0.21**	0.07–0.63	0.60*	0.39–0.92
Education (ref = general)				
Vocational	0.70	0.17–2.90	0.59°	0.34–1.04
Technical	0.32	0.07–1.52	1.15	0.48–2.75
Age	0.60°	0.36–1.00	0.94	0.73–1.19
Ethnicity (ref = Belgium)	0.71	0.25–2.00	0.84	0.53–1.37
Sport club membership (ref = yes)	0.54	0.19–1.59	1.18	0.74–1.88

VPA vigorous-intensity physical activity, *OR* odds ratio, *CI* confidence interval, *Exp. B* exponent of B, *POS* public open space, *ref* reference category, *min* minutes, ° = α < 0.1 = trend towards significance

*α < 0.05; **α < 0.01

[a] The logistic regression model estimated the association of the independent factors with the odds of having used a POS for VPA

[b] The Gamma models (Exp. B) estimated the proportional difference in min of VPA in POS associated with a one-unit difference in the independent variables for adolescents that had used a POS. Analyses were controlled for mean temperature, residence, POS visits/day, total wear time (mean min/day), total time in POS, total time in VPA/day and amount of days. All Gamma models were fitted using the log link function

variable associated with time spent in POS was accompaniment by siblings.

Surprisingly, there was limited variability in the POS locations used by the participants in this study as 70% of all POS visits were located at a public transportation stop/station. This suggests that public transportation stops/stations are frequently visited by adolescents in Flanders (Belgium), but these locations are not very suitable for physical activity. POS such as parks, a playground/

sport field and squares are very suitable for physical activity, but were not often used by adolescents. Only 3.5% of the POS events was located at a square, 2.9% at a sport field/playground and 2.9% in a park. However, when the POS visits that took place at a public transportation stop/station are not taken into account, 12.0% of POS visits were located at squares; 10.3% at sport fields/playgrounds and 10.2% at parks. These findings are of importance for interventions aiming at the promotion of POS use among adolescents in Flanders, as we now know that POS such as parks, sport fields/playgrounds and squares are not often used and extra initiatives are warranted to encourage their use. Additionally, when public transportation routes are (re)designed, it is recommended to place public transportations stops close to locations suitable for physical activity (such as a park of square). Our results differ from previous Danish research where GPS measures revealed that 40% of the adolescents had used a playground, 97% had used urban green space and 32% had visited a shopping centre at 1 day during the data collection period [68]. It is difficult to compare the results of our study with these of this Danish study as the results are presented differently (i.e. % of events located at specific location, compared to % of participants that used a location), however, clearly some differences exist. On the one hand, some methodological differences between the studies could have caused these differences. In the Danish study, GIS was used to categorize the events into subdomains (i.e. locations such as playgrounds or urban green space) used during leisure time. It has been acknowledged that sometimes GIS layers lack details [45] which could have led to misclassification of events. For example, when a participant was waiting at the bus stop near a park, this could have been misclassified as an event in the park. Additionally, in the Danish study, the subdomain "public transportation stop/station" was not included, and 1–4 days of data were included whereas in our study only 1–2 days. On the other hand, these differences between studies could possibly be attributed to cultural differences between countries meaning that POS use is more integrated in Danish adolescents' life [68].

This study provided new insight into the associations between the accompaniment and time, sedentary time and physical activity in POS. Results from the one-on-one interviews revealed that adolescents used POS most often with friends/classmates, followed by siblings, parents and alone. Previous research using ecological momentary assessment indicated that most 14-year-old adolescents reported to be physically active in the company of friends, followed by classmates and family members. Furthermore, the company with whom the greatest proportion of walking occurred was with friends or alone [74, 75]. In this study, only the accompaniment with siblings was associated with more time in POS, whereas no associations were found between the accompaniment and physical activity in POS. These contradicting results indicate that additional research on this topic is needed and that interventions targeting all children within a family could possibly be more effective. One explanation for this result could be that adolescents are allowed to stay longer outside when their parents know they are not alone, but in the company of a sibling.

It is known that total physical activity levels decline when adolescents grow older [76–78]. This study has added upon this knowledge by demonstrating that this age-dependent decrease also exist for POS physical activity. In this study, an increase in age with 1 year, was associated with a 40% lower odds of having engaged in VPA in POS. From previous qualitative research it became apparent that the playgrounds and facilities present in POS are often designed for younger children causing a lack of age appropriate facilities for (older) adolescents [27]. Creating POS with attractive facilities for older adolescents (such as sport fields [27] and adventurous playgrounds with high swings and big slides [79]) could possibly counteract this age-dependent decline in physical activity levels.

Total physical activity levels among adolescent girls have been shown to be lower than adolescent boys' physical activity levels [77, 78, 80]. Additionally, our results revealed that also in POS, girls accumulate less physical activity compared to boys. Analyses revealed that boys spent more time in MVPA and VPA in POS compared to girls. This is in line with previous research from the US using GPS and accelerometers in a sample of 11- to 14-year-olds. It was reported that more physical activity was accumulated at playgrounds by boys compared to girls and boys had higher odds of spending time in MVPA at parks compared to girls [30]. Furthermore, previous observational research reported lower use of parks by girls (children and adolescents) and lower energy expenditure levels among girls compared to boys [26, 34, 81, 82]. Additionally, previous studies have shown that safety related factors (such as the presence of sufficient lighting [83], traffic safety [84], number of violent crimes [85]) were related to physical activity in parks and in the neighbourhood among girls. It is thus possible that safety issues contribute to gender differences in POS use. However, safety related factors are very context-specific and can differ between countries. In Belgium, the overall victimisation rate (= percentage of people victimised once or more) was significantly higher than the average of the 18 EU countries in 2004 [86].

Additionally, these results suggest that urban planners should consider adding attractive characteristics and features, in order to attract more girls to POS. It has been shown that adolescent girls prefer individual, non-competitive activities such as dancing or running or group activities with the focus on fun, such as netball [87–89]. Including features suitable for such activities could be a useful strategy to attract more girls to POS. However, additional research is needed to define what POS characteristics could specifically attract or repel girls for physical activity in POS.

Our study revealed ethnicity to be associated with time spent in POS among adolescents. The odds for having used a POS was higher among non-western-European adolescents compared to participants with a western-European ethnicity. However, it could be possible that adolescents with non-western-European ethnicity used public transportation more often, which could have influenced our results (because of the high number of POS visits that were located at public transportations stops/stations). This is an important result, as adolescents with a non-western-European ethnicity are often hard to reach for interventions. However, our results were only borderline significant and research on this topic among adolescents is lacking and, therefore, these results should be interpreted with caution.

Furthermore, this study revealed that participants enrolled in technical education were more likely to spent time in POS and participants enrolled in vocational education spent less min in VPA in POS compared to participants enrolled in general education. In Flanders (Belgium) technical education is focussed on practice lessons and technical-theoretical courses, whereas vocational education is focussed on learning a profession [90]. Not much is known about the association between education and time in POS among adolescents, but our findings are consistent with previous Australian research on adults' individual factors associated with park use. This Australian study revealed that park users had less educational qualifications compared to non-park users [91]. However, adolescents enrolled in vocational education accumulated less min of VPA in POS compared to participants enrolled in general education. Currently, it is not known which POS characteristics invite adolescents to engage in VPA in POS and it is possible that differences exist according to educational level. Another explanation could be that adolescents enrolled in vocational education visit other types of POS what are less inviting for VPA (such as a train station). These findings have important social relevance as people with low educational level and low SES are at risk for low levels of physical activity [92] and are target populations that are hard to reach by standard physical activity initiatives from sport clubs or school sport. Therefore, interventions taking place in POS could have the ability to reach the target groups most in need for physical activity promotion. However, additional research is needed to define how adolescents could be encouraged to engage in physical activity in POS.

To our knowledge, this was the first study to look into the associations with sedentary time in POS. However, no associations were found with the individual nor with the social environmental factors. This could indicate that other factors are more important for sedentary time in POS. In this study, no environmental factors were included in the analyses, however, it is possible that the environmental characteristics of a POS (e.g., the presence of benches), are associated with sedentary time in POS. These factors should be included in future research.

This study emphasized the need for further research into the factors associated with time, sedentary time and physical activity in POS among adolescents. Within this study a social ecological approach was pursued. However, due to lacking variability in the POS locations that were used it was not possible to study the associations for the different types of POS locations that were used with time, sedentary time and physical activity in POS. Future studies could prevent this issue by assessing a larger sample from different cities and gathering data on more than 2 days. For larger samples, using data collected by the participants' smartphones using mobile object trajectory analysis, could be a cost-effective and time-efficient option. Furthermore, it is recommended to develop a method in which subjective measurements can be obtained in a less time consuming manner. For example, using ecological momentary assessment via a smartphone application in combination with GPS and accelerometers could be a useful method [93]. Such an application can prompt questions about the accompaniment or about the characteristics of the public open

space, when the smartphone detects that a participant is present at a public open space of interest. This way the use of a smartphone application could lessen the burden on the researchers and allow the researcher to collect data on more than 2 days. However, developing such an application poses some technical difficulties and is very expensive. In this study, no specific spatial analyses were performed such as spatial clustering or spatial time services. We suggest including such analyses in future research as these were outside the scope of this paper.

Strengths and limitations

One of the major strengths of this study was the use of objective measurement methods for both locations and physical activity measures. By using these methods it was possible to investigate the locations that were actually used by the adolescents. Furthermore, these objectively measured data were combined with subjective interview data, to provide conclusive data and avoid the weaknesses of using solely qualitative or quantitative measurement methods [94]. Another strength was the broad definition of POS that was used in this study, whereas in other research often narrow definitions of POS were used. For example Edwards defined POS as "spaces reserved for the provision of green space and natural environments, accessible to the general public free of charge" and thereby excluded all non-green POS [95]. In this study, sedentary time and physical activity accumulated during trips to and from POS were included in analyses which, to our knowledge, has never been done before and provides a more comprehensive view on POS' contribution to sedentary time and physical activity compared to previous studies that only included sedentary time and physical activity accumulated after arriving at the POS. Furthermore, it was attempted to include factors associated with POS use from different layers of the socio-ecological model in order to provide a more comprehensive insight into the use of POS. However, only individual and social environmental factors could be included into the analyses, because of the low levels of POS use and the low variability in POS locations that were used. This could be due to the fact that only 1 or 2 days of data were included for analyses, which was the biggest limitation of this study. Furthermore, also events that were more "transport" related (e.g., when participants were waiting for a bus at a bus stop, with the sole intention to take the bus) were included in our study and this could be considered as a limitation. Due to the structure of the data it was not possible to solely select the events located at a public transportation stop/station that could actually be classified as leisure time (e.g., when participants used a station as a meeting place). It is possible that the high number of POS visits located at public transportations stops/stations has altered the results. Another limitation of the study was that the data were collected from September to December, a period that is characterized by lower temperatures in this part of the world. This could have elicited different results compared to a period with generally better weather conditions. However, by including weather information (sun, rain and temperature) as covariates in the statistical analyses, we tried to tackle this barrier. Only three questions were included in the personal interviews and no questions were asked concerning the reasons for not engaging in physical activity. This could also be considered as a limitation of this study. The data were only collected in one city in Flanders (Belgium), inclusion of other cities could have provided different results and would have increased the generalizability of the current findings.

Conclusion

Our research showed that ethnicity, education, gender, age and accompaniment are associated with time and physical activity in POS but not with sedentary time in POS among adolescents. Identifying the population groups that are currently least using POS (for physical activity) is important in order to guide interventions. In this study it was found that boys, younger adolescents, non-western-European adolescents and lower educated adolescents used POS more often (for physical activity). Additionally, the accompaniment by siblings in POS was shown to be associated with more time spent in POS. Understanding the use of POS is necessary in order to develop POS that are attractive to all adolescents and provide opportunities to engage in physical activity alone or in company. Additional research is warranted to elaborate on the current knowledge about the use of POS among adolescents.

Abbreviations

BMI: body mass index; CSV: comma separated value; GIS: geographical information system; GPS: global positioning system; LPA: light-intensity physical activity; MPA: moderate-intensity physical activity; MVPA: moderate- to vigorous-intensity physical activity; PALMS: personal activity and location movement system; POS: public open spaces; SES: socio-economic status; US: United States; VPA: vigorous-intensity physical activity; WHO: World Health Organisation.

Authors' contributions

Design of the study: LVH, HV, PC, DVD, NVDW, JVC, BD; Data collection: LVH, HV, TB; Data processing, analyse and interpretation: LVH, HV, TB, JVC; Drafting the article: LVH; Critical revision of the article: LVH, HV, PC, DVD, NVDW, TB, JVC, BD; All authors read and approved the final manuscript.

Author details

[1] Department of Public Health, Faculty of Medicine and Health Sciences, Ghent University, Ghent, Belgium. [2] Physical Activity, Nutrition and Health Research Unit, Department of Movement and Sport Sciences, Faculty of Physical Education and Physical Therapy, Vrije Universiteit Brussel, Brussels, Belgium. [3] Fund for Scientific Research Flanders (FWO), Brussels, Belgium. [4] Department of Movement and Sport Sciences, Faculty of Medicine and Health Sciences, Ghent University, Ghent, Belgium. [5] Department of Geography – CartoGIS, Faculty of Sciences, Ghent University, Ghent, Belgium.

Acknowledgements

None.

Competing interests

The authors declare that they have no competing interests.

Funding

Linde Van Hecke and Hannah Verhoeven are funded by the Research Foundation Flanders: http://www.fwo.be/en/ (FWO, 54488-G0A8514N). Delfien Van Dyck is funded by the Research Foundation Flanders: http://www.fwo.be/en/ (FWO: post-doctoral mandate FWO12/PDO/158). Jelle Van Cauwenberg is supported by a Postdoctoral Fellowship of the Research Foundation Flanders: http://www.fwo.be/en/ (FWO: 12I1117N).

References

1. WHO. Global recommendations on physical activity for health. Geneva: World Health Organisation; 2010.
2. Bauman AE. Updating the evidence that physical activity is good for health: an epidemiological review 2000–2003. J Sci Med Sport/Sports Med Aust. 2004;7(1 Suppl):6–19.
3. Hallal PC, et al. Adolescent physical activity and health: a systematic review. Sports Med. 2006;36(12):1019–30.
4. Janssen I, Leblanc AG. Systematic review of the health benefits of physical activity and fitness in school-aged children and youth. Int J Behav Nutr Phys Act. 2010;7:40.
5. Janssen I, et al. Comparison of overweight and obesity prevalence in school-aged youth from 34 countries and their relationships with physical activity and dietary patterns. Obes Rev. 2005;6(2):123–32.
6. Tremblay MS, et al. Sedentary behavior research network (SBRN)—terminology consensus project process and outcome. Int J Behav Nutr Phys Act. 2017;14(1):75.
7. Tremblay MS, et al. Systematic review of sedentary behaviour and health indicators in school-aged children and youth. Int J Behav Nutr Phys Act. 2011;8:98.
8. Braithwaite I, et al. The worldwide association between television viewing and obesity in children and adolescents: cross sectional study. PLoS ONE. 2013;8(9):e74263.
9. Dumith SC, et al. Physical activity change during adolescence: a systematic review and a pooled analysis. Int J Epidemiol. 2011;40(3):685–98.
10. Basterfield L, et al. Longitudinal study of physical activity and sedentary behavior in children. Pediatrics. 2011;127(1):e24–30.
11. Wickel EE, Belton S. School's out… now what? objective estimates of afterschool sedentary time and physical activity from childhood to adolescence. J Sci Med Sports. 2016;19(8):654–8.
12. Telama R. Tracking of physical activity from childhood to adulthood: a review. Obes Facts. 2009;2(3):187–95.
13. Van Hecke L, et al. Variation in population levels of physical activity in European children and adolescents according to cross-European studies: a systematic literature review within DEDIPAC. Int J Behav Nutr Phys Act. 2016;13:70.
14. Cooper AR, et al. Objectively measured physical activity and sedentary time in youth: the International children's accelerometry database (ICAD). Int J Behav Nutr Phys Act. 2015;12:113.
15. Verloigne M, et al. Variation in population levels of sedentary time in European children and adolescents according to cross-European studies:

a systematic literature review within DEDIPAC. Int J Behav Nutr Phys Act. 2016;13:69.

16. Telama R, et al. Physical activity from childhood to adulthood: a 21-year tracking study. Am J Prev Med. 2005;28(3):267–73.

17. Kjonniksen L, Torsheim T, Wold B. Tracking of leisure-time physical activity during adolescence and young adulthood: a 10-year longitudinal study. Int J Behav Nutr Phys Act. 2008;5:69.

18. Biddle SJ, et al. Tracking of sedentary behaviours of young people: a systematic review. Prev Med. 2010;51(5):345–51.

19. Glanz K, Rimer BK, Viswanath K. Health behavior and health education—theory, research and practice. Berlin: Jossey-Bass A Wiley Imprint; 2008.

20. Sallis JF, et al. An ecological approach to creating active living communities. Annu Rev Public Health. 2006;27:297–322.

21. Bauman AE, et al. Correlates of physical activity: why are some people physically active and others not? Lancet. 2012;380(9838):258–71.

22. Godbey GC, et al. Contributions of leisure studies and recreation and park management research to the active living agenda. Am J Prev Med. 2005;28(2 Suppl 2):150–8.

23. Grow HM, et al. Where are youth active? roles of proximity, active transport, and built environment. Med Sci Sports Exerc. 2008;40(12):2071–9.

24. Bedimo-Rung AL, Mowen AJ, Cohen DA. The significance of parks to physical activity and public health: a conceptual model. Am J Prev Med. 2005;28(2 Suppl 2):159–68.

25. Kaczynski A. Environmental correlates of physical activity: a review of evidence about parks and recreation. Leisure Sci. 2007;29:315–54.

26. Cohen DA, et al. Contribution of public parks to physical activity. Am J Public Health. 2007;97(3):509–14.

27. Van Hecke L, et al. Social and physical environmental factors influencing adolescents' physical activity in urban public open spaces: a qualitative study using walk-along interviews. PLoS ONE. 2016;11(5):e0155686.

28. Day R, Wager F. Parks, streets and "just empty space": the local environmental experiences of children and young people in a Scottish study. Local Environ. 2010;15(6):509–23.

29. Veitch J, et al. Adolescents' ratings of features of parks that encourage park visitation and physical activity. Int J Behav Nutr Phys Act. 2016;13:73.

30. Oreskovic NM, et al. Adolescents' use of the built environment for physical activity. BMC Public Health. 2015;15(1):251.

31. Klinker CD, et al. Context-specific outdoor time and physical activity among school-children across gender and age: using accelerometers and GPS to advance methods. Front Public Health. 2014;2:20.

32. Klinker CD, et al. Using accelerometers and global positioning system devices to assess gender and age differences in children's school, transport, leisure and home based physical activity. Int J Behav Nutr Phys Act. 2014;11(1):8.

33. Rainham DG, et al. Spatial classification of youth physical activity patterns. Am J Prev Med. 2012;42(5):e87–96.

34. Van Hecke L, et al. Active use of parks in flanders (Belgium): an exploratory observational study. Int J Environ Res Public Health. 2017;14(1):35.

35. Besenyi GM, et al. Demographic variations in observed energy expenditure across park activity areas. Prev Med. 2013;56(1):79–81.

36. Floyd MF, et al. Park-based physical activity in diverse communities of two US cities. An observational study. Am J Prev Med. 2008;34(4):299–305.

37. Shores KA, West ST. The relationship between built park environments and physical activity in four park locations. J Public Health Manag Pract JPHMP. 2008;14(3):e9–16.

38. Ding D, et al. Neighborhood environment and physical activity among youth a review. Am J Prev Med. 2011;41(4):442–55.

39. Ferreira I, et al. Environmental correlates of physical activity in youth—a review and update. Obes Rev. 2007;8(2):129–54.

40. Giles-Corti B, Donovan RJ. Socioeconomic status differences in recreational physical activity levels and real and perceived access to a supportive physical environment. Prev Med. 2002;35(6):601–11.

41. Timperio A, et al. Features of public open spaces and physical activity among children: findings from the CLAN study. Prev Med. 2008;47(5):514–8.

42. Duncan MJ, Mummery WK. GIS or GPS? a comparison of two methods for assessing route taken during active transport. Am J Prev Med. 2007;33(1):51–3.

43. Badland H, et al. Examining commute routes: applications of GIS and GPS technology. Environ Health Prev Med. 2010;15(4):723–41.

44. Stopher P, FitzGerald C, Xu M. Assessing the accuracy of the Sydney household travel survey with GPS. Transportation. 2007;34(6):723–41.

45. Kerr J, Duncan S, Schipperjin J. Using global positioning systems in health research a practical approach to data collection and processing. Am J Prev Med. 2011;41(5):532–40.

46. United Nations Development Program. 2017. http://hdr.undp.org/en/composite/HDI. Accessed on 21 Dec. 2015.

47. Statbel. Statistics Belgium—Bodemgebruik. België, gewesten en gemeenten (1834–2017).

48. Statbel. Statistics Belgium—Structuur van de bevolking volgens woonplaats: grootste gemeenten.

49. Boussauw K. City profile: Ghent, Belgium. Cities. 2014;40:32–43.

50. City of Ghent (2017). https://gent.buurtmonitor.be/. 12, 21.

51. http://www.steunpuntwerk.be/node/2779, 2017, 12, 21.

52. Statistics Belgium 2016. http://statbel.fgov.be/nl/binaries/1801_nl%20gent_en_gentgebruikers_digitaal_tcm325-244558.pdf. Accessed on 28 Dec. 2017.

53. Shaw C, Brady L-M, Davey C. Guidelines for research with children and young people. New York: NCB Research Centre; 2011.

54. Ruiz-Canela M, Lopez-del-Burgo C, Carlos S, Calatrava M, Beltramo C, Osorio A, et al. Observational research with adolescents: a framework for the management of the parental permission. BMC Med Ethics. 2013;14(2):2 **(Research Support, Non-U.S. Gov't)**.

55. Belgium, Belgian Official Journal. The privacy act. 2015;12:8, T.C.f.t.P.o. Privacy, Editor 1993.

56. Lenders, S. Afbakening van het Vlaamse platteland - een statistische analyse 4:1. 2005. Available from: http://www2.vlaanderen.be/landbouw/downloads/volt/38.pdf.

57. Lien N, Friestad C, Klepp KI. Adolescents' proxy reports of parents socioeconomic status: how valid are they? J Epidemiol Commun Health. 2001;55:731–7.

58. Government F. Het Vlaamse beleid naar etnisch-culturele minderheden: jaarrapport 2004–2005. Accessed on 08 Mar. 2017.

59. Aadland E, Ylvisaker E. Reliability of the actigraph GT3X + accelerometer in adults under free-living conditions. PLoS ONE. 2015;10(8):e0134606.

60. Kelly LA, et al. Validity of actigraphs uniaxial and triaxial accelerometers for assessment of physical activity in adults in laboratory conditions. BMC Med Phys. 2013;13(1):5.

61. Santos-Lozano A, et al. Actigraph GT3X: validation and determination of physical activity intensity cut points. Int J Sports Med. 2013;34(11):975–82.

62. Chen KY, Bassett DR Jr. The technology of accelerometry-based activity monitors: current and future. Med Sci Sports Exerc. 2005;37(11 Suppl):S490–500.

63. Sanders T, Cliff DP, Lonsdale C. Measuring adolescent boys' physical activity: bout length and the influence of accelerometer epoch length. PLoS ONE. 2014;9(3):e92040.

64. Ainsworth BE, et al. Compendium of physical activities: a second update of codes and MET values. Med Sci Sports Exerc. 2011;43(8):1575–81.

65. Ainsworth BE, et al. Compendium of physical activities: classification of energy costs of human physical activities. Med Sci Sports Exerc. 1993;25(1):71–80.

66. Ainsworth BE, et al. Compendium of physical activities: an update of activity codes and MET intensities. Med Sci Sports Exerc. 2000;32(9 Suppl):S498–504.

67. Trost SG, et al. Comparison of accelerometer cut points for predicting activity intensity in youth. Med Sci Sports Exerc. 2011;43(7):1360–8.

68. Klinker CD, et al. When cities move children: development of a new methodology to assess context-specific physical activity behaviour among children and adolescents using accelerometers and GPS. Health Place. 2015;31:90–9.

69. Carlson JA, et al. Locations of physical activity as assessed by GPS in young adolescents. Pediatrics. 2016;137(1):e20152430.

70. Dunton GF, et al. Locations of joint physical activity in parent-child pairs based on accelerometer and GPS monitoring. Ann Behav Med. 2013;45:S162–72.

71. Schipperijn J, et al. Dynamic accuracy of GPS receivers for use in health research: a novel method to assess GPS accuracy in real-world settings. Front Public Health. 2014;2:21.

72. Carlson JA, et al. Validity of PALMS GPS scoring of active and passive travel compared with SenseCam. Med Sci Sports Exerc. 2015;47(3):662–7.

73. Bates D, Maechler M, Bolker B, Walket S. R package Lme4. 2016. Available from: https://cran.r-project.org/web/packages/lme4/index.html.

74. Dunton GF, et al. Mapping the social and physical contexts of physical activity across adolescence using ecological momentary assessment. Ann Behav Med. 2007;34(2):144–53.

75. Dunton GF, et al. Adolescents' sports and exercise environments in a US time use survey. Am J Prev Med. 2010;39(2):122–9.

76. Biddle S, et al. Correlates of participation in physical activity for adolescent girls: a systematic review of recent literature. J Phys Act Health. 2005;2(4):423–34.

77. Sallis JF, Prochaska JJ, Taylor WC. A review of correlates of physical activity of children and adolescents. Med Sci Sports Exerc. 2000;32(5):963–75.

78. Trost SG, et al. Age and gender differences in objectively measured physical activity in youth. Med Sci Sports Exerc. 2002;34(2):350–5.

79. Veitch J, Salmon J, Deforche B, Ghekiere A, Van Cauwenberg J, Bangay S, Timperio A. Park attributes that encourage park visitation among adolescents: a conjoint analysis. Landsc Urban Plan. 2017;161:52–8.

80. Van Der Horst K, et al. A brief review on correlates of physical activity and sedentariness in youth. Med Sci Sports Exerc. 2007;39(8):1241–50.

81. Baran PK, et al. Park use among youth and adults: examination of individual, social, and urban form factors. Environ Behav. 2014;46(6):768–800.

82. Reed J, et al. A descriptive examination of the most frequently used activity settings in 25 community parks using direct observation. J Phys Act Health. 2008;5(Supp 1):S183–95.

83. Reis RS, et al. Association between physical activity in parks and perceived environment: a study with adolescents. J Phys Act Health. 2009;6(4):503–9.

84. Carver A, Timperio A, Crawford D. Perceptions of neighborhood safety and physical activity among youth: the CLAN study. J Phys Act Health. 2008;5(3):430–44.

85. Gomez JE, et al. Violent crime and outdoor physical activity among inner-city youth. Prev Med. 2004;39(5):876–81.

86. Van Dijk J, et al. The burden of crime in the EU-research report: a comparative analysis of the european crime and safety survey (EU ICS) 2005: Brussels.

87. Aaron DJ, et al. Longitudinal study of the number and choice of leisure time physical activities from mid to late adolescence: implications for school curricula and community recreation programs. Arch Pediat Adolesc Med. 2002;156(11):1075–80.

88. Scheerder J, Seghers J. Jongeren in beweging—over bewegingsbeleid, sportparticipatie, en fysieke activiteit bij schoolgaande jongeren in Vlaanderen, 2011.

89. Casey MM, et al. Using a socioecological approach to examine participation in sport and physical activity among rural adolescent girls. Qual Health Res. 2009;19(7):881–93.

90. Flemish Government, Studiegebieden in het secundair onderwijs, accessed at 01/08/2017. Available from: https://data-onderwijs.vlaanderen.be/onderwijsaanbod/structuur.aspx?vorm=TSO&hs=311.

91. Lin BB, et al. Opportunity or orientation? who uses urban parks and why. PLoS ONE. 2014;9(1):e87422.

92. Hanson MD, Chen E. Socioeconomic status and health behaviors in adolescence: a review of the literature. J Behav Med. 2007;30(3):263–85.

93. Dunton GF, et al. Investigating children's physical activity and sedentary behavior using ecological momentary assessment with mobile phones. Obesity. 2011;19(6):1205–12.

94. Johnson R, Onwuegbuzie A. Mixed methods research: a research paradigm whose time has come. Educ Res. 2004;33(7):14–26.

95. Edwards N, et al. Development of a public open space desktop auditing tool (POSDAT): a remote sensing approach. Appl Geogr. 2013;38:22–30.

A direct observation method for auditing large urban centers using stratified sampling, mobile GIS technology and virtual environments

Sean J. V. Lafontaine[1], M. Sawada[2,3]* and Elizabeth Kristjansson[3,4]

Abstract

Background: With the expansion and growth of research on neighbourhood characteristics, there is an increased need for direct observational field audits. Herein, we introduce a novel direct observational audit method and systematic social observation instrument (SSOI) for efficiently assessing neighbourhood aesthetics over large urban areas.

Methods: Our audit method uses spatial random sampling stratified by residential zoning and incorporates both mobile geographic information systems technology and virtual environments. The reliability of our method was tested in two ways: first, in 15 Ottawa neighbourhoods, we compared results at audited locations over two subsequent years, and second; we audited every residential block (167 blocks) in one neighbourhood and compared the distribution of SSOI aesthetics index scores with results from the randomly audited locations. Finally, we present interrater reliability and consistency results on all observed items.

Results: The observed neighbourhood average aesthetics index score estimated from four or five stratified random audit locations is sufficient to characterize the average neighbourhood aesthetics. The SSOI was internally consistent and demonstrated good to excellent interrater reliability. At the neighbourhood level, aesthetics is positively related to SES and physical activity and negatively correlated with BMI.

Conclusion: The proposed approach to direct neighbourhood auditing performs sufficiently and has the advantage of financial and temporal efficiency when auditing a large city.

Keywords: Direct observation, Auditing, Large urban centers, Methodological approach, Stratified sampling, Technology, Virtual environments

Background

The impact of qualitative characteristics of the built environment (BE) on health and well-being has become well established in health geography [1–3]. At the neighbourhood level, the impact of the built environment on physical and mental health has provided evidence of the link between urban disorder and social status [4, 5]. Establishing such linkages forms the basis for evidence based decision making that can improve neighbourhoods and the well-being of residents. Given the potential importance of such evidence for neighbourhood renewal efforts and policy formulation, there is a fundamental need to evaluate the methods, context, and manner through which such research is completed. There have been recent efforts to evaluate new methods of qualitative observations of neighbourhood BEs using new approaches and technologies [6–12]. This study adds to those efforts by presenting an efficient and effective method of undertaking qualitative neighbourhood observations over large urban areas using mobile GIS technology.

Neighbourhood level BE audits use a wide range of data collection techniques to gather information about

*Correspondence: msawada@uottawa.ca
[2] Laboratory for Applied Geomatics and GIS Science (LAGGISS),
Department of Geography, Environment and Geomatics, University
of Ottawa, Ottawa, ON K1N 6N5, Canada
Full list of author information is available at the end of the article

the contextual factors that can affect residents. Common data collection techniques include observations of resident perceptions (via phone interviews or mailed questionnaires) or secondary use of census data. However, results based on resident perceptions can contain response bias and census data are limited to information on neighbourhood socio-economic structure and rarely capture information on the BE qualitative characteristics [13–15]. The most effective approach to BE auditing is direct observational research. Direct observation of the BE allows for the collection of fine-grained details at various spatial scales. However, few studies have used direct observational data collection techniques to evaluate neighbourhood characteristics over entire urban centers [5]. Auditing large urban centers is a daunting task; direct observational field audits require auditors (two or more for reliability assessment) to be physically present to evaluate and observe the built environment at multiple locations. Large-scale spatial audits can be time and cost intensive [5, 16, 17]. For example, in one of the largest direct observation studies in Canada, researchers physically audited a total of 176 block faces across six Toronto neighbourhoods over 3 months (August–October) [5]. Even such a relatively modest sized direct observational study presents considerable financial and temporal constraints. Thus, extending a direct audit to an entire large urban center, block-by-block, is beyond the financial capacity of modestly funded research projects. Time and financial expediency underline the need to develop more efficient methods for direct field audit studies.

In response to such practical limitations on direct observation, and with varying degrees of success, some studies have employed vehicles or vehicle-mounted video recordings to achieve rapid auditing of the BE [18–20]. The use of a virtual environment (VE) such as Google Street View or Microsoft StreetSide is increasingly being explored in lieu of real-time built environment audits [1, 11, 15–17, 19, 21–26]. For example, a systematic social observation instrument (SSOI) applied using both Google Street View and a direct field audit for 143 items across 37 block faces in New York City, found strong concordance for some dimensions of walkability, but only modest agreement for aesthetics and physical disorder [23]. In other cases, strong correlations between virtual and field audits for items such as recreation, the food environment and land use have been observed [1]. VE audits using Google Street View, panoramic imagery or video footage do show high interrater reliability [21, 26]. Even crowd sourcing is being explored as a means to distinguish between perceived safety, class and uniqueness of city blocks [27]. Some research has employed machine based learning to assess perceived qualities of the BE such as safety and walkability [28].

Although BE virtual audits have met with some success, they cannot match the depth and comprehensiveness of direct real-time observations [11]. Why? Because VEs do not feed a number of sensory inputs [16, 29] including noise levels, soundscape and scent among others. Moreover, within a VE like Google Street View, the date of image acquisition can change suddenly and unpredictably, particularly across intersections [22] and cause temporal discrepancies (year or season) that bias audit results—either human or machine based. Virtual audits are also limited in measuring fine-grained or micro-level detail in images [1, 15–17, 23]. A balance between direct and virtual BE audits may be achieved by mixed methods that utilize technology to achieve temporal and financial efficiency, while maintaining the integrity and comprehensiveness of real-time observation methods.

To what degree can a combination of mobile GIS technology and limited spatial sampling adequately assess, with minimal time and effort, qualitative neighbourhood characteristics across large urban areas? To address this question, this study presents and evaluates a novel direct observation method that employs a simple SSOI to assesses urban aesthetics. However, the focus of this research is not on the instrument itself. Rather, this study focuses on the performance of a BE audit method that combines VEs for auditor training and mobile GIS technology for real-time data collection at randomly audited locations within neighbourhoods. We assess whether our audit method is sufficient to measure the qualitative variability of the BE across neighbourhoods in a large urban center. The accuracy of the random sampling design is assessed by comparing results to a complete block-by-block audit of 167 block faces in one of the neighbourhoods. Internal consistently and interrater reliability are calculated for all raters. The proposed method holds considerable promise as a means to conduct spatial large-scale audits of the BE that can add important independent variables for health geographic studies.

Methods

Audit instrument

Our goal was not to produce an exhaustive systematic social observation instrument (SSOI), rather, we simply wanted to produce an SSOI scale that would be sufficient in measuring the variation in aesthetic quality across the BE. The items were selected and the scale was developed after reviewing literature that used measurement scales aimed to assess components of the environment. To increase the breadth and depth of measures and approaches to measurement scale development, we included studies that were not solely focused on aesthetics. Relevant studies [5, 18, 30–36] were examined and organized by reviewing content, domains, measures, items, data collection, and psychometric properties. We also included research conducted in North America and Europe in our review of the literature that provided a diversity of geographic locations [4, 5, 30, 31]. Furthermore, we used an approach employed by Caughy et al. [18] and Parsons et al. [5] among others, in which pilot testing was used to further refine the SSOI items. This process lead to the development of a 10 item scale (Table 1) with each item having five Likert response values.

The creation of descriptors for the Likert response values for each item was a vital step in the development of an SSOI for many reasons, but most importantly because of the subjective nature of observations [1, 5]. Each item's Likert response scale contained three descriptor definitions (a descriptor for the maximum value, middle value and lowest value) together with reference photos for each value. The instrument itself was entered on a mobile GIS device so that data would be collected and validated in real-time.

Mobile GIS technology

Mobile devices with GPS receivers provide a platform for rapid and comprehensive data collection [37]. An Apple iPad 2 + cellular was chosen for this research because the '+cellular' models contain the hardware-based GPS receiver required to record positions of field audit points without an internet connection (off-line mode). We used GIS Kit Pro by GARAFA software for mobile mapping and data collection on Apple's iOS (Fig. 1). The GIS Kit application is a mobile Geographic Information System (GIS) software that combines data management with a mapping engine for an effective mobile data solution

(see http://www.garafa.com). The single-use license fee for GIS Kit was $299 per user and an iPad + cellular was ~$599. The aesthetics SSOI was entered into GIS Kit as a feature class.

The process of collecting, transferring and processing data using a mobile device takes 50% less time when compared to traditional paper-based methods [24, 38]. While time is not reduced when undertaking observations, the expediency originates from the reduced data processing and handling provided by an all-digital approach. As such, field audit data requires no post-field transcription or geo-referencing. In comparison to a complete VE audit, the only appreciable difference is the time taken to travel between audit locations with the mobile GIS technology. In this research, the data collected within GIS Kit were exported as shapefiles and directly opened in a desktop GIS, Google Earth or within a statistical analysis package.

Sampling strategy

Field audits took place within 15 neighbourhoods (Fig. 2) selected from the Ottawa Neighbourhood Study (ONS) (www.neighbourhoodstudy.ca). We based this selection on neighbourhood SES quintile; we selected 5 high, medium, and low neighbourhoods. Audit points within each of these neighbourhoods were located based on residential zones defined by City of Ottawa by-laws: R1—Residential First Density (detached dwellings), R2—Residential Second Density (two unit dwellings), R3—Residential Third Density (multiple attached dwellings), R4—Residential Fourth Density (low rise apartments), R5—Residential Fifth Density (mid/high-rise apartments) and the RM-Mobile Home (Retrieved from http://www.ottawa.ca/residents/bylaw/a_z/zoning/parts/pt_06/index_en.html) (Fig. 3). Within Ottawa, high density zoning (tower blocks and multiunit apartments, R4 and R5 in Fig. 3) can be indicative of lower income areas when compared to low density residential zoning (single family homes to town homes, R1–R3 in Fig. 3). In the absence of highly resolved socioeconomic data at the sub-neighbourhood block-level that could be used to guide the determination of audit locations within neighbourhoods, the probability of selecting an audit point was made directly proportional to the area occupied by each residential zone type within a neighbourhood. Here, we are loosely assuming that residential zoning density is a proxy variable for within-neighbourhood variation in SES. Within each of the 15 neighbourhoods, four (2011) or five (2012) audit points were located. Overall, there were 60 (2011) and 90 (2012) audit points across the 15 Ottawa neighbourhoods. At each audit point, a 100 m buffer (radius of circle) was created within a desktop GIS and the buffers were loaded into the mobile GIS

Table 1 Each SSOI item contained five Likert response values: extremely poor, below average, average, above average, and excellent (for qualitative items) or none, few, some, many and lots (for quantitative items)

Item	Auditor 1	Auditor 2	Mean
Cleanliness of streets and properties	0.100	0.152	0.126
Presence of trees	0.038	0.091	0.064
Quality of trees	0.049	0.050	0.049
Landscaping	0.220	0.086	0.153
Flowers and shrubs	0.079	0.047	0.063
Houses well-spaced	0.085	0.204	0.144
Upkeep of homes	0.284	0.244	0.264
Presence of outdoor furniture	0.037	0.032	0.034
Quality of outdoor furniture	0.051	0.034	0.042
Pedestrian infrastructure	0.058	0.061	0.059

Item weightings used in deriving the aesthetics index score, s_i, for each audit location were determined as the mean value from both auditors—see text for details

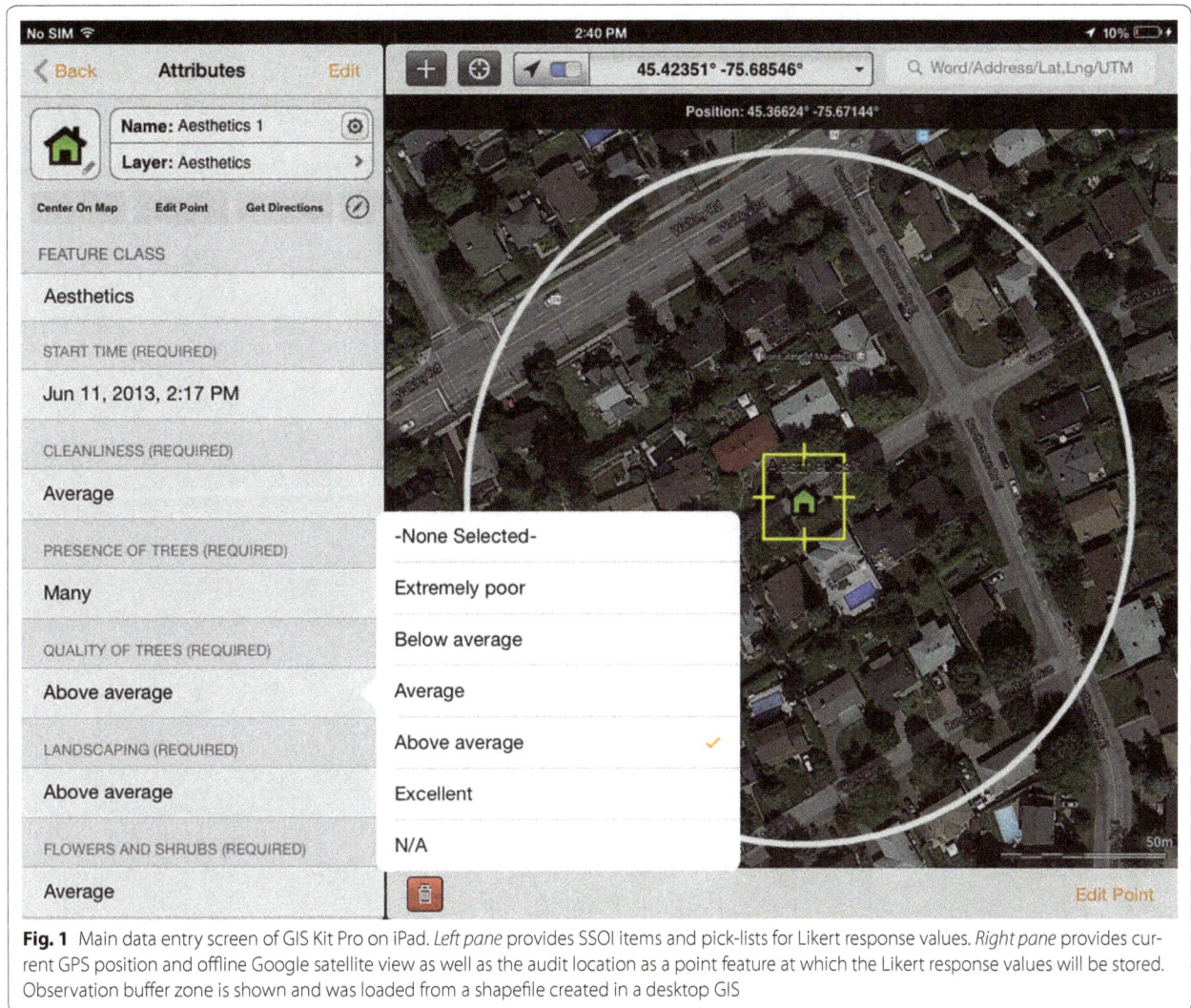

Fig. 1 Main data entry screen of GIS Kit Pro on iPad. *Left pane* provides SSOI items and pick-lists for Likert response values. *Right pane* provides current GPS position and offline Google satellite view as well as the audit location as a point feature at which the Likert response values will be stored. Observation buffer zone is shown and was loaded from a shapefile created in a desktop GIS

Kit. These buffers represent the audit locations within which observations are made. The GPS capability of the iPAD + Cellular allowed the auditor to actively monitor their position on the mobile map within GIS Kit and thereby determine when they arrived at the edge of an audit location to begin observations (Fig. 1). To control for the variability in block length and observation time across the urban area, observations were only made within the audit location (e.g., within each audit point's buffer zone).

To validate the sensitivity of results to the number of audited locations in a neighbourhood, in 2013 every residential block (167 blocks) within one neighbourhood was audited (Fig. 4). We then compared the average and frequency distribution of aesthetics index scores (derivation explained below) from the 167 audit locations in 2013 to the neighbourhood average aesthetics index score from the 2011 and 2012 audit locations

in that neighbourhood. Additionally, for visualization purposes, the 167 block observations were used to calculate 102 average block aesthetics index scores. Pycnophylactic interpolation [39, 40], a volume preserving technique, was used to create a surface of average block aesthetics index score variation within the neighbourhood. Because our needs were only visual, a simple pycnophylactic areal interpolation technique honors the discontinuous nature of observations that apply to an entire block, while at the same time, smoothing the hard discontinuities between blocks that share block-face aesthetics index scores. However, a number of techniques for interpolation of areal data have been developed [41–44]. Many of these techniques provide estimates of uncertainty and would be more appropriate when the purpose of mapping is area-based estimation at unknown locations of a social surface or for transferring data from one zonal geography to another.

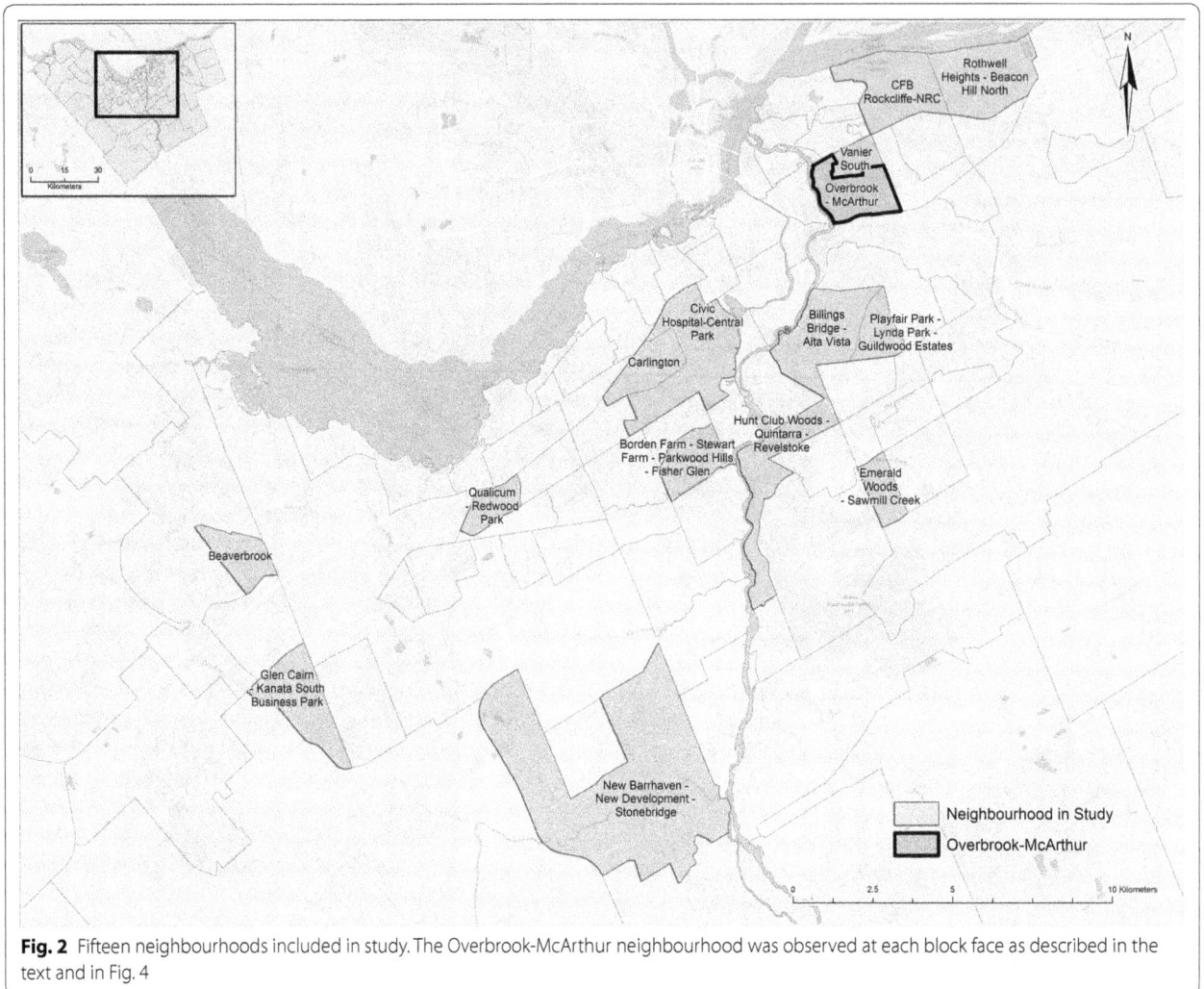

Fig. 2 Fifteen neighbourhoods included in study. The Overbrook-McArthur neighbourhood was observed at each block face as described in the text and in Fig. 4

Finally, for the 15 neighbourhoods, we compared the neighbourhood average aesthetics index score results to select health determinants in order to provide impetus for research situating urban aesthetics within an ecological framework for geographic health determinants.

Audit timing

In 2011, audits were completed between November and December on Saturday's between 9:00 am and 5:00 pm. Each week, three or four neighbourhoods were observed. In 2012, audits were collected for 79 neighbourhoods (a subset of 15 are included here for comparison with 2011) between June and August each weekday, ensuring that data collection did not take place the day prior to, or of, garbage pick-up. Complete VE audits of the BE cannot control for the timing of garbage collection. In 2013, audits took place daily from mid-July to mid-August for each of 167 blocks in one neighbourhood (Overbrook-McArthur).

Observational method

At each audit location, two independent observers were used in each year. Overall, six different observers were used over the three year period, two independent observers in each year. Once at the end an audit location, the two auditors would cross to the other side of the street and continue walking back to the original starting point. Immediately after walking, both auditors, independently and without discussion or debrief, completed the SSOI separately on their individual iPads. Once complete, GIS Kit saved the completed audit as a point feature together with the associated SSOI attribute data. The data was exported daily to a Dropbox account or emailed directly from GIS Kit as both *kml* and shapefiles. This method of data collection was practiced and applied consistently to all neighbourhood observations each year.

Additionally, while walking the audit location, the auditors would document certain aspects by taking geotagged photographs that were stored as attributes

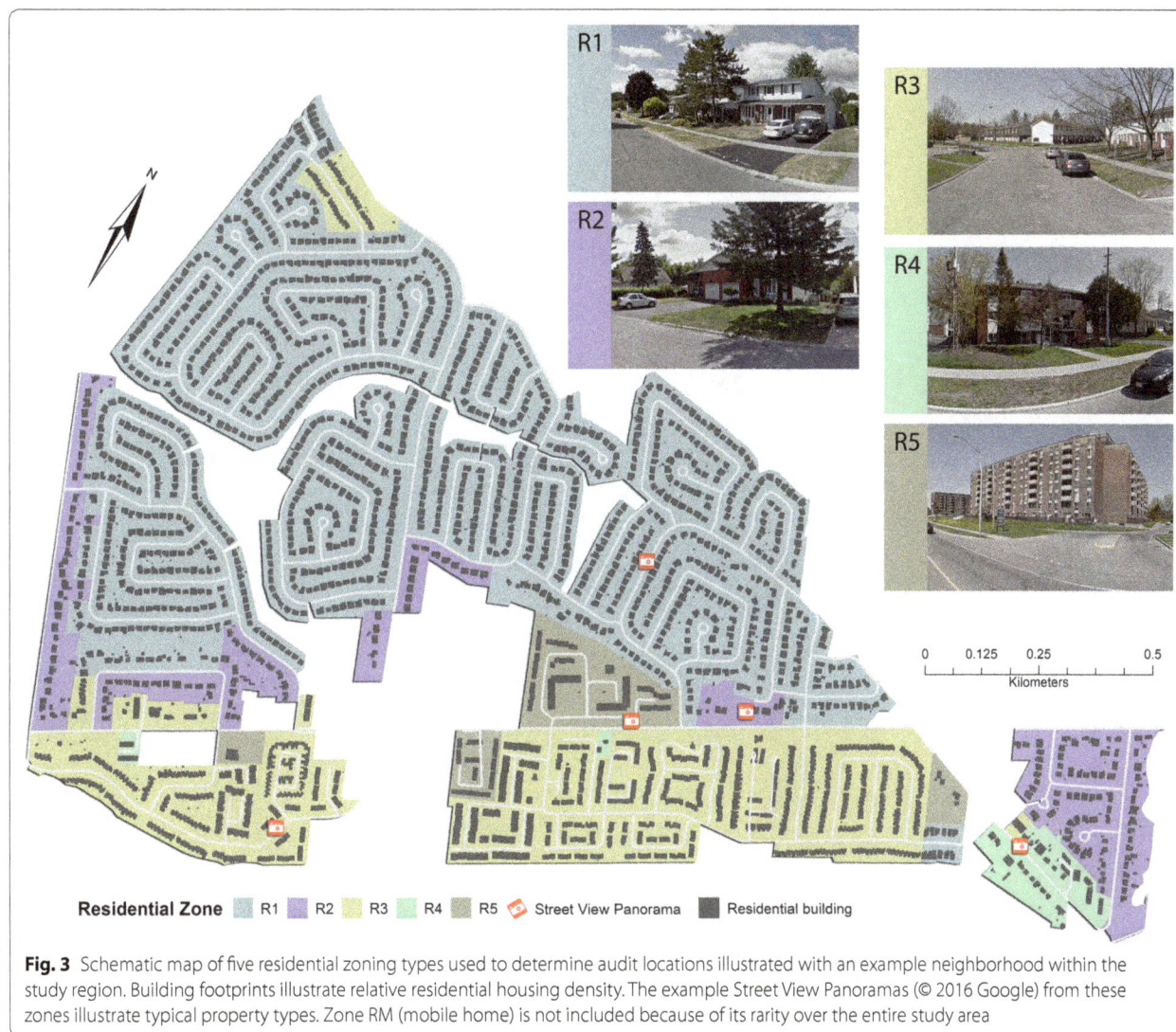

Fig. 3 Schematic map of five residential zoning types used to determine audit locations illustrated with an example neighborhood within the study region. Building footprints illustrate relative residential housing density. The example Street View Panoramas (© 2016 Google) from these zones illustrate typical property types. Zone RM (mobile home) is not included because of its rarity over the entire study area

within the feature table for each audit point within GIS Kit. For instance, if there was an exceptional or poorly maintained property or an attractive arrangement of flowers and shrubs, one of the auditors would take a picture. This allowed the auditors to collect tangible photographic evidence of neighbourhood characteristics in addition to the Likert response values for each audit location. All photographs were collected for research purposes only; no images are made public. Additionally, no identifying features, such as addresses, were captured.

Virtual environment training

In all years, Google Street View was used to train the auditors. Practice observation sessions (excluding the neighbourhoods in the study sample) were completed using the same SSOI and tools (iPad with GIS Kit) used for real-time field observations. A two week period of training was utilized. During the first week of training,

both auditors examined the SSOI item definitions and reference images for each item's Likert response value. Then, the raters used Google Street View to undertake practice audits at predetermined locations. Virtual training was followed by calculation of inter-rater reliability measures and an intervention session for free discussion of items that showed poor agreement. Following approximately three to four rounds of virtual practice, the auditors undertook field trials in a neighbourhood close to the University of Ottawa (Sandy Hill) before beginning real-time field data collection.

Aesthetics index scores

Aesthetics index scores for each neighbourhood were derived as weighted averages to address the issue of the relative or subjective significance of certain items compared to others (e.g., upkeep of homes versus the presence of outdoor furniture). Weighted averages

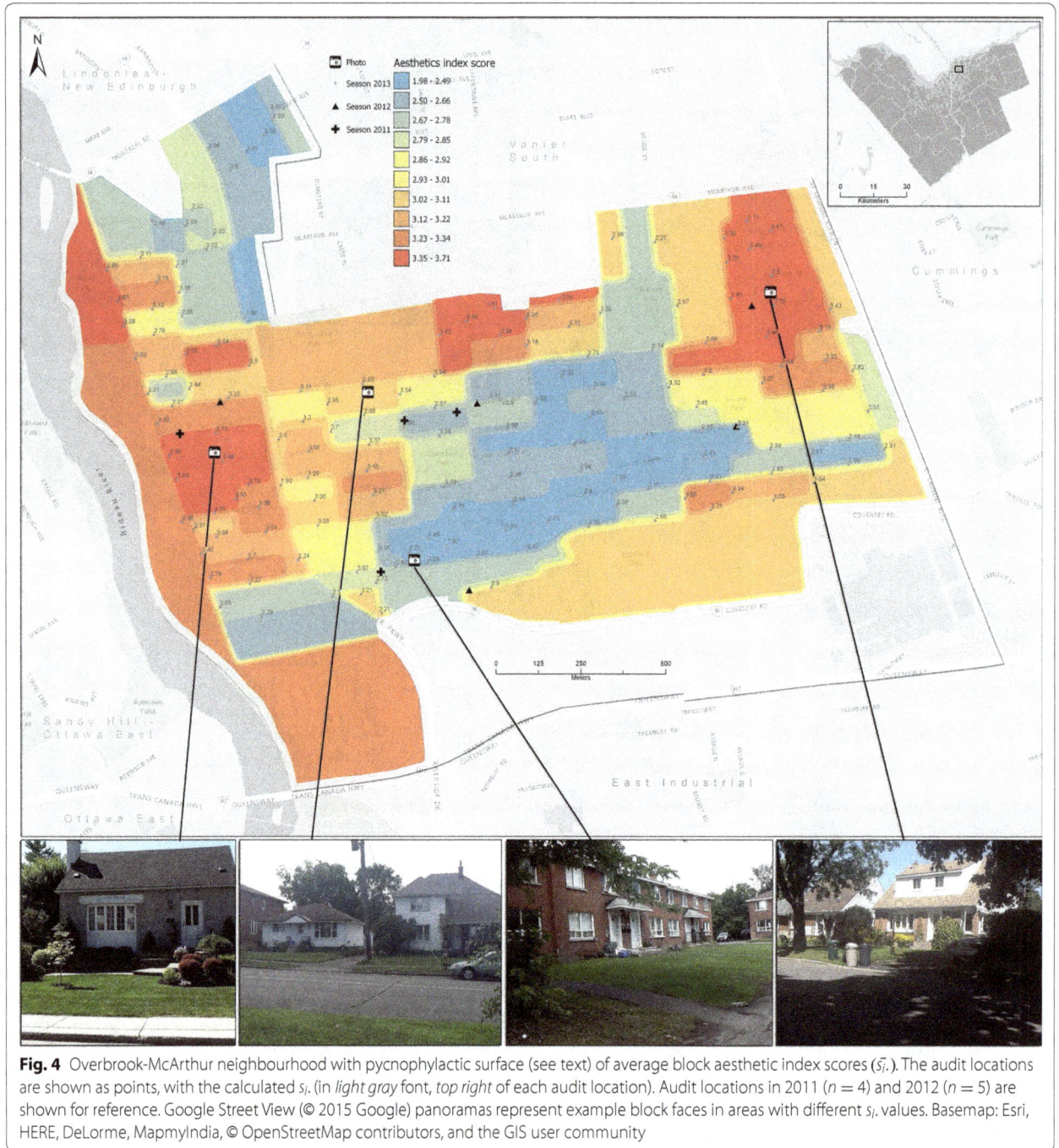

Fig. 4 Overbrook-McArthur neighbourhood with pycnophylactic surface (see text) of average block aesthetic index scores ($\bar{s_l}$). The audit locations are shown as points, with the calculated s_l (in *light gray* font, *top right* of each audit location). Audit locations in 2011 ($n = 4$) and 2012 ($n = 5$) are shown for reference. Google Street View (© 2015 Google) panoramas represent example block faces in areas with different s_l values. Basemap: Esri, HERE, DeLorme, MapmyIndia, © OpenStreetMap contributors, and the GIS user community

provide an additional step to reduce potential biases or preferences of different auditors. Weights were derived through the use of a pairwise comparison matrix for each of the SSOI items [45]. This comparison matrix was completed by each of the auditors after discussion and consideration. For instance, the upkeep of homes is given more weight because it has a greater impact on the aesthetics of a neighbourhood than does the presence of outdoor furniture (Table 1).

Given a rectangular matrix of a neighbourhood's Likert response values across all SSOI items, x, and an equally sized matrix of row-standardized weights, w, a *neighbourhood average aesthetics index score*, Q_s, is calculated as:

$$s_{i\cdot} = \frac{C}{N_i} \sum_{j=1}^{N_i} w_{ij} x_{ij} \left\{ \begin{array}{c} 0 \leq w_i \leq 1; \sum_{i=1}^{n} w_i = 1 \\ x \in \{1, 2, \ldots, 5\} \end{array} \right.$$

$$Q_s = \frac{1}{n} \sum_{i=1}^{n} s_{i\cdot} . \{i \in \{1, 2, \ldots, 15\}\}$$

where $s_{i\cdot}$ is the *aesthetics index score* for audit location i in neighbourhood s, C is the number of SSOI items, $C = 10$ in this study, N_i is number of numbers in the ith row (e.g., the number of applicable items for an audit location), w_{ij} is the weight for SSOI item i column j, x_{ij} is the ordinal value of SSOI Likert response item i, column j. This aesthetics index score, $s_{i\cdot}$, calculation includes only N_i so that the neighbourhood average aesthetics index score, Q_s, is not penalized for non-applicable SSOI items at a given audit location. The aesthetics index score, $s_{i\cdot}$, is normalized to range between 1 and 5 by the constant C.

Internal consistency

Using the weighted matrix of auditor's observations, we examined the internal consistency of the data to ensure validity. Internal consistency is defined as the degree of reliability within a test; the extent to which different items are assessing the same construct [46]. For the aesthetics SSOI, internal consistency was measured using Cronbach's α with bootstrapped confidence intervals calculated using the R library 'psych' [47].

Interrater reliability

Interrater reliability (IRR) measures the degree of similarity/agreement of observations made by different auditors on the same set of objects after controlling for disagreement due to observational error [48]. IRR was assessed using a two-way mixed, absolute, average-measures intraclass correlation coefficient (ICC), r [49]. IRR was calculated using the R library 'irr' [50].

Comparison with health determinants

We compare the neighbourhood average aesthetics index score, Q_s, to three health determinants: Neighbourhood SES, self-reported overweight or obese BMI and physical activity. Neighbourhood SES was calculated for 96 Ottawa Neighbourhoods using five age-sex standardized variables from the 2006 Canadian long-form Census [51]: percent of households below the low-income cut-off, average household income, percent of unemployed residents, percent of residents with less than a high school education, and percent of single-parent families. The SES index was t-scored to represent a mean of 50 with a standard deviation of 10 and values for the 15 neighbourhoods were ranked from highest (1) to (15) lowest for comparison with the ranked Q_s. Physical activity was evaluated with data from previous research

(unpublished) using International Physical Activity Questionnaire (IPAQ) and included self-reported overweight or obese BMI and physical activity (moderately or highly active) [52]. Relations between Q_s in 2011 and 2012 and health determinants were established using Spearman's rank correlation coefficient, ρ, using the R library 'Hmisc' [53]. Given the small sample size of $n = 15$ neighbourhoods, empirical p-values were calculated to assess the significance of correlation coefficients with health determinants using 9999 permutations of the independent variable (Q_s in 2011, 2012). Bias corrected (BCa) rank correlation confidence intervals at the 95% level were determined using nonparametric ordinary bootstrapping with 10,000 iterations within the R library 'boot' [54, 55]. All other confidence intervals for variables presented in this paper are based on 2000 bootstrapped iterations.

All statistical analyses were undertaken in R v3.2 [56] and SPSS 22 [57] (for SES).

Results
Internal consistency

The reliability of all SSOI items was, in 2011, α = 0.73 (95% CI [0.63, 0.79]) and, in 2012, α = 0.64 (95% CI [0.57, 0.69]). In 2013, the full block-by-block audit in one neighbourhood yielded an α = 0.72 (95% CI [0.69, 0.75]). One SSOI item, pedestrian infrastructure, showed a very low item-total correlation in both years for the 15 neighbourhood audit (Table 2). In 2012, cleanliness, the presence of trees and quality of trees have lower item-total correlations than in the other two years (Table 2).

Interrater reliability

Considering only statistically significant values, average Intraclass Correlation Coefficients (ICC) across all SSOI items in 2011 was $r = 0.85$, in 2012, $r = 0.72$ and in 2013, $r = 0.71$. In 2012, cleanliness, presence of trees and quality of trees were not significant and pedestrian infrastructure was not significant in 2013. Quality of trees in 2013 is significant with a fair IRR. The ICC values are good to excellent for all other SSOI items in all years (Table 3) [48].

Neighbourhood average aesthetics index scores (Q_s) in 2011 and 2012

The relative ranking of Q_s varied between 2011 and 2012 (Table 4). However, across both years, five of the neighbourhoods are consistently ranked in the lower half of the Q_s ranks (Table 4). Alternatively, three were consistently ranked in the top five (Table 4).

Discrepancies between the 2011 and 2012 Q_s rankings included CFB—Rockliffe-NRC which had the lowest rank in 2012 but a much higher rank in 2011. Beaverbrook was also discrepant due to the lower landscaping

Table 2 SSOI items and comparison of internal consistency: α is Cronbach's alpha if an item is dropped; ITC is the item-total correlation corrected for item overlap and scale reliability

Item	2011		2012		2013	
	α	ITC	α	ITC	α	ITC
Cleanliness of streets and properties	0.69	0.47	0.60	0.45	0.64	0.71
Presence of trees	0.70	0.61	0.64	0.27	0.72	0.28
Quality of trees	0.71	0.71	0.64	0.31	0.72	0.34
Landscaping	0.66	0.79	0.53	0.82	0.61	0.86
Flowers and shrubs	0.70	0.69	0.58	0.87	0.67	0.83
Houses well-spaced	0.72	0.43	0.64	0.35	0.74	0.24
Upkeep of homes	0.69	0.66	0.60	0.61	0.65	0.73
Presence of outdoor furniture	0.73	0.40	0.65	0.09	0.73	0.19
Quality of outdoor furniture	0.73	0.50	0.63	0.47	0.70	0.66
Pedestrian infrastructure	0.75	0.12	0.64	0.19	0.74	0.05

Table 3 Interrater reliability results as intraclass correlation coefficients, r, for all three field seasons for 10 SSOI items retained after 2011

Item	2011			2012			2013		
	n	r	95% CI	n	r	95% CI	n	r	95% CI
Cleanliness of streets and properties	56	0.66**	[0.44,0.89]	73	0.30#	[−0.08,0.55]	167	0.81	[0.75,0.86]
Presence of trees	59	0.89	[0.78,0.94]	74	0.48#	[0.30,0.62]	167	0.75	[0.66,0.82]
Quality of trees	59	0.77	[0.59,0.87]	74	0.09#	[−0.31,0.32]	167	0.40**	[0.21,0.54]
Landscaping	57	0.79	[0.61,0.90]	74	0.69	[0.54,0.79]	167	0.79	[0.74,0.84]
Flowers and shrubs	57	0.78	[0.59,0.89]	74	0.66	[0.46,0.78]	165	0.80	[0.75,0.85]
Houses well-spaced	59	0.89	[0.76,0.95]	74	0.77**	[0.62,0.89]	158	0.73	[0.60,0.82]
Upkeep of homes	58	0.88	[0.80,0.93]	74	0.77	[0.64,0.84]	160	0.78	[0.71,0.84]
Presence of outdoor furniture	51	0.97	[0.93,0.99]	72	0.67	[0.48,0.79]	167	0.62	[0.47,0.72]
Quality of outdoor furniture	59	0.96	[0.88,0.99]	54	0.67	[0.47,0.81]	123	0.67	[0.57,0.76]
Pedestrian infrastructure	58	0.87	[0.76,0.94]	73	0.80	[0.66,0.88]	165	0.34#	[0.26,0.42]

Not significant at p < 0.05, ** significant at p < 0.01, all others significant at p < 0.001

Likert response values in 2012 compared to 2011. A similar explanation was apparent for Glen Cairn—Kanata South Business Park. However, the rank correlation between Q_s in both years is positive and significant 0.51 (p = 0.0241), 95% CI [0.0273, 0.8226].

Validation of sampling approach

The full neighbourhood audit in 2013 (of Overbrook-McArthur) shows the variability and spatial structure of the aesthetics index scores, $s_{i\cdot}$, among the 167 block observations (Fig. 4).

The univariate distribution of $s_{i\cdot}$ exhibits bimodality in 2013 (Fig. 5a). Spatially, this bimodality is evident in the map of $s_{i\cdot}$ (Fig. 4). In 2013, the observed Q_s was 2.897. The observed Q_s was 3.097 in 2011 and 3.094

in 2012 (Fig. 5b). Extracting $s_{i\cdot}$ from the 2013 dataset at the same block locations that were audited in 2011 and 2012, yields Q_s values of 2.73 and 2.86 respectively (Fig. 5b).

Simulating 100,000 random draws of 5 without replacement from the 167 audit locations in 2013, the range of possible Q_s is $2.00 \leq s_{i\cdot} \leq 3.66$ with ninety-five percent falling in the interval of $2.44 \leq s_{i\cdot} \leq 3.34$. The observed Q_s in 2013 was 2.897 (±0.224). To assess the representativeness of the 2012 random sampling method, the observed Q_s of 3.094 would occur at least 19.6% of the time when taking 5 random audit locations in that neighbourhood. Likewise, with draws of 4 samples, the 2011 Q_s of 3.097 would be exceeded 22.1% of the time. In general, the observed Q_s in 2011–2012 based on four or five random samples of $s_{i\cdot}$ are very likely to occur for this

Table 4 Neighbourhoods ranked according to neighbourhood average aesthetic index scores (Q_s) (values are rounded to two decimal places)

Field season 2011	Q_s	Field season 2012	Q_s
Carlington	2.92	CFB Rockcliffe—NRC	2.83
Vanier South	3.02	Vanier South	2.90
Overbrook—McArthur	3.10	Glen Cairn—Kanata South Business Park	2.91
Emerald Woods—Sawmill Creek	3.28	Carlington	3.02
Civic Hospital—Central Park	3.50	Emerald Woods—Sawmill Creek	3.07
Qualicum—Redwood Park	3.61	Overbrook—McArthur	3.09
Borden Farm—Stewart Farm—Parkwood Hills—Fisher Glen	3.63	Civic Hospital—Central Park	3.19
Glen Cairn—Kanata South Business Park	3.71	Beaverbrook	3.22
Playfair Park—Lynda Park—Guildwood Estates	3.73	Hunt Club Woods—Quintarra—Revelstoke	3.29
CFB Rockcliffe-NRC	3.81	Qualicum—Redwood Park	3.31
Rothwell Heights—Beacon Hill North	3.85	New Barrhaven—New Development—Stonebridge	3.37
Hunt Club Woods—Quintarra—Revelstoke	3.89	Borden Farm—Stewart Farm—Parkwood Hills—Fisher Glen	3.38
Billings Bridge—Alta Vista	4.05	Rothwell Heights—Beacon Hill North	3.54
Beaverbrook	4.23	Billings Bridge—Alta Vista	3.56
New Barrhaven—Stonebridge	4.29	Playfair Park—Lynda Park—Guildwood Estates	3.74

neighbourhood using the sampling methodology based on zoning density.

Comparison with health determinants

In both years, Q_s exhibits a positive significant correlation with both SES and, in 2012, with moderate or high physical activity (IPAQ) (Table 5). The correlation between Q_s and self-reported overweight or obese (BMI) is significant and negative in both years (Table 5). In both 2011 and 2012, neighbourhoods ranking higher aesthetically are more likely to also possess high SES. Likewise, a highly aesthetic neighbourhood was associated with lower BMI and to a lesser extent a higher IPAQ.

Discussion

Internal consistency

The aesthetics SSOI possesses acceptable to good internal consistency and the SSOI items within the neighbourhood aesthetics observational tool are sufficiently measuring and evaluating the same construct. Item-total correlation (ITC) values were acceptable to good in all years. The quality of pedestrian infrastructure had a weak ITC in all field seasons. The weak ITC may reflect the idea that pedestrian infrastructure is more indicative of physical disorder, rather than a direct indicator of aesthetics. The lower ITC values for cleanliness, the presence of trees and quality of trees in 2012 is most likely due to the timing of the field audit in that year. The observations in August of 2012 were during a prolonged drought with the driest July on record and the driest year on record in Ottawa. The condition of lawns

and trees were affected by significant browning and/or leaf loss and this in-turn affected the perceptions of overall cleanliness and tree quality. These same items also exhibit the lowest and non-significant interrater reliability in 2012. The auditors had some difficulty in assessing these items based on their reference photos and VE training using non-drought conditions. Overall, however, the SSOI is capturing and evaluating the same construct(s).

Interrater reliability

Overall, interrater reliability was greater for most SSOI items in 2011. We believe that this effect is due to the intervention methods applied in 2011. Three neighbourhoods were observed each week and prior to the next observation session, IRR was calculated to determine which SSOI items required improvement and subsequently followed up with mock training using Google Street View. The cumulative effect of these interventions was gradual improvement in IRR for SSOI items that showed improved consensus building. Thus, sequential interventions may be more effective than a single pre-audit period of training. Pedestrian infrastructure was problematic in 2013 where one auditor found the SSOI item not applicable far more often than the other.

Neighbourhood average aesthetics index scores (Q_s) in 2011 and 2012

Except for two neighbourhoods, a total of five neighbourhoods with lowest SES also have the lowest

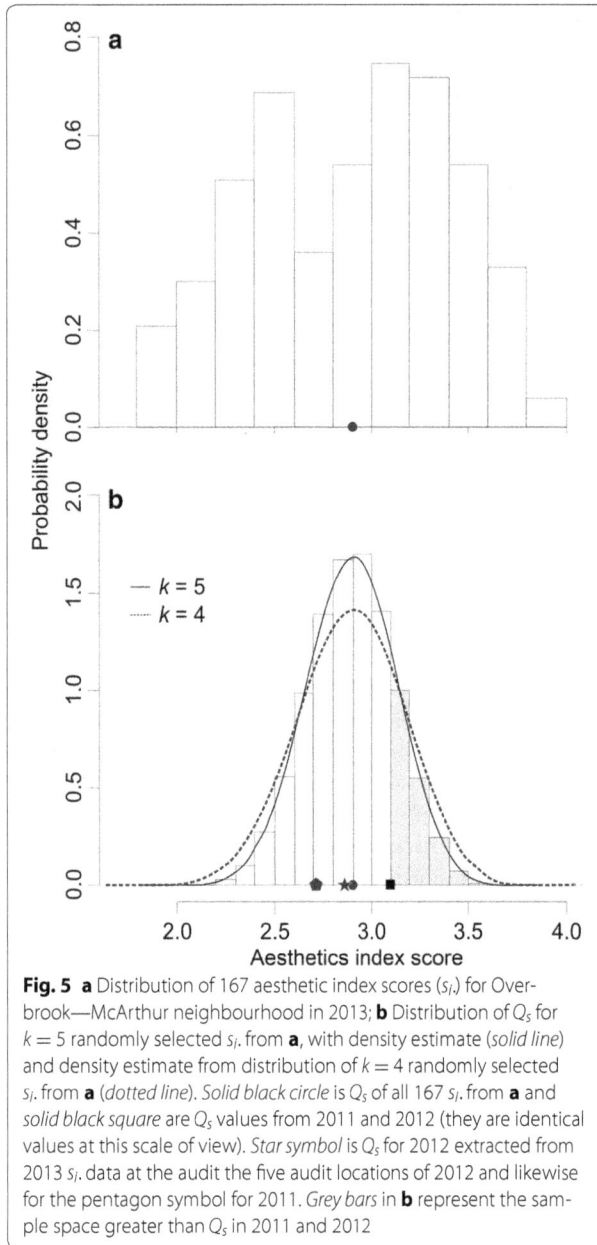

Fig. 5 **a** Distribution of 167 aesthetic index scores (s_i) for Over-brook—McArthur neighbourhood in 2013; **b** Distribution of Q_s for $k = 5$ randomly selected s_i. from **a**, with density estimate (*solid line*) and density estimate from distribution of $k = 4$ randomly selected s_i. from **a** (*dotted line*). *Solid black circle* is Q_s of all 167 s_i. from **a** and *solid black square* are Q_s values from 2011 and 2012 (they are identical values at this scale of view). *Star symbol* is Q_s for 2012 extracted from 2013 s_i. data at the audit the five audit locations of 2012 and likewise for the pentagon symbol for 2011. *Grey bars* in **b** represent the sample space greater than Q_s in 2011 and 2012

important information. For example, Billings Bridge, a neighbourhood in the bottom half of SES rankings, unexpectedly received high Q_s values in both audits. That result suggests that SES may not always be indicative of a neighbourhood's aesthetic appeal. In contrast, the neighbourhood of Borden Farm—Stewart Farm—Parkwood Hills—Fisher Glen, ranked much higher in 2012 despite having lower SES. The neighbourhood of Glen Cairn—Kanata South Business Park ranked highly in 2011 and much lower in 2012. In this case, examination of the field reference photos in the two years pointed out that the audit locations in 2012 were hard-hit by the 2012 drought in Ottawa, affecting landscaping and trees.

Sampling approach

Despite having different auditors in all three years, Q_s values within the neighbourhood with 167 block observations (Overbrook-McArthur) were very similar and show that the observed Q_s values from the random sampling in 2011–2012 are not significantly different from the 2013 Q_s across 167 full blocks. This suggests that taking 4 or 5 random audit locations within a neighbourhood stratified by residential zoning type can sufficiently characterize neighbourhood aesthetics.

We choose to observe all 167 blocks in the Overbrook-McArthur neighbourhood to validate our sampling regime because this neighbourhood is heterogeneous. Overbrook-McArthur's spatial variability in s_i. (Fig. 4) is typical of a neighbourhood that has been undergoing gentrification. Over the past two decades, gentrification began with the western portion of the neighbourhood adjacent to the Rideau River and has more recently increased in the section east of the Vanier Parkway and west of St. Laurent Boulevard. These gentrified regions have the highest s_i.. Lower s_i. values are apparent within the center of the neighbourhood, a region that contains row housing and low-income housing units (two middle panoramas in Fig. 4). The spatial variability of s_i. is reflected in the bimodality of the frequency distribution of s_i. (Fig. 5a) and this bimodality is caused by the pattern of gentrification.

The Q_s ranking of CFB Rockcliffe-NRC in 2011 and 2012 was drastically different and requires explanation. Exceptionally in 2011, only three residential locations were audited. The fourth location was within a former

neighbourhood average aesthetics index scores (Q_s). Moreover, three neighbourhoods which have high SES were ranked in the top five Q_s values in both years. However, there were several exceptions that provide

Table 5 Spearman's rank correlation coefficients, ρ, with bootstrapped 95% confidence intervals in brackets, between Q_s in (2011, 2012) and SES, self-reported overweight or obese (BMI) and moderately or highly active (IPAQ)

	SES (n = 15)	BMI (n = 13)	IPAQ (n = 12)
Q_s 2011	0.72 (*0.0012*) [0.2500, 0.9449]	−0.50 (*0.0425*) [−0.8571, 0.0467]	0.45 (*0.0752*) [−0.1739, 0.9091]
Q_s 2012	0.60 (*0.0079*) [0.1320, 0.8448]	−0.65 (*0.0098*) [−0.9222, 0.0196]	0.69 (*0.0083*) [0.0571, 0.9423]

Empirical *p* values are in parentheses and were determined by 9999 permutations of Q_s

medium-density residential military housing unit that was undergoing demolition. That fact was unknown when establishing the audit locations. In 2012, four of five audit locations were in the high density zoning areas, whereas in 2011 the audit locations occurred equally within high, medium and low density zoning. Moreover, much of this neighbourhood is largely green space that was reclaimed from a former Royal Canadian Air Force base.

Comparison with health determinants

The neighbourhood average aesthetics index score (Q_s) relations with health determinants are generally consistent with expectations. However, given the small sample size of 15 neighbourhoods these observations largely provide impetus for further research and hypothesis testing with a larger number of neighbourhoods. Specifically, the efficient and effective method of auditing described herein can facilitate future research wishing to conduct spatially large scale studies in a temporally and financially responsible manner. In addition, with a larger sample, determination of MAUP induced zoning and spatial scale effects on Q_s variation could be assessed [58].

Support from other research lends further strength to the comparison of aesthetics and health determinants (i.e., BMI and physical activity) and offers opportunities for future research. The connection between aesthetics and health is commonly observed in research on physical activity, such as walkability, which, at the ecologic level, can be directly correlated with health outcomes [13, 35, 59, 60]. Walkability is the extent to which the built environment supports and encourages walking and has been linked to physical health with benefits such as improved BMI and cardiovascular fitness [59]. Neighbourhood aesthetics were found to be a significant predictor of walkability and physical activity in a study spanning 11 countries [13]. For instance, people are more likely to walk and be otherwise physically active in aesthetically appealing neighbourhoods [19, 61, 62].

Efficiency of the mobile GIS equipment

The mobile GIS technology proved to be an extremely valuable, efficient, and effective combination. Mobile technology provides a medium that enables auditors to efficiently travel to and observe each of the randomly selected audit locations, thereby streamlining data collection and data entry. As such, more time can be invested in subsequent data analysis.

The SSOI only had to be entered into one iPad and then shared as a GIS Kit feature class among everyone within the audit team. That process allowed for standardization of the SSOI across all devices. Moreover, because all data was digitally stored on the iPad in a GIS friendly format, data could be uploaded or e-mailed at the end of each audit session thereby minimizing risks of data loss or corruption if a device was damaged. The capture of geotagged photographs within each audit location and stored within the geographic feature table of each point were useful in understanding the effects of drought in 2012 on some SSOI items.

The iPad contains many other applications that were valuable to the current study and aided in the efficiency and effectiveness of data collection. One of the biggest advantages of using the iPad is its use of task-specific applications and software. The capability of GIS Kit to cache Google Maps and satellite imagery, along with its GPS navigator, provided an easy to use method of navigation which enabled the auditors to efficiently travel to audit locations without an internet connection. GPS navigation was particularly useful for the spatially random sampling design used in this study, since audit locations are scattered across urban space. The auditors could easily ask for directions to the next audit location and follow the computed route. Furthermore, during training sessions, the ability to modify items and SSOI descriptions in the field during an audit and then sharing the modified feature class was convenient in preparing the devices for use in the sampling.

There are a range of other options for georeferenced field data collection, and, while they cannot all be reviewed here, some common options are ArcPad for ArcGIS (http://www.esri.com/software/arcgis/arcpad); however, a licensing fee and ArcGIS desktop are required as well custom development in ArcPad. ArcGIS Collector and, in particular, Survey123 (https://survey123.arcgis.com/) by ESRI Inc. can work in either Android and iOS or a web browser but do require a paid institutional subscription to ArcGIS Online. Maptionairre (https://maptionnaire.com/) is a software as a service (SaaS) that can be purchased by project or on a continuous basis. Similar functionality can be achieved using open source software such as the web form based Kobo Toolbox (http://www.kobotoolbox.org/) or QField (http://www.qfield.org/) for Android that operates within the QGIS ecosystem but does have a larger learning curve.

Generalization

There is an increased need for built environment audits that consider non-US contexts (where a large number of observational audits originate) [63]. Highlighting this need are the many cultural and social differences between the US and other parts of the world including both Canada and Europe. For instance, using Canada as an example, there is a significant difference in the levels of crime and minority segregation in neighbourhoods and both tend to be higher in the United States [5]. Furthermore, Canadian differences in the experience of low income households, for example, presents a challenge when applying U.S. based neighbourhood studies [64]. Our study is applicable to other Canadian contexts, particularly regarding the underlying mechanisms and implications (e.g., policy formulation), and the methods can equally be applied to other countries and regions in the Northern and Southern Hemisphere with similar populations, urban development, built environments, and land use features.

Limitations

A common limitation of neighbourhood observational field audits is weather conditions [5]. To ensure high reliability and validity, it is best to observe neighbourhoods under the same environmental conditions; however, this can be difficult, especially at certain times of the year. The observations in 2011 took place during the month of November; a time when the weather is cooler, trees have less leaves, and snow can be common. In 2012, the field audit took place during the final stages of a major drought. Although steps were taken to prevent bias due to weather, it is recommended that future studies evaluate aesthetics in different seasons (e.g. spring or summer) to determine the variability of aesthetic features at different times of the year and their potential impact on perception and measurement. In a Canadian context, SSOIs that account for winter require considerable research. One advantage of VE audits, such as those using Google Street View, is that they can minimize some weather induced biases because almost all imagery is from the summer months in the Northern Hemisphere. It may be advantageous to utilize both virtual and field audits simultaneously to assess seasonal biases if temporal discrepancies in street view imagery can be controlled.

Although there are many benefits to utilizing the iPad in the current study, there were also minor limitations with the GIS Kit application. For instance, formatting long SSOI item titles to fit the GIS Kit data entry column was difficult (Fig. 1). The SSOI item called "cleanliness" was actually "cleanliness of streets and properties", but placing long titles on the data entry column in GIS Kit made data entry cumbersome. Another limitation of GIS Kit involves the clarity and relevancy of the Google Street or Satellite caches (maps). Although rare, reliance on 3rd party mapping systems, like Google Maps, meant that some audit locations were within sections of a neighbourhood that contained new developments that were not yet integrated into Google Maps. Thus, on occasion, the ability of the auditor to efficiently travel to the predetermined area was affected. Another minor concern, while not unique to the iPad, is the touch screen. This technology is extremely sensitive; therefore, auditors must be very aware of when they are touching the screen because they could unintentionally alter the collected data with an unintended touch of a finger or knuckle. A final concern, more so than a limitation, is the learning curve required to use an iPad and the GIS Kit application. The iPad, and more so GIS Kit, requires some familiarity and training to be able to use both efficiently and effectively. Although there are some limitations to utilizing the iPad and GIS Kit in the current study, the benefits and potential of this technology far outweigh the limitations. Future studies are recommended and encouraged to utilize mobile GIS technologies and applications to improve the efficiency of research design execution.

Conclusion

With the expansion and growth of research on neighbourhood characteristics in recent years there is an increased need for direct observational field audits, and specifically, research that focuses on the aesthetic features of neighbourhoods [2–4, 19]. This focus will also provide a more complete and contextual perspective for neighbourhood research. The current study addressed the need for direct observational research by showing that a simple SSOI together with minimal sampling and mobile GIS technology can be effective for rapid BE audits and evaluation. The need for direct observational research is not only relevant to Canadian settings [5] but is applicable to other countries and regions in the Northern and Southern Hemisphere with similar populations, urban development, built environments, and land use features.

The current study evaluates a new and effective collection method that is relevant to several disciplines and presents many potential research opportunities. A manifestation of this interdisciplinary relationship has already occurred. For example, the City of Ottawa Crime Stoppers program expressed interest in utilizing the new direct observation method and SSOI to examine neighbourhood aesthetic levels in relation to crime rates in Ottawa neighbourhoods. Based on the outcome, efforts to restore or improve neighbourhood aesthetics could be implemented and these policies may create more enjoyable neighbourhoods for residents, which in turn would actively promote the mental and physical well-being of residents.

Abbreviations

GIS: geographic information systems; SSOI: systematic social observation instrument; SES: socioeconomic status; BMI: body mass index; GPS: global positioning system; KML files: Keyhole Markup Language, an open source ASCII format for geographic data; R1 to R5: types of residential dwellings; IRR: interrater reliability; ICC: intraclass correlation coefficient; ITC: item-total correlation; IPAQ: International Physical Activity Questionnaire; CFB Rockcliffe NRC: Canadian Forces Base Rockcliffe, National Research Council; MAUP: modifiable areal unit problem; ArcPad: ESRI Inc. mobile windows CE, windows phone application for mobile geographic data collection; iOS: an operating system for mobile devices used by Apple Inc..

Authors' contributions

SJVL developed, pilot tested, and implemented the original measurement instrument (SSOI), participated in data collection, drafted and edited the manuscript, and coordinated and organized the drafting of the manuscript. MS performed statistical analyses, mapping, sampling development, and drafted and significantly edited the manuscript as well as participated in its design. EK participated in the design of the study, performed statistical analysis, and helped to edit the manuscript. All authors read and approved the final manuscript.

Author details

¹ School of Psychology, University of Ottawa, Ottawa, ON K2L 1K9, Canada. ² Laboratory for Applied Geomatics and GIS Science (LAGGISS), Department of Geography, Environment and Geomatics, University of Ottawa, Ottawa, ON K1N 6N5, Canada. ³ Ottawa Neighbourhood Study (ONS), University of Ottawa, Vanier 5023, 136 Jean Jacques Lussier, Ottawa, ON K1N 6N5, Canada. ⁴ School of Psychology and Institute of Population Health, University of Ottawa, Ottawa, ON K2L 1K9, Canada.

Acknowledgements

We thank Colin Ellis, Mija Azdajic, Melissa Weber, Arno van Dijk and Annabelle Boudreault for their participation in data collection. We are also indebted to Nathalie Paquette for proof-reading the manuscript.

Competing interests

The authors declare that they have no competing interests.

Funding

This work was funded by a grant from the United Way, Ottawa to the Ottawa Neighbourhood Study. The United Way had no input into the design of this study, analysis or interpretation of the data nor in writing, reviewing or approving the manuscript.

References

1. Clarke P, Ailshire J, Melendez R, Bader M, Morenoff J. Using Google Earth to conduct a neighborhood audit: reliability of a virtual audit instrument. Health Place. 2010;16:1224–9.
2. O'Campo P. Invited commentary: advancing theory and methods for multilevel models of residential neighborhoods and health. Am J Epidemiol. 2003;157:9–13.
3. Sampson RJ, Morenoff JD, Gannon-Rowley T. Assessing, "Neighborhood Effects": social processes and new directions in research. Annu Rev Sociol. 2002;28:443–78.
4. Cohen D, Spear S, Scribner R, Kissinger P, Mason K, Wildgen J. "Broken windows" and the risk of gonorrhea. Am J Public Health. 2000;90:230–6.
5. Parsons JA, Singh G, Scott AN, Nisenbaum R, Balasubramaniam P, Jabbar A, et al. Standardized observation of neighbourhood disorder: does it work in Canada? Int J Health Geogr. 2010;9(6):1–19.
6. Kahila-Tani M, Broberg A, Kyttä M, Tyger T. Let the citizens map—public participation GIS as a planning support system in the Helsinki master plan process. Plan Pract Res. 2016;31:195–214.
7. Pánek J, Pászto V, Marek L. Mapping emotions: spatial distribution of safety perception in the City of Olomouc. In: Ivan I, Singleton A, Horák J, Inspektor T, editors. Rise Big Spat. Data [internet]. Cham: Springer International Publishing; 2017 [cited 2016 Nov 29]. p. 211–24. http://link.springer.com/10.1007/978-3-319-45123-7_16.
8. Pánek J, Pászto V. Emotional mapping in local neighbourhood planning: case study of Příbram, Czech Republic. Int J E-Plan Res. 2017;6:1–22.
9. MacKerron G, Murato S. Mappiness, the happiness mapping app [internet]. [cited 2016 Nov 29]. http://www.mappiness.org.uk/.
10. Huck JJ, Whyatt JD, Coulton P. Spraycan: a PPGIS for capturing imprecise notions of place. Appl Geogr. 2014;55:229–37.
11. Clews C, Brajkovich-Payne R, Dwight E, Ahmad Fauzul A, Burton M, Carleton O, et al. Alcohol in urban streetscapes: a comparison of the use of Google Street View and on-street observation. BMC Public Health [internet]. 2016 [cited 2016 Dec 6];16. http://bmcpublichealth.biomedcentral.com/articles/10.1186/s12889-016-3115-9.
12. Jankowski P, Czepkiewicz M, Młodkowski M, Zwoliński Z. Geo-questionnaire: a method and tool for public preference elicitation in land use planning. Trans GIS. 2016;20(6):903–24.
13. Cerin E, Saelens BE, Sallis JF, Frank LD. Neighborhood environment walkability scale: validity and development of a short form. Med Sci Sports Exerc. 2006;38:1682–91.
14. Ewing R, Handy S. Measuring the unmeasurable: urban design qualities related to walkability. J Urban Des. 2009;14:65–84.
15. Odgers CL, Caspi A, Bates CJ, Sampson RJ, Moffitt TE. Systematic social observation of children's neighborhoods using Google Street View: a reliable and cost-effective method. J Child Psychol Psychiatry. 2012;53:1009–17.
16. Ben-Joseph E, Lee JS, Cromley EK, Laden F, Troped PJ. Virtual and actual: relative accuracy of on-site and web-based instruments in auditing the environment for physical activity. Health Place. 2013;19:138–50.
17. Badland HM, Opit S, Witten K, Kearns RA, Mavoa S. Can virtual streetscape audits reliably replace physical streetscape audits? J Urban Health. 2010;87:1007–16.
18. Caughy MO, O'Campo PJ, Patterson J. A brief observational measure for urban neighborhoods. Health Place. 2001;7:225–36.
19. Foster S, Giles-Corti B, Knuiman M. Creating safe walkable streetscapes: does house design and upkeep discourage incivilities in suburban neighbourhoods? J Environ Psychol. 2011;31:79–88.
20. Mills JW, Curtis A, Kennedy B, Kennedy SW, Edwards JD. Geospatial video for field data collection. Appl Geogr. 2010;30:533–47.
21. Kelly CM, Wilson JS, Baker EA, Miller DK, Schootman M. Using Google Street View to audit the built environment: inter-rater reliability results. Ann Behav Med. 2013;45:S108–12.
22. Curtis JW, Curtis A, Mapes J, Szell AB, Cinderich A. Using google street view for systematic observation of the built environment: analysis of spatio-temporal instability of imagery dates. Int J Health Geogr. 2013;12(53):1–10.
23. Rundle AG, Bader MDM, Richards CA, Neckerman KM, Teitler JO. Using Google Street View to audit neighborhood environments. Am J Prev Med. 2011;40:94–100.
24. Ploeger SK, Sawada M, Elsabbagh A, Saatcioglu M, Nastev M, Rosetti E. Urban RAT: new tool for virtual and site-specific mobile rapid data collection for seismic risk assessment. J Comput Civ Eng. 2016;30:4015006.
25. Hwang J, Sampson RJ. Divergent pathways of gentrification: racial inequality and the social order of renewal in chicago neighborhoods. Am Sociol Rev. 2014;79:726.
26. Wilson JS, Kelly CM, Schootman M, Baker EA, Banerjee A, Clennin M, et al. Assessing the built environment using omnidirectional imagery. Am J Prev Med. 2012;42:193–9.
27. Schootman M, Nelson EJ, Werner K, Shacham E, Elliott M, Ratnapradipa K, et al. Emerging technologies to measure neighborhood conditions in public health: implications for interventions and next steps. Int J Health Geogr. 2016;15:1–9.
28. Naik N, Philipoom J, Raskar R, Hidalgo C. Streetscore—predicting the perceived safety of one million streetscapes. In: CVPRW 14 Proceedings of 2014 IEEE conference on computer vision pattern recognition workshop. IEEE; 2014. p. 793–9.
29. Salesses P, Schechtner K, Hidalgo CA. The collaborative image of the city: mapping the inequality of urban perception. PLoS ONE. 2013;8:e68400.
30. Rioux L, Werner C. Residential satisfaction among aging people living in place. J Environ Psychol. 2011;31:158–69.

31. Dunstan F, Weaver N, Araya R, Bell T, Lannon S, Lewis G, et al. An observa-
     tion tool to assist with the assessment of urban residential environments.
     J Environ Psychol. 2005;25:293–305.

32. Hoehner CM, Brennan Ramirez LK, Elliott MB, Handy SL, Brownson RC.
     Perceived and objective environmental measures and physical activity
     among urban adults. Am J Prev Med. 2005;28:105–16.

33. Raudenbush SW, Sampson RJ. Ecometrics: toward a science of assessing
     ecological settings, with application to the systematic social observation
     of neighborhoods. Sociol Methodol. 1999;29:1–41.

34. Brownson RC, Chang JJ, Eyler AA, Ainsworth BE, Kirtland KA, Saelens BE,
     et al. Measuring the environment for friendliness toward physical activity:
     a comparison of the reliability of 3 questionnaires. Am J Public Health.
     2004;94:473–83.

35. Saelens BE, Sallis JF, Black JB, Chen D. Neighborhood-based differences
     in physical activity: an environment scale evaluation. Am J Public Health.
     2003;93:1552–8.

36. Jirovec RL, Jirovec MM, Bosse R. Environmental determinants of
     neighborhood satisfaction among urban elderly men. Gerontologist.
     1984;24:261–5.

37. Aanensen DM, Huntley DM, Feil EJ, Al-Own F, Spratt BG. EpiCollect: Link-
     ing smartphones to web applications for epidemiology, ecology and
     community data collection. PLoS ONE. 2009;4(9):1–7.

38. Kennedy R, McLeman R, Sawada M, Smigielski J. Use of smartphone
     technology for small-scale silviculture: a test of low-cost technology in
     Eastern Ontario. Small-Scale For. 2014;13:101–15.

39. Tobler WR. Smooth pycnophylactic interpolation for geographical
     regions. J Am Stat Assoc. 1979;74:519.

40. Rase W-D. Volume-preserving interpolation of a smooth surface from
     polygon-related data. J Geogr Syst. 2001;3:199–213.

41. Yoo E-H, Kyriakidis PC, Tobler W. Reconstructing population density
     surfaces from areal data: a comparison of Tobler's pycnophylactic
     interpolation method and area-to-point kriging. 面状数据的人口密度
     面重构: Tobler's pycnophylactic 插值法和面到点克里金插值法的对比:
     reconstructing population density surfaces from areal data. Geogr Anal.
     2010;42:78–98.

42. Kyriakidis PC. A geostatistical framework for area-to-point spatial interpo-
     lation. Geogr Anal. 2004;36:259–89.

43. Kyriakidis PC, Yoo E-H. Geostatistical prediction and simulation of point
     values from areal data. Geogr Anal. 2005;37:124–51.

44. Goodchild MF, Anselin L, Deichmann U. A framework for the areal inter-
     polation of socioeconomic data. Environ Plan A. 1993;25:383–97.

45. Dodgson JS, Spackman M, Pearman A, Phillips LD. Multi-criteria analysis:
     a manual. London: Department for Communities and Local Government;
     2009.

46. Dozois DJA, Seeds PM, Firestone P. Psychological assessment and
     research methods. In: Dozois DJA, Firestone P, editors. Abnormal psychol-

ogy: Perspectives (DSM-5 Edition). 4th ed. Toronto: Pearson; 2010. p. 59.

47. Revelle W. psych: procedures for personality and psychological research
     [internet]. Evanston, Illinois, USA: Northwestern University; 2016. https://
     CRAN.R-project.org/package=psych.

48. Hallgren KA. Computing inter-rater reliability for observational data: an
     overview and tutorial. Tutor Quant Methods Psychol. 2012;8:23.

49. McGraw KO, Wong SP. Forming inferences about some intraclass correla-
     tion coefficients. Psychol Methods. 1996;1:30–46.

50. Gamer M, Lemon J, Fellows I, Singh P. irr: various coefficients of interrater
     reliability and agreement [internet]. 2015. https://cran.r-project.org/
     package=irr.

51. Statistics Canada. 2006 Canadian long-form census. 2006.

52. Hagströmer M, Oja P, Sjöström M. The international physical activity
     questionnaire (IPAQ): a study of concurrent and construct validity. Public
     Health Nutr. 2006;9:755–62.

53. Harrell FEJ, Dupont C. Hmisc: Harrell miscellaneous [internet]. 2014.
     https://cran.r-project.org/package=Hmisc.

54. Canty A, Ripley B. Boot: Bootstrap R (S-Plus) Functions. [internet]. 2016.
     https://cran.r-project.org/package=boot.

55. Davison AC, Hinkley DV. Bootstrap methods and their application. Cam-
     bridge: Cambridge University Press; 1997.

56. R Core Team. R: A language and environment for statistical computing
     [internet]. Vienna, Austria: R Foundation for Statistical Computing; 2014.
     http://www.R-project.org/.

57. IBM. IBM SPSS statistics for Windows. 2013.

58. Strominger J, Anthopolos R, Miranda ML. Implications of construction
     method and spatial scale on measures of the built environment. Int J
     Health Geogr. 2016;15(15):1–13.

59. Southworth M. Designing the walkable city. J Urban Plan Dev.
     2005;131:246–57.

60. Kolbe-Alexander TL, Pacheco K, Tomaz SA, Karpul D, Lambert EV. The
     relationship between the built environment and habitual levels of physi-
     cal activity in South African older adults: a pilot study. BMC Public Health.
     2015;15(518):1–9.

61. Pikora TJ, Giles-Corti B, Knuiman MW, Bull FC, Jamrozik K, Donovan RJ.
     Neighborhood environmental factors correlated with walking near
     home: using SPACES. Med Sci Sports Exerc. 2006;38:708–14.

62. Sugiyama T, Giles-Corti B, Summers J, du Toit L, Leslie E, Owen N. Initiating
     and maintaining recreational walking: a longitudinal study on the influ-
     ence of neighborhood green space. Prev Med. 2013;57:178–82.

63. Quintas R, Raggi A, Bucciarelli P, Franco MG, Andreotti A, Caballero FF,
     et al. The COURAGE built environment outdoor checklist: an objective
     built environment instrument to investigate the impact of the environ-
     ment on health and disability: COURAGE built environment outdoor
     checklist outcomes. Clin Psychol Psychother. 2014;21:204–14.

64. Oreopoulos P. Neighbourhood effects in Canada: a critique. Can Public
     Policy. 2008;34:237–58.

7

Evaluating neighborhood structures for modeling intercity diffusion of large-scale dengue epidemics

Tzai-Hung Wen[1*], Ching-Shun Hsu[1] and Ming-Che Hu[2]

Abstract

Background: Dengue fever is a vector-borne infectious disease that is transmitted by contact between vector mosquitoes and susceptible hosts. The literature has addressed the issue on quantifying the effect of individual mobility on dengue transmission. However, there are methodological concerns in the spatial regression model configuration for examining the effect of intercity-scale human mobility on dengue diffusion. The purposes of the study are to investigate the influence of neighborhood structures on intercity epidemic progression from pre-epidemic to epidemic periods and to compare definitions of different neighborhood structures for interpreting the spread of dengue epidemics.

Methods: We proposed a framework for assessing the effect of model configurations on dengue incidence in 2014 and 2015, which were the most severe outbreaks in 70 years in Taiwan. Compared with the conventional model configuration in spatial regression analysis, our proposed model used a radiation model, which reflects population flow between townships, as a spatial weight to capture the structure of human mobility.

Results: The results of our model demonstrate better model fitting performance, indicating that the structure of human mobility has better explanatory power in dengue diffusion than the geometric structure of administration boundaries and geographic distance between centroids of cities. We also identified spatial–temporal hierarchy of dengue diffusion: dengue incidence would be influenced by its immediate neighboring townships during pre-epidemic and epidemic periods, and also with more distant neighbors (based on mobility) in pre-epidemic periods.

Conclusions: Our findings suggest that the structure of population mobility could more reasonably capture urban-to-urban interactions, which implies that the hub cities could be a "bridge" for large-scale transmission and make townships that immediately connect to hub cities more vulnerable to dengue epidemics.

Keywords: Dengue, Epidemic diffusion, Spatial regression, Human mobility, Taiwan

Background

Dengue fever is a vector-borne infectious disease that is transmitted by contact between vector mosquitoes and susceptible hosts [1]. Since the 1970s, dengue fever has been gradually spreading throughout tropical and sub-tropical countries, and its transmission involves interactions among carriers, mosquitoes, and healthy humans.

More than 125 countries are impacted by the disease, and it is an increasingly serious threat to global public health due to climate change. Previous studies showed meteorological and social–economic risk factors that facilitate the disease transmission, including temperature, rainfall, population density, demographic composition, urbanized levels and more [2–4]. The Fifth Assessment Report (AR5) of the Intergovernmental Panel on Climate Change (IPCC) also confirmed that global warming would create more suitable habitats for vector mosquitoes in sub-tropical regions and speed up the geographic expansion of dengue epidemic areas due to global mobility including

*Correspondence: wenthung@ntu.edu.tw
[1] Department of Geography, National Taiwan University, No. 1, Sec. 4, Roosevelt Road, Taipei City 10617, Taiwan
Full list of author information is available at the end of the article

to some high-latitude countries such as France and Japan [5–12].

Due to the limited flight range of mosquitoes [13], it is impossible for the virus to be transmitted to distant areas by dengue vectors. Population movement across countries by air traffic is the major driver of the international spread of the disease [12–17]. Via air travel, disease importation from dengue-endemic countries is a trigger point for initiating indigenous epidemics in some dengue-epidemic countries or regions, such as Tokyo, Japan; south-east France; and southern Taiwan [14, 18]. Routine mobility behaviors, such as daily commutes, are also drivers of large-scale intercity transmission [19]. Therefore, understanding the spatial structure of population mobility is crucial for assessing the possible mechanisms of dengue diffusion and identifying the geographic characteristics of high-risk areas [20].

Recent studies on assessing the influence of human mobility on dengue transmission can be categorized into three approaches. The first is to construct simulation or statistical models that incorporate human mobility as the mechanism of dengue diffusion [21]. For example, Barmak et al. [22] showed that the long-distance mobility pattern is an efficient pathway for dengue transmission. Another study used survival analysis to show that daily routine commuters facilitate the large-scale spatial–temporal diffusion of the epidemic in a city [19]. The second perspective is to collect human mobility or behavior data to analyze the spread of dengue. Stoddard et al. [15] showed that small-scale mobility behavior among households also played an important role in dengue epidemics in Iquitos, Peru. Wesolowski et al. [16] used the Call Detail Records (CDRs) from mobile phones to analyze the spatial behaviors of humans in Pakistan for predicting diffusion of dengue in time and space. Airline traffic data are also available for studying the international spread of dengue epidemics and assessing the disease importation risk from dengue-endemic countries [23, 24]. The third perspective is to analyze geometric structures of geography to measure geospatial similarity or neighborhoods as a surrogate for human mobility. Spatial regression modeling is the major approach for measuring the neighborhood effects on dengue risk after controlling for environmental factors [4, 25].

The above studies showed that human mobility could be the main risk factor for dengue transmission on both the regional and global scales. However, methodological concerns remain for examining the effect of intercity human mobility. First, spatial settings in the regression model often examine the geometric relationships of geography as a surrogate for spatial interactions and human interactions. For example, the weights of spatial contiguity can be defined as administration boundaries with common borders and points [26] or areas based on k-nearest neighbors within a specific distance [25]. These definitions may simplify the complex interactions of humans because the geometry of spatial contiguity cannot comprehensively reflect these human interactions due to topographical or social–economic barriers across the study area [27]. Moreover, the spatial heterogeneity of human interactions or mobility may not be captured by the geometry of the boundaries alone. In addition, it is difficult to differentiate the effect of urban-to-urban or rural-to-rural mobility on epidemic diffusion if these areas share similar geometric structures. Some studies suggest that the use of real population flow could act as a spatial weight that captures more realistic spatial interactions [27, 28]. Therefore, approaches that use Global Positioning System (GPS) logs, cell phone records or geotags from social media for tracking moving trajectories of individuals have become emerging methods for studying human mobility and dengue risk [29, 30]. However, massive cell phone data provided by telecommunication companies are often difficult to access in the research community. Tracking collective behaviors from cell phone data may also violate location privacy, and this approach could be controversial in most developed countries. Due to these concerns, mathematical models, such as gravity, spatial interaction or radiation models, are used to estimate population flow across cities. Spatial models have become widely used approaches to study the geography of human mobility and disease transmission [29, 31, 32]. Among these models, the radiation model is a parameter-free algorithm that is robust in estimating the flow of intercity human mobility [32].

To clarify the role of intercity human mobility, we used the radiation model to capture the structure of spatial mobility as a possible mechanism. We examined the effect of neighborhood structures on the spatial–temporal spread of dengue epidemics in southern Taiwan from 2014 to 2015, the most severe outbreaks over the course of 70 years in Taiwan, and identified the common social-demographic features in these high-epidemic regions. By profiling the neighborhood effects on the spatial–temporal structures of disease spread, we proposed a study framework for interpreting possible pathways of intercity diffusion of dengue epidemics. The purposes of the study are (1) to investigate the influence of neighborhood structures on epidemic progression from the pre-epidemic to epidemic periods and (2) to compare the definitions of different neighborhood structures for interpreting the spread of dengue epidemics.

Data and methods

Study area

Southeast Asia is one of the major dengue-endemic regions in the world [33–36]. Taiwan is located in the border region of Southeast and East Asia. Southern Taiwan, which is passed through by the Tropic of Cancer, has a tropical monsoon climate; it is dry in the winter and hot and wet in the summer and autumn. The population has grown quickly, reaching 5.5 million in 2014. With an average of 683 persons/km^2, metropolitan areas of southern Taiwan have become one of the most densely populated areas in the world. Due to its climatic and demographic characteristics, the region is a severe dengue-epidemic region of Taiwan, which annually covers more than 85% of the total confirmed dengue cases in Taiwan. Therefore, this region, including Tainan and Kaohsiung Cities and Pin-tung County, was used as the study area. A township was used as the unit for analysis, which is the basic unit for regional master planning and national policy implementation. Our study analyzed the dengue incidence and profiled the social–economic structures of spatial diffusion

in 108 townships from 2014 to 2015. To differentiate between the social–economic statuses of each township, we categorized the urbanization levels into seven types, including highly or middle-developed, emerging, general, aging, rural, and non-developed areas as shown in Fig. 1. These types were determined by sociodemographic variables, including population density, population ratio of people with college or above educational levels, population ratio of elder people over 65 years old, population ratio of people of agriculture workers, and the number of physicians per 100,000 people from Taiwan census database [37].

Dengue epidemics in study area

Dengue fever is a notifiable infectious disease in Taiwan. The dengue surveillance data from the Taiwan Centers for Disease Control (Taiwan CDC) are based on institutional reporting and border surveillance. The confirmed dengue cases reported by the Taiwan CDC are laboratory-positive dengue cases, which indicates a suspected dengue case with anti-dengue IgM seroconversion or single anti-dengue IgM positivity or a case with

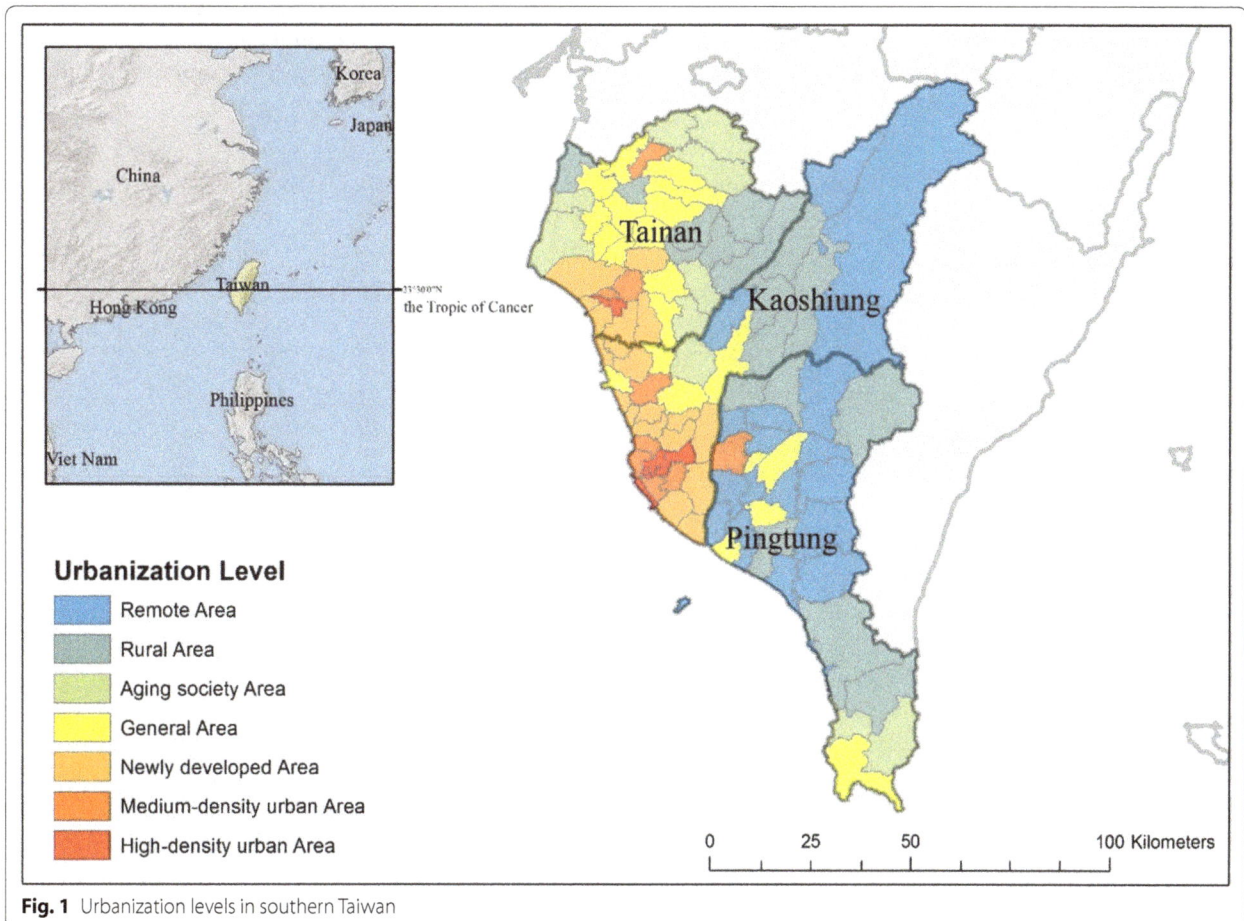

Fig. 1 Urbanization levels in southern Taiwan

dengue virus identification through RT-PCR [38]. Their residences of cases were also aggregated as counts in townships for public announcement. Figure 2 shows the temporal trend of dengue epidemics from 1998 to 2015 in Taiwan. The figure indicates that, in the last 2 years, the number of confirmed cases reached 15,732 and 43,784, and 233 people dead, respectively, which are the most severe outbreaks over the course of 70 years in Taiwan. Most high-epidemic areas were concentrated in Tainan and Kaohsiung Cities (Fig. 3). Moreover, the southern Taiwan is located in the border of tropical and sub-tropical climatic zones (Fig. 1). Therefore, the dengue epidemics in Taiwan can be regarded as one of dengue sentinel indicators in Southeast and East Asia, which monitors geographic expansion of dengue epidemics to middle or high-latitude countries.

Figure 4 shows the monthly variations of dengue cases in southern Taiwan, 2014 and 2015, and it indicates that there were significant epidemic seasons in these 2 years. We defined the month with the highest dengue cases as the start of epidemic season. Therefore, we categorized the periods of October to December of 2014 and September to December of 2015 as epidemic seasons. We further investigated the association of neighborhood structures and dengue diffusion between pre-epidemic and epidemic seasons in these 2 years.

Table 1 summarizes the population density, number of townships and dengue incidence during the pre-epidemic and epidemic periods in 7 urbanization stratifications, including remote, rural, ageing, general, new-developed, medium-density and high-density areas. It shows that dengue cases were concentrated in medium- and high-density areas in both the pre-epidemic and epidemic stages. Therefore, human mobility between townships with high urbanization levels could be critical routes of spatial transmission.

Spatial weights and neighborhood structures
Spatial proximity and human mobility may influence neighborhood diffusion of dengue epidemics. Different definitions of neighborhood structures reflect the effects of spatial interactions. We defined three neighborhood structures, including Queen Contiguity, Distance-threshold weights and matrix of human mobility, for investigating the influence of different types of neighborhood structures on dengue diffusion.

Queen contiguity weights
The queen contiguity is one of the standard contiguity-based spatial weighting methods in geographic analysis. It determines neighboring units as those that have any point in common, including both common boundaries

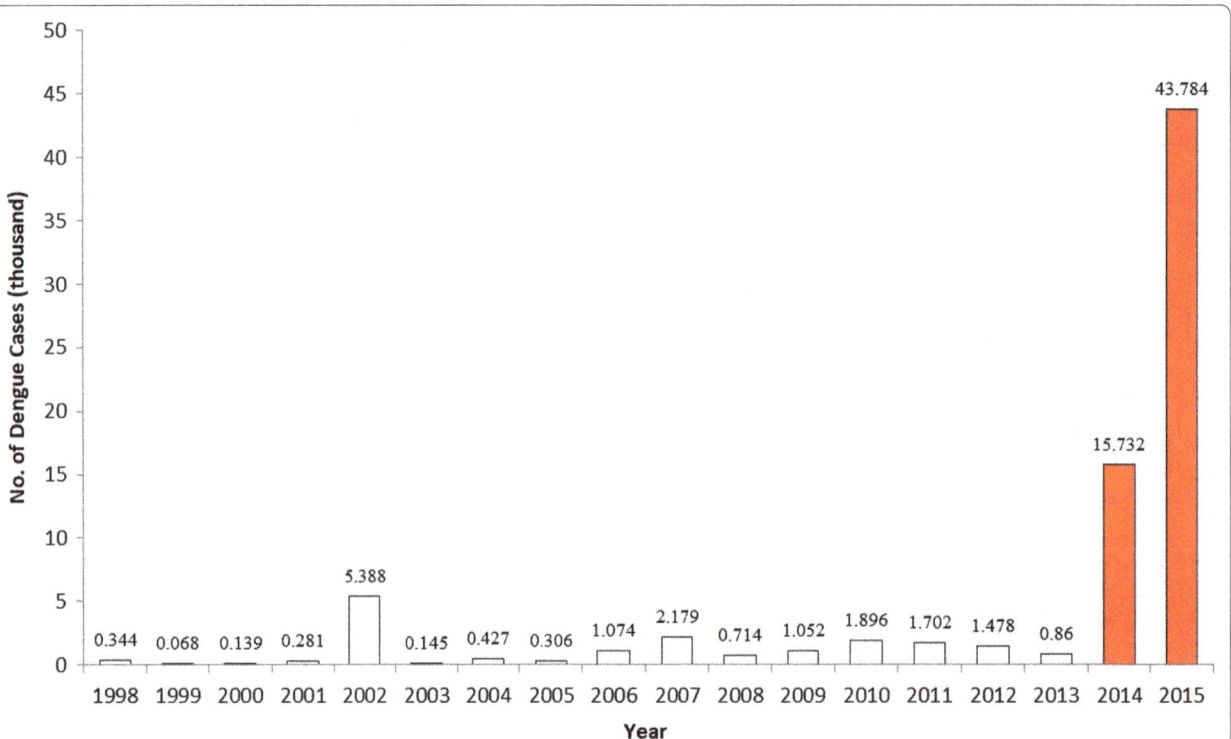

Fig. 2 Number of dengue cases in Taiwan (1998–2015)

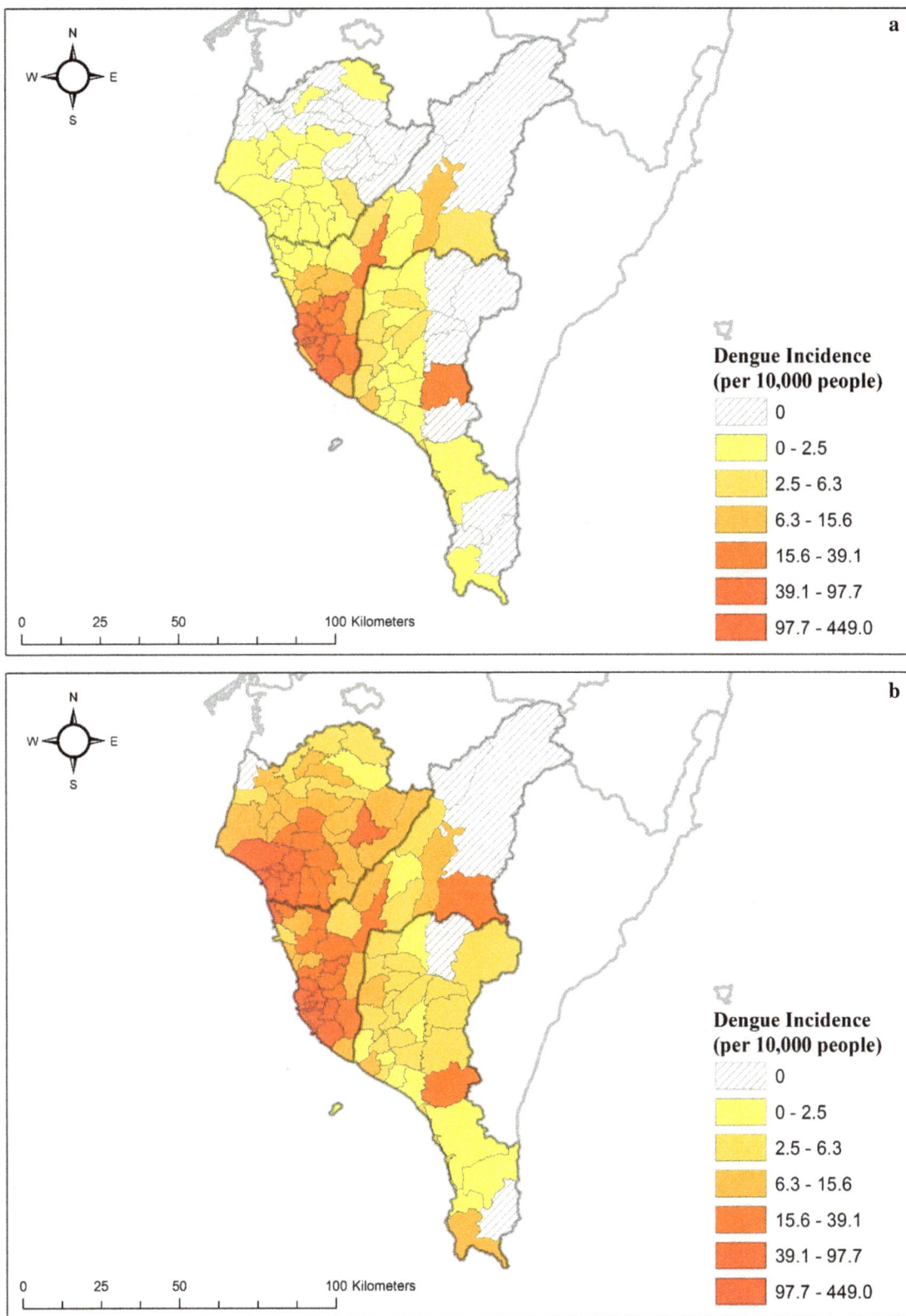

Fig. 3 Spatial distributions of dengue incidence in **a** 2014 and **b** 2015

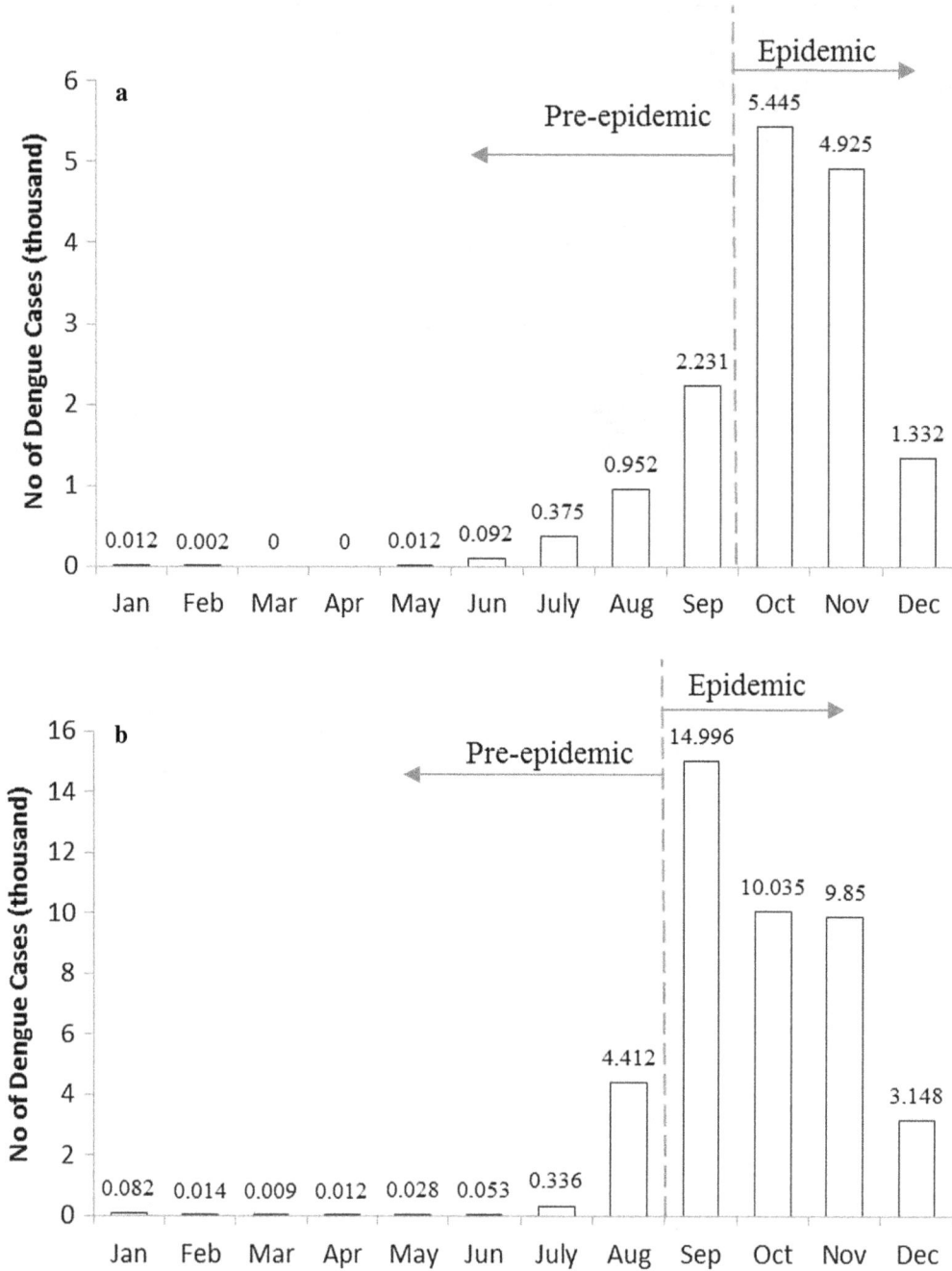

Fig. 4 Monthly number of dengue cases in **a** 2014 and **b** 2015. In 2014, the period of Jan.–Sep. is defined as pre-epidemic and Oct.–Dec. as epidemic; in 2015, the period of Jan.–Aug. is defined as pre-epidemic and Sep.–Dec. as epidemic stage

and common corners. The spatial weights in a queen contiguity matrix (W_Q) represent townships that share administration boundaries and have higher possibilities of interacting with each other. Based on queen contiguity, each township has an average of 5.14 neighboring townships in our study.

Distance-threshold weights

The distances among townships could influence the extent of daily mobility. The queen contiguity cannot incorporate the effect of distance on spatial interaction. The extent of daily mobility is measured by the journeys someone takes from home to work and back again. The

Table 1 Summarized Statistics in urbanization levels

Township stratification	Counts of towns	Avg. population density, person/km²	Dengue incidence rate, per 10,000 people	
			Pre-epidemic	Epidemic
Remote area	22	132.9	1.07	5.5
Rural area	18	121.5	0.81	7.24
Aging society area	10	163.1	0.64	4.01
General area	21	616.2	2.52	14.08
Newly developed area	19	1870.8	13.56	72.5
Medium-density urban area	9	5421.5	24.69	116.23
High-density urban area	9	10,746.7	24.97	196.16

Institute of Transportation identified 20 km as the average daily journey distance for urban trips [39]. Therefore, we measured distances between centroids of townships for establishing a spatial weight matrix (W_D) that defined the townships within 20 km as the criteria of a neighborhood for modeling spatial interactions. In other words, the distance-threshold weights can reflect spatial interactions between townships within 20 km.

Matrix of human mobility

The weights of Queen Contiguity and Distance-threshold reflect geometric characteristics of neighborhood structures rather than the patterns of human mobility. In other words, these definitions cannot differentiate the directions and volumes of population flow between urban-to-urban and urban-to rural areas. Therefore, we adopted the concept of radiation model proposed by Simini et al. [32] for quantifying spatial interaction between townships (Eq. 1). The radiation model can estimate routine human mobility, which reflects daily commute [32]. Therefore, we used the proportions of commuters from one to another location as the spatial weight matrix for quantifying spatial associations among locations.

$$T_{ij} = m_i \frac{m_j}{(m_i + s_{ij})(m_i + m_j + s_{ij})} \tag{1}$$

where T_{ij} is the proportion of the commuters in township i travelling to township j; m_i and m_j are the populations in townships i and j, respectively; and s_{ij} is the total population in the circle centered at i and touching j, excluding the source and destination population as shown Fig. 5a. The population in the circle (s_{ij}) represents attraction (e.g., opportunity of jobs) to mi. If s_{ij} is larger, it indicates that the population in the m_i has more mobility alternatives, which decreases the mobility propensity from m_i to m_j. The parameter-free model is validated in various

behaviors of human mobility, including journeys with a short travel time, daily commute, and migration [32]. We used the model to estimate the trips for constructing an Original-Destination Matrix W, W(i,j) is the estimated trips from township i to j and the transpose matrix $W^T(i,j)$ is then the estimated trips from j to i. Therefore, we generated a fully connected symmetric matrix $W_F = W + W^T$, which can capture the spatial interactions between townships, and W_F is the spatial weights we used to measure the human mobility between townships (Fig. 5b). Township population statistical data for the radiation model is from the Department of Household Registration, Ministry of the Interior in Taiwan.

Figure 6 illustrates an example of the neighborhood structures of Fongshan District in Kaohsiung City based on these three criteria. The neighborhood structures in Fig. 6a, b reflect the geometric characteristics of the administration boundary, and the spatial interactions in Fig. 6c capture the spatial variations of human mobility and characteristics of urbanization.

Statistical analysis

We used spatial regression modeling for investigating the neighborhood effects on spatial–time diffusion of dengue incidence between a township and its neighboring area. Spatial lag model, one of spatial regression specifications, adds a spatial lag operator to the outcome variable (e.g. disease incidence) for investigating neighboring effects as diffusion process [40, 41]. Therefore, by integrating dengue cases in different periods, in this study, spatial lag model was used for quantitatively measuring dengue diffusion effects in different periods.

We developed three statistical model specifications: Model 1 only measures the neighboring effect of the pre-epidemic period (t1), and Model 2 considers the diffusion effect of dengue incidence in neighboring townships during both the pre-epidemic (t1) and epidemic (t2) periods. Comparing these two models can differentiate diffusion

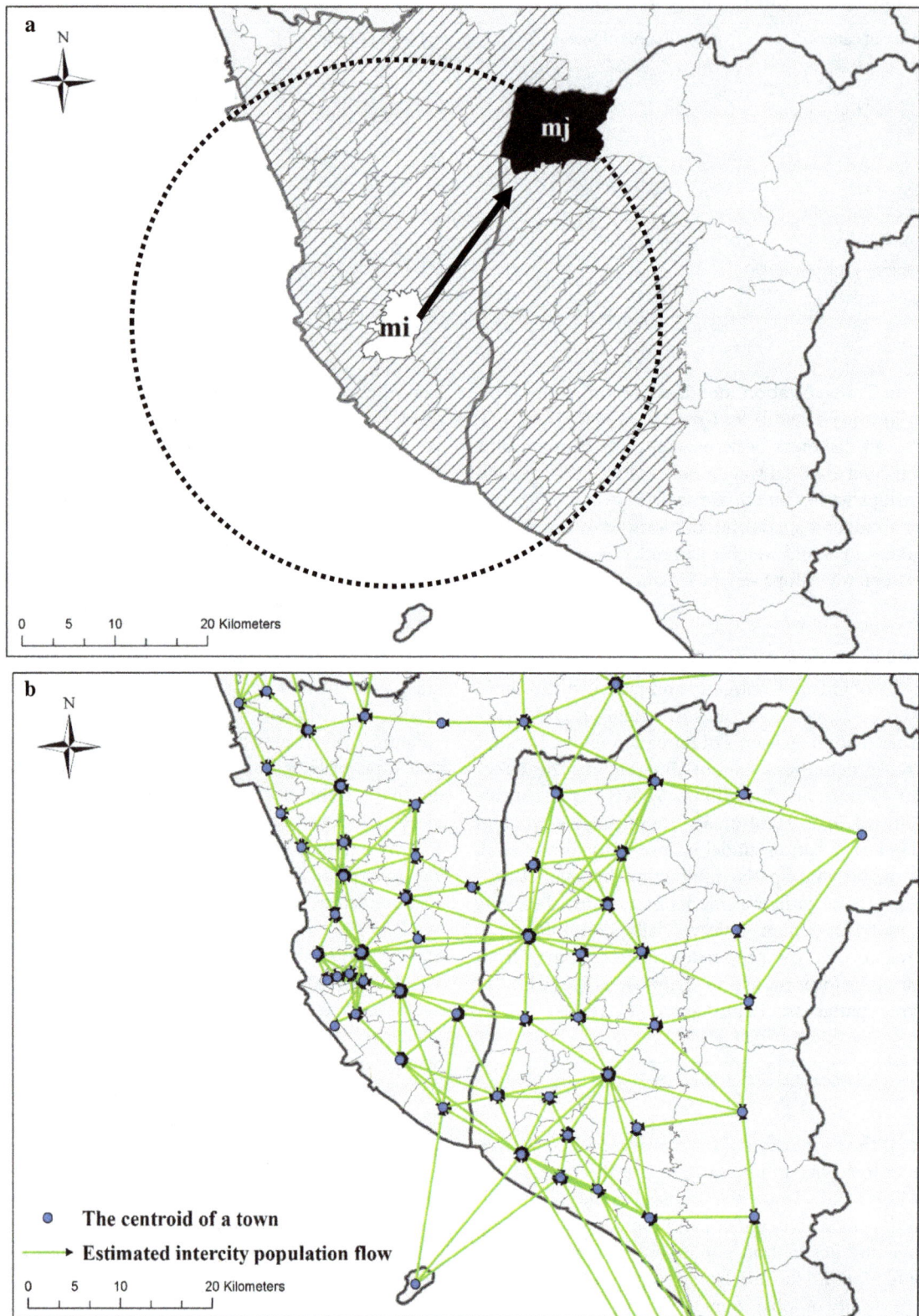

Fig. 5 Illustrations of **a** an example of using a radiation mode to estimate population flow from m_i (source) to m_j (destination), which considers total population in the circle centered at m_i and touching m_j excluding the source (m_i) and the destination (m_j) population. More population in the circle represent people in the mi have more attractive (e.g. opportunity of jobs), and it decreases mobility propensity from mi to m_j; **b** network connectivity structure of human mobility estimated by a radiation model to represent spatial interaction

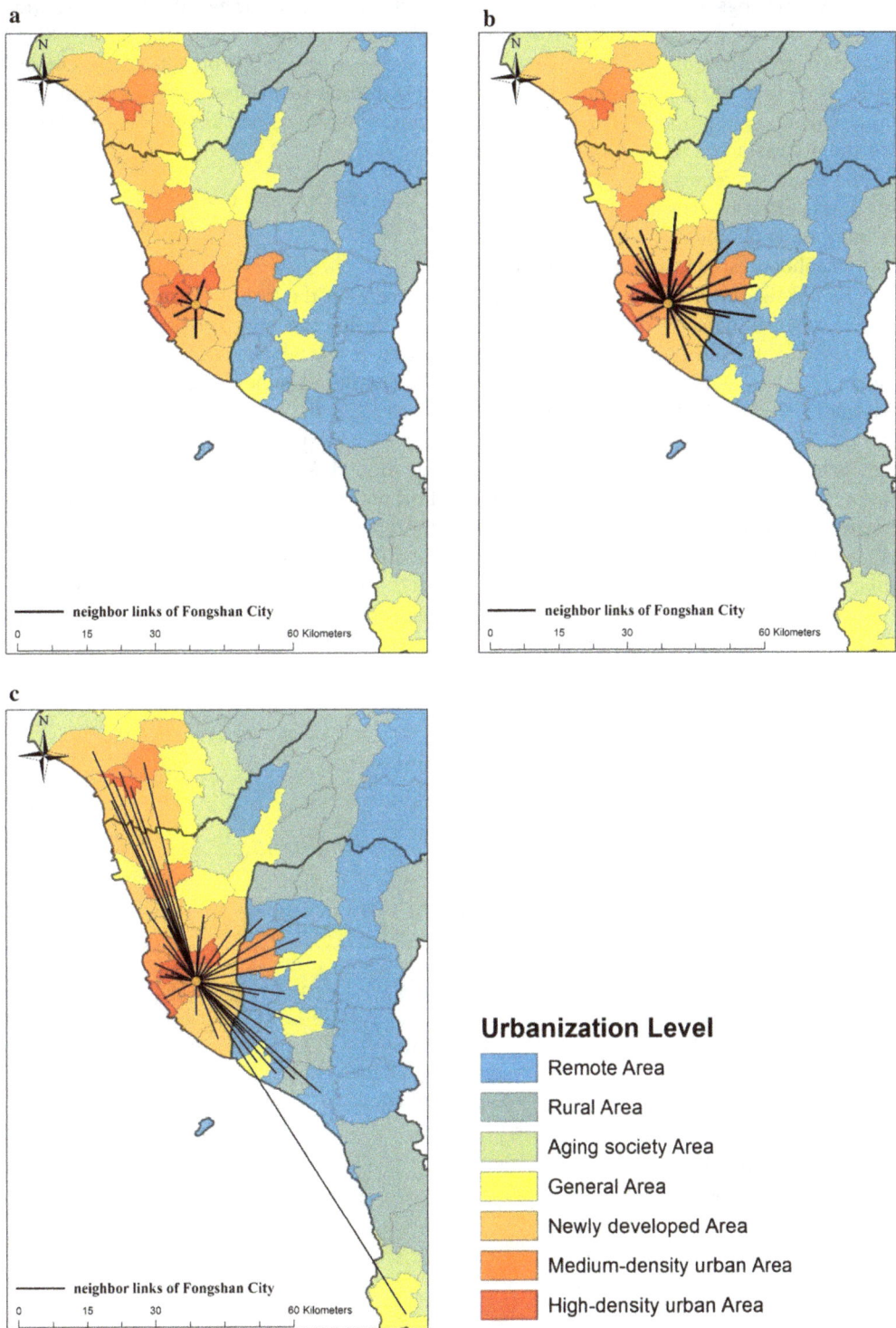

Fig. 6 An example of neighborhood structures of Fongshan District of Kaohsiung City based on three definitions: **a** queen contiguity, **b** distance-threshold weights and **c** structure of human mobility

effects from the pre-epidemic (t1) and epidemic (t2) periods to investigate the influence of neighborhood structures on epidemic progression. Model 3 considers the

second-order neighboring townships of the pre-epidemic period (t1) for quantifying the relatively long-distance diffusion effect during the period.

Moreover, different settings of neighborhood structures, including Queen Contiguity, distance-threshold weights and structure of human mobility, are compared in each model for each year so that we could systematically understand which neighborhood structure is more appropriate for the discussion on spatial autocorrelation of dengue and the result we found would be more convinced. Models 1 was fitted to data using ordinary least squares (OLS) method and Models 2 and 3 were fitted using maximum likelihood estimation (MLE) with the R package spdep. The Akaike information criterion (AIC) is used as the performance indicator of model fitting. A model with a lower AIC value has a better explanation for dengue diffusion.

The model framework of statistical analysis is shown in Fig. 7. Different colors of the layers represent different-order neighborhood structures. The variables in the first layer (blue) represent a township i; the second layer (green) represent the 1-order neighborhood (immediate neighbors), and the third layer (pink) represent the 2-order neighborhood (distant neighbors). The arrows represents influence relations between these variables. Detailed model specifications are described as follows.

Model 1: pre-epidemic neighborhood effect model
We used ordinary least squares (OLS) Regression to investigate the diffusion effect of dengue incidence in neighboring townships during the pre-epidemic period, controlling for urbanization levels, as shown in Eq. 2

$$Y_{t2} = \sum_{a=1}^{6} \beta_a x_a + \rho_{t1} W y_{t1} + \varepsilon \qquad (2)$$

where y_{t2} is the logarithmic dengue incidence of a township during the epidemic period (t2) and x is the urbanization level, which is a categorical variable. There are six dummy variables used to capture seven urbanization levels. β_a is the marginal effect for one urbanization type (a). W is a spatial weight matrix, including the abovementioned W_Q, W_D and W_F, for investigating the neighborhood structures. $W y_{t1}$ measures dengue incidence in pre-epidemic period (t1) and its coefficient ρ_{t1} is the marginal neighboring effect during the pre-epidemic period (t1), which can capture diffusion process of dengue epidemics from t1 to t2. ε is the regression residual.

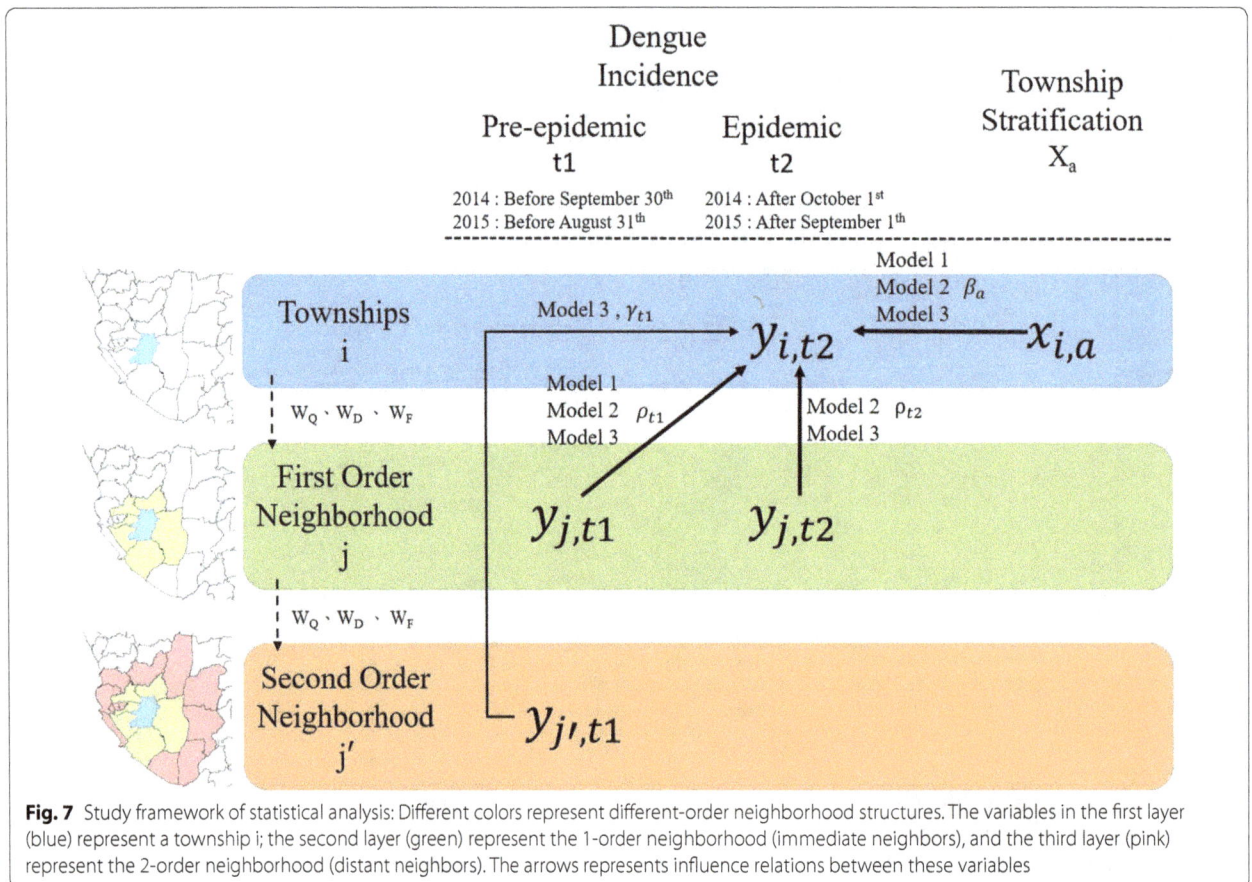

Fig. 7 Study framework of statistical analysis: Different colors represent different-order neighborhood structures. The variables in the first layer (blue) represent a township i; the second layer (green) represent the 1-order neighborhood (immediate neighbors), and the third layer (pink) represent the 2-order neighborhood (distant neighbors). The arrows represents influence relations between these variables

Model 2: current neighborhood effect model

We used spatial lag models (SLM) to investigate the diffusion effect of dengue incidence in neighboring townships during both the pre-epidemic (t1) and epidemic (t2) periods, controlling for urbanization levels, as shown in Eq. 3.

$$y_{t2} = \rho_{t2}\mathrm{W}y_{t2} + \sum_{a=1}^{6} \beta_a x_a + \rho_{t1} W y_{t1} + \varepsilon \qquad (3)$$

where β_a is the marginal effect for one urbanization type (a). W is a spatial weight matrix, including the above-mentioned $\mathrm{W_Q}$, $\mathrm{W_D}$ and $\mathrm{W_F}$, for investigating the neighborhood structures. Similar as Model 1, $\rho_{t2}\mathrm{W}y_{t2}$ measures diffusion effect of dengue incidence in epidemic period (t2). ρ_{t2} is the marginal neighboring effect during the epidemic period (t2), and ρ_{t1} is the effect during the pre-epidemic period (t1), and ε is the regression residual.

Model 3: long distance model

We used spatial Durbin models (SDM) to investigate the 2-order neighborhood effect in the pre-epidemic period as shown in Eq. 4. The 2-order neighborhood for a township refers to the neighbors of neighboring townships. In other words, the 2-order neighboring effect can capture the effect of relatively long-distance diffusion. Model 3 is the same as Model 2, except for the term $\gamma_{t1} W \left(W y_{t1} \right)$, which captures 2-order neighboring townships.

$$y_{t2} = \rho_{t2}\mathrm{W}y_{t2} + \sum_{a=1}^{6} \beta_a x_a + \rho_{t1} W y_{t1} + \gamma_{t1} W \left(W y_{t1} \right) + \varepsilon \qquad (4)$$

where β_a is the marginal effect for one urbanization type (a). W is a spatial weight matrix, including the above-mentioned $\mathrm{W_Q}$, $\mathrm{W_D}$ and $\mathrm{W_F}$, for investigating the neighborhood structures. ρ_{t2} is the marginal neighboring effect during the epidemic period (t2); ρ_{t1} is the effect during the pre-epidemic period (t1); γ_{t1} is the marginal 2-order neighboring effect during the pre-epidemic period (t1); and ε is the regression residual.

Results

Tables 2 and 3 summarize the effects of different model configurations and epidemic progression on dengue incidence in 2014 and 2015.

Our findings show consistent results for the dengue epidemics of 2014 and 2015.

Table 4 summarized the model-fitting performances (AIC values) for different settings of neighborhood structures and spatial model configurations for dengue diffusion in 2014 and 2015. It shows that Model 3 (long distance model) with structure of human mobility has the lowest AIC value. (Detailed statistical results for all of the models can be found in Additional file 1: Tables S1–S4). This finding indicates that population mobility as the neighborhood structure can better explain the relatively

Table 2 Model results of 2014 dengue epidemic using the matrix of population mobility as spatial weights

Independent variables	Model 1	Model 2	Model 3
Intercept	1.527(0.79)	1.149(0.69)	3.039***(0.75)
Spatial-lag of dengue incidence			
1st order neighbors in pre-epidemic period ρ_{t1}	1.107***(0.08)	0.671***(0.11)	− 0.002(0.17)
1st order neighbors in epidemic period ρ_{t2}	–	0.428***(0.09)	0.306**(0.10)
2nd order neighbors in pre-epidemic period γ_{t1}	–	–	1.001***(0.20)
Urbanization levels[a]			
Rural area β_1	− 0.229(0.24)	− 0.099(0.21)	0.015(0.198)
Aging society area β_2	0.641*(0.31)	0.569*(0.27)	0.384(0.25)
General area β_3	0.236(0.24)	0.26(0.21)	0.465*(0.20)
Newly developed area β_4	0.964***(0.24)	0.647**(0.22)	0.771***(0.20)
Medium-density urban area β_5	0.791*(0.30)	0.595*(0.27)	0.639*(0.24)
High-density urban area β_6	0.521(0.33)	0.313(0.29)	0.456(0.27)
Performance of model fitting			
AIC	259.54	247.11	226.01
R-square	0.72	–	–

The value in parentheses is standard error

*p value < 0.05; **p value < 0.01; ***p value < 0.001

[a] "Remote area" as reference category

Table 3 Model results of 2015 dengue epidemic using the matrix of population mobility as spatial weights

Independent variables	Model 1	Model 2	Model 3
Intercept	-3.08***(0.90)	-1.56(0.81)	-0.53(0.92)
Spatial-lag of dengue incidence			
1st order neighbors in pre-epidemic period $\rho t1$	0.50***(0.09)	0.27*(0.08)	-0.007(0.16)
1st order neighbors in epidemic period $\rho t2$	–	0.47***(0.08)	0.467***(0.08)
2nd order neighbors in pre-epidemic period $\gamma t1$	–	–	0.40*(0.19)
Urbanization levels[a]			
Rural area β_1	-0.11(0.25)	-0.10(0.21)	-0.14(0.20)
Aging society area β_2	-0.37(0.30)	-0.45(0.25)	-0.53(0.25)
General area β_3	0.42(0.24)	0.40(0.21)	0.33(0.20)
Newly developed area β_4	1.34***(0.26)	0.77**(0.24)	0.66*(0.24)
Medium-density urban area β_5	1.94***(0.32)	1.31***(0.29)	1.21***(0.29)
High-density urban area β_6	2.47***(0.33)	1.44***(0.33)	1.36***(0.32)
Performance of model fitting			
AIC	259.25	239.52	237.17
R-square	0.708	–	–

The value in parentheses is standard error

*p value < 0.05; **p value < 0.01; ***p value < 0.001

[a] "Remote area" as reference category

long-distance (2nd-order) and immediate (1st-order) neighboring dengue diffusion in different periods.

Regarding urbanization levels in the models with population mobility structures, in Tables 2 and 3, Model 3 shows areas that are newly developed, medium-density and high-density are associated with significantly higher dengue incidence relative to remote areas. Interestingly, the results of Model 3 also indicate that the dengue incidence during the epidemic period is significantly associated with 1st-order neighbors during the epidemic period (t2) and 2nd-order neighbors which are relatively distant townships compare with 1st-order neighbors during the pre-epidemic period (t1) since the coefficient of ρ_{t2} and γ_{t1} in Model 3 are significant. Our results show the spatial–temporal hierarchy of dengue diffusion: the dengue incidence in a township would be impacted by immediate neighbors during pre-epidemic and epidemic periods, and also with more distant neighbors (based on mobility) in pre-epidemic periods.

Discussion

Recent literature has indicated that one of the major driving forces of geographic expansion of dengue is human mobility on different scales, including within-city, intercity in a region, and international travels [13, 15, 16]. To quantify the effects of mobility on the spatial diffusion of dengue epidemics, previous literature replaced spatial mobility structures with geometric relationships in spatial regression models [4, 25]. However, these geometric relationships cannot fully reflect realistic spatial interactions [27, 28]. On the other hand, large-scale intercity individual mobility routes are difficult to collect, track, and access in most countries. Therefore, our study proposed a framework for model configuration to profile intercity dengue diffusion. First, we used a radiation model to construct the structure of human mobility as neighborhood weight in the spatial regression model. Second, we categorized the pre-epidemic and epidemic periods for investigating the time-lag effect on dengue

Table 4 AIC values for different settings of neighborhood structures and spatial model configurations for dengue diffusion

Neighborhood structures	2014			2015		
	Model 1	Model 2	Model 3	Model 1	Model 2	Model 3
Queen contiguity	328.4	319.7	320.6	278.0	278.1	275.7
Distance-threshold weights	256.0	254.3	255.0	270.7	268.0	269.9
Structure of human mobility	259.5	247.1	226.0	259.3	239.5	237.2

Model 1: pre-epidemic neighborhood effect model, Model 2: current neighborhood effect model, and Model 3: long distance model

diffusion. Lastly, we incorporated 2nd-order and 1st-order neighboring structures in our model to quantify relatively long-distance and immediate diffusion effects. Compared with conventional model configuration in spatial regression analysis, our proposed radiation model specification demonstrates better model fitting performance in both 2014 and 2015, which indicates that the structure of human mobility has better explanatory power in dengue diffusion than geometric relationships. The model results in the 2014 and 2015 dengue epidemics have consistent findings, indicating that intercity mobility and urbanization could be driving forces of large-scale epidemic expansion of dengue [12, 14, 17, 19].

Our findings show that highly-urbanized areas are positively associated with dengue incidence in 2014 and 2015, which is consistent with the literature, such as in [3, 4, 42]. In southern Taiwan, household plant plotting in townhouse buildings and small-area flooding water in yards after an extensive rainfall provide appropriate habitats for dengue vector mosquitoes in urbanized areas. Meanwhile, areas with high population densities could help mosquitoes bite people more easily [4]. On the other hand, female *Aedes aegypti*, a major dengue vector mosquito, are most active during the daytime, which means that there is a high frequency of biting by *A. aegypti* for people gathering in public places, which increases the risk of dengue outbreak [43–45].

Regarding geographic expansion of epidemics, our study identifies a significant neighboring diffusion effect on dengue epidemics. The dengue incidence in a township would be impacted by neighboring townships during either the pre-epidemic or epidemic period. This finding implies that the potential sources of diffusion for the township might be its neighboring townships with high dengue incidence. The result reflects the structure of human mobility as spatial interactions causing epidemic expansion [4, 25]. Moreover, the 2nd-order neighboring structure also has a significant effect on the township during the pre-epidemic period, which reflects the relatively long-distance diffusion effect. In other words, our results demonstrate a "ripple" process of dengue diffusion, which means that the immediate (first-order) neighboring effect occurs in the initial epidemic wave and that the wider geographic expansion occurs in a later epidemic wave, which is affected by the distant (second-order) neighboring effect.

Cliff et al. [46] categorized spatial diffusion patterns into three major types. Contagion results from direct contact for spreading. Relocation describes diffusion source shifts to another distant location. Hierarchy refers to transmission through an ordered sequence of settlements rather than following a distance-based neighborhood structure. Numerous studies have interpreted the epidemiological implications of these diffusion patterns [47–49]. In most cases, the structure of epidemic diffusion is often a mixture of these patterns [13, 49, 50], and relocation and hierarchical patterns cause long-distance dispersion [51]. Our proposed model has profiled possible mechanisms for these patterns. Conventional geometric relationships, such as contiguity-based and distance-threshold weighting schemes, are based on a distance-decayed structure, which could capture the characteristics of contagious diffusion. However, geometric relationships do not reflect topographic variability and long-distance interactions due to transportation. A radiation model considered in our study captures the structure of intercity interactions, reflecting patterns of human mobility. For example, in Fig. 6c, population flows from Fongshan city (high-density urbanized areas) are not only to neighboring townships, but there are also flows to other distant high-density cities in Tainan. This means that our model can capture realistic urban-to-urban interactions partially, which could cause relocation and hierarchical diffusion. Brockmann and Helbing [23] also proposed a concept of "effective distance," which replaces conventional geographic distance with the matrix of passenger flux through air traffic between cites for predicting global disease arrival times. In summary, large-scale geographic expansion of epidemic propagation is difficult to explain only by the geometric structure of administration boundaries or geographic distances of centroids between cities. Population mobility or passenger flows could more reasonably capture the structure of spatial interactions and long-distance diffusion patterns. In other words, hub cities could play a role as a "bridge" for large-scale transmission and make townships connecting to hub cities more vulnerable to dengue epidemics.

The study has some limitations. First, the mobility structure was estimated by a parameter-free radiation model, which only considers the population size of a city rather than the empirical or surveyed mobility data. Although the estimated mobility structure captures urban-to-urban interactions, we did not consider the detailed mobility behaviors of individuals or even dengue patients, such as choices of transportation modes or purposes of the trip. Further investigation on more detailed intercity mobility structure is warranted. Second, in addition to human mobility, dengue diffusion is a complex process in terms of the spatial–temporal variability in mosquito density, effectiveness of control measures, pathogen activity and host immunity [43, 52]. However, most of these factors are not available for intercity-scale studies. It is necessary to develop reliable sampling schemes for collecting these data in further investigations. Thirdly, we only used the most severe epidemics in Taiwan as case study. Although the findings are consistent in both years, it does not imply the findings still valid in other years. It would be worth to incorporate long-term longitudinal epidemic data for investigating the influence of human mobility on dengue diffusion. Our findings may suggest that, in severe epidemic years, human mobility plays a significant role in intercity dengue diffusion. Finally, the spatial heterogeneity of intercity diffusion effect should also be considered in further investigation. For example, a geographic weighted regression (GWR) can be further used to differentiate the effect of human mobility on dengue incidence in each township. Spatially-varying relationships of neighboring effects on dengue incidence could provide the heath authority for implementing better adopt specific control and prevention strategies to specific areas.

Conclusions

The study proposed a study framework for investigating relatively long-distance and immediate neighboring diffusion effects on epidemic propagation and clarified the role of intercity-scale human mobility structure and urbanization levels as driving forces in large-scale dengue transmission. Our findings suggest that the intercity mobility structure reflects urban-to-urban interactions, which causes a mixture of relocation and hierarchical diffusion patterns for large-scale dengue epidemics in southern Taiwan. This can be identified as a "ripple" process wherein an immediate neighboring effect occurs in the first stage and wider geographic expansion occurs in a later stage, which is influenced by the distant neighboring diffusion effect.

Abbreviations

AIC: Akaike information criterion; AR5: The Fifth Assessment Report; CDC: Centers of Disease Control; CDRS: call detail records; IPCC: Intergovernmental Panel on Climate Change; GPS: Global Positioning System; GWR: geographically weighted regression; OLS: ordinary least squares; SDM: spatial Durbin model; SLM: spatial lag model.

Authors' contributions

THW conceived the experiments. THW and CSH conducted the experiments and analyzed the data. THW, CSH and MCH interpreted the results and wrote the paper. All authors read and approved the final manuscript.

Author details
[1] Department of Geography, National Taiwan University, No. 1, Sec. 4, Roosevelt Road, Taipei City 10617, Taiwan. [2] Department of Bioenvironmental Systems Engineering, National Taiwan University, No. 1, Sec. 4, Roosevelt Road, Taipei City 10617, Taiwan.

Acknowledgements
None.

Competing interests
The authors declare that they have no competing interests.

Funding
The research was supported by Grants from the Ministry of Science and Technology in Taiwan (MOST 105-2627-M-002-018 and MOST 105-2410-H-002-150-MY3). The authors also acknowledge the financial support provided by the Infectious Diseases Research and Education Center, the Ministry of Health and Welfare (MOHW) and National Taiwan University (NTU) and NTU Research Center for Future Earth (NTU-107L9010). The funders had no role in the study design, data collection and analysis, or manuscript preparation.

References

1. Galvani AP, May RM. Epidemiology: dimensions of superspreading. Nature. 2005;438(7066):293.
2. Bhatt S, Gething PW, Brady OJ, Messina JP, Farlow AW, Moyes CL, Drake JM, Brownstein JS, Hoen AG, Sankoh O. The global distribution and burden of dengue. Nature. 2013;496(7446):504.
3. Qi X, Wang Y, Li Y, Meng Y, Chen Q, Ma J, Gao GF. The effects of socioeconomic and environmental factors on the incidence of dengue fever in the Pearl River Delta, China, 2013. PLoS Negl Trop Dis. 2015;9(10):e0004159.
4. Wu P-C, Lay J-G, Guo H-R, Lin C-Y, Lung S-C, Su H-J. Higher temperature and urbanization affect the spatial patterns of dengue fever transmission in subtropical Taiwan. Sci Total Environ. 2009;407(7):2224–33.
5. Åström C, Rocklöv J, Hales S, Béguin A, Louis V, Sauerborn R. Potential distribution of dengue fever under scenarios of climate change and economic development. EcoHealth. 2012;9(4):448–54.
6. Bouzid M, Colón-González FJ, Lung T, Lake IR, Hunter PR. Climate change and the emergence of vector-borne diseases in Europe: case study of dengue fever. BMC Public Health. 2014;14(1):781.
7. Hales S, De Wet N, Maindonald J, Woodward A. Potential effect of population and climate changes on global distribution of dengue fever: an empirical model. Lancet. 2002;360(9336):830–4.
8. Kutsuna S, Kato Y, Moi ML, Kotaki A, Ota M, Shinohara K, Kobayashi T, Yamamoto K, Fujiya Y, Mawatari M. Autochthonous dengue fever, Tokyo, Japan, 2014. Emerg Infect Dis. 2015;21(3):517.
9. Patz JA, Martens W, Focks DA, Jetten TH. Dengue fever epidemic potential as projected by general circulation models of global climate change. Environ Health Perspect. 1998;106(3):147.
10. Stocker TF, Qin D, Plattner G-K, Tignor M, Allen SK, Boschung J, Nauels A, Xia Y, Bex V, Midgley PM: Climate change 2013: the physical science basis. In: Contribution of working group I to the fifth assessment report of the intergovernmental panel on climate change. Cambridge University Press, Cambridge; 2013.
11. Sutherst RW. Global change and human vulnerability to vector-borne diseases. Clin Microbiol Rev. 2004;17(1):136–73.
12. Thai KT, Anders KL. The role of climate variability and change in the transmission dynamics and geographic distribution of dengue. Exp Biol Med. 2011;236(8):944–54.
13. Kan C-C, Lee P-F, Wen T-H, Chao D-Y, Wu M-H, Lin NH, Huang SY-J, Shang C-S, Fan I-C, Shu P-Y. Two clustering diffusion patterns identified from the 2001–2003 dengue epidemic, Kaohsiung, Taiwan. Am J Trop Med Hyg. 2008;79(3):344–52.
14. Itoda I, Masuda G, Suganuma A, Imamura A, Ajisawa A, Yamada K-I, Yabe S, Takasaki T, Kurane I, Totsuka K. Clinical features of 62 imported cases of dengue fever in Japan. Am J Trop Med Hyg. 2006;75(3):470–4.
15. Stoddard ST, Forshey BM, Morrison AC, Paz-Soldan VA, Vazquez-Prokopec GM, Astete H, Reiner RC, Vilcarromero S, Elder JP, Halsey ES. House-to-house human movement drives dengue virus transmission. Proc Natl Acad Sci. 2013;110(3):994–9.
16. Wesolowski A, Qureshi T, Boni MF, Sundsøy PR, Johansson MA, Rasheed SB, Engø-Monsen K, Buckee CO. Impact of human mobility on the emergence of dengue epidemics in Pakistan. Proc Natl Acad Sci. 2015;112(38):11887–92.
17. Wesolowski A, Eagle N, Tatem AJ, Smith DL, Noor AM, Snow RW, Buckee CO. Quantifying the impact of human mobility on malaria. Science. 2012;338(6104):267–70.

18. Shang C-S, Fang C-T, Liu C-M, Wen T-H, Tsai K-H, King C-C. The role of imported cases and favorable meteorological conditions in the onset of dengue epidemics. PLoS Negl Trop Dis. 2010;4(8):e775.

19. Wen T-H, Lin M-H, Fang C-T. Population movement and vector-borne disease transmission: differentiating spatial–temporal diffusion patterns of commuting and noncommuting dengue cases. Ann Assoc Am Geogr. 2012;102(5):1026–37.

20. Vazquez-Prokopec GM, Stoddard ST, Paz-Soldan V, Morrison AC, Elder JP, Kochel TJ, Scott TW, Kitron U. Usefulness of commercially available GPS data-loggers for tracking human movement and exposure to dengue virus. Int J Health Geogr. 2009;8(1):68.

21. de Castro Medeiros LC, Castilho CAR, Braga C, de Souza WV, Regis L, Monteiro AMV. Modeling the dynamic transmission of dengue fever: investigating disease persistence. PLOS Negl Trop Dis. 2011;5(1):e942.

22. Barmak DH, Dorso CO, Otero M, Solari HG. Dengue epidemics and human mobility. Phys Rev E. 2011;84(1):011901.

23. Brockmann D, Helbing D. The hidden geometry of complex, network-driven contagion phenomena. Science. 2013;342(6164):1337–42.

24. Gardner LM, Sarkar S. Risk of dengue spread from the Philippines through international air travel. Transp Res Rec J Transp Res Board. 2015;2501:25–30.

25. Tipayamongkholgul M, Lisakulruk S. Socio-geographical factors in vulnerability to dengue in Thai villages: a spatial regression analysis. Geospat Health. 2011;5(2):191–8.

26. Almeida ASD, Medronho RDA, Valencia LIO. Spatial analysis of dengue and the socioeconomic context of the city of Rio de Janeiro (Southeastern Brazil). Rev Saude Publica. 2009;43(4):666–73.

27. Chi Y, Jhou M, Hsieh Y. Spatial analysis of foreign brides in Taiwan. J Popul Stud. 2009;38(3):67–113.

28. Rincke J. A commuting-based refinement of the contiguity matrix for spatial models, and an application to local police expenditures. Reg Sci Urban Econ. 2010;40(5):324–30.

29. Tizzoni M, Bajardi P, Decuyper A, King GKK, Schneider CM, Blondel V, Smoreda Z, González MC, Colizza V. On the use of human mobility proxies for modeling epidemics. PLoS Comput Biol. 2014;10(7):e1003716.

30. Vazquez-Prokopec GM, Bisanzio D, Stoddard ST, Paz-Soldan V, Morrison AC, Elder JP, Ramirez-Paredes J, Halsey ES, Kochel TJ, Scott TW. Using GPS technology to quantify human mobility, dynamic contacts and infectious disease dynamics in a resource-poor urban environment. PLoS ONE. 2013;8(4):e58802.

31. de Dios OrtÃozar J, Willumsen LG. Modelling transport. New York: Wiley; 2011.

32. Simini F, González MC, Maritan A, Barabási A-L. A universal model for mobility and migration patterns. Nature. 2012;484(7392):96.

33. Corbel V, Nosten F, Thanispong K, Luxemburger C, Kongmee M, Chareon-viriyaphap T. Challenges and prospects for dengue and malaria control in Thailand, Southeast Asia. Trends Parasitol. 2013;29(12):623–33.

34. World Health Organization (WHO) Regional Office for South-East Asia. Comprehensive guidelines for prevention and control of dengue and

dengue haemorrhagic fever: Revised and expanded edition. New Delhi: WHO; 2011.

35. Shepard DS, Undurraga EA, Halasa YA. Economic and disease burden of dengue in Southeast Asia. PLoS Negl Trop Dis. 2013;7(2):e2055.

36. Undurraga EA, Halasa YA, Shepard DS. Use of expansion factors to estimate the burden of dengue in Southeast Asia: a systematic analysis. PLoS Negl Trop Dis. 2013;7(2):e2056.

37. Liu C-Y, Hung Y, Chuang Y, Chen Y, Weng W, Liu J, Liang K. Incorporating development stratification of Taiwan townships into sampling design of large scale health interview survey. J Health Manag. 2006;4(1):1–22.

38. King C-C, Wu Y-C, Chao D-Y, Lin T-H, Chow L, Wang H-T, Ku C-C, Kao C-L, Chien L-J, Chang H-J. Major epidemics of dengue in Taiwan in 1981–2000: related to intensive virus activities in Asia. Dengue Bull. 2000;24:1–10.

39. Lin K, Su C, Chang C, Leu H, Chang S, Yang Y. The demand model of intercity transportation systems under national sustainable development in Taiwan (2/4). Taipei: Ministry of Transportation and Communications, Institute of Transportation; 2006.

40. Abreu M, de Groot HL, Florax RJ. Spatial patterns of technology diffusion: an empirical analysis using TFP, Discussion Paper No. 04079/3. Amsterdam-Rotterdam: Tinbergen Institute; 2004.

41. Ng I-C, Wen T-H, Wang J-Y, Fang C-T. Spatial dependency of tuberculosis incidence in Taiwan. PLoS ONE. 2012;7(11):e50740.

42. Vallée J, Dubot-Pérès A, Ounaphom P, Sayavong C, Bryant JE, Gonzalez JP. Spatial distribution and risk factors of dengue and Japanese encephalitis virus infection in urban settings: the case of Vientiane, Lao PDR. Trop Med Int Health. 2009;14(9):1134–42.

43. Chadee D, Shivnauth B, Rawlins S, Chen A. Climate, mosquito indices and the epidemiology of dengue fever in Trinidad (2002–2004). Ann Trop Med Parasitol. 2007;101(1):69–77.

44. Gubler DJ. Dengue and dengue hemorrhagic fever. Clin Microbiol Rev. 1998;11(3):480–96.

45. Wen T-H, Lin M-H, Teng H-J, Chang N-T. Incorporating the human-Aedes mosquito interactions into measuring the spatial risk of urban dengue fever. Appl Geogr. 2015;62:256–66.

46. Cliff AD. Spatial diffusion: an historical geography of epidemics in an island community, vol. 14. Cambridge: CUP Archive; 1981.

47. Cohen J, Tita G. Diffusion in homicide: exploring a general method for detecting spatial diffusion processes. J Quant Criminol. 1999;15(4):451–93.

48. Meade MS, Emch M. Medical geography. New York: Guilford Press; 2010.

49. Hsueh Y-H, Lee J, Beltz L. Spatio-temporal patterns of dengue fever cases in Kaoshiung City, Taiwan, 2003–2008. Appl Geogr. 2012;34:587–94.

50. Ruan S, Wang W, Levin SA. The effect of global travel on the spread of SARS. Math Biosci Eng. 2006;3(1):205.

51. Yang Y, Atkinson PM. Individual space–time activity-based model: a model for the simulation of airborne infectious-disease transmission by activity-bundle simulation. Environ Plan. 2008;35(1):80–99.

52. Sanchez L, Vanlerberghe V, Alfonso L, del Carmen Marquetti M, Guzman MG, Bisset J, Van Der Stuyft P. Aedes aegypti larval indices and risk for dengue epidemics. Emerg Infect Dis. 2006;12(5):800.

8

Mapping outdoor habitat and abnormally small newborns to develop an ambient health hazard index

Charlene C. Nielsen[1,2], Carl G. Amrhein[1], Alvaro R. Osornio-Vargas[2]* and the DoMiNO Team[1,2]

Abstract

Background: The geography of where pregnant mothers live is important for understanding outdoor environmental habitat that may result in adverse birth outcomes. We investigated whether more babies were born small for gestational age or low birth weight at term to mothers living in environments with a higher accumulation of outdoor hazards.

Methods: Live singleton births from the Alberta Perinatal Health Program, 2006–2012, were classified according to birth outcome, and used in a double kernel density estimation to determine ratios of each outcome per total births. Individual and overlay indices of spatial models of 136 air emissions and 18 land variables were correlated with the small for gestational age and low birth weight at term, for the entire province and sub-provincially.

Results: There were 24 air substances and land sources correlated with both small for gestational age and low birth weight at term density ratios. On the provincial scale, there were 13 air substances and 2 land factors; sub-provincial analysis found 8 additional air substances and 1 land source.

Conclusion: This study used a combination of multiple outdoor variables over a large geographic area in an objective model, which may be repeated over time or in other study areas. The air substance-weighted index best identified where mothers having abnormally small newborns lived within areas of potential outdoor hazards. However, individual air substances and the weighted index provide complementary information.

Keywords: Small for gestational age, Low birth weight at term, Pollution, GIS, Index

Background

A truly ecologically-based study of health integrates habitat, population, and behavior—encompassing a more complete geography as framed by Meade's triangle of human ecology [1, 2]. Three vertices conceptualize what is known about an important pediatric topic: maternal exposure to outdoor pollution and neonatal outcomes (Fig. 1). Here we focus on the lesser studied habitat vertex, specifically the outdoor environment, since less attention is traditionally given to incorporating ecological factors in understanding disease [1]. The location aspect

of habitat—where pregnant women live, where industry and services are situated, where demographic groups congregate—is important because where one lives and where one starts out in life, even during fetal development, ultimately influences lifelong health [3–6].

Toxicant exposures and environmental influences on mothers during crucial stages of pregnancy may result in newborns that are too small or born too early. Adverse birth outcomes (ABO) are important markers of infant survival, development and future health. Our research focuses on being born too small, clinically defined as Small for Gestational Age (SGA) when newborns are below the 10th percentile weight based on sex and weeks of pregnancy, or Low Birth Weight at Term (LBWT) when newborns are less than 2500 g weight at term, 37 or more weeks gestation [7].

*Correspondence: osornio@ualberta.ca
[2] Department of Pediatrics, University of Alberta, 3-591 ECHA, 11,405 87th Avenue, Edmonton, AB T6G 1C9, Canada
Full list of author information is available at the end of the article

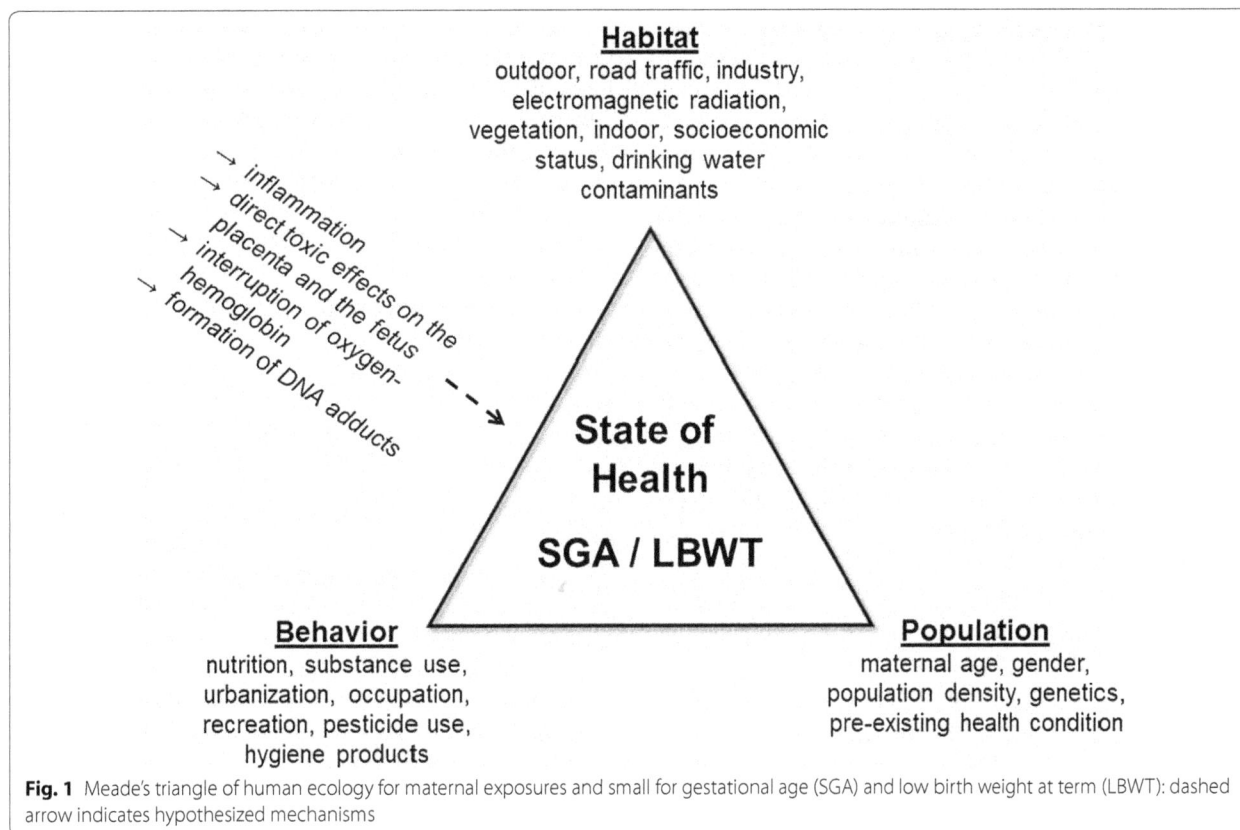

Fig. 1 Meade's triangle of human ecology for maternal exposures and small for gestational age (SGA) and low birth weight at term (LBWT): dashed arrow indicates hypothesized mechanisms

The province of Alberta, Canada, had a population of 3,645,257 at the 2011 Census [8]. That was a 10.8% increase from 2006 while the national average increase was 5.9%. For a land area of 640,082 km^2, the population density was 5.7 persons/km^2, where 83% of the population lived in or near urban centers. Alberta's economic activities were focused on agriculture, natural resources, and nonrenewable energy—having a higher number of industrial facilities reporting to the National Pollutant Release Inventory (NPRI) than any other province or territory [9]. The NPRI is a valuable data source on industrial-based pollutants [10]. Alberta also has higher ABOs: SGA was 8.8% (Canada was 8.4%); and low birth weight for all gestational ages was 6.7% (Canada was 6.0%) [11]. Alberta rates also increased during 2000–2014: SGA from 10 to 11.5%; and low birth weight for all gestational ages from 6.1 to 6.7% [12].

ABO complications include death, physical and cognitive disabilities, and chronic health problems later in life, costing emotional stress and the majority of the health care expenses among all newborns [13]. Disorders related to short gestation and low birth weight are consistently ranked as the 2nd leading cause of infant death (congenital deformation is the leading cause) [14]—and have increased in Canada since the year 2000 [11, 12].

Abnormally small newborns are the result of growth restriction, which may be due to environmental pollutants thought to cause inflammation in mothers, direct toxic effects on the placenta and the fetus, interruption of oxygen-hemoglobin, or DNA damage represented by the formation of DNA adducts [15, 16].

The environment includes social, built, and natural features. Individual risks are also very important to ABOs, but are neither readily available nor easily mapped. These include personal, behavioral, social, and indoor exposures, such as: adequate prenatal care; food type and contaminants; rest, stress, and pre-existing health conditions; occupation and socioeconomic status; smoking and other substance use; drinking water contaminants. Our focus is on the outdoor environmental habitat because it is a common source of shared exposures susceptible to regulation (biology and behavior are not). These include air, water, human-constructed, and natural outdoor hazards, such as: industrial emissions; traffic pollution; agricultural chemical inputs of pesticides, herbicides, and fertilizers; electromagnetic radiation; proximity to oil and gas extraction activities; wildfire smoke.

Environmental health research has found many environmental factors to be associated with various health outcomes [17–25]. However, these are typically explored singly: one exposure or category of exposure at a time. A unified environmental measure may be constructed across multiple variables to encompass the complex nature of the overall environment.

Environmental indices have history: Inhaber had proposed an integrated national index for Canada in the 1970s [26]. Rather than relying on individual pollutants to reflect the state-of-the-environment, Inhaber mathematically combined such indicators for the purpose of resource allocation, ranking of locations, enforcement of standards, trend analysis, public information, or scientific research [27]. Under that premise, Messer et al. [28] developed a California county-level environmental quality index using principal components analysis (PCA) to calculate 5 environmental domains (air, water, land, built, and sociodemographic), which were then combined into a single index using PCA on the first components, and stratified by rural–urban continuum codes. Similarly, Messer et al.'s CalEnviroScreen 2.0 [29, 30] superimposed 19 individual indicators that related to pollution exposures, environmental conditions, and population characteristics, weighted and summed each set of indicators, and then multiplied together pollution and population (i.e. Threat × Vulnerability = Risk). We have not found similar environmental health indices available for Canada, or the province of Alberta, and especially none focused primarily on maternal exposures associated with ABO.

Using a Geographical Information System (GIS), we developed a simplified and reproducible index for Alberta by estimating and aggregating pollutants from communal outdoor factors. GIS supports the inclusion of diverse data and enables modelling of hazard-exposure-dose–response processes in space [31, 32]. To capture the relevant pollutant estimates, spatially and temporally appropriate GIS data files were overlaid to develop a vulnerability map of combined disparate (in theme and measurement units) environmental factors, similar to Messer et al. [28, 29]. The index will aid our examination of maternal ambient health hazards and abnormally small newborns by providing a relative ranking of locations across the province that are not limited by administrative boundaries.

Our research is part of the Data Mining and Neonatal Outcomes (DoMiNO) project that is exploring the collocation of adverse birth outcomes and environmental variables in Canada [33]. For our geographical perspective on the project we hypothesized that SGA or LBWT babies are more likely to be born to mothers living in environments with a higher number of outdoor hazards (especially pollutants) than in relatively healthier habitats with fewer exposure hazards. Our objective was to examine how the separate and combined exposures to

the outdoor built-up, natural, and social environments of pregnant mothers coincided with patterns in adverse birth outcomes (ABO). We also expected that the large Alberta province would have regional variations in the outdoor environment and investigated this effect on the associations.

Methods
GIS parameters
We used Esri's ArcGIS Desktop 10.5 software to perform all spatial database processing, management, distribution analyses, hazard estimations, and index calculations [34]. Proximity was extremely important in our spatial analysis; therefore, we customized an Alberta-focused map projection, based on the following parameters: name Azimuthal Equidistant; central meridian − 113.5; latitude of origin 53.5; linear unit meter (1.0); and geographic coordinate system (GCS) datum North American 1983 (NAD 1983). We projected all GIS data to this distance-preserving spatial reference.

For raster files we used a 250 m by 250 m cell size to reasonably represent both urban and rural areas in the very large study area, and to match the coarsest dataset: MODIS Terra satellite [35].

Because Alberta is landlocked, we included data features within 50 km surrounding the provincial boundary where available: by doing so, any potential pollutant source close to the outer edge of the province was included.

Regional attribution
We produced sub-provincial maps of the percent ratios for each ABO to facilitate comparisons more meaningful to health care and environmental management. We assigned administrative attributes to postal code locations. This allowed grouping by health region [36] or airshed zone [37] because both are health-related administrative boundaries that help identify where there may be different outdoor factors of importance.

Health regions are designated by the provincial Ministry of Health to identify geographic areas where hospital boards or regional health authorities administer and deliver public health care, and are subject to change [38]. At the start of our study period, there were 9 health regions for Alberta (Table 2): Chinook Regional Health Authority (4821); Palliser Health Region (4822); Calgary Health Region (4823); David Thompson Regional Health Authority (4824); East Central Health (4825); Capital Health (4826); Aspen Regional Health Authority (4827); Peace Country Health (4828); and Northern Lights Health Region (4829).

Airshed zones are endorsed by the multi-stakeholder Clean Air Strategic Alliance (CASA) to identify geographic areas where the air quality is similar in emission sources, volumes, impacts, dispersion and administrative characteristics [39]. Because Alberta has several unique topographical, meteorological, or ecological conditions for resolving air quality, there are 9 airsheds currently recognized (Table 2): Alberta Capital Airshed Alliance (ACAA); Calgary Region Airshed Zone (CRAZ); Fort Air Partnership (FAP); Lakeland Industry and Community Association (LICA); Palliser Airshed Society (PAS); Parkland Airshed Management Zone (PAMZ); Peace Airshed Zone Association (PASZA); West Central Airshed Society (WCAS); and Wood Buffalo Environmental Association (WBEA). It is important to note that the entire province is not monitored by airshed zones, with the southwest corner, east-central, and majority of the north having no airshed (NA).

Dependent variables

The Alberta Perinatal Health Program (APHP) provided anonymized data for the province of Alberta, from 2006 to 2012 [40]. We obtained ethics approval from the Research Ethics Board at the University of Alberta and the APHP.

We selected for live single births between 22 and 42 weeks gestation, and geocoded them to the centroid of the 6-character postal code of the mothers' residences at the time of the birth registration. DMTI Spatial's Platinum Postal Code Suite [41] provided the longitude and latitude coordinates for the years 2001–2013, which we uniquely selected to guarantee static locations through the entire study period. 95% of the original data had valid coordinates for use in spatial analyses. Using the previous definitions, we classified the birth records as binary variables identifying SGA or LBWT. Details are available in Serrano et al. [42].

To eliminate the confines of arbitrary administrative boundaries, we followed the double kernel density (DKD) method [43–48] to calculate distributions of SGA and LBWT, normalized by all births. DKD involves kernel density estimation—a non-parametric method that spreads point values across a surface by calculating the magnitude-per-unit area from points (representing the counts of birth events), fitted to a smoothly tapered function that spreads the values within a specified distance (25 km for this study) around each point [49]. Points within the radius that are further from the center are weighted lower than those closer, and helps indicate "hot spots". Dividing each ABO by the kernel density of total births yielded ratios of the birth outcome that also masked locations of the residences, helping protect privacy.

Independent variables

Personal maternal monitoring data were not available for this retrospective study. We used landscape features as spatial proxies of exposure hazards, as done in previously published research [32]. In total, we chose 18 outdoor sources, identified in published studies [17–23] or added for novel exploration (10 built; 5 social; 3 natural) plus 136 industrial air substance emissions. Table 1 lists the environmental variables and indicates specific characteristics and processing details.

We applied kernel density to spread industrial emissions from the NPRI database as tonnes per area within a 10 km radius (based on distances determined from the project's data mining algorithm [33]). We used the count of other point features—industrial facilities, gas stations, waste/landfills, oil/gas well pads, food stores, and health care/hospitals—in kernel density to calculate the number per area within a 3-km radius. We also applied kernel density to roads and electrical power lines to calculate length per area within a 3-km radius. A main advantage of using kernel density is it accounts for distance decay (features have less influence further away). When linear features are the input it also helps to approximate the number of intersections—important when analyzing pollution sources from roads because vehicles idle at intersections.

For areal features, we used focal statistics, also known as moving-window or neighborhood analyses, on binary surfaces of feedlots, mine sites, cultivated lands, aboriginal lands, water/blue space, and wildfires. The mean statistic on binary values of 1, indicating presence of the feature, and 0, indicating absence, yielded proportions. For vegetation/naturalness, the mean statistic returned the mean Normalized Difference Vegetation Index (NDVI), where higher values identify more chlorophyll-producing healthy green vegetation captured by the satellite imagery pixels. Except for the 50-km wildfire radius, all others had a 3-km radius. We accepted the original values for the coarser resolution nighttime lights and area-based, neighborhood-level socioeconomic index.

Spearman's rank correlation

We joined values from the DKD distributions and each independent variable surface extracted to unique postal codes where births occurred. Our data were non-normally distributed due to many zero values in both the dependent and independent variables. We used Python 2.7 software [50] with the pandas 0.16 site package [51] to calculate Spearman's rank correlations among ABO and each environmental variable. To test the association of the combined environmental factors, we calculated a second set of Spearman's rank correlations using DKD

Table 1 Outdoor environmental factors mapped for association with adverse birth outcomes

Category	Variable	Year	Feature	Method	Radius (km)	Units	Source
Built	136 air substances	Average 2006–2012	Point	Kernel density	10	tonnes or kg/km^2	EnvCan [9]
	Industrial facilities	Unique 2006–2012	Point		3	#/km^2	
	Roads	2012	Line			km/km^2	StatsCan [69]
	Electrical power lines	2012	Line			km/km^2	AltaLIS [70]
	Gas stations	2015	Point			#/km^2	DMTI Spatial [41]
	Waste/landfills	2015	Point			#/km^2	
	Oil/gas well pads	2012	Point			#/km^2	ABMI [71]
	High density livestock operations	2012	Area	Focal statistics		#/km^2	
	Mine sites	2012	Area			km^2/km^2	
	Cultivated lands	2012	Area			km^2/km^2	
	Nighttime lights	Average 2006–2012	Raster	None	0	index	NOAA [72]
Social	Food stores	2015	Point	Kernel density	3	#/km^2	DMTI Spatial [41]
	Health care	2015	Point			#/km^2	
	Hospitals	2015	Point			#/km^2	
	Aboriginal lands	2016	Area	Focal statistics		km^2/km^2	NRCan [73]
	Neighborhood socioeconomic index	2006	Raster	None	0	index	Chan [74]
Natural	Vegetation/naturalness	Maximum 2006–2012	Raster	Focal statistics	3	index/km^2	NASA [35]
	Water	2013	Area			km^2/km^2	NRCan [73]
	Wildfires	Average 2006–2012	Area		50	km^2/km^2	AgFor [75]

The time (year), distance threshold (radius in meters), units, and source are indicated for each

values to test the indices. Correlation was calculated for the entire province and aggregated by sub-provincial unit.

Overlay analysis

Overlay analysis is a simple and reproducible method to combine several inputs into a single output [52]. It is most common for optimal site selection and suitability modeling, especially for mapping habitat. The class values represent rankings from higher to lower suitability or risk. In our study, we applied it to essentially map "reverse suitability" to identify maternal ambient health hazards.

Because the values of continuous surfaces varied in measurement units, we standardized them into a similar ratio scale by reclassifying the environmental variables into five standard classes using quintiles. The ordering of the reclassification corresponded with the direction of the correlation: most were straightforward but if the variable was negatively correlated then the reclassification was applied in a backwards fashion; e.g. vegetation, water, and socioeconomic status classes were ranked 5–1 because lower original values were considered to be more hazardous. We calculated the sub-indices as weighted sum overlays with equal weightings on air substances and land-based sources separately, which were then overlaid together. We were interested in preserving the combined

effects of the industrial air substances; therefore, in addition to an equal weighted sum of both, we also approximated a conservative two-thirds (0.7) weighting to the air substances summed with a one-third (0.3) weighting of the land-based sources. In the two different indices—Overlay Equal and Overlay 0.7/0.3—the class rankings were accumulations that represent where the study area had more environmental hazards.

Overall, the reverse suitability indices were calculated by modeling each individual pollutant surface using distance-centered analyses (i.e. kernel densities and focal statistics), reclassified into quintiles of class rankings, and overlaid as weighted sums. The detailed GIS methods for the map-based calculations of all the independent variables and subsequent indices are specified in Table 1 (i.e. features, methods, and radii) and shown graphically in Fig. 2.

Results

Spatial distribution of adverse birth outcomes

Table 2 shows raw counts of births, SGA, and LBWT, based on valid postal codes. For 2006–2012, the entire province of Alberta had 333,247 births with a valid spatial location (95% of total registered), allocated to 53,399 postal codes. 29,679 geocoded births were classified as SGA (8.9%) and 5485 were classified as LBWT at term (1.6%).

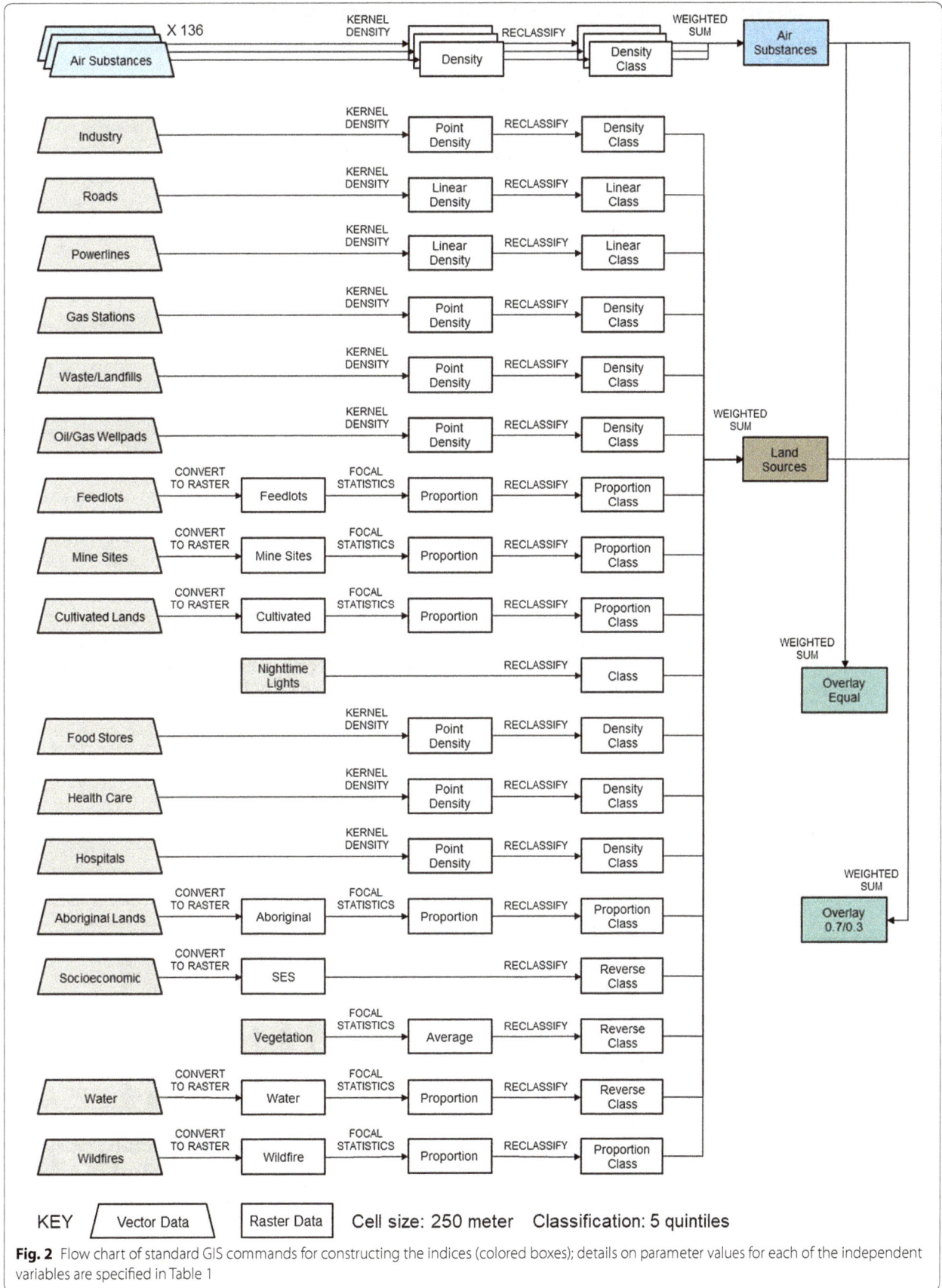

Fig. 2 Flow chart of standard GIS commands for constructing the indices (colored boxes); details on parameter values for each of the independent variables are specified in Table 1

Table 2 Alberta's sub-provincial units and descriptive statistics, in descending order of birth number

Unit	Map code	Name	Area (km²)	Postal codes	Geolocated births	SGA	LBWT
Province	none	Alberta	663,563	53,399	333,247	29,679	5485
Health Region	4823	Calgary Health Region	39,350	20,537	121,965	12,543	2339
	4826	Capital Health	11,883	20,004	99,691	8596	1566
	4824	David Thompson Regional Health Authority	61,578	3325	29,766	2394	476
	4827	Aspen Regional Health Authority	137,639	1440	18,004	1252	222
	4821	Chinook Regional Health Authority	26,062	2406	16,639	1342	233
	4828	Peace Country Health	123,870	1580	16,428	1188	215
	4829	Northern Lights Health Region	189,696	1073	11,097	808	147
	4822	Palliser Health Region	39,772	1723	9920	858	147
	4825	East Central Health	33,812	1311	9737	698	140
Airshed Zone	CRAZ	Calgary Regional Airshed Zone	32,372	20,530	120,392	12,409	2310
	ACAA	Alberta Capital Airshed Alliance	4933	19,474	95,085	8284	1503
	NA	No Airshed Zone	362,439	4867	47,527	3509	647
	PAMZ	Parkland Airshed Management Zone	40,936	2774	24,896	1978	387
	PASZA	Peace Airshed Zone Association	45,892	1409	12,475	927	175
	PAS	Palliser Airshed Society	39,900	1723	9920	858	147
	WBEA	Wood Buffalo Environmental Association	69,214	1061	7540	627	115
	WCAS	West Central Airshed Society	47,142	612	7386	559	107
	LICA	Lakeland Industrial Community Association	16,215	455	4479	293	43
	FAP	Fort Air Partnership	4519	494	3547	235	51

Figure 3 depicts the percentages of ABO for each sub-provincial unit relative to Alberta (marked by *). For health regions, SGA ranged from 7.0 to 10.3% and LBWT ranged from 1.2 to 1.9%. Health region 4823 had the highest number of births (n = 121,965), highest SGA (n = 12,543, 10.3%), and highest LBWT (n = 2339, 1.9%); 4825 had the lowest number of births (n = 9737), SGA (n = 698, 7.2%), and LBWT (n = 140, 1.4%); but 4827 had

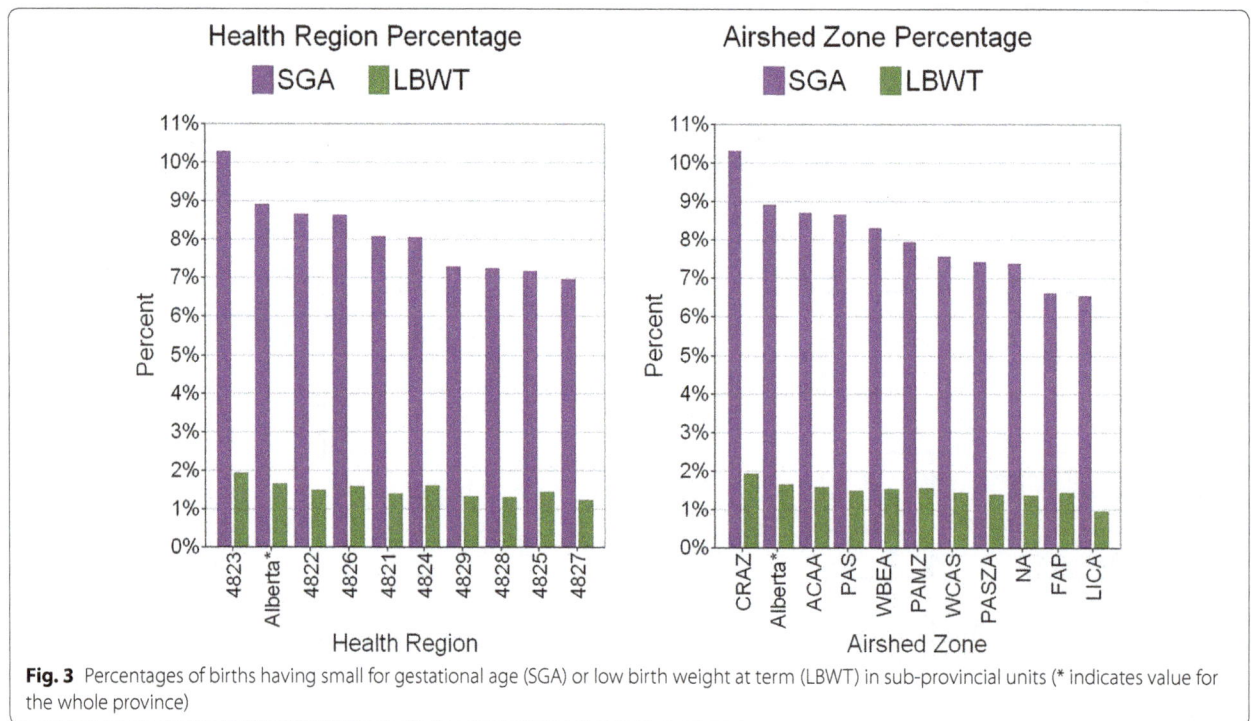

Fig. 3 Percentages of births having small for gestational age (SGA) or low birth weight at term (LBWT) in sub-provincial units (* indicates value for the whole province)

the lowest SGA (n = 1252, 7.0%) and LBWT (n = 222, 1.2%). For airshed zones, SGA ranged from 6.5 to 10.3% and LBWT ranged from 1.0 to 1.9%. Airshed zone CRAZ had the highest number of births (n = 120,392), SGA (n = 12,409, 10.3%), and LBWT (n = 2310, 1.9%); FAP had the lowest number of births (n = 3.547) and LICA had the lowest SGA (n = 293, 6.5%) and lowest LBWT (n = 43, 1.0%).

The distributions of births per area in Fig. 4 show higher concentrations of more than 3 births per km^2 in the sub-provincial units containing the major cities of Edmonton and Calgary, with medium densities in the adjacent units and in the airshed zones containing Grande Prairie (west-central) and Cold Lake (east-central).

The patterns differ by sub-provincial unit for ABOs mapped as numbers per births (Fig. 5). SGA is highest in the units containing Edmonton and along the west–east Banff–Calgary-Brooks corridor. Health regions have medium SGA adjacent to the high SGA. Airsheds also show medium SGA in the west and north-east. LBWT is highest in the north–south Edmonton-Red Deer-Calgary corridor. Medium LBWT is adjacent to the higher units, except for the northern health regions containing Grande

Prairie-Peace River and Fort McMurray-Fox Lake. The lower LBWT in the central health region 4827 separates the province; LBWT in the airshed containing Cold Lake is the lowest in the province.

Figure 6 maps the results of the DKD method for each ABO. Both ABOs cover the same areas of the province and the darker colors indicate higher values for SGA (purple) and LBWT (green). The result of DKD is a continuous value, but the maps classified with tertiles visually enhance the slightly different distributions for SGA and LBWT: urban (Edmonton and Calgary) areas shared highest values for both ABO; central areas had more LBWT; and southeast areas had more SGA.

Hazard mapping

The Spearman's rank correlation values were sorted in descending order for each of the independent variables (Table 3). Provincially, variables having correlations greater than 0.40 (low value accepted since data were not adjusted for epidemiological factors because they were not available for mapping) with SGA were: i-Butyl alcohol (rho = 0.56); Asbestos; Nighttime Light; Toluenediisocyanate; Toluene-2,4-diisocyanate;

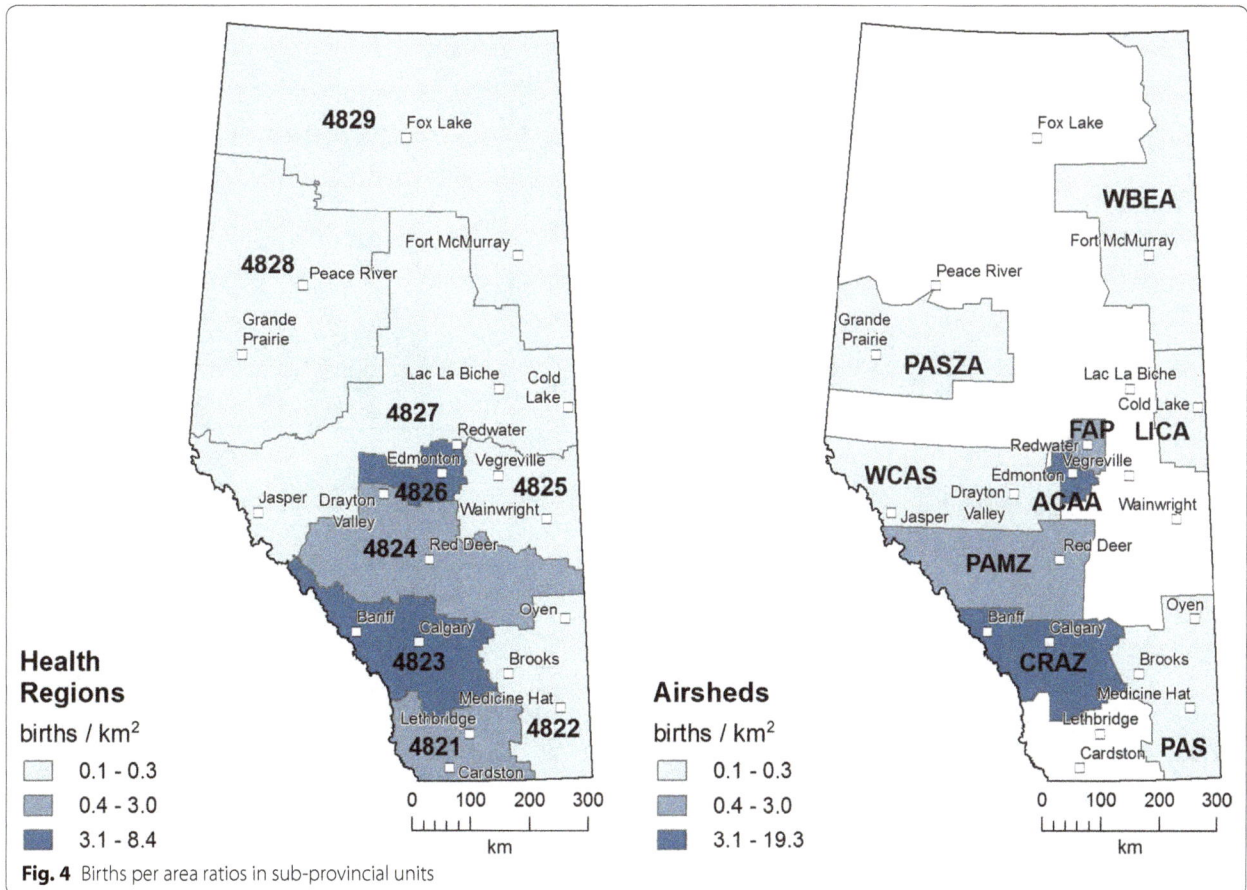

Fig. 4 Births per area ratios in sub-provincial units

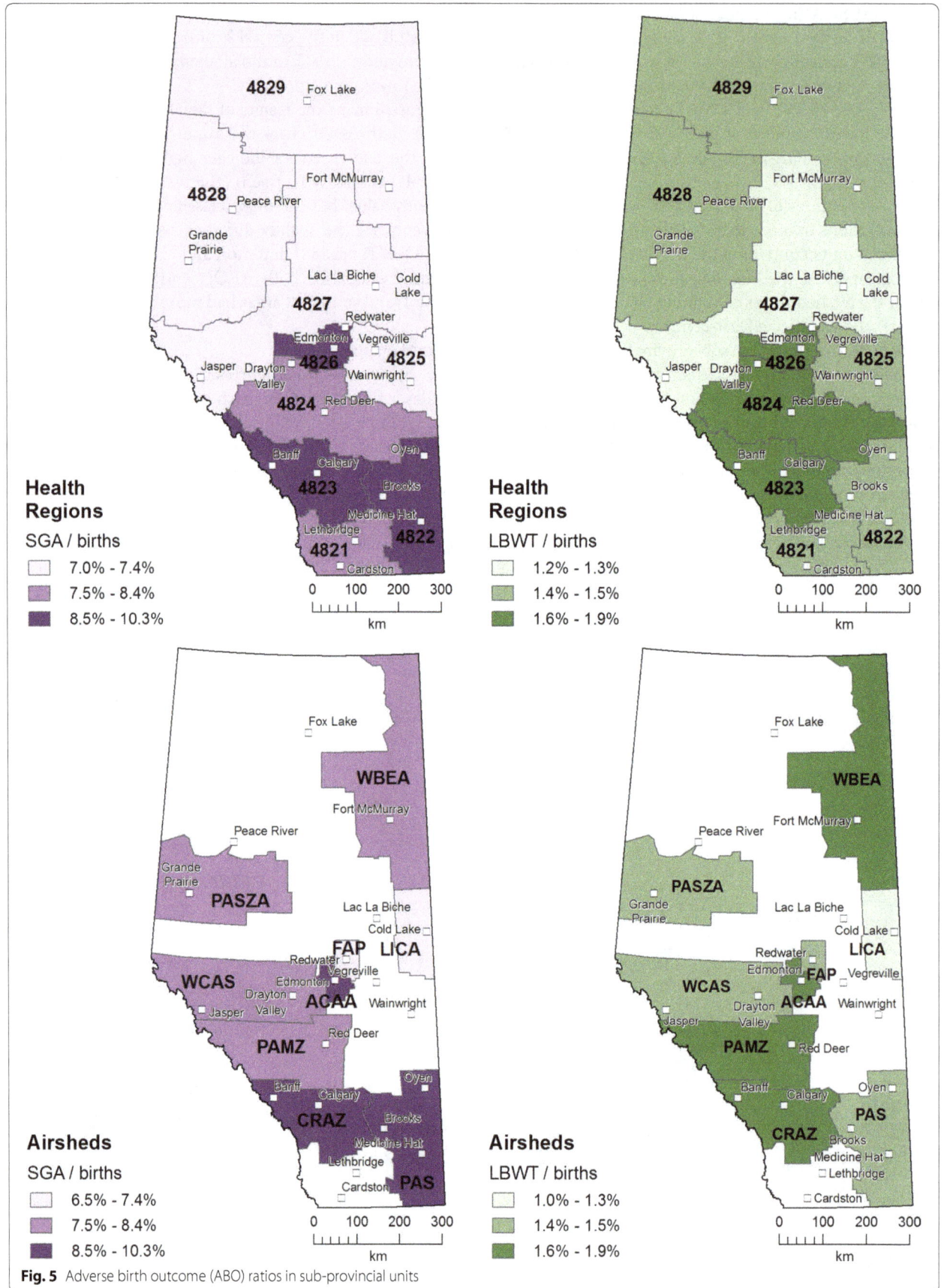

Health Regions

SGA / births
- ☐ 7.0% - 7.4%
- ☐ 7.5% - 8.4%
- ☐ 8.5% - 10.3%

Health Regions

LBWT / births
- ☐ 1.2% - 1.3%
- ☐ 1.4% - 1.5%
- ☐ 1.6% - 1.9%

Airsheds

SGA / births
- ☐ 6.5% - 7.4%
- ☐ 7.5% - 8.4%
- ☐ 8.5% - 10.3%

Airsheds

LBWT / births
- ☐ 1.0% - 1.3%
- ☐ 1.4% - 1.5%
- ☐ 1.6% - 1.9%

Fig. 5 Adverse birth outcome (ABO) ratios in sub-provincial units

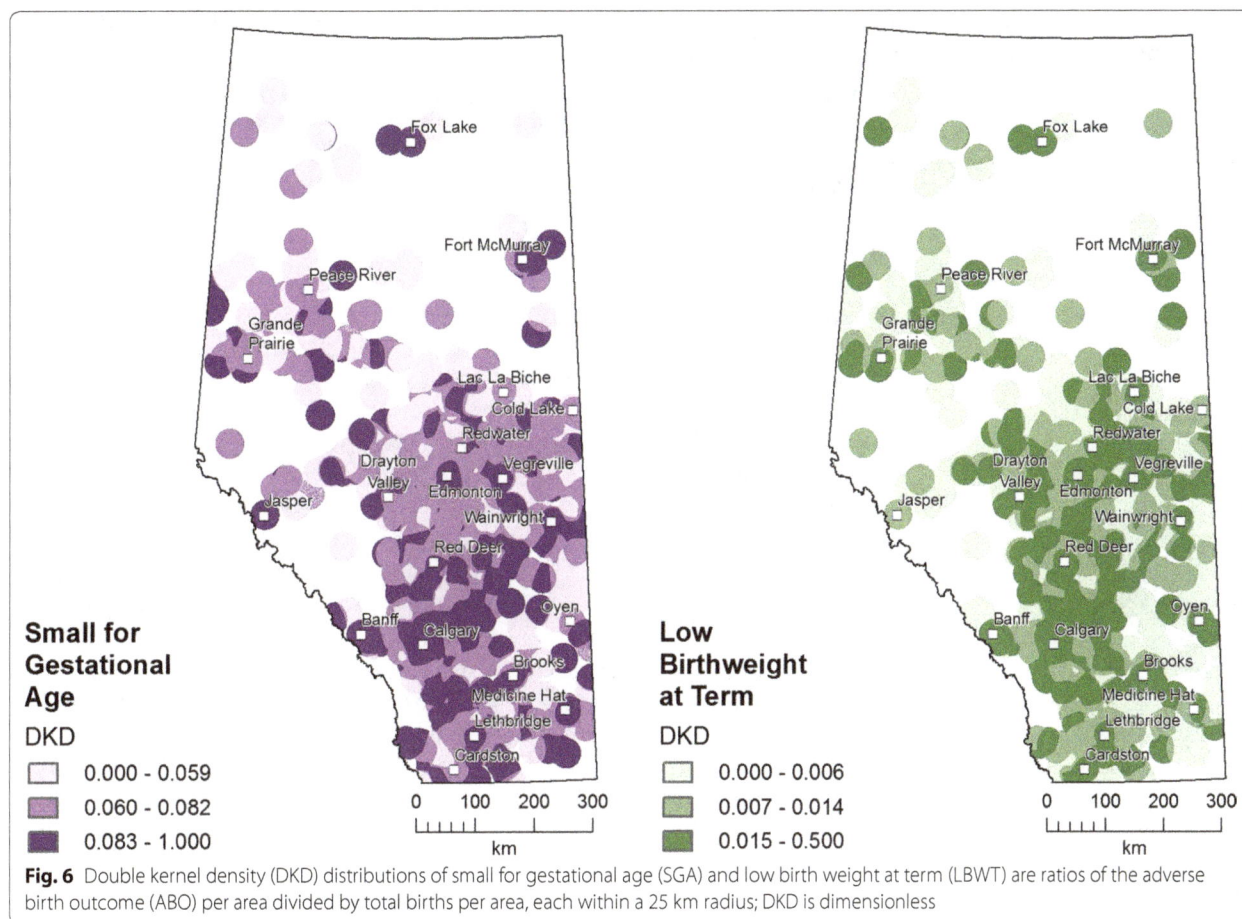

Fig. 6 Double kernel density (DKD) distributions of small for gestational age (SGA) and low birth weight at term (LBWT) are ratios of the adverse birth outcome (ABO) per area divided by total births per area, each within a 25 km radius; DKD is dimensionless

Toluene-2,6-diisocyanate; Chromium Aluminum; Hydrogen sulphide; Road; 2-Ethoxyethanol; *Nickel; Quinoline; Aniline; Cyclohexane; Acetaldehyde; and *Phosphorus ($rho = 0.42$). Variables with correlations greater than 0.40 with LBWT were: i-Butyl alcohol ($rho = 0.54$); Asbestos; Toluenediisocyanate; Toluene-2,4-diisocyanate; Toluene-2,6-diisocyanate; Aluminum; Chromium; Nighttime Light; Hydrogen sulphide; 2-Ethoxyethanol; Quinoline; Aniline; Road; Cyclohexane; Acetaldehyde; *Isopropyl alcohol; and *Ethylene oxide ($rho = 0.41$). Both ABOs were strongly associated with 15 air substances (the asterisk * marks those that differed: Nickel and Phosphorous for SGA; Ethylene oxide and Isopropyl alcohol for LBWT) and 2 land sources (both Nighttime Light and Road). Both ABOs had negative correlations (< -0.40) with Vegetation (SGA $rho = -0.56$; LBWT $rho = -0.48$), Oil/Gas Wellpad (SGA $rho = -0.53$; LBWT $rho = -0.49$), and Cultivated Land (SGA $rho = -0.47$; LBWT $rho = -0.41$).

The dilution effect of spreading the hazards across the large study area highlighted regional importance. Using the criteria of four or more health regions having a rho greater than 0.40 indicated the importance of Nitrogen oxides, Sulphur dioxide, Particulate Matter less than or equal to 2.5 μ ($PM_{2.5}$), and Acetaldehyde with SGA. The same criteria identified Xylene, Mine Site, Manganese, and Lead for LBWT. Four or more airshed zones having a rho greater than 0.40 highlighted Sulphur dioxide and Acetaldehyde with SGA, and Xylene, Particulate Matter less than or equal to 10 microns (PM_{10}), and $PM_{2.5}$ for LBWT.

The number of unique environmental variables having rho values greater than 0.40 province-wide or within four or more sub-provincial units totaled 30 (24 air substances and 6 land-based).

Spatial distribution of the indices

Figure 7 maps the results from the weighted overlay sum of the five class rankings for 136 emitted air substances, 18 land sources, the overlay equal weighting of both, and the Overlay 0.7/0.3 weighting of air substances and land. The distribution of the higher rankings spatially coincides with Alberta's populated places, except for higher values along the foothills, the Fort McMurray oil sands area in the north, and some scattered areas in the northeast.

Table 3 Spearman's rank correlations of small for gestational age (SGA) and low birth weight at term (LBWT) with air substances and land sources (*), in descending correlation *rho* values

Variable	Province *rho*		Health Region count (*rho* range)		Airshed Zone count (*rho* range)	
	SGA	LBWT	SGA	LBWT	SGA	LBWT
i-Butyl alcohol	**0.56**	**0.54**	1 (0.02 to 0.81)	3 (0.42 to 0.80)	1 (0.32 to 0.81)	2 (0.45 to 0.80)
Asbestos (friable form)	**0.54**	**0.52**	1 (0.73 to 0.73)	1 (0.67 to 0.67)	1 (0.73 to 0.73)	1 (0.67 to 0.67)
*Nighttime Light	**0.51**	**0.47**	2 (− 0.17 to 0.48)	1 (− 0.50 to 0.42)	2 (− 0.40 to 0.51)	3 (− 0.50 to 0.52)
Toluenediisocyanate (mixed isomers)	**0.49**	**0.51**	0 (0.26 to 0.26)	1 (0.42 to 0.42)	0 (0.26 to 0.26)	1 (0.42 to 0.42)
Toluene-2,4-diisocyanate	**0.49**	**0.50**	0 (0.26 to 0.26)	1 (0.41 to 0.41)	0 (0.26 to 0.26)	1 (0.41 to 0.41)
Toluene-2,6-diisocyanate	**0.49**	**0.50**	0 (0.26 to 0.26)	1 (0.41 to 0.41)	0 (0.26 to 0.26)	1 (0.41 to 0.41)
Chromium (and its compounds)	**0.48**	**0.47**	2 (− 0.07 to 0.68)	2 (− 0.07 to 0.77)	2 (− 0.23 to 0.68)	2 (− 0.26 to 0.77)
Aluminum (fume or dust)	**0.48**	**0.49**	1 (0.20 to 0.67)	1 (0.25 to 0.76)	1 (− 0.18 to 0.67)	1 (− 0.20 to 0.76)
Hydrogen sulphide	**0.47**	**0.47**	4 (− **0.09 to 0.59**)	3 (− 0.06 to 0.67)	3 (− 0.34 to 0.59)	3 (− 0.35 to 0.67)
*Road	**0.46**	**0.42**	2 (− 0.11 to 0.47)	0 (− 0.37 to 0.38)	3 (− 0.01 to 0.60)	2 (− 0.37 to 0.51)
2-Ethoxyethanol	**0.44**	**0.46**	0 (0.25 to 0.25)	1 (0.41 to 0.41)	0 (0.25 to 0.25)	1 (0.41 to 0.41)
Nickel (and its compounds)	**0.44**	**0.39**	2 (− 0.20 to 0.66)	3 (− 0.88 to 0.75)	2 (− 0.24 to 0.66)	2 (− 0.88 to 0.75)
Quinoline (and its salts)	**0.43**	**0.46**	0 (0.25 to 0.25)	1 (0.40 to 0.40)	0 (0.25 to 0.25)	1 (0.40 to 0.40)
Aniline (and its salts)	**0.43**	**0.45**	0 (0.25 to 0.25)	1 (0.40 to 0.40)	0 (0.25 to 0.25)	1 (0.40 to 0.40)
Cyclohexane	**0.42**	**0.42**	3 (− 0.07 to 0.81)	3 (− 0.07 to 0.81)	3 (− 0.27 to 0.81)	3 (− 0.30 to 0.81)
Acetaldehyde	**0.42**	**0.42**	4 (− **0.41 to 0.60**)	3 (− 0.07 to 0.59)	4 (− **0.34 to 0.60**)	3 (− 0.34 to 0.59)
Phosphorus (total)	**0.42**	0.38	1 (− 0.20 to 0.49)	1 (− 0.88 to 0.44)	1 (− 0.49 to 0.52)	1 (− 0.88 to 0.46)
Isopropyl alcohol	0.40	**0.41**	2 (− 0.40 to 0.52)	3 (− 0.47 to 0.53)	2 (− 0.60 to 0.77)	2 (− 0.67 to 0.52)
PAHs, Total unspeciated	0.40	0.40	0 (0.30 to 0.32)	1 (0.33 to 0.43)	0 (0.26 to 0.32)	1 (0.29 to 0.43)
Ethylene oxide	0.36	**0.41**	0 (− 0.43 to 0.25)	1 (− 0.20 to 0.41)	0 (− 0.30 to 0.25)	1 (− 0.32 to 0.41)
Ammonia (total)	0.36	0.34	1 (− 0.41 to 0.63)	1 (− 0.75 to 0.73)	1 (− 0.50 to 0.53)	1 (− 0.75 to 0.66)
Phosphorus (yellow or white)	0.35	0.37	0 (− 0.14 to 0.05)	0 (− 0.14 to 0.23)	0 (− 0.15 to 0.05)	0 (− 0.14 to 0.23)
Methylenebis(phenylisocyanate)	0.34	0.38	0 (− 0.43 to 0.23)	0 (− 0.49 to 0.38)	0 (0.13 to 0.23)	1 (0.38 to 0.72)
PM$_{10}$—Particulate Matter <= 10 Microns	0.33	0.30	3 (− 0.33 to 0.89)	3 (− 0.83 to 0.62)	3 (− 0.75 to 0.93)	4 (− **0.83 to 0.68**)
n-Butyl alcohol	0.31	0.32	1 (− 0.71 to 0.79)	1 (− 0.75 to 0.81)	1 (0.19 to 0.79)	1 (0.36 to 0.81)
Dichloromethane	0.31	0.31	1 (0.27 to 0.72)	2 (0.42 to 0.74)	1 (− 0.22 to 0.71)	2 (− 0.25 to 0.73)
Ethylene	0.30	0.33	3 (0.02 to 0.80)	3 (0.02 to 0.79)	3 (− 0.32 to 0.80)	3 (− 0.33 to 0.79)
Styrene	0.30	0.31	1 (0.00 to 0.81)	1 (− 0.01 to 0.82)	1 (− 0.32 to 0.83)	1 (− 0.32 to 0.85)
Lead (and its compounds)	0.30	0.30	3 (− 0.07 to 0.68)	4 (− **0.26 to 0.76**)	3 (− 0.23 to 0.87)	3 (− 0.65 to 0.76)
*Food Store	0.28	0.28	1 (− 0.18 to 0.58)	1 (− 0.23 to 0.57)	2 (− 0.18 to 0.58)	1 (− 0.17 to 0.57)
Cumene	0.27	0.27	1 (0.29 to 0.58)	2 (0.44 to 0.61)	1 (− 0.14 to 0.57)	2 (− 0.09 to 0.60)
Methyl isobutyl ketone	0.25	0.26	1 (0.07 to 0.69)	1 (0.25 to 0.73)	1 (0.07 to 0.67)	1 (0.08 to 0.71)
Xylene (mixed isomers)	0.24	0.26	1 (− 0.71 to 0.54)	5 (− **0.74 to 0.59**)	2 (− 0.65 to 0.74)	5 (− **0.47 to 0.87**)
Sulphur dioxide	0.24	0.20	5 (− **0.27 to 0.88**)	3 (− 0.87 to 0.74)	4 (− **0.35 to 0.91**)	2 (− 0.87 to 0.68)
Manganese (and its compounds)	0.24	0.21	3 (− 0.03 to 0.68)	4 (− **0.34 to 0.72**)	3 (− 0.50 to 0.65)	3 (− 0.71 to 0.70)
Fluorene—PAH	0.23	0.13	2 (− 0.32 to 0.50)	2 (− 0.89 to 0.55)	2 (− 0.49 to 0.52)	2 (− 0.89 to 0.53)
2-Butoxyethanol	0.22	0.23	1 (− 0.69 to 0.66)	1 (− 0.70 to 0.66)	1 (0.11 to 0.64)	1 (0.11 to 0.64)
*Gas Station	0.20	0.20	1 (− 0.23 to 0.58)	0 (− 0.25 to 0.30)	2 (− 0.41 to 0.56)	1 (− 0.42 to 0.58)
Naphthalene	0.20	0.14	1 (− 0.21 to 0.59)	2 (− 0.89 to 0.63)	1 (− 0.40 to 0.61)	2 (− 0.89 to 0.65)
Propylene	0.18	0.19	1 (− 0.11 to 0.68)	1 (− 0.01 to 0.71)	1 (− 0.30 to 0.70)	1 (− 0.31 to 0.73)
*Health Care	0.17	0.17	2 (− 0.21 to 0.51)	0 (− 0.36 to 0.24)	2 (− 0.22 to 0.53)	0 (− 0.49 to 0.28)
Volatile Organic Compounds (VOCs)	0.17	0.15	3 (− 0.45 to 0.88)	2 (− 0.74 to 0.67)	2 (− 0.45 to 0.92)	1 (− 0.74 to 0.69)
Toluene	0.17	0.19	1 (− 0.05 to 0.68)	2 (− 0.35 to 0.72)	2 (− 0.66 to 0.74)	3 (− 0.46 to 0.89)
Formic acid	0.14	0.15	0 (− 0.50 to 0.39)	1 (− 0.50 to 0.52)	0 (− 0.49 to 0.39)	1 (− 0.50 to 0.52)
PM$_{2.5}$—Particulate Matter <= 2.5 Microns	0.14	0.11	4 (− **0.57 to 0.88**)	3 (− 0.73 to 0.59)	3 (− 0.57 to 0.91)	4 (− **0.73 to 0.61**)
1,2,4-Trimethylbenzene	0.13	0.18	1 (− 0.05 to 0.57)	2 (− 0.07 to 0.60)	2 (− 0.38 to 0.67)	1 (− 0.47 to 0.60)
Formaldehyde	0.12	0.10	2 (− 0.41 to 0.70)	3 (− 0.81 to 0.71)	3 (− 0.29 to 0.83)	3 (− 0.81 to 0.70)

Table 3 continued

Variable	Province rho		Health Region count (rho range)		Airshed Zone count (rho range)	
	SGA	LBWT	SGA	LBWT	SGA	LBWT
Vanadium (except when in an alloy) and its compounds	0.11	0.12	1 (− 0.05 to 0.49)	1 (0.05 to 0.54)	1 (− 0.21 to 0.47)	1 (− 0.16 to 0.52)
Carbon disulphide	0.10	0.10	1 (− 0.21 to 0.41)	1 (− 0.28 to 0.52)	1 (− 0.26 to 0.75)	0 (− 0.32 to 0.30)
Benzo(g,h,i)perylene—PAH	0.10	0.05	2 (− 0.27 to 0.60)	2 (− 0.89 to 0.65)	2 (− 0.49 to 0.59)	2 (− 0.89 to 0.64)
Indeno(1,2,3-c,d)pyrene—PAH	0.09	0.05	2 (− 0.27 to 0.61)	2 (− 0.89 to 0.65)	2 (− 0.49 to 0.59)	2 (− 0.89 to 0.64)
Pyrene—PAH	0.09	0.03	2 (− 0.27 to 0.62)	2 (− 0.89 to 0.66)	2 (− 0.49 to 0.61)	2 (− 0.89 to 0.65)
Perylene—PAH	0.09	0.04	2 (− 0.27 to 0.60)	2 (− 0.89 to 0.64)	2 (− 0.49 to 0.59)	2 (− 0.89 to 0.64)
Benzo(a)phenanthrene—PAH	0.09	0.04	2 (− 0.27 to 0.61)	2 (− 0.89 to 0.64)	2 (− 0.49 to 0.60)	2 (− 0.89 to 0.64)
Benzo(e)pyrene—PAH	0.08	0.04	2 (− 0.27 to 0.61)	2 (− 0.89 to 0.65)	2 (− 0.27 to 0.59)	2 (− 0.89 to 0.64)
Benzo(a)anthracene—PAH	0.08	0.04	2 (− 0.27 to 0.61)	2 (− 0.89 to 0.65)	2 (− 0.27 to 0.59)	2 (− 0.89 to 0.64)
Fluoranthene—PAH	0.08	0.02	2 (− 0.27 to 0.61)	2 (− 0.89 to 0.65)	2 (− 0.27 to 0.60)	2 (− 0.89 to 0.64)
Methyl ethyl ketone	0.08	0.08	1 (− 0.21 to 0.80)	1 (− 0.31 to 0.82)	1 (− 0.32 to 0.79)	1 (− 0.32 to 0.81)
Benzene	0.07	0.09	0 (− 0.12 to 0.29)	1 (− 0.08 to 0.54)	1 (− 0.66 to 0.70)	2 (− 0.31 to 0.88)
Benzo(k)fluoranthene—PAH	0.07	0.02	2 (− 0.27 to 0.60)	2 (− 0.89 to 0.65)	2 (− 0.49 to 0.59)	2 (− 0.89 to 0.64)
*Aboriginal Land	0.07	0.05	0 (− 0.35 to 0.00)	0 (− 0.29 to 0.03)	0 (− 0.64 to − 0.04)	0 (− 0.29 to 0.23)
Diethanolamine (and its salts)	0.07	0.06	1 (0.00 to 0.41)	1 (− 0.01 to 0.46)	1 (− 0.25 to 0.44)	1 (− 0.25 to 0.49)
Benzo(a)pyrene—PAH	0.06	0.02	2 (− 0.27 to 0.57)	2 (− 0.89 to 0.61)	2 (− 0.49 to 0.56)	2 (− 0.89 to 0.60)
Aluminum oxide (fibrous forms)	0.06	0.05	1 (0.81 to 0.81)	1 (0.80 to 0.80)	1 (0.81 to 0.81)	1 (0.81 to 0.81)
Benzo(j)fluoranthene—PAH	0.06	0.01	2 (− 0.27 to 0.57)	2 (− 0.89 to 0.61)	2 (− 0.49 to 0.56)	2 (− 0.89 to 0.60)
Benzo(b)fluoranthene—PAH	0.06	0.01	2 (− 0.27 to 0.57)	2 (− 0.89 to 0.61)	2 (− 0.49 to 0.56)	2 (− 0.89 to 0.60)
n-Hexane	0.04	0.05	2 (− 0.09 to 0.63)	2 (− 0.31 to 0.65)	2 (− 0.36 to 0.53)	2 (− 0.47 to 0.85)
Calcium fluoride	0.03	0.02	1 (0.67 to 0.67)	1 (0.71 to 0.71)	1 (0.08 to 0.67)	1 (0.08 to 0.70)
Carbonyl sulphide	0.03	0.03	1 (0.04 to 0.41)	2 (− 0.28 to 0.52)	2 (− 0.26 to 0.75)	1 (− 0.31 to 0.48)
*Mine site	0.02	0.00	2 (− 0.35 to 0.43)	**4 (− 0.41 to 0.50)**	1 (− 0.21 to 0.53)	2 (− 0.60 to 0.57)
Biphenyl	0.01	0.00	1 (0.60 to 0.60)	1 (0.64 to 0.64)	1 (− 0.16 to 0.59)	1 (− 0.11 to 0.63)
*Waste/Landfill	0.01	0.05	0 (− 0.29 to 0.30)	1 (− 0.31 to 0.42)	1 (− 0.29 to 0.80)	1 (− 0.27 to 0.42)
Ethylene glycol	0.00	0.00	1 (− 0.69 to 0.41)	2 (− 0.85 to 0.53)	1 (− 0.44 to 0.75)	1 (− 0.85 to 0.49)
Hydrogen fluoride	0.00	0.00	1 (0.04 to 0.55)	1 (− 0.05 to 0.59)	1 (− 0.09 to 0.54)	1 (− 0.01 to 0.58)
Methyl tert-butyl ether	0.00	− 0.01	1 (0.77 to 0.77)	1 (0.78 to 0.78)	1 (0.15 to 0.76)	1 (0.15 to 0.77)
n,n-Dimethylformamide	0.00	− 0.02	1 (0.72 to 0.72)	1 (0.74 to 0.74)	1 (0.15 to 0.71)	1 (0.15 to 0.73)
Vinyl acetate	0.00	− 0.01	1 (0.56 to 0.56)	1 (0.58 to 0.58)	1 (0.54 to 0.54)	1 (0.57 to 0.57)
N-Methyl-2-pyrrolidone	0.00	− 0.01	1 (0.53 to 0.53)	1 (0.57 to 0.57)	1 (0.15 to 0.52)	1 (0.15 to 0.56)
Isoprene	0.00	0.00	0 (0.00 to 0.00)	0 (− 0.01 to − 0.01)	0 (− 0.01 to − 0.01)	0 (− 0.01 to − 0.01)
Titanium tetrachloride	0.00	0.00	0 (0.00 to 0.00)	0 (− 0.01 to − 0.01)	0 (− 0.01 to − 0.01)	0 (− 0.01 to − 0.01)
Methanol	− 0.01	− 0.01	1 (− 0.39 to 0.52)	1 (− 0.79 to 0.48)	0 (− 0.39 to 0.30)	1 (− 0.79 to 0.48)
Cresol (all isomers and their salts)	− 0.01	− 0.02	1 (0.00 to 0.55)	1 (− 0.32 to 0.59)	1 (− 0.49 to 0.54)	1 (− 0.72 to 0.58)
Carbon monoxide	− 0.01	− 0.04	2 (− 0.41 to 0.89)	1 (− 0.82 to 0.60)	2 (− 0.41 to 0.92)	2 (− 0.82 to 0.48)
Trichloroethylene	− 0.01	− 0.01	1 (0.49 to 0.49)	1 (0.53 to 0.53)	1 (− 0.24 to 0.51)	1 (− 0.27 to 0.56)
p-Phenylenediamine (and its salts)	− 0.02	− 0.01	0 (− 0.03 to − 0.03)	0 (− 0.03 to − 0.03)	0 (− 0.18 to − 0.18)	0 (− 0.13 to − 0.13)
Acrolein	− 0.02	− 0.10	1 (0.06 to 0.70)	1 (0.00 to 0.67)	1 (0.05 to 0.75)	0 (0.05 to 0.20)
Hexavalent chromium (and its compounds)	− 0.02	0.02	0 (− 0.07 to 0.31)	0 (− 0.32 to 0.17)	0 (− 0.50 to 0.08)	0 (− 0.71 to 0.25)
Dibenzo(a,i)pyrene—PAH	− 0.02	− 0.09	1 (− 0.21 to 0.54)	1 (− 0.89 to 0.59)	1 (− 0.21 to 0.53)	1 (− 0.89 to 0.58)
7H-Dibenzo(c,g)carbazole—PAH	− 0.02	− 0.11	1 (− 0.21 to 0.55)	1 (− 0.89 to 0.59)	1 (− 0.21 to 0.54)	1 (− 0.89 to 0.58)
tert-Butyl alcohol	− 0.02	− 0.03	0 (0.31 to 0.31)	0 (0.35 to 0.35)	0 (0.17 to 0.29)	0 (0.17 to 0.34)
Molybdenum trioxide	− 0.03	− 0.11	1 (− 0.20 to 0.44)	1 (− 0.88 to 0.49)	1 (− 0.20 to 0.43)	1 (− 0.88 to 0.48)
Acenaphthene—PAH	− 0.03	− 0.11	2 (− 0.21 to 0.63)	2 (− 0.89 to 0.66)	2 (− 0.49 to 0.61)	2 (− 0.89 to 0.66)
Chlorine	− 0.04	− 0.02	2 (− 0.55 to 0.54)	3 (− 0.32 to 0.57)	2 (− 0.55 to 0.56)	3 (− 0.72 to 0.60)
Phenanthrene—PAH	− 0.05	− 0.11	1 (− 0.27 to 0.49)	2 (− 0.89 to 0.44)	1 (− 0.49 to 0.52)	1 (− 0.89 to 0.46)
*Industrial facility	− 0.05	− 0.02	1 (− 0.18 to 0.43)	0 (− 0.46 to 0.29)	1 (− 0.62 to 0.47)	1 (− 0.59 to 0.40)

Table 3 continued

Variable	Province rho		Health Region count (rho range)		Airshed Zone count (rho range)	
	SGA	LBWT	SGA	LBWT	SGA	LBWT
*Hospital	− 0.05	− 0.03	1 (− 0.19 to 0.44)	0 (− 0.30 to 0.19)	2 (− 0.33 to 0.70)	0 (− 0.47 to 0.19)
5-Methylchrysene—PAH	− 0.06	− 0.22	0 (− 0.21 to − 0.21)	0 (− 0.89 to − 0.89)	0 (− 0.21 to − 0.21)	0 (− 0.89 to − 0.89)
1-Nitropyrene—PAH	− 0.06	− 0.22	0 (− 0.21 to − 0.21)	0 (− 0.89 to − 0.89)	0 (− 0.21 to − 0.21)	0 (− 0.89 to − 0.89)
Dibenzo(a,e)fluoranthene—PAH	− 0.06	− 0.22	0 (− 0.21 to − 0.21)	0 (− 0.89 to − 0.89)	0 (− 0.21 to − 0.21)	0 (− 0.89 to − 0.89)
Dibenzo(a,h)pyrene—PAH	− 0.06	− 0.22	0 (− 0.21 to − 0.21)	0 (− 0.89 to − 0.89)	0 (− 0.21 to − 0.21)	0 (− 0.89 to − 0.89)
Dibenzo(a,l)pyrene—PAH	− 0.06	− 0.22	0 (− 0.21 to − 0.21)	0 (− 0.89 to − 0.89)	0 (− 0.21 to − 0.21)	0 (− 0.89 to − 0.89)
Dibenz(a,h)acridine—PAH	− 0.06	− 0.22	0 (− 0.21 to − 0.02)	0 (− 0.89 to − 0.01)	0 (− 0.21 to − 0.02)	0 (− 0.89 to − 0.01)
Dibenzo(a,e)pyrene—PAH	− 0.06	− 0.22	0 (− 0.21 to − 0.02)	0 (− 0.89 to − 0.01)	0 (− 0.21 to − 0.02)	0 (− 0.89 to − 0.01)
Anthracene	− 0.06	− 0.22	0 (− 0.21 to − 0.03)	0 (− 0.89 to − 0.03)	0 (− 0.21 to − 0.19)	0 (− 0.89 to − 0.14)
Dibenz(a,j)acridine—PAH	− 0.06	− 0.13	1 (− 0.21 to 0.55)	1 (− 0.89 to 0.59)	1 (− 0.21 to 0.54)	1 (− 0.89 to 0.58)
Sulphuric acid	− 0.06	− 0.10	2 (− 0.21 to 0.52)	2 (− 0.89 to 0.56)	2 (− 0.50 to 0.54)	2 (− 0.89 to 0.58)
Ethylbenzene	− 0.07	− 0.05	2 (− 0.71 to 0.46)	3 (− 0.74 to 0.55)	2 (− 0.37 to 0.69)	1 (− 0.47 to 0.49)
Dibenzo(a,h)anthracene—PAH	− 0.07	− 0.14	2 (− 0.21 to 0.55)	2 (− 0.89 to 0.59)	2 (− 0.49 to 0.54)	2 (− 0.89 to 0.58)
Hydrochloric acid	− 0.08	− 0.07	1 (− 0.01 to 0.49)	2 (− 0.32 to 0.61)	0 (− 0.50 to 0.39)	2 (− 0.71 to 0.49)
*High Density Livestock Operation	− 0.08	− 0.08	0 (− 0.41 to 0.14)	0 (− 0.39 to 0.13)	0 (− 0.41 to 0.14)	0 (− 0.18 to 0.14)
Polymeric diphenylmethane diisocyanate	− 0.09	− 0.10	1 (− 0.15 to 0.41)	1 (− 0.15 to 0.53)	1 (− 0.15 to 0.75)	0 (− 0.15 to 0.20)
7,12-Dimethylbenz(a)anthracene—PAH	− 0.10	− 0.25	1 (− 0.21 to 0.48)	1 (− 0.89 to 0.43)	1 (− 0.49 to 0.51)	1 (− 0.89 to 0.45)
3-Methylcholanthrene—PAH	− 0.10	− 0.25	1 (− 0.21 to 0.49)	1 (− 0.89 to 0.44)	1 (− 0.49 to 0.52)	1 (− 0.89 to 0.46)
*Power Line	− 0.10	− 0.04	1 (− 0.84 to 0.41)	3 (− 0.31 to 0.67)	0 (− 0.86 to 0.26)	2 (− 0.31 to 0.53)
1,1,2-Trichloroethane	− 0.10	− 0.08	0 (− 0.20 to − 0.20)	0 (− 0.20 to − 0.20)	0 (− 0.26 to − 0.01)	0 (− 0.29 to − 0.01)
HCFC-142b	− 0.10	− 0.08	0 (− 0.20 to − 0.20)	0 (− 0.20 to − 0.20)	0 (− 0.26 to − 0.01)	0 (− 0.29 to − 0.01)
1,1,2,2-Tetrachloroethane	− 0.10	− 0.08	0 (− 0.20 to − 0.20)	0 (− 0.20 to − 0.20)	0 (− 0.26 to − 0.01)	0 (− 0.29 to − 0.01)
Carbon tetrachloride	− 0.10	− 0.08	0 (− 0.20 to − 0.20)	0 (− 0.20 to − 0.20)	0 (− 0.26 to − 0.01)	0 (− 0.29 to − 0.01)
Pentachloroethane	− 0.10	− 0.08	0 (− 0.20 to − 0.20)	0 (− 0.20 to − 0.20)	0 (− 0.26 to − 0.01)	0 (− 0.29 to − 0.01)
Dicyclopentadiene	− 0.10	− 0.08	0 (− 0.20 to 0.00)	0 (− 0.20 to − 0.01)	0 (− 0.26 to − 0.01)	0 (− 0.29 to − 0.01)
1,3-Butadiene	− 0.10	− 0.08	0 (− 0.20 to 0.00)	0 (− 0.20 to − 0.01)	0 (− 0.26 to − 0.01)	0 (− 0.29 to − 0.01)
Chloroethane	− 0.10	− 0.08	0 (− 0.20 to − 0.20)	0 (− 0.20 to − 0.20)	0 (− 0.28 to − 0.01)	0 (− 0.31 to − 0.01)
Chloroform	− 0.10	− 0.08	0 (− 0.20 to − 0.20)	0 (− 0.20 to − 0.20)	0 (− 0.31 to − 0.01)	0 (− 0.31 to − 0.01)
Vinyl chloride	− 0.10	− 0.08	0 (− 0.20 to − 0.20)	0 (− 0.20 to − 0.20)	0 (− 0.32 to − 0.01)	0 (− 0.34 to − 0.01)
Zinc (and its compounds)	− 0.11	− 0.17	2 (− 0.19 to 0.54)	3 (− 0.86 to 0.58)	2 (− 0.50 to 0.54)	2 (− 0.86 to 0.59)
Arsenic (and its compounds)	− 0.11	− 0.13	1 (− 0.18 to 0.55)	1 (− 0.32 to 0.59)	1 (− 0.50 to 0.52)	1 (− 0.71 to 0.57)
Tetrachloroethylene	− 0.12	− 0.12	1 (0.42 to 0.42)	1 (0.47 to 0.47)	1 (− 0.24 to 0.41)	1 (− 0.27 to 0.46)
Dioxins and furans—total	− 0.12	− 0.12	2 (− 0.10 to 0.66)	1 (− 0.32 to 0.70)	2 (− 0.50 to 0.67)	1 (− 0.71 to 0.71)
Nitrogen oxides (expressed as NO$_2$)	− 0.13	− 0.19	**6 (− 0.26 to 0.90)**	2 (− 0.83 to 0.61)	3 (− 0.27 to 0.91)	1 (− 0.83 to 0.48)
Chlorine dioxide	− 0.13	− 0.15	1 (− 0.15 to 0.49)	1 (− 0.32 to 0.44)	1 (− 0.49 to 0.52)	1 (− 0.72 to 0.46)
Hexachlorobenzene	− 0.13	− 0.14	2 (− 0.03 to 0.49)	2 (− 0.32 to 0.48)	2 (− 0.50 to 0.52)	2 (− 0.71 to 0.52)
*Socioeconomic Index	− 0.14	− 0.14	0 (− 0.59 to 0.21)	0 (− 0.58 to 0.17)	0 (− 0.59 to 0.26)	0 (− 0.58 to 0.24)
1,2-Dichloroethane	− 0.15	− 0.08	0 (− 0.42 to − 0.20)	0 (− 0.20 to 0.12)	0 (− 0.26 to − 0.01)	0 (− 0.29 to − 0.01)
Acetonitrile	− 0.15	− 0.15	0 (0.13 to 0.13)	0 (0.18 to 0.18)	0 (0.08 to 0.15)	0 (0.14 to 0.15)
1,4-Dioxane	− 0.15	− 0.08	0 (− 0.42 to − 0.20)	0 (− 0.20 to 0.12)	0 (− 0.30 to − 0.30)	0 (− 0.32 to − 0.32)
HCFC-22	− 0.15	− 0.08	0 (− 0.42 to − 0.20)	0 (− 0.20 to 0.12)	0 (− 0.30 to − 0.01)	0 (− 0.32 to − 0.01)
*Water body	− 0.17	− 0.12	1 (− 0.62 to 0.49)	0 (− 0.55 to 0.14)	1 (− 0.70 to 0.49)	0 (− 0.63 to 0.22)
Phenol (and its salts)	− 0.17	− 0.18	1 (− 0.13 to 0.41)	1 (− 0.10 to 0.53)	1 (− 0.18 to 0.75)	0 (− 0.19 to 0.20)
Triethylamine	− 0.17	− 0.18	0 (0.06 to 0.06)	0 (0.11 to 0.11)	0 (0.02 to 0.15)	0 (0.07 to 0.15)
Acenaphthylene—PAH	− 0.18	− 0.26	1 (− 0.21 to 0.49)	1 (− 0.89 to 0.44)	1 (− 0.49 to 0.52)	1 (− 0.89 to 0.46)
Nitrilotriacetic acid (and its salts)	− 0.19	− 0.19	0 (− 0.35 to − 0.35)	0 (− 0.35 to − 0.35)	0 (− 0.40 to − 0.40)	0 (− 0.40 to − 0.40)
Mercury (and its compounds)	− 0.19	− 0.21	0 (− 0.18 to 0.37)	1 (− 0.33 to 0.42)	0 (− 0.50 to 0.23)	0 (− 0.71 to 0.28)
Nitrate ion in solution at pH > = 6.0	− 0.19	− 0.19	0 (− 0.33 to − 0.33)	0 (− 0.31 to − 0.31)	0 (− 0.38 to − 0.38)	0 (− 0.37 to − 0.37)

Table 3 continued

Variable	Province *rho*		Health Region count (*rho* range)		Airshed Zone count (*rho* range)	
	SGA	LBWT	SGA	LBWT	SGA	LBWT
Nitric acid	− 0.19	− 0.19	0 (− 0.34 to − 0.34)	0 (− 0.34 to − 0.34)	0 (− 0.40 to − 0.40)	0 (− 0.39 to − 0.39)
Selenium (and its compounds)	− 0.19	− 0.21	1 (− 0.06 to 0.56)	1 (− 0.43 to 0.61)	1 (− 0.16 to 0.53)	1 (− 0.67 to 0.58)
Silver (and its compounds)	− 0.20	− 0.20	0 (− 0.36 to − 0.36)	0 (− 0.35 to − 0.35)	0 (− 0.42 to − 0.42)	0 (− 0.41 to − 0.41)
Antimony (and its compounds)	− 0.20	− 0.20	0 (− 0.37 to − 0.37)	0 (− 0.36 to − 0.36)	0 (− 0.42 to − 0.18)	0 (− 0.41 to − 0.13)
Cadmium (and its compounds)	− 0.20	− 0.21	3 (− 0.09 to 0.53)	2 (− 0.03 to 0.60)	1 (− 0.34 to 0.44)	2 (− 0.66 to 0.49)
Copper (and its compounds)	− 0.20	− 0.23	1 (− 0.18 to 0.62)	2 (− 0.34 to 0.65)	1 (− 0.21 to 0.61)	1 (− 0.35 to 0.64)
*Wildfire	− 0.24	− 0.28	1 (− 0.35 to 0.57)	0 (− 0.64 to 0.39)	3 (− 0.47 to 0.57)	1 (− 0.71 to 0.75)
Cobalt (and its compounds)	− 0.30	− 0.39	0 (− 0.43 to − 0.03)	1 (− 0.88 to 0.46)	0 (− 0.42 to − 0.11)	0 (− 0.88 to 0.00)
*Cultivated Land	**− 0.47**	**− 0.41**	0 (− 0.33 to 0.17)	1 (− 0.34 to 0.49)	1 (− 0.61 to 0.81)	2 (− 0.62 to 0.54)
*Oil/Gas Wellpad	**− 0.53**	**− 0.49**	0 (− 0.45 to 0.31)	0 (− 0.34 to 0.33)	2 (− 0.81 to 0.80)	2 (− 0.74 to 0.79)
*Vegetation	**− 0.56**	**− 0.48**	2 (− 0.50 to 0.80)	3 (− 0.52 to 0.48)	1 (− 0.48 to 0.83)	3 (− 0.52 to 0.58)

In the right half of the table, the count of units exceeding *rho* > 0.40 and the range are shown for the data aggregated by health regions and airshed zones. Variables having a rho > 0.4 for the province or for 4 or more sub-provincial units are indicated by bold font

Quantile class breaks were used to visualize the contrast of higher to lower areas.

Associations with the hazards and indices

The actual index values were used for the correlations with ABO DKD (Table 4). The correlations of the overlay indices with ABOs were very low for the entire province. The Air Substances were highest for both SGA (*rho* = 0.21) and LBWT (*rho* = 0.16). Land Factor correlations were slightly negative for SGA (*rho* = − 0.26) and LBWT (*rho* = − 0.23). Both overlay indices were lower than the Air Substances for SGA: Overlay Equal had a *rho* = 0.18 and Overlay 0.7/0.3 had a *rho* = 0.15. Overlay Equal was lower for LBWT (*rho* = 0.13) but Overlay 0.7/0.3 was higher (*rho* = 0.20).

Figure 8 displays index correlations with ABOs, by health region and airshed zone. In the graph symbols, longer bars mean greater association and bar direction designates positive (up) or negative (down). The air substances and land-based sources were included to demonstrate how much of an effect each had on the indices. The following indices had correlations greater than 0.40 with an ABO:

- Air Substances with SGA in four health regions—4829 (*rho* = 0.85), 4828 (*rho* = 0.67), 4826 (*rho* = 0.55), 4823 (*rho* = 0.42); and with LBWT in three health regions—4828 (*rho* = 0.73), 4826 (*rho* = 0.59), and 4823 (*rho* = 0.56).
- Air Substances with SGA in four airshed zones—WBEA (*rho* = 0.89), PASZA (*rho* = 0.57), ACAA (*rho* = 0.55) and CRAZ (*rho* = 0.42); and with LBWT in four airshed zones—LICA (*rho* = 0.85),

PASZA (*rho* = 0.66), ACAA (*rho* = 0.60), and CRAZ (*rho* = 0.56).

- Land sources were weakly associated with both SGA and LBWT in most health regions and airshed zones.
- Overlay Equal index with SGA in four health regions—4828 (*rho* = 0.58), 4826 (*rho* = 0.54), 4823 (*rho* = 0.42), and 4827 (*rho* = 0.42); and with LBWT in four health regions—4828 (*rho* = 0.0.63), 4826 (*rho* = 0.0.59), 4821 (*rho* = 0.57), and 4823 (*rho* = 0.57).
- Overlay Equal index with SGA in three airshed zones—ACAA (*rho* = 0.55), PASZA (*rho* = 0.45), and CRAZ (*rho* = 0.42); and with LBWT in three airshed zones—ACAA (*rho* = 0.60), CRAZ (*rho* = 0.57), and PASZA (*rho* = 0.51).
- Overlay 0.7/0.3 index with SGA in four health regions—4829 (*rho* = 0.75), 4828 (*rho* = 0.62), 4826 (*rho* = 0.55), and 4823 (*rho* = 0.42); and with LBWT in four health regions—4828 (*rho* = 0.68), 4826 (*rho* = 0.59), 4823 (*rho* = 0.57), and 4821 (*rho* = 0.51).
- Overlay 0.7/0.3 index with SGA in four airshed zones—WBEA (*rho* = 0.78), ACAA (*rho* = 0.55), PASZA (*rho* = 0.50), and CRAZ (*rho* = 0.42); and with LBWT in four airshed zones—LICA (*rho* = 0.60), ACAA (*rho* = 0.60), PASZA (*rho* = 0.59), and CRAZ (*rho* = 0.57).

The health regions having the least association with SGA were 4821, 4822, 4824, and 4825; with LBWT these were 4822, 4824, 4827, and 4829. The airshed zones having the least association with SGA were FAP, PAMZ, PAS, and WCAS; with LBWT these were FAP, PAMZ, PAS, and WBEA.

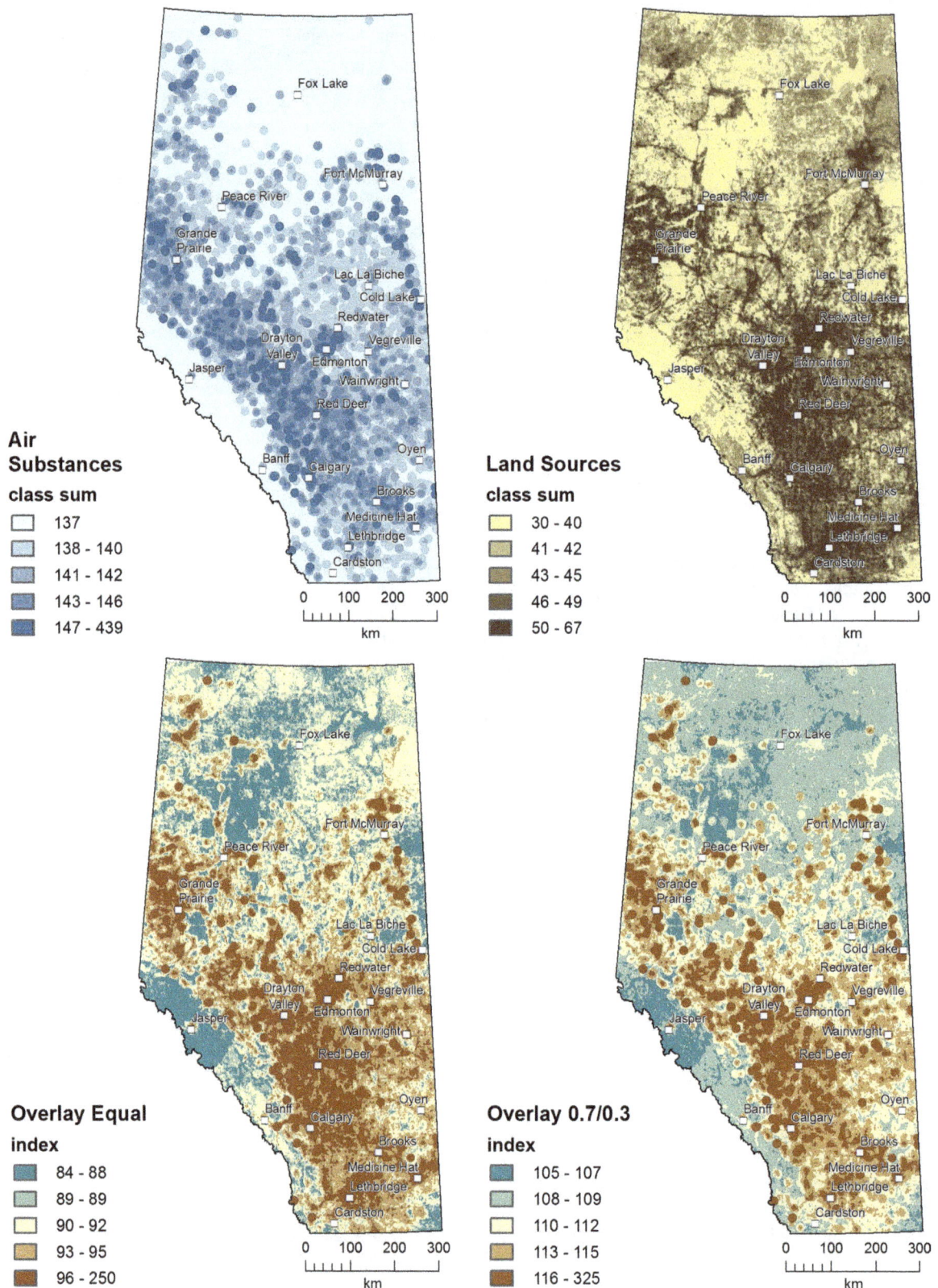

Fig. 7 Weighted sum overlays for air substances and land-based sources were combined as equal and 0.7/0.3 weighted indices to identify the most hazardous locations

Table 4 Spearman's rank correlations of small for gestational age (SGA) and low birth weight at term (LBWT) with air substances, land sources, and weighted sum overlay indices for the entire province of Alberta

Index name	Inputs	SGA rho	LBWT rho
Air substances	Sum of 136 variables classified to 5 quantiles	0.21	0.16
Land sources	Sum of 18 variables classified to 5 quantiles	− 0.26	− 0.23
Overlay equal	Air substances + land sources	0.18	0.13
Overlay 0.7/0.3	0.7 * air substances + 0.3 * land sources	0.15	0.20

SGA and LBWT were negatively correlated with *all* indices in health region 4822 and two airshed zones (PAS, FAP). The negative association also occurred in health region 4825 and airshed zone WCAS, but a higher positive correlation occurred with the Land Sources.

Using the criteria of correlations higher than 0.40, the Overlay 0.7/0.3 index had the highest overall count of sub-provincial units—both ABOs represented by at least 4 health regions and 4 airshed zones.

Discussion
Individual hazards
Of 136 NPRI substances reported in Alberta, 24 air-emitted substances had moderate correlations with one or both ABO DKD ratios. Of these, 2-Ethoxyethanol and Lead are recognized developmental toxicants [53, 54]. Acetaldehyde, Aluminum, Ethylene oxide, Isopropyl alcohol, Nickel, Nitrogen oxides, PM_{10}, $PM_{2.5}$, Sulphur dioxide, Xylene, Chromium, Hydrogen sulphide, Manganese, Phosphorus, and Quinoline are suspected developmental toxicants, with more than half of the air substances associated with decreased fetal/offspring weight in animal studies [53, 54]. The following air substances are neither recognized or suspected as no studies were reported: Aniline, Asbestos, Cyclohexane, i-Butyl alcohol, Toluene-2,4-diisocyanate, Toluene-2,6-diisocyanate, and Toluenediisocyanate (note: the latter three have been combined in later versions of the NPRI database [9]).

Of the 18 land sources mapped, 6 had moderate correlations with one or both ABOs. Provincially, Cultivated Land was negatively associated with SGA and LBW (likely because residences were not inside agricultural fields), but some regions were positive, similar to the Almberg et al. [55] study on proximity to pesticide-treated agricultural fields. Proximity to Mine Sites were associated for 2–3 health regions or airsheds; a related study found positive association for a single mine site indicating this is likely a more localized factor [56].

Nighttime Lights have not been explored with ABOs; however, breast cancer, which has other similar exposures, has a positive association [44, 57]. The smaller area airsheds showed high correlations of ABOs with Oil/Gas Wellpads, but was negative for the entire province and by health regions; mixed associations were also reported by Mckenzie et al. [58] and Casey et al. [59]. The moderate to higher correlations of Roads match much published research on the effect of maternal proximity to roads [60, 61]. Green or natural Vegetation was negatively correlated at the provincial level, but very mixed within health regions and airsheds; the sub-provincial dissimilarity with other studies [62, 63] was likely affected by the radii, resolution of the satellite sources, and the widely varying ecoregions in the province.

Ambient hazard indices
Both indices identified where there was an accumulation of hazards and therefore directly addressed the hypothesis that there were more small newborns where there were more outdoor hazards during the mothers' pregnancies. Since we were interested in preserving combined effects that the industrial air substances contributed to the outdoor environment, we weighted the sum of those more highly than the sum of all the land-based sources. Province-wide, the Overlay Equal index better identified SGA and the Overlay 0.7/0.3 better identified LBWT.

Differences in index associations were likely due to the spatial distributions (i.e. DKD) of the ABOs. Both SGA and LBWT showed that hot spots did not occur strictly within the large urban centers. Calgary and Edmonton exhibited higher ratio classes, but not for their entire core. The peripheral edges of the Calgary-Red Deer corridor, the communities along the Banff-Calgary-Brooks corridor, the Fort McMurray surroundings, and the northern Fox Creek area were high for both SGA and LBWT. Jasper and south-east Alberta had higher SGA, while the communities west and east of Edmonton had higher LBWT. The distributions of the type of ABO spatially varied across the province—differences that may have been due in part to population and behavior, but also visually collocated with the higher amounts of outdoor hazard mapping.

Separately, the air substances and land sources varied in association with the ABO distributions. On the provincial scale, there were 13 hazards spatially related to both the SGA and LBWT ratios. Assessing the relationships sub-provincially found many more factors involved, including those already supported in the scientific literature, including: nitrogen oxides, particulate matter ($PM_{2.5}$ and PM_{10}), and sulphur dioxide.

Despite the disparate boundaries, spatially corresponding health regions (HR) and airshed zones (AZ) had

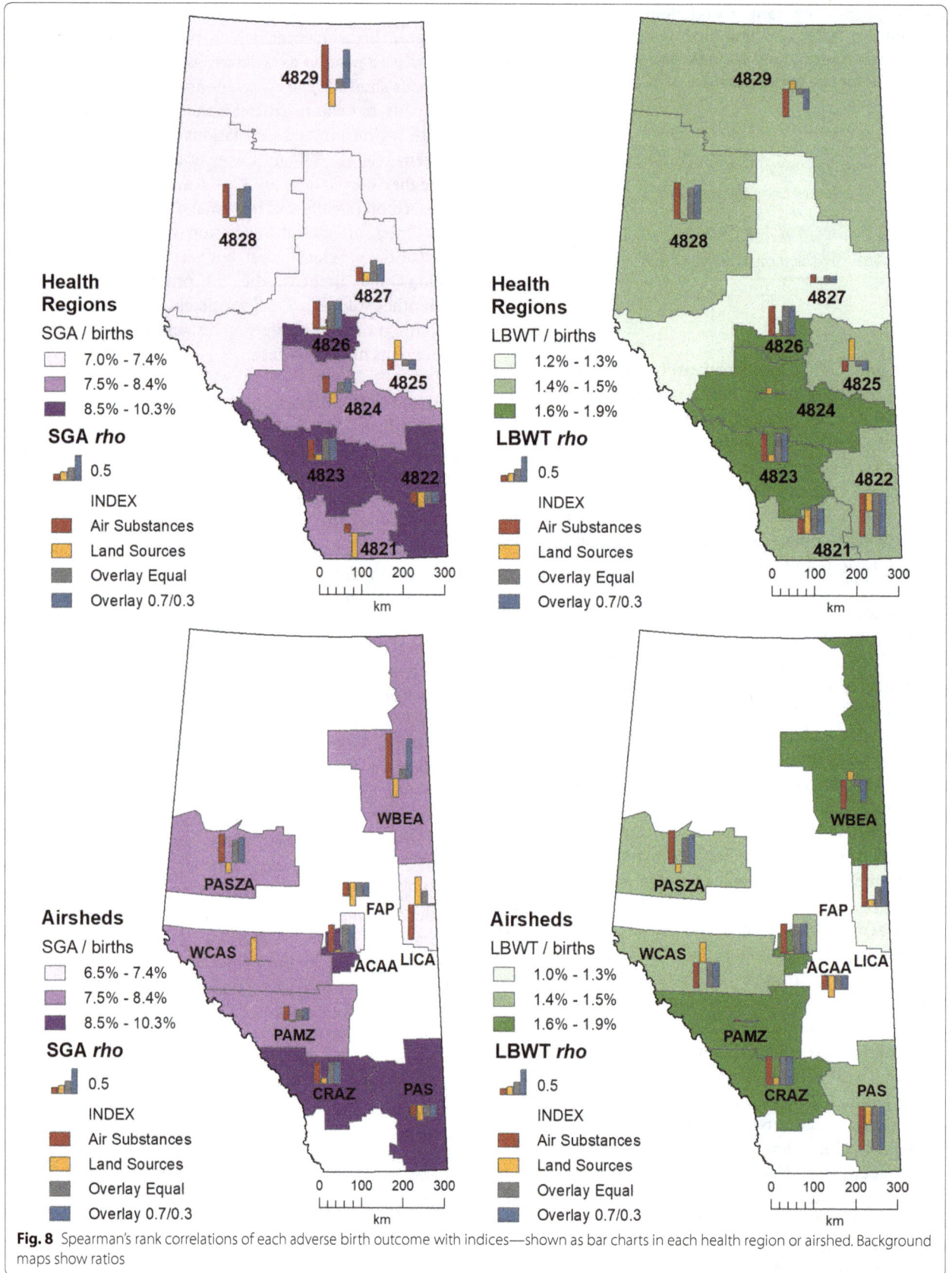

Fig. 8 Spearman's rank correlations of each adverse birth outcome with indices—shown as bar charts in each health region or airshed. Background maps show ratios

comparable patterns in spatial relationships to the hazard indices. HR 4822/AZ PAS had highly negative correlations with all indices, suggesting that factors other than the outdoor environment may be more important in these regions. HR 4829/AZ WBEA exhibited opposite correlations with indices: SGA was positive and LBWT was negative. HR 4826/AZ ACAA and FAP and HR 4823/AS CRAZ for SGA and LBWT were positively correlated with the indices—these are the more populated regions. 4828/PASZA also had positive index correlations with SGA and LBWT. HR 4824/AZ PAMZ for SGA was positive with the indices, but for LBWT had no association. The reverse was found in HR 4821 (no corresponding AZ), where SGA was negative and LBWT was positive. HR 4825 had no relationship with the ABOs, and AZ LICA had no association with SGA and a positive one with LBWT. HR 4827 and AZ WCAS are too large and diverse to compare. Inconsistent relationships for each ABO with the indices may be due to: (1) the variable geography within the administrative boundaries; (2) differences in etiology of the ABOs; and/or (2) the actual distribution of each ABO exhibiting slightly different patterns: SGA and LBWT appear to be more of a heartland issue.

The combination of the outdoor hazards into a single index were very weakly associated with SGA and LBWT provincially. This was not surprising given Alberta includes forestry, agriculture, and energy extraction activities, thus yielding diverse "pockets" of different pollutants. Analyzing smaller geographic areas, based on health regions or airsheds, helped recognize possible differences in the outdoor environmental factors.

The large area of some units may capture populations that are more similar in size to the smaller units, but the environmental variability may have diluted the effects of hazards. The sub-provincial units that had negative correlations will need further analysis to determine the regionally important hazards. Relationships found here show that province-wide (i.e. large region) approaches to outdoor hazards may be inappropriate or inefficient. Where health regions and airshed zones are more similar, policy and monitoring may be more agreeable.

Existing ambient hazard indices are not available for comparison. Environmental Quality Indices (EQI), such as those developed by Messer et al. [28] and Stieb et al. [64] depict the state-of-the-environment from actual measured conditions [27]. The Air Quality Health Index (AQHI) by Stieb et al. does a very good job at aggregating the monitored criteria air contaminants for risk communication. Messer's EQI was associated with pre-term birth [65], but still has the limitation of fixed administrative units. And because a main goal was a continuous index, we were unable to incorporate an effective rural classification without the introduction of administrative boundaries, as done by Messer et al. Our more ecologically-encompassing index incorporated industrial air pollutants and land-based sources, similar to the holistic model developed for a single urban area by Tarocco et al. [66].

Limitations

We analyzed the entire registered birth population for the study period that had valid locations. The 6-character postal codes provided good accuracy for urban neighborhoods, especially within the context of the 250-m cell size, but the rural residences were not as exact. DMTI Spatial had applied algorithms to weight the postal code local delivery area centroid toward the more populated communities [41], but that did not guarantee an actual residence contained within the cell. The problem of rural resolution was exhibited by oil–gas wellpads and agricultural land that may be closer to actual residences, but postal codes were not accurate enough due to too large of delivery areas for the centroids.

Although there is concern that the mother did not live at that postal code for the entire pregnancy, previous research determined low mobility during pregnancy and any relatively short distances moved did not substantially change the exposure assignment [67].

The spatial data for the independent variables were restricted to publicly available sources that may not have had the most temporally appropriate capture date of the mapped features. We also did not have access to reliable province-wide data for other possible environmental factors, such as water quality, noise, or non-industrial pollution sources. And as suitable as the NPRI data were, the values were annually reported estimates and not actual measurements [9]. Despite these shortcomings, the available data provided an as inclusive as possible foundation for the index.

Many of the GIS methods involved the selection of radius distances. The size of the radius used in calculating the DKD affected how "hot" an area appeared, and may have exaggerated the extent for large distances; the 25-km radius may have been too large for rural communities with diverse topographies. When estimating air-emitted pollutants, wind would have varied by season and throughout the years; therefore, the use of circular shapes in calculating the tonnes per area may not have accurately reflected wind-dispersion for some areas. The conservative 10 km radius for spreading the air substances may have remedied this for upwind locations, but potentially underrepresented it for downwind locations. For the index, not all variables may be equally important, but the use of expert judgment would have introduced subjectivity that was not reproducible. Therefore, the equal treatment of the air substances and land sources in the overlay analyses was used.

The correlation threshold value of 0.40 may have over-represented the inclusion of some of the independent variables. The choice of this statistical threshold was based on inspection of the data to ensure that a wide variety of hazards would be represented and not erroneously overlooked due to the modifiable areal unit problem introduced by the boundaries of the sub-provincial units [68].

It is important to stress that our research was not able to find causal relationships, but identified where outdoor environmental hazards collocate with residences of mothers who gave birth to abnormally small newborns.

Strengths

The calculations of the outdoor environmental variables were continuous and covered the entire study area. Therefore, the DKD calculation of the SGA and LBWT ratios was appropriately consistent because it also was not confined to arbitrary geographical boundaries. Aggregation early in the analysis would have produced an inflexible distribution of the ABOs. The introduction of health regions and airsheds afterward allowed for scenario investigations relevant to health care administration, policy implications, and airshed monitoring.

The primary outdoor pollutants associated with abnormally small newborns agreed with published research, but additional unstudied air substances were discovered. For many regions, the reduction of data into a single index was achievable.

The development and application of the ambient health hazard indices for any study area, any time period, and where relevant data are available is simplified by the reverse suitability approach in a standard GIS. The distance-centered methods and weighted sum overlay, commonly used in wildlife habitat studies, are also relevant to human habitat related to various environmental health outcomes.

Conclusion

This is to date the first study on abnormally small newborns that used a combination of multiple outdoor variables over a large geographic area. Our results showed that SGA and LBWT varied sub-provincially with outdoor environmental factors, suggesting that provincial government should be aware of multiple sources of place-dependent exposures. Summing up class rankings of hazards provided a simple model for correlating with the sub-provincial distributions of ABO. There were regions/airsheds that were higher than the national and provincial rates. The temporal nuances had been masked by combining all years: spatial patterns in the hazards and birth outcomes likely varied through time; therefore, future research should consider the timing of exposures. Research should also combine the vertices of habitat, population, and behavior to investigate the complex interactions of the outdoor hazards found here by including maternal characteristics revealed in traditional epidemiological studies. We found that the industrial air substances were important—and the Overlay 0.7/0.3 weighted index had the most associations in the sub-provincial units. Therefore, both the individual air substance associations and the convenient single-measure index provide complementary information to move us toward a better understanding of the links between the outdoor environment and birthweight. Mapping the outdoor environmental hazards for mothers giving birth to abnormally small newborns provides insight for preventative or remedial recommendations *where* they may be needed to help determine healthier futures.

Abbreviations
ABO: adverse birth outcome; APHP: Alberta perinatal health program; AZ: airshed zone; DoMiNO: data mining and neonatal outcomes; DKD: double kernel density; GIS: geographical information systems; HR: health region; LBWT: low birth weight at term; NPRI: national pollutant release inventory; SGA: small for gestational age.

Authors' contributions
CN conceived the study, developed the methodology, designed and carried out the analyses, and drafted the manuscript. CA provided expertise in developing the methodology, and reviewed and edited the manuscript. AOV oversaw the data collection, provided expertise in developing the methodology, and reviewed and edited the manuscript. All authors read and approved the final manuscript.

Author details
[1] Department of Earth and Atmospheric Sciences, University of Alberta, Edmonton, Canada. [2] Department of Pediatrics, University of Alberta, 3-591 ECHA, 11,405 87th Avenue, Edmonton, AB T6G 1C9, Canada.

Acknowledgements
This research is part of the Data Mining and Neonatal Outcomes (DoMiNO) interdisciplinary collaborative project using spatial data mining to explore the colocation of adverse birth outcomes and environmental variables; team members: Aelicks N, Arbour L, Aziz K, Blagden P, Buka I, Chan E, Chandra S, Demers P, Erickson A, Jabbar S, Hystad P, Kumar M, Li J, Nicol A, Nielsen C, Phipps E, Serrano-Lomelin J, Setton E, Shah P, Stieb D, Villeneuve P, Wine O, Yuan Y, Zaiane O, and Osornio-Vargas A. The authors wish to thank summer students, Rusk B and Silverman E, for their assistance in acquiring some of the environmental data, as well as anonymous reviewers and Griffith D for their suggestions to improve the manuscript.

Competing interests
The authors declare they have no competing interests.

Funding
Funding is courtesy of the Canadian Institutes of Health Research (CIHR) and The Natural Sciences and Engineering Research Council of Canada (NSERC) Collaborative Health Research Program (Application Number 290275).

References

1. Meade MS, Emch M. Medical geography. 3rd ed. New York: Guilford Press; 2010.

2. Meade MS. Medical geography as human ecology: the dimension of population movement. Geogr Rev. 1977;64:379–93.

3. Barker DJ. The fetal and infant origins of adult disease. BMJ Br Med J. 1990;301:1111.

4. Barker DJP. Maternal nutrition, fetal nutrition, and disease in later life. Nutrition. 1997;13:807–13.

5. Barker DJP. The developmental origins of chronic adult disease. Acta Paediatr Suppl. 2004;93:26–33.

6. Barker DJP, Osmond C. Infant mortality, childhood nutrition, and ischaemic heart disease in England and wales. Lancet. 1986;327:1077–81.

7. Kramer MS. The epidemiology of adverse pregnancy outcomes: an overview. J Nutr. 2003;133:1592S–6S.

8. Statistics Canada. Population, urban and rural, by province and territory, Alberta [digital data]. Statistics Canada, Government of Canada; 2011. Available from: http://www.statcan.gc.ca/tables-tableaux/sum-som/l01/cst01/demo62j-eng.htm.

9. Environment Canada. National pollutant release inventory, 2005–2012 [digital data]. Natl Pollut Release Invent. 2014. Available from: https://www.ec.gc.ca/inrp-npri/.

10. Wine O, Hackett C, Campbell S, Cabrera-Rivera O, Buka I, Zaiane O, et al. Using pollutant release and transfer register data in human health research: a scoping review. Environ Rev. 2014;22:51–65.

11. Statistics Canada. Table 102-4318—Birth-related indicators (low and high birth weight, small and large for gestational age, pre-term births), by sex, three-year average, Canada, provinces, territories, census metropolitan areas and metropolitan influence zones, occasional. Can Socio-Econ Inf Manage Syst. 2014. Available from: http://www5.statcan.gc.ca/cansim/a05?lang=eng&id=01024318.

12. Alberta Health. Alberta interactive health data application—reproductive health—singleton small for gestational age percent by geography and low birth weight percent by geography, 2000–2014 [digital data]. Interact Heal Data Appl. 2016. Available from: http://www.ahw.gov.ab.ca/IHDA_Retrieval/ihdaData.do.

13. Canadian Institute for Health Information (CIHI). Too early, too small: a profile of small babies across Canada. 2009. Available from: https://secure.cihi.ca/free_products/too_early_too_small_en.pdf.

14. Statistics Canada. Table 102-0562—Leading causes of death, infants, by sex, Canada, annual, 2006–2012 [digital data]. Can Socio-Economic Inf Manage Syst 2012. Available from: http://www5.statcan.gc.ca/cansim/pick-choisir?lang=eng&searchTypeByValue=1&id=1020562.

15. Shah PS, Balkhair T. Air pollution and birth outcomes: a systematic review. Environ Int. 2011;37:498–516.

16. Vadillo-Ortega F, Osornio-Vargas A, Buxton MA, Sánchez BN, Rojas-Bracho L, Viveros-Alcaráz M, et al. Air pollution, inflammation and preterm birth: a potential mechanistic link. Med Hypotheses. 2014;82:219–24.

17. Maisonet M, Correa A, Misra D, Jaakkola JJK. A review of the literature on the effects of ambient air pollution on fetal growth. Environ Res. 2004;95:106–15.

18. Weselak M, Arbuckle TE, Foster W. Pesticide exposures and developmental outcomes: the epidemiological evidence. J Toxicol Environ Heal Part B, Crit Rev. 2007;10:41–80.

19. Triche EW, Hossain N. Environmental factors implicated in the causation of adverse pregnancy outcome. Semin Perinatol. 2007;31:240–2.

20. Koranteng S, Osornio-Vargas AR, Buka I. Ambient air pollution and children's health: a systematic review of Canadian epidemiological studies. Paediatr Child Health. 2007;12:225–33.

21. Windham G, Fenster L. Environmental contaminants and pregnancy outcomes. Fertil Steril. 2008;89:e111–6.

22. Dadvand P, Parker J, Bell ML, Bonzini M, Brauer M, Darrow LA, et al. Maternal exposure to particulate air pollution and term birth weight: a multi-country evaluation of effect and heterogeneity. Environ Health Perspect. 2013;121:367–73.

23. Stieb DM, Chen L, Eshoul M, Judek S. Ambient air pollution, birth weight and preterm birth: a systematic review and meta-analysis. Environ Res. 2012;117:100–11.

24. Meng G, Thompson ME, Hall GB. Pathways of neighbourhood-level socio-economic determinants of adverse birth outcomes. Int J Health Geogr. Int J Health Geogr. 2013;12:1–16.

25. Meng G, Hall GB, Thompson ME, Seliske P. Spatial and environmental impacts on adverse birth outcomes in Ontario. Can Geogr. 2013;57:154–72.

26. Inhaber H. Environmental quality: outline for a national index for Canada. Science. 1974;186:798–805.

27. Ott WR. Environmental indices: theory and practice. Ann Arbor, MI: Ann Arbor Science Publishers, Inc.; 1978.

28. Messer LC, Jagai JS, Rappazzo KM, Lobdell DT. Construction of an environmental quality index for public health research. Environ Heal. 2014;13:1–22.

29. Office of Environmental Health Hazard Assessment. Draft California communities environmental health screening tool (CalEnviroScreen). 2014. Available from: http://oehha.ca.gov/ej/pdf/CES20PublicReview04212014.pdf.

30. Messer LC, Vinikoor LC, Laraia BA, Kaufman JS, Eyster J, Holzman C, et al. Socioeconomic domains and associations with preterm birth. Soc Sci Med. 2008;67:1247–57.

31. Cromley EK, McLafferty SL. GIS and public health. 2nd ed. New York: Guilford Press; 2012.

32. Nuckols JR, Ward MH, Jarup L. Using geographic information systems for exposure assessment in environmental epidemiology studies. Environ Health Perspect. 2004;112:1007–15.

33. Osornio-Vargas AR, Zaiaine O, Wine O. Domino project: data mining and newborn outcomes exploring environmental variables, abstract number 2187. Int Soc Environ Epidemiol. Seattle, WA: National Institute of Environmental Health Sciences; 2015. pp. 3–607. Available from: http://ehp.niehs.nih.gov/isee/p3-607/.

34. Esri. ArcGIS Desktop, Release 10.5 [software]. Esri Inc; 2016. Available from: www.esri.com.

35. NASA EOSDIS Land Processes DAAC, Didan K. MOD13Q1: MODIS/Terra Vegetation Indices 16-Day L3 Global 250 m Grid SIN V006 [digital data]. MOD13Q1 Version 6. 2014. Available from: https://lpdaac.usgs.gov/dataset_discovery/modis/modis_products_table/mod13q1_v006.

36. Statistics Canada. Health region boundary files, ArcInfo, Alberta, 2007, Catalog no. 82-402-X [digital data]. 82-402-X. 2008. Available from: http://www.statcan.gc.ca/pub/82-402-x/82-402-x2009001-eng.htm.

37. Alberta Environment and Sustainable Resource Devlopment. Alberta Airsheds [digital data]. GeoDiscover Alberta. 2010. Available from: https://genesis.srd.alberta.ca/genesis_tokenauth/rest/services/Air-Layers/Latest/MapServer/generatekml.

38. Statistics Canada. Health regions: boundaries and correspondence with census geography 2007 (updates). 2009. Available from: http://www.statcan.gc.ca/pub/82-402-x/82-402-x2009001-eng.pdf.

39. Clean Air Strategic Alliance. Airshed Zones Guidelines. Edmonton, Alberta; 2004. Available from: http://www.casahome.org/.

40. Alberta Health Services. Alberta Perinatal Health Program, 2006–2012 [digital data]. Alberta Perinat Heal Progr 2014. Available from: http://aphp.dapasoft.com.

41. DMTI Spatial. CanMap content suite—platinum postal code and enhanced points of interest, 2001–2013 [digital data]. Markham, Ontario: DMTI Spatia Incl; 2014. Available from: http://www.dmtispatial.com/canmap/.

42. Serrano-Lomelin J, Nielsen C, Aziz K, Kumar M, Chandra S, Aelicks N, et al. Co-occurrence of maternal risk factors and neighborhood socio-economic status profiles associated with adverse birth outcomes in Alberta, Canada.

43. Davarashvili S, Zusman M, Keinan-Boker L, Rybnikova N, Kaufman Z, Silverman BG, et al. Application of the double kernel density approach to the analysis of cancer incidence in a major metropolitan area. Environ Res. 2016;150:269–80.

44. Kloog I, Haim A, Portnov BA. Using kernel density function as an urban analysis tool: investigating the association between nightlight exposure and the incidence of breast cancer in Haifa, Israel. Comput Environ Urban Syst. 2009;33:55–63.

45. Müller AH, Stadtmüller U, Tabnak F, Moller H, Stadtmuller U, Tabnak F. Spatial smoothing of geographically aggregated data, with application to the construction of incidence maps. J Am Stat Assoc. 2016;92:61–71.

46. Portnov BA, Dubnov J, Barchana M. Studying the association between air pollution and lung cancer incidence in a large metropolitan area using a kernel density function. Socioecon Plann Sci. 2009;43:141–50.

47. Zusman M, Broitman D, Portnov BA. Application of the double kernel density approach to the multivariate analysis of attributeless event point datasets. Lett Spat Resour Sci. 2015;3:1–20.

48. Zusman M, Dubnov J, Barchana M, Portnov BA. Residential proximity to petroleum storage tanks and associated cancer risks: Double Kernel Density approach vs. zonal estimates. Sci Total Environ. 2012;441:265–76.

49. Silverman BW. Density estimation for statistics and data analysis. New York: Chapman and Hall; 1997.

50. Python Software Foundation. Python Language Reference, Version 2.7. 2016. Available from: www.python.org.

51. PyData Development Team. pandas 0.16 [software]. 2015. Available from: http://pandas.pydata.org/pandas-docs/version/0.16.0/.

52. Mitchell A. The Esri guide to GIS analysis, volume 3: modeling suitability, movement, and interaction. Redlands: Esri Press; 2012.

53. GoodGuide. Chemical profiles. Scorec Pollut Inf Site. 2011. Available from: http://scorecard.goodguide.com/chemical-profiles/.

54. Air Toxics Assessment Group. Health effects notebook for hazardous air pollutants. Environ Prot Agency. 2017. Available from: https://www.epa.gov/haps/health-effects-notebook-hazardous-air-pollutants.

55. Almberg KS, Turyk M, Jones RM, Anderson R, Graber J, Banda E, et al. A study of adverse birth outcomes and agricultural land use practices in Missouri. Environ Res. 2014;134:420–6.

56. Ahern M, Mullett M, MacKay K, Hamilton C. Residence in coal-mining areas and low-birth-weight outcomes. Matern Child Health J. 2011;15:974–9.

57. Curtis A, Leitner M. Geographic information systems and public health: eliminating perinatal disparity. Hershey: IRM Press; 2006.

58. Mckenzie LM, Guo R, Witter RZ, Savitz DA, Newman LS, Adgate JL. Birth outcomes and maternal residential proximity to natural gas development in rural Colorado. Environ Health Perspect. 2014;122(4):412–17.

59. Casey JA, Savitz DA, Rasmussen SG, Ogburn EL, Pollak J, Mercer DG, et al. Unconventional natural gas development and birth outcomes in Pennsylvania, USA. Epidemiology. 2016;27:163–72.

60. Miranda ML, Edwards SE, Chang HH, Auten RL. Proximity to roadways and pregnancy outcomes. J Expo Sci Environ Epidemiol. 2012;23:32–8.

61. Wilhelm M, Ritz B. Residential proximity to traffic and adverse birth outcomes in Los Angeles County, California, 1994–1996. Environ Health Perspect. 2003;111:207–16.

62. Donovan GH, Michael YL, Butry DT, Sullivan AD, Chase JM. Urban trees and the risk of poor birth outcomes. Health Place. 2011;17:390–3.

63. Hystad P, Davies HW, Frank L, Van Loon J, Gehring U, Tamburic L, et al. Residential greenness and birth outcomes: evaluating the influence of spatially correlated built-environment factors. Environ Health Perspect. 2014;122:1095–102.

64. Stieb DM, Burnett RT, Smith-Doiron MH, Brion O, Shin HH, Economou

V. A new multipollutant, no-threshold air quality health index based on short-term associations observed in daily time-series analyses. J Air Waste Manage Assoc. 2008;58:435–50.

65. Rappazzo KM, Messer LC, Jagai JS, Gray CL, Grabich SC, Lobdell DT. The associations between environmental quality and preterm birth in the United States, 2000–2005: a cross-sectional analysis. Environ Health. 2015;14:50.

66. Tarocco S, Amoruso I, Caravello G. Holistic model-based monitoring of the human health status in an urban environment system: pilot study in Verona city, Italy. J Prev Med Hyg. 2011;52:73–82.

67. Chen L, Bell EM, Caton AR, Druschel CM, Lin S. Residential mobility during pregnancy and the potential for ambient air pollution exposure misclassification. Environ Res. 2010;110:162–8.

68. Amrhein CG. Searching for the elusive aggregation effect: evidence from statistical simulations. Environ Plan A. 1995;27:105–19.

69. Statistics Canada. Census and intercensal road network. Statistics Canada Catalogue no. 92-500-X [digital data]. 92-500-X. 2012. Available from: http://www12.statcan.gc.ca/census-recensement/2011/geo/RNF-FRR/index-eng.cfm.

70. AltaLIS. 20 K Alberta Base Features [digital data]. AltaLIS, Agent Alberta Data Partnerships Ltd. 2012. Available from: http://www.altalis.com/products/base/20k_base_features.html.

71. Alberta Biodiversity Monitoring Institute. ABMI Human Footprint Inventory for 2012 conditions Version 3 [digital data]. Alberta Biodivers Monit Inst. 2012. Available from: http://www.abmi.ca/home/data/gis-data/human-footprint-download.html?scroll=true.

72. National Oceanic and Atmospheric Administration. DMSP-OLS nighttime lights time series, 2005–2012, Version 4 [digital data]. Def Meteorol Satel Progr Oper Linescan Syst (OLS), Natl Ocean Atmos Adm Natl Centers Environ Inf 2012. Available from: https://ngdc.noaa.gov/eog/dmsp/downloadV4composites.html.

73. Natural Resources Canada. Free Data—GeoGratis: Atlas of Canada National Frameworks Data, Aboriginal Lands, and CanVec [digital data]. Nat Resour Canada (NRCan), Gov. Canada. 2013. Available from: https://www.nrcan.gc.ca/earth-sciences/geography/topographic-information/free-data-geogratis/download-directory-documentation/17215.

74. Chan E, Serrano J, Chen L, Stieb DM, Jerrett M, Osornio-Vargas A. Development of a Canadian socioeconomic status index for the study of health outcomes related to environmental pollution. BMC Public Health. 2015;15:714.

75. Alberta Agriculture and Forestry. Historical wildfire information—spatial wildfire data, 2005–2012 [digital data]. Alberta Agric For (AgFor), Gov Alberta, Agric For Prov For Fire Cent. 2016. Available from: http://wildfire.alberta.ca/wildfire-maps/historical-wildfire-information/default.aspx.

9

Social and physical environmental correlates of independent mobility in children: a systematic review taking sex/gender differences into account

Isabel Marzi[1*], Yolanda Demetriou[2] and Anne Kerstin Reimers[1]

Abstract

Background: Children's independent mobility (CIM) is an important contributor to physical activity and health in children. However, in the last 20 years CIM has significantly decreased. To develop effective intervention programs to promote CIM, the impact of the environment on CIM must be identified. This review seeks to provide an overview of sex/gender-specific socio-ecological correlates of CIM.

Methods: A systematic literature search of five databases (PubMed, PsycInfo, Scopus, Medline, Web of Science) was conducted with a priori defined eligibility criteria and identified 1838 potential articles published between January 1990 and November 2017. Two independent reviewers screened the literature and identified and rated methodological quality of the studies. Related factors of CIM were summarized separately for CIM license (parental permission to travel independently) and CIM destination (destinations to which a child travels independently), and separately for boys and girls using a semi-quantitative method.

Results: Twenty-seven peer-reviewed journal articles were identified which examined the relationship between the social and physical environment and CIM. Only seven studies reported results divided by sex/gender. Most associations between the environment and CIM were found in the expected direction (positive or negative) or not associated at all. The social environment seemed to be more influential for ensuring CIM than the physical environment. Neighborhood safety, fear of crime and stranger, parental support, and perception of traffic were important social environmental factors influencing CIM, while car ownership, distance, and neighborhood design were relevant physical environmental attributes. Few studies examined sex/gender-related environmental correlates of independent mobility, and those findings were inconsistent.

Conclusion: The findings of this systematic review serve as suggestions for intervention programs to increase CIM and to identify future directions in research. To establish a robust comprehension of the impact of the social and physical environment on CIM, further sex/gender-sensitive studies using comparable measurements for CIM and environmental correlates are needed.

Keywords: Independent mobility, Social environment, Physical environment, Children, Sex/gender differences

*Correspondence: isabel.marzi@hsw.tu-chemnitz.de
[1] Faculty of Behavioral and Social Sciences, Chemnitz University
of Technology, Chemnitz, Germany
Full list of author information is available at the end of the article

Background

Physical activity is associated with numerous health benefits [1, 2]. However, in 2010 more than 80% of school-aged children worldwide did not to meet the World Health Organization recommendation of 60 min of moderate to vigorous-intensity physical activity daily [3, 4]. Walking or cycling for transport, otherwise known as 'active travel', is one way in which children can increase their levels of physical activity. A number of studies have examined the contribution of active travel to overall activity levels and health [5] and have generally found that children who walk to school are more likely to engage in physical activity overall and are more likely to meet physical activity guidelines than children who travel motorized. Additionally, children who walk or cycle to school have a lower BMI than those who are passive travelers [6].

Children's independent mobility (CIM) defined as "the freedom of children to travel around their neighborhood or city without adult supervision" [7] is one important contributor to active travel and underscores the relationship between active travel behavior and physical activity. For both boys and girls, CIM is positively associated with physical activity on weekdays and, furthermore, for girls on weekends [8].

In addition to these health outcomes, CIM is associated with cognitive and motor development as well as social competencies of children [9–12]. Rissotto and Tonucci [13] showed that CIM has positive effects on cognitive development of children due to social and environmental experience. Furthermore, children who are independently mobile have more social competencies as they spend more time with peers than others [12]. In contrast, a lower CIM level predicts greater feelings of loneliness [14].

However, CIM has significantly decreased over the past 20 years [15, 16]. In Australia, the proportion of children travelling to school independently was 61% in 1991 but this proportion declined to 32% by 2012 [15]. Increased car use corresponding to a decline in independent mobility was recorded in several countries [17]. In Denmark, car use doubled between 1978 and 2000; within the same period the number of children walking to school fell by almost 40% [17]. Although Finnish children still enjoy the highest amount of independent mobility [18], CIM significantly decreased over a period of 20 years in Finland as well [16]: In the inner city of Helsinki, the proportion of children travelling independently to and from school decreased from 82 to 50%.

Socio-ecological models postulate multiple environmental influences on health behavior [19]. Children in particular are less autonomous concerning their physical activity and mobility and are more likely to be influenced by their environment than are adults [20]. Thus, understanding social and physical environmental correlates of independent mobility among children is an important prerequisite to develop effective interventions to increase the number of children engaging in independent mobility. Empirical studies examined various physical environmental (e.g., walkability, and urbanity) and social environmental (e.g., parental fear, perception of danger, and social support) factors that influence CIM. Changes in children's physical environments over the past 20 years, such as more car traffic and fewer playgrounds, affect active travel behaviors and deter CIM [17, 21, 22]. Access to organized leisure activities determines the extent of CIM as Fyhri, Hjorthol [17] reported that children are often taken to leisure activities by car, because activities take place outside the immediate neighborhood. Additionally, due to an increasing crime rate, high urbanization, and long distances to school, parents limit CIM by prohibition [17, 23]. Moreover, the neighborhood environment and the local social network determine CIM [24]. Mothers' perception of social danger and traffic around school has also been found to inhibit independent active travel [25, 26]. In contrast, older siblings or dog ownership are associated with greater CIM as older siblings and dogs provide parents an increased sense of safety [27].

Accounting for sex/gender differences with regard to independent mobility is important. Gender theories postulate that such differences are due to socially determined gender roles; gender-typed patterns of behavior occur based on socialization processes [28, 29]. Generally, girls tend to be less physically active than boys and less inclined to participate in organized sports [3, 30, 31]. Regarding CIM, sex/gender differences appear to exist, with girls having less freedom to travel around without parental supervision than boys [24, 32, 33]. Furthermore, boys seem to become independently mobile earlier than girls: Brown et al. [34] showed that 60% of boys between 4 and 6 years living in England are allowed to go out alone whereas the proportion of girls stands around 44%. As CIM is related to physical activity, knowing the reasons for low levels of CIM and considering them in intervention programs could be one way to increase physical activity in girls. There is evidence for different mechanisms explaining sex/gender differences in CIM: The higher protectiveness of parents about their daughters than about their sons and higher safety concerns can limit girls' independent mobility level [25, 34–36].

Health promotion programs are increasingly designed based on the socio-ecological perspective, thus identifying various levels of contextual influences on children's independent mobility is required [37, 38]. Nevertheless, to the best of our knowledge no comprehensive overview of socio-ecological correlates of independent mobility in children has yet been published. For active—but not independent—travel a review published by Panter et al. [39] pointed out the importance of environmental determinants of active travel behaviors. However, for CIM no such summary is available as a recent meta-analytical review by Sharmin and Kamruzzaman [40] focused solely on the association between the built environment and CIM. A systematic review by Qui and Zhu [41] focused on housing and community environments and its impact on CIM. Nevertheless, this review has its limitations, because no distinction was made between different types of CIM, i.e., range, destination, time or license and no quality assessment was conducted to identify current research gaps. Additionally, sex/gender-related differences concerning the correlates of CIM have not been incorporated in previous reviews [40, 41]. Thus, this systematic review aims to provide an overview of socio-ecological correlates of CIM with a particular focus on differences between boys and girls and categorized by different CIM types.

Methods

This systematic review was conducted and is reported based on the Preferred Reporting Items for Systematic Reviews and Meta-Analyses (PRISMA) guidelines [42].

Search strategy

The literature search was conducted on 7 November 2017 using the databases PubMed, Medline, Scopus, PsycInfo and Web of Science Core Collection. The search strategy included a combination of terms for independent mobility ("independent mobil*"), correlates (environment* OR neighborhood OR family OR families OR home OR parent* OR mother* OR father* OR sibling* OR urban* OR park*) and children (kids* OR child* OR girl* OR boy*). Additional articles were sought by reviewing reference lists of included full text articles and citations of full text articles using the Web of Science "Citation Network" statistics of each study.

Eligibility criteria

Studies were deemed eligible if they met all following inclusion criteria: (1) subjects of the study were healthy children (age 3–12 years or the average age was in this range); (2) at least one association between CIM and an environmental (social and physical) correlate was examined; (3) an appropriate study design was used (cross-sectional or longitudinal; no case or intervention study); (4) the study employed a quantitative design; (5) the study was published in a peer-reviewed journal, written in English or German language; (6) the study was published after 1990, because in that year Hillman et al. [22]

introduced the term "children's independent mobility", in their seminal study on this topic. An exception was made for some intervention studies if a cross-sectional analysis of the association of interest was reported.

If the study examined attitudes towards independent mobility instead of CIM itself, it was excluded. Studies referring to active commuting to school or active travel were only included if they clearly defined whether children travelled independently.

Environmental correlates

Social and physical correlates were selected based on the socio-ecological model of Sallis et al. [19]. Correlates of the social environment were categorized into three subcategories: children's perceived neighborhood environment (e.g., fear of stranger), parents' perceived neighborhood environment (e.g., neighborhood friendliness), and social cultural environment (e.g., parental rules towards CIM). To categorize correlates of the physical environment the following five domains were established based on Sallis et al. [19] and Ding et al. [43]: home environment (e.g., car ownership), school environment (e.g., school-specific walkability), recreational environment (e.g., access to parks and playground), neighborhood design (e.g., degree of urbanization), and transport environment (e.g., traffic). Studies with only socio-demographic characteristics of the child, the family and/or household were excluded.

Study selection

The study selection occurred in three steps compromising (1) title-screening, (2) abstract-screening, and (3) full-text-screening by two independent researchers (IM, CS). Studies were included or excluded depending on the eligibility criteria. During each step of the screening process, all references that could not be conclusively excluded were kept for further screening in the next step. Disagreement between the two reviewers on final inclusion was resolved by discussion with a third researcher (AKR). The selection process was documented using the reference management software EndNote X7 [44].

Data extraction

The following data was extracted from each article: author(s); year of publication; country; study design; sample description (number of participants, age, sex/gender); definition, measurement, and instrument of CIM; type, measurement, and instruments of examined correlates; and main study results on the relationship between social and physical environmental factors and CIM (see Additional file 1). CIM was classified as CIM range, CIM time, CIM destination, or CIM license [40]. CIM range describes the distance children can travel independently from their home. CIM time defines how many minutes children can travel outside of their home independently. Destinations a child independently travels to are included in the term CIM destination. Whether parents allow children to travel independently is defined as CIM license.

Quality assessment

The methodological quality of the studies included was evaluated by two independent reviewers (IM, KB) using 11 a priori defined quality criteria based on existing quality assessments published by Downes et al. [45] and Uijtdewilligen et al. [46]. Each criterion was either coded as "no" or "unclear" (0) if the study either did not meet the criterion or the criterion was not mentioned. If the study provided information on the quality item but only in parts, the criterion was coded as "partial" (0.5), while if the study completely met the criterion it was coded as "yes" (1). If a study referred to another publication containing relevant information for scoring the quality items, the study of interest was consulted. However, if the additional source did not provide the requested information or just in parts, the criterion was coded—according to the defined coding system—with "no" or "unclear", respectively. As many studies included multiple correlates (e.g., social factors, and physical factors), criterion eight was scored on a scale ranging from 0 to 1. For example, if a study analyzed four different types of correlates of which three were measured with a reliable tool, a score of 0.75 was calculated. The methodological quality score of each study was calculated by the percentage of fulfilled criteria relative to the sum of all criteria (11 points in total). A quality score of $\geq 70\%$ was considered high methodological quality, while a score of $< 70\%$ was considered insufficient methodological quality [46]. The quality assessment for each study is presented in Additional file 2.

Synthesis of results

Due to the heterogeneity of social and physical environmental correlates and outcome measures of CIM a meta-analysis of the selected studies was considered inappropriate. The results of all selected studies were analyzed using a semi-quantitative method. In addition to associations between the social and physical environment and independent mobility in children in general, associations were considered separately for both, girls and boys, with appropriate studies. Bivariate associations between CIM and environmental correlates (19 studies) and multivariate regression models (20 studies) were considered separately as various socio-demographic, social, and physical environmental correlates were integrated into multiple regression models. As no study evaluated CIM time and only three CIM range, the results

were only analyzed separately for CIM destination and CIM license.

The strength of evidence was adapted from previously published scoring systems [11, 43, 47]. If 0–33% of studies showed a significant association ($p \leq 0.05$) of CIM and social or physical environmental correlates, the findings were classified as no association (0). If 34–59% of studies demonstrated significant associations, the findings were classed as being inconsistent (?). If 60–100% reported significant associations between CIM and the social or physical environment, the findings were categorized as positive (+) or negative (−), depending on the direction of the relationship. For less than four available studies for positive or negative associations the evidence was rated as limited (small +, −). Additionally, the methodological quality of the studies was included in scoring the strength of evidence. If 60–100% of high quality studies showed a significant correlation, the findings were considered strong evidence for a positive (++) or negative (−) correlation.

As the publications of Foster et al. [36], Villanueva et al. [48] and Villanueva et al. [33] analyzed the same study population, some social and physical environmental correlates were doubled in the results. For that reason significant associations of doubled correlates of these publications were considered as one study result for scoring the strength of evidence.

Results
Flow chart

A total of 1838 potentially relevant articles (2165 including duplicates) were identified by the database search and screened based on title and abstract. Next, the full texts of 59 studies were retrieved for detailed review. As 34 studies were excluded due to inappropriate age range, aim of study, study design or for multiple reasons, 25 studies identified by the database screenings have been included in this systematic review. Two additional relevant publication were identified by backward reference tracking, yielding a total of 27 papers included in this systematic review (Fig. 1).

Characteristics of included studies

General study characteristics are summarized in Table 1. An additional file shows more details of the studies included (see Additional file 1). More than 80% of the selected studies were cross-sectional, two were longitudinal and another two studies were longitudinal including cross-section analyses. The sample sizes ranged from 181 children [49] to a study population of 2110 children [50]. Nearly half of the studies were conducted in Europe, with 10 from either Australia or New Zealand, five from North America or Canada and one from Asia. Most studies

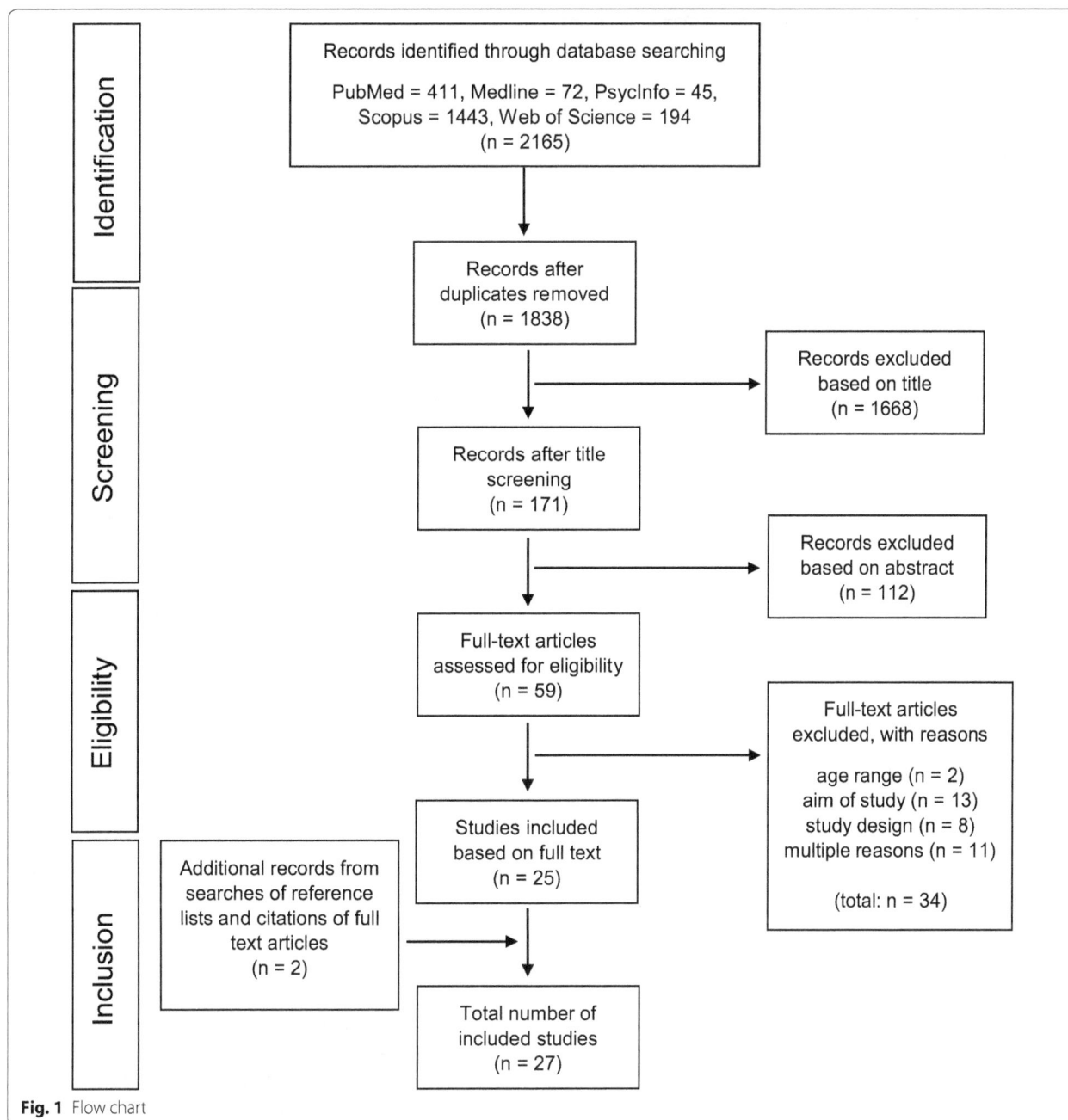

Fig. 1 Flow chart

(85%) were published between 2010 and 2017 with the earliest publication in 2001 [12].

In the majority of studies, the mean age of the sample population ranged from 9 to 12 years [12, 23–25, 27, 32, 33, 35, 36, 48, 49, 51–61]. Fewer studies focused on younger children aged 6 to 9 years [26, 50, 59, 62–64]. All studies targeted girls and boys, but merely seven studies separated results by sex/gender [33, 35, 36, 48, 52–54]. Of all studies, eighteen described CIM by destinations a child traveled independently to. Fewer studies examined

CIM licenses. CIM range was evaluated by another three studies. No study evaluated CIM as independent time outside. Ten studies utilized solely parent-report measures of CIM, and a further six studies applied children's self-reporting. Another ten studies combined child and parental report measurements of CIM. Twenty-one studies [12, 23–25, 32, 33, 35, 36, 48, 49, 52–57, 60–64] examined both social and physical environmental correlates of CIM. Three studies [50, 51, 58] focused on the relationship between the physical environment and CIM and

Table 1 Characteristics of studies included (n = 27 studies)

Characteristics	N (%)	Study source
Study design		
Cross-sectional	23 (85)	[12, 23–26, 32, 33, 35, 36, 48, 50, 51, 53–59, 61–64]
Longitudinal including cross-sectional analyses	2 (8)	[27, 49]
Longitudinal	2 (8)	[52, 60]
Sample size		
< 500	14 (52)	[12, 25, 27, 49, 53, 55–61, 63, 64]
> 500	13 (48)	[23, 24, 26, 32, 33, 35, 36, 48, 50–52, 54, 62]
Geographic origin		
Europe	11 (41)	[12, 23, 25, 35, 51, 52, 56, 58, 59, 62, 64]
North America/Canada	5 (18)	[24, 26, 32, 61, 63]
Australia/New Zealand	10 (37)	[27, 33, 36, 48, 49, 53–55, 57, 60]
Asia	1 (4)	[50]
Publication year		
2010–2017	23 (85)	[23–27, 32, 33, 35, 36, 48–55, 57–61, 63]
1990–2009	4 (15)	[12, 56, 62, 64]
IM definition[a]		
CIM range	3 (11)	[35, 56, 63]
CIM time	0	
CIM destination	18 (67)	[23, 25, 26, 32, 33, 36, 48, 51–55, 57–60, 62, 64]
CIM license	10 (37)	[12, 23, 24, 27, 49, 53, 56, 58, 61, 64]
No response	1 (4)	[50]
IM Measurement		
Child reported	6 (22)	[51, 52, 55, 59, 60, 62]
Parent reported	10 (37)	[12, 24–27, 35, 49, 56, 61, 63]
Child and parent reported	10 (37)	[23, 32, 33, 36, 48, 53, 54, 57, 58, 64]
No response	1 (4)	[50]
Correlates measurement		
Objective	1 (4)	[51]
Subjective	10 (37)	[12, 24–27, 35, 56, 59, 62, 63]
Objective and subjective	16 (59)	[23, 32, 33, 36, 48–50, 52–55, 57, 58, 60, 61, 64]

[a] More than 100% possible due to multiple types of CIM in one study

two further studies [26, 59] reported only the association between social environmental factors and CIM. For social and physical environmental factors most studies combined objective and subjective measurements. Ten studies applied only subjective measurements and one study used solely objective measurements.

Results of methodological quality assessment

The study quality was rated high in 12 studies [25, 27, 32, 36, 49, 51, 52, 55, 59–61, 64] and low in 15 studies [12, 23, 24, 26, 33, 35, 48, 50, 53, 54, 56–58, 62, 63]. The agreement between the two reviewers in the methodological quality of included studies (IM and KB) was 75% (Cohen's kappa $\kappa = 0.752$). In discussion of individual study quality scores, a final agreement of 100% was achieved. The methodological quality criteria and the number and proportion of studies fulfilling the criteria are presented in Table 2; more detailed quality assessments of each study included is presented in an additional file (see Additional file 2). All 27 studies contained clearly defined aims. As the aim of the majority of the studies was to identify causal relationships between the social and physical environment and CIM, most studies did not fulfil the criterion regarding study design. Twenty-five studies failed to meet criteria for response rate, since the response rate was less than 80% or not clearly defined. Only three studies undertook measures to address and categorize nonresponders. Standardized methods of acceptable quality were used to measure CIM and correlates in more than 50% of the studies. One study lacked clearly defined statistical methods and internally consistent results. More than 80% of the studies presented results for all the analyses described in the methods; four studies were missing some data.

Table 2 Criteria for methodological quality assessment and number (%) of studies scoring points for each criterion

		Studies fulfilling the criteria n (%)	
		Yes	Partial
Criteria			
1	Were the aims/objectives of the study clear?	27 (100)	0 (0)
Methods			
2	Was the study design appropriate for the stated aims?	6 (22)	21 (78)
3	Were the main features of the study population stated (description of sampling frame, distribution by age and sex/gender)?	14 (52)	13 (48)
4	Was the response rate at least 80%?	2 (8)	0 (0)
5	Were measures undertaken to address and categorize non-responders?	3 (11)	0 (0)
6	Were the exposure and outcome variables measured appropriate to the aims of the study?	17 (63)	10 (37)
7	Were standardized methods of acceptable quality used to measure IM?[a]	12 (44)	6 (22)
8	Were standardized methods of acceptable quality used to measure correlates?[a]	18 (69)	6 (22)
9	It is clear what was used to determine statistical significance and/or precision estimated (e.g., p values, confidence intervals)?	23 (85)	2 (8)
Results			
10	Were the results internally consistent?	26 (96)	1 (4)
11	Were the results presented for all the analyses described in the methods?	23 (85)	4 (15)

[a] Reliability: ICC > 0.70; Cronbach's alpha > 0.65, pilot testing, published previously

Social environment and CIM destination

A total of 48 associations of social environmental correlates and independent mobility to different destinations were reviewed in 10 studies. Some studies investigated similar constructs but employed different terminologies. Thus, these variables (e.g., safe for children, and safe place) were collected and an umbrella term was used (e.g., neighborhood safety) yielding a total sum of 23 social environmental correlates (Table 3). Three of four correlates describing children's perceived neighborhood environment were significantly associated with CIM destination in the expected direction: fear of strangers (67%), neighborhood safety (100%), and many other children residing within their area (100%). Concerning the parental perceived neighborhood environment, 75% of all comparisons showed significant associations with CIM destination, including fear of strangers (100%), fear of crime (100%), neighborhood friendliness (100%), perception of traffic (63%), informal social control (100%), and people out on walks in the neighborhood (100%). Less evidence existed for associations between the social cultural environment and CIM destination; four of eight variables had more than 60% of significant associations. Mobility licenses (100%), confidence in children's abilities (100%), a child's personal safety (100%), and having friends (100%) were positively associated with CIM destination. Several relationships of social environmental correlates and CIM destination were categorized as inconsistent, including neighborhood friendliness (children; 50%), neighborhood safety (parents; 40%), parental rules (50%), and parent encouragement (50%). No association showed strong evidence with 60–100% of high quality studies reporting the association in the expected direction.

Physical environment and CIM destination

The evidence for associations between the physical environment and CIM destination was much weaker than for social environmental correlates. Only 11 of 23 variables demonstrated evidence for significant associations with CIM destination, reviewed in 14 studies (Table 3). Car ownership (60%), dog ownership (100%), distance to school (100%), school density (100%), remote places (100%), population density (100%), degree of urbanization (71%), urban structure (100%) were consistently associated with CIM destination in the expected direction, but with little evidence. Furthermore, different neighborhood designs, such as mainly single-family housing, densely built up residential areas and big buildings were associated with CIM. Inconsistent associations were reported for five physical environmental variables, including bike ownership (50%), school-specific walkability (40%), access to parks (33%), street connectivity (38%), and land use mix (50%). Transport attributes, including walking facilities, biking facilities, streetlight density and traffic (objective), were also not consistently associated with CIM destination.

Table 3 Social and physical environmental correlates of CIM Destination

Correlates	Study source	Association with CIM +	Association with CIM 0	Association with CIM −	Strength of evidence Association[a]	n/N (%)[b]
Social environment						
Perceived neighborhood environment (children)						
Fear of strangers	[32, 33]		[33] F	[33] M; [32]	−	2/3 (67)
Neighborhood friendliness	[33]	[33] M	[33] F		?	1/2 (50)
Neighborhood safety	[32, 33]; [62]c	[33] M, F; [32]		[62]c	+	4/4 (100)
Many other children within their area	[33, 36]	{[33] M, F; [36] M, F}e			+	2/2 (100)
Perceived neighborhood environment (parents)						
Sense of community	[52]		[52] (M, F)		0	0/2 (0)
Fear of strangers	[32, 36]			[32]; [36] M, F	−	3/3 (100)
Fear of crime	[63]			[63]	−	1/1 (100)
Neighborhood friendliness	[33, 36, 60]	{[33] M, F; [36] M, F}e; [60]			+	3/3 (100)
Neighborhood safety	[52, 63]; [52]c	[52] F; [63]	[52] M; [52]c M, F		?	2/5 (40)
Perception of traffic	[36, 52, 62, 63]; [32, 33]d(2); [33, 60, 63]c	[33]c M, F; [63]c	[33] M, F; [52]M, F; [36] M; [60]c	[62, 63]; [32]d(2); [36] F; [33] M, F	−	10/16 (63)
Often people out on walks in the neighborhood	[33]	[33] M, F			+	2/2 (100)
Informal social control	[36]	[36] M, F			+	2/2 (100)
Social cultural environment						
Mobility license	[53–55, 64]	[53] M, F; [54] M, F; [55, 64]			+	6/6 (100)
Parental rules (towards IM) walking	[52]		[52] M, F		0	0/2 (0)
Parental rules (towards IM) play outside	[52]	[52] M	[52] F		?	1/2 (50)
Parent encourage for walking/cycling	[52]		[52] M	[52] F	?	1/2 (50)
Friend encourage for walking/cycling	[52]		[52] M, F		0	0/2 (0)
Confidence in children's abilities	[33, 60]	[33] M, F; [60]			+	3/3 (100)
Child's personal safety	[33, 60]	[33] M, F; [60]			+	3/3 (100)
Fearful of child engaging in antisocial behavior	[33]		[33] M, F		0	0/2 (0)
Parental physical activity	[63]		[63]		0	0/1 (0)
Parent activity with child	[63]		[63]		0	0/1 (0)
Many children we know walk or cycle to school	[60]		[60]		0	0/1 (0)
Having friends	[33]	[33] M, F			+	2/2 (100)
Physical environment						
Home environment						
Car ownership	[32, 50, 52, 62]		[32]; [52] F	[50, 62]; [52] M	−	3/5 (60)
Dog ownership	[27]	[27]			+	1/1 (100)
Bike ownership	[33]	[33] F	[33] M		?	1/2 (50)
Size of backyard	[33]		[33] M, F		0	0/2 (0)
School environment						
Distance	[32, 50, 51, 62]			[32, 50, 51, 62]	−	4/4 (100)

Table 3 (continued)

Correlates	Study source	Association with CIM			Strength of evidence	
		+	0	−	Association[a]	n/N (%)[b]
School-specific walk-ability	[33, 36, 52, 62]	{[33] F; [36] F}[e]; [62]	{[33] M; [36] M}[e]; [52] M, F		?	2/5 (40)
School characteristics	[52]		[52] M, F		0	0/2 (0)
School density	[50]	[50]			+	1/1 (100)
Recreational environment						
Parks	[33, 60]	[33] M	[33] F; [60]		?	1/3 (33)
Quality and quantity of public open spaces	[55]		[55]		0	0/1 (0)
Remote places	[51]	[51]			+	1/1 (100)
Neighborhood design						
Street connectivity	[32, 50]; [52][d (3)]		[52] M, F; [52] (M); [52] M, F	[32, 50]; [52] F	?	3/8 (38)
Neighborhood walk-ability	[52]		[52] M, F		0	0/2 (0)
Land use mix	[32, 50, 52]		[52] M; [50]	[32]; [52] F	?	2/4 (50)
Population density	[50]			[50]	−	1/1 (100)
Degree of urbanization (ref: urban)	[23, 50, 53, 54, 58, 62, 64]	[54]	[53]	[23, 50, 58, 62, 64]	−	5/7 (71)
Urban structure (new)	[32]	[32]			+	1/1 (100)
Street-trees	[32]		[32]		0	0/1 (0)
Densely built up residential areas	[51]	[51]			+	1/1 (100)
Mainly single-family housing	[51]	[51]			+	1/1 (100)
Big building and public transport hubs	[51]			[51]	−	1/1 (100)
Transport environment						
Walking facilities	[52]; [60]; [32][c]	[60]	[52] M, F	[32][c]	?	2/4 (50)
Biking facilities	[60]		[60]		0	0/1 (0)
Streetlight density	[52]		[52] M, F		0	0/2 (0)
Traffic (objective)	[50, 51]; [32][d (2)]		[32, 51]	[32, 50]	?	2/4 (50)

Effects which are specific to different sex/gender groups are noted separately: M (male); F (female)

CIM children's independent mobility

[a] No evidence: no studies were identified; no association (0): 0–33% of studies showed a significant association; inconsistent association (?): 34–59% of studies reported significant associations; positive (+) or negative (−) association: 60–100% of studies demonstrated significant associations; limited evidence for a positive or negative association (small +, −): <4 studies available for the associations of interest; strong evidence (++) or (−−) association: 60–100% of high quality studies showed a significant association

[b] n = number of studies/measures reporting associations in the expected direction; N = number of identified studies/measures on the association of interest; (%) = percentage of studies reporting associations in the expected direction

[c] Items are reversed

[d(x)] The same study may occur twice or more often within a topic if different measures are used and show different associations; x = number of measures

[e] {…} = study results of two studies with the same population were considered as one study

Social environment and CIM license

With regard to children's license to be independently mobile, fewer correlates were examined due to a limited number of studies (7 studies). In total eight correlates regarding the parental perceived neighborhood environment and social cultural environment were reviewed (Table 4). Perceived neighborhood attributes, such as fear of strangers (100%), neighborhood friendliness (66%), and neighborhood safety (100%), were significantly associated with CIM license. Additionally, social norms (100%) and parents' travel attitudes (100%) showed associations with CIM license. All associations demonstrated little evidence. The associations between CIM license and parents perceived fear of crime (34%) and traffic (34%) were inconsistent.

Table 4 Social and physical environmental correlates of CIM License

Correlates	Study source	Association with CIM			Strenght of evidence	
		+	0	–	Association[a]	n/N (%)[b]
Social environment						
Perceived neighborhood environment (parents)						
Fear of strangers	[24][c]	[24][c]			+	1/1 (100)
Fear of crime	[61][c;] [49][d (2)]	[61][c]	[49][d (2)]		?	1/3 (33)
Neighborhood friendliness	[24, 61]; [49][c]	[24, 61]	[49][c]		+	2/3 (66)
Neighborhood safety	[24, 61]; [49][c]	[24, 61]		[49][c]	+	3/3 (100)
Perception of traffic	[24, 49]; [61][c]	[61][c]	[24, 49]		?	1/3 (33)
Neighborhood maintenance	[49][d(4)]		[49][d(4)]		0	0/4 (0)
Social cultural environment						
Social norms (no support of IM)	[49]			[49]	–	1/1 (100)
Parents' attitudes toward active travel modes	[24]	[24]			+	1/1 (100)
Child-centered social control	[61]		[61]		0	0/1 (0)
Physical environment						
Home environment						
Car ownership	[61]			[61]	–	1/1 (100)
Recreational environment						
Park availability	[49][d (2)]		[49][d (2)]		0	0/2 (0)
Park attractiveness	[49]	[49]			+	1/1 (100)
Playgrounds	[49][d (2)]		[49][d (2)]		0	0/2 (0)
School environment						
School density	[49][d (2)]		[49][d (2)]		0	0/2 (0)
Neighborhood design						
Housing unit density	[61]		[61]		0	0/1 (0)
Degree of Urbanization	[23, 53, 58, 64]		[53]	[23, 58, 64]	–	3/4 (75)
Neighborhood Walkability	[24][d(6)]		[24][d(6)]		0	0/6 (0)
Transport environment						
Traffic (objective)	[49]		[49]		0	0/1 (0)

CIM children's independent mobility

[a] No evidence: no studies were identified; no association (0): 0–33% of studies showed a significant association; inconsistent association (?): 34–59% of studies reported significant associations; positive (+) or negative (–) association: 60–100% of studies demonstrated significant associations; limited evidence for a positive or negative association (small +, –): <4 studies available for the associations of interest; strong evidence (++) or (––) association: 60–100% of high quality studies showed a significant association

[b] n = number of studies/measures reporting associations in the expected direction; N = number of identified studies/measures on the association of interest; (%) = percentage of studies reporting associations in the expected direction

[c] Items are reversed

[d(x)] The same study may occur twice or more often within a topic if different measures are used and show different associations; x = number of measures

Physical environment and CIM license

Similar to CIM destination less significant associations existed for physical environmental attributes and CIM license; only three of nine variables demonstrated significant associations. As shown in Table 4, car ownership (100%), park attractiveness (100%), and degree of urbanization (75%) were associated with CIM license in the expected direction. Strong evidence was not found for any association with physical environment. No variable of the school environment and transport environment was associated with CIM licenses and neither was availability of parks and playgrounds.

Results from multivariate regression models

The results of the multivariate regression models of 12 studies, including these models in addition to univariate associations, and of eight studies solely presenting multivariate regression models were also analyzed in this systematic review (Table 5). These results highlight the evidence of bivariate associations between the environment and CIM. Nevertheless, socio-demographic characteristics such as age and sex/gender remained significant in nearly all regression models and tended to be important predictors of CIM. Additionally, having siblings was significantly associated with CIM in four models.

Concerning the social environment, perceived neighborhood attributes, such as neighborhood safety and fear of strangers, remained significant correlates of CIM. Moreover, parental rules and attitudes towards independent mobility showed associations with CIM. Three physical environmental attributes were consistently associated with CIM: distance to school, car ownership and traffic. There is less evidence for neighborhood design (e.g., walkability) and degree of urbanization, but many models were controlled for urban setting and, thus, did not report this association.

Sex/gender differences in CIM correlates

Due to a limited number of studies reporting results separately for boys and girls and the heterogeneity of correlates, no evidence can be found for sex/gender-specific correlates of independent mobility. Mobility licenses were positively associated with CIM for boys and girls. Two further correlates analyzed in two different studies [36, 52] were school-specific walkability and parental perception of traffic, which yielded inconsistent results for girls and boys (Table 3). Concerning the results of multivariate regression models, only for physical environmental attributes differences were reviewed between boys and girls. For girls only, neighborhood design, such as walkability and land use mix as well as access to a bike, was associated with girls' independent mobility [48, 52]. Car ownership and destination accessibility (e.g., parks, shopping centers, and recreation venues) were significant correlates of independent mobility in boys but not in girls [48, 52]. Inconsistent associations were reported for traffic with studies reporting associations for boys and girls and only for girls [33, 35, 48].

Discussion

The aim of this systematic review was to identify social and physical environmental correlates of independent mobility in children with a special focus on sex/gender. Associations of CIM destination and license and social environment were consistently positive, except for fear of strangers and crime. Car ownership and urban setting showed consistently negative associations with CIM License and CIM destination, respectively. However, five physical environmental attributes (dog ownership, shorter distance to school, school density, remote places, and new urban structure) were positively associated with CIM destination. Differences in correlates of independent mobility in boys and girls were found solely for the physical environment, with neighborhood design and bike ownership influencing girls' independent mobility and associations of destination accessibility and car ownership with boys' independent mobility.

CIM is related to physical activity, e.g., if children are walking or cycling without adult accompaniment. However, correlates of CIM seem to be slightly different to correlates of physical activity [43]. CIM tends to be more determined by the social environment than the physical environment. In comparison, physical activity is more associated with objectively measured environmental attributes such as walkability and traffic speed/volume [43]. For CIM other factors may be important to address when developing intervention programs, such as social norms, parents' perceptions of neighborhood, and parental rules. Particularly, CIM license depends on parents' perception of neighborhood environment [24, 49, 61]. As many studies have demonstrated that CIM increases with children's age [23, 25, 62], parental restrictions on CIM probably decrease with children's age while physical environmental attributes which support independent active travel may gain in importance.

Previous reviews of the physical environment and children's travel behavior reported inconsistent results and non-occurring associations for several physical attributes as well [39, 65]. For children, the impact of the physical environment is potentially influenced by granting (or not) of mobility licenses by their parents who are literally the gatekeepers of their travel behavior. For adults a variety of neighborhood physical features, such as walkability, street connectivity and access to services, are consistently associated with active travel behavior [66, 67].

The two constructs "parental perception of traffic" and "traffic (objective)" supported the conclusion that social environmental attributes determine CIM more than those of the physical environment: traffic perception was consistently associated with CIM; inconsistent associations were reported for objectively measured traffic. Nevertheless, physical environmental correlates with inconsistent results (e.g., school-specific walkability, access to parks, street connectivity, and land use mix) need to be addressed in future research as some studies have shown that activity-friendly environments can promote active travel behavior [68].

Results of multivariate regression models of studies included in this review underline the differing relevance of the social and physical environment for CIM. Age, sex/gender and parental perceived neighborhood environment tend to be represented as significant correlates of CIM [12, 25, 26, 32, 49, 50, 61, 62]. On the other hand, few physical environmental correlates (e.g., car ownership, and distance) remained significant in multivariate regression models [26, 32, 50, 52, 56, 57, 62]. Although these models help to identify the actual effects of different correlates on CIM, the comparison

Table 5 Results of multivariate regression models showing only significant correlates of CIM (n = 20 studies)

Study source	Socio-demographic and psychosocial characteristics	Social environment	Physical environment
Alparone et al. [25]	Age, birth order	fear of strangers Perception of positive potentiality of outdoor autonomy	n. s.
Buliung et al. [32] (to school)	Age, sex/gender Flexible work schedule	Neighborhood safety	Distance Traffic
Buliung et al. [32] (from school)	Age, sex/gender, Flexible work schedule, fathers' employment status	Neighborhood safety	Traffic
Christian et al. [49]	Age, older siblings	Neighborhood safety Social norms	n. s.
Cordovil et al. [23]	Age	Mobility license	Car ownership Distance
Fyhri et al. [62]	Age, sex/gender	Neighborhood safety Fear of strangers	Parents car use frequency Distance
Janssen et al. [63]	Age	Neighborhood safety Fear of crime	n. s.
Johannson [56] CIM license	Age, maturity, siblings	Neighborhood safety Traffic perception Need to protect	n. s.
Johannson [56] CIM range	Age, maturity, siblings	Attitude towards CIM	Car ownership Traffic
Kytta [16] (Finnish data)	n. s.	Mobility license	Urbanization
Kytta [64] (Belrushian data)	Sex/gender	n. s.	Urbanization
Lam and Loo [50]	Age Household income, family structure, mothers' employment status, domestic helpers at home	n. s.	Distance Urbanization School density
Lin et al. [57]	Siblings	n.s.	Car ownership Distance
Mammen et al. [26]	Age Language spoken at home	Fear of strangers Traffic perception	Car ownership Distance
Prezza et al. [12]	Age, sex/gender	Neighborhood Friendliness	Park accessibility Urban structure Courtyard
Santos et al. [59][a]	n. r.	Neighborhood safety Parents' physical activity	
Veitch et al. [60][b] school	Child enjoys walking	child's personal safety	Walking facilities
Veitch et al. [60][b] local destinations	n. s.	Many other children with in the neighborhood	n.s.
Wolfe and McDonald [61]	Age, race	Neighborhood safety	Housing unit density
Multivariate regressions models with separate results for boys and girls			
Carver et al. [52][d] girls	n. r.	Parent encouragement for walking	Street connectivity Land use mix
Carver et al. [52][d] boys	n. r.	Parental rules towards outdoor play	Car ownership
Foster et al. [36] girls	n. r.	Fear of strangers Informal social control	n. r.
Foster et al. [36] boys	n. r.	Fear of strangers	n. r.
Ghekiere et al. [35] girls	Grade Cycle skills Traffic skills	n. s.	traffic
Ghekiere et al. [35] boys	Grade Cycle skills Traffic skills	n. s.	n. s.
Villanueva et al. [35][e] girls	Child's confidence	Neighborhood safety Traffic perception Confidence in child's ability	Bike ownership School-specific walkability

Table 5 (continued)

Study source	Socio-demographic and psychosocial characteristics	Social environment	Physical environment
Villanueva et al. [48][e] boys	Child's confidence	Neighborhood friendliness Traffic perception confidence in child's ability	Distance to green space Count of shopping centers, recreation venues, community services and retail shops Park attractiveness
Villlanueva et al. [48][e] girls	Child's confidence	Neighborhood safety People on walks in the neighborhood Confidence in child's ability	Bike ownership School-specific walkability
Villlanueva et al. [48][e] boys	Child's confidence	Neighborhood safety Many other children with in the neighborhood Traffic perception confidence in child's ability	

Abbreviations: *CIM* children's independent mobility, *n. r.* not reported, *n. s.* not significant

[a] Adjusted for child's age and gender

[b] Controlled for sex and age of child, urban/rural location, maternal education and employment, distance to school, whether the child changed school between T1 and T2, and clustering within suburbs

[c] Controlled for sex and age of child, urban/rural location, maternal education and employment, and clustering within suburbs

[d] Controlled for parental education level, distance from home to school, urban/rural

[e]Adjusted for socio-economic status, age, maternal education, child's school year, whether or not child was sick last week, school clustering

of findings should be interpreted carefully as all regression models integrated a wide range of socio-demographic, social and physical environmental correlates and adjusted for different variables.

Only three studies focused on parental physical activity and parents' and friends' encouragement for walking, but the results were inconsistent [52, 59, 63]. However, family and peer support and modeling seemed to be relevant for CIM as in other studies having siblings and friends was positively related to CIM [33, 49, 56, 57]. Previous reviews showed that parental physical activity and physical activity of peers is associated with youth activity behaviors [47, 69, 70] . Additionally, a study by Mackett et al. [71] demonstrated that girls in particular were only allowed to go out if they were accompanied by other children. In order to promote CIM, future research should specially focus on parent and peer related correlates of CIM, such as social support and social modelling. Furthermore, parent perceived environmental factors, such as fear of crime and neighborhood safety which were inconsistently associated with CIM, demand further research.

In physical activity, sport participation and CIM sex/gender differences are consistently reported, with girls tending to be less active or rather mobile than boys [3, 12, 72]. To overcome these sex/gender gaps, intervention programs need to be sex/gender-sensitive and take sex/gender-specific situations into account. A study by Reimers et al. [72] pointed out that girls residing longer destinations from the nearest sport facilities are less likely to take part in club sport activities. This relationship has not been observed in boys in this study. Promoting independent mobility in girls could therefore increase both their physical activity on the way to sports facilities and other physical activities by enabling girls to get access to other physical activity facilities or locations. CIM could be a door opener to get access to physical activity facilities and locations, such as gyms, playgrounds, parks etc., where children can participate in various physical activities and are able to meet other children to actively play with. This could be true for girls and boys. Promoting CIM in girls and boys could contribute to physical activity as active living behavior. Since an active living behavior is often established in childhood and adolescence, it could also affect physical activity and health in adulthood [73, 74].

Thus, this systematic review was the first to investigate sex/gender-related correlates of CIM for the development of effective intervention programs. Sex/gender differences with regard to the extent of independent mobility are consistently reported as being lower for girls than for boys [12, 34, 58]. To promote CIM, especially in girls, it is necessary to sufficiently understand the impact of social and environmental influences on girls' and boys' independent travel behaviors. However, only seven studies were identified that reported results separately for boys and girls [33, 35, 36, 48, 52–54]. Due to heterogeneity in the correlates and differing statistical methods, the results of the studies did not provide evidence of sex/gender-related correlates of CIM. This marks a research gap which must be addressed in future studies to develop effective sex/gender-specific intervention programs for boys and girls.

In this systematic review all studies with a quantitative design were included, irrespective of whether they were cross-sectional analyses or longitudinal analyses. Thus, the objective was to identify correlates of CIM because the number of high quality longitudinal studies was very limited. However to identify causal relationships between the environment and CIM, more longitudinal studies are needed.

According to Sharmin and Kamruzzaman [40], in the present systematic review, CIM was categorized into four different types: CIM destination, CIM license, CIM time, and CIM range. However, the majority of studies examined CIM destination and CIM license, and the results were solely presented for these two definitions of CIM. A study by Bhosale et al. [75] showed that CIM license and destination access are significantly correlated, which explains the similarities in the social and physical environmental correlates of both CIM types.

Apart from similarities between CIM license and CIM destination, some studies [49, 61] reported that the correlates of independent mobility differ between visited destinations. For example distance to park [49] and social control [61] were correlated with specific destinations (i.e., a park and a friend's house, respectively) but not with overall independent mobility. Due to a lack of comparability, in this systematic review, the results were only analyzed for overall independent mobility. More research is required to separate correlates by visited destination.

CIM range was analyzed in merely three studies and CIM time not at all. Time and range may be insufficient indicators for CIM or simply rarely used at this stage. Using GPS as an objective measure of CIM could provide a more comprehensive understanding of CIM time and CIM range as indicator of CIM [76].

Based on the results of the methodological quality assessment, the lack of a standardized definition and measurement of independent mobility and environmental correlates limited the comparison of the included studies. In fact, a wide variety of measurements were used to determine CIM. Although results were separated for CIM license and CIM destination, measurements differed for child and parental report, with no study employing objective measures. To compare studies Bates and Stone [76] recommended using a standardized methodological design and a combination of subjective and objective measurements of CIM in future research.

Additionally, a wide selection of social and physical environmental correlates was used in the studies to evaluate the relationship between the environment and CIM.

Thus, some correlates appeared only in one study, which provided only limited evidence. Furthermore, terminological differences were observed between researchers. For example, "stranger danger" was paraphrased as "trust in strangers" [24], "worried about strangers" [32, 33], and "fear of strangers" [32], which based on the description and measurement evaluated the same construct or the contrary. Due to such differences the comparison of various studies might be limited. Thus, future research should aim to create and apply standardized terms. Moreover, the heterogeneity of applied measurements for the same social and physical construct in different studies and the lack of reliable tools could lead to inconsistent findings as well.

The lack of generalizability of study results is caused by insufficient response rates in almost all studies. Acceptable response rates should to be at least 80% [46]. The response rate of included studies ranged between 18% [53] and 100% [64] with merely two studies above the recommended 80% [25, 64].

To analyze the influence of the methodological quality of studies on strength of evidence and the associations evaluated, differences in the results between high and low quality studies were considered. However, no systematic differences were found for positive, negative and non-existing associations in high and low quality studies. Thus, the methodological quality has no potential influence on inconsistent associations.

Strengths and limitations

A strength of this review is the systematic search of relevant primary studies employing several search engines and a comprehensive list of search terms. Furthermore, the reference lists of all studies included were reviewed for additional sources. Another strength is that two independent reviewers (IM, CS) systematically screened relevant articles in three steps. Additionally, to evaluate the risk of bias a quality assessment was developed based on existing criteria lists for cross-sectional studies focusing on the methodological quality of the studies included. All results (bivariate and multivariate associations) were included in this systematic review, but analyzed separately as the multivariate associations integrated different correlates and, thus, were not directly comparable with the bivariate associations. Nevertheless, including both statistical methods helps to provide a further understanding of the relationship between socio-demographic characteristics, the social environment, and the physical environment with CIM. Stratifications of results by CIM definition provided additional information on the relationship between the environment and CIM.

A first limitation of this systematic review is the lack of evidence for causal relationships between the environment and CIM, because only two studies contained a longitudinal study design. Secondly, associations were only considered by significance and direction, not by effect size. Thirdly, conclusions may be heavily influenced by the low methodological quality of the studies and by individual findings of single studies, because many conclusions were based only on the result of one study. Additionally, no association demonstrated strong evidence, i.e., associations with at least four studies of high quality reporting the significant association in the expected direction. The fourth limitation is that only English- and German-language articles were considered for this review. Finally, as few studies reported sex/gender-specific results, sex/gender-related correlates could not be analyzed in detail.

Conclusion

This systematic review provides an overview of social and environmental correlates of independent mobility in children and highlights important research gaps.

Based on the socio-ecological perspective, this systematic review pointed out important social and physical environmental correlates which could be considered when developing intervention programs to halt the decline of CIM, especially in girls. Overall, the synthesis of existing studies revealed that neighborhood safety, fear of crime and strangers, parental support and perception of traffic are significant social correlates. Furthermore, car ownership, distance, and neighborhood design belong to physical environmental attributes, which influence CIM. To possibly address factors, such as neighborhood safety or fear of crime, which are limitedly modifiable and more determined by political decisions concerning the domestic security, intervention programs should focus on the interaction between social and physical environment [77]. Promoting children to walk or cycle to school together with other children instead of walking alone and promoting their competence to travel safely could be one way to deter parent's concerns about safety in the neighborhood and to expand mobility licenses [78].

Additionally, this systematic review identified future directions of research and suggests that the influence of the environment on CIM has not yet been fully understood. One important aspect is the implementation of longitudinal studies focusing on children's independent mobility to get insights into causal relationships of the social and physical environment and CIM. Additionally, to foster a robust understanding of the impact of the social and physical environment on CIM, more studies employing comparable measuring standards for CIM and environmental predictors are needed.

Furthermore, this systematic review showed that sex/gender-related correlates are limitedly evaluated in literature until now. Promoting independent mobility, especially in girls, could additionally promote their physical activity and thus, contributes to healthy development in children [11]. To consider social inequalities in sport participation between boys and girls and the sex/gender gap in CIM future research should evaluate sex/gender-specific correlates of CIM.

Additional files

Additional file 1. Characteristics of studies included on association of CIM and the social and physical environment The table shows the extracted data separated for all studies included, consisting of author(s); year of publication; country; study design; sample description (number of participants, age, sex/gender); definition, measurement, and instrument of CIM; type, measurement, and instruments of examined correlates; and main study results on the relationship between social and physical environmental factors and CIM.

Additional file 2. Quality Assessment for all studies included. The table shows the methodological quality rating of each criteria and the total quality score for all included studies.

Abbreviation
CIM: children's independent mobility.

Authors' contributions
IM drafted the manuscript, conducted the review, and synthesized the findings. AKR supervised the project. YD and AKR contributed to the concept of the paper and provided edits to the paper. All authors read and approved the final manuscript.

Author details
[1] Faculty of Behavioral and Social Sciences, Chemnitz University of Technology, Chemnitz, Germany. [2] Department of Sport and Health Sciences, Technical University of Munich, Munich, Germany.

Acknowledgements
The authors thank Christine Schmidt (CS) and Karolina Boxberger (KB) for their assistance in the screening of the literature and the rating of methodological quality.

Competing interests
The authors declare that they have no competing interests.

Funding
The publication costs of this article were funded by the German Research Foundation/DFG and the Technische Universität Chemnitz in the funding programme Open Access Publishing.

References
1. Warburton DER, Nicol CW, Bredin SSD. Health benefits of physical activity: the evidence. Can Med Assoc J. 2006. https://doi.org/10.1503/cmaj.051351.
2. Janssen I, LeBlanc AG. Systematic review of the health benefits of physical activity and fitness in school-aged children and youth. Int J Behav Nutr Phys Act. 2010. https://doi.org/10.1186/1479-5868-7-40.

3. Hallal PC, Andersen LB, Bull FC, Guthold R, Haskell W, Ekelund U. Global physical activity levels: surveillance progress, pitfalls, and prospects. Lancet. 2012. https://doi.org/10.1016/S0140-6736(12)60646-1.

4. WHO. Prevalence of insufficient physical activity. Geneva: WHO; 2010. http://www.who.int/gho/ncd/risk_factors/physical_activity_text/en/. Accessed 05 Apr 2018.

5. Larouche R, Saunders TJ, Faulkner GEJ, Colley R, Tremblay M. Associations between active school transport and physical activity, body composition, and cardiovascular fitness: a systematic review of 68 studies. J Phys Act Health. 2014. https://doi.org/10.1123/jpah.2011-0345.

6. Gordon-Larsen P, Nelson MC, Beam K. Associations among active transportation, physical activity, and weight status in young adults. Obes Res. 2005. https://doi.org/10.1038/oby.2005.100.

7. Tranter P, Whitelegg J. Children's travel behaviours in Canberra: car-dependent lifestyles in a low-density city. J Transp Health. 1994. https://doi.org/10.1016/0966-6923(94)90050-7.

8. Page AS, Cooper AR, Griew P, Davis L, Hillsdon M. Independent mobility in relation to weekday and weekend physical activity in children aged 10–11 years: the PEACH Project. Int J Behav Nutr Phys Act. 2009. https://doi.org/10.1186/1479-5868-6-2.

9. Mackett RL, Lucas L, Paskins J, Turbin J. The therapeutic value of children's everyday travel. Transp Res Part A Policy Pract. 2004. https://doi.org/10.1016/j.tra.2004.09.003.

10. Davis A, Jones LJ. Children in the urban environment: an issue for the new public health agenda. Health Place. 1996. https://doi.org/10.1016/1353-8292(96)00003-2.

11. Schoeppe S, Duncan MJ, Badland H, Oliver M, Curtis C. Associations of children's independent mobility and active travel with physical activity, sedentary behaviour and weight status: a systematic review. J Sci Med Sport. 2013. https://doi.org/10.1016/j.jsams.2012.11.001.

12. Prezza M, Pilloni S, Morabito C, Sersante C, Alparone FR, Giuliani MV. The influence of psychosocial and environmental factors on children's independent mobility and relationship to peer frequentation. J Community Appl Soc. 2001. https://doi.org/10.1002/casp.643.

13. Rissotto A, Tonucci F. Freedom of movement and environmental knowledge in elementary school children. J Environ Psychol. 2002. https://doi.org/10.1006/jevp.2002.0243.

14. Pacilli MG, Giovannelli I, Prezza M, Augimeri ML. Children and the public realm: antecedents and consequences of independent mobility in a group of 11-13-year-old Italian children. Child Geogr. 2013. https://doi.org/10.1080/14733285.2013.812277.

15. Schoeppe S, Tranter P, Duncan MJ, Curtis C, Carver A, Malone K. Australian children's independent mobility levels: secondary analyses of cross-sectional data between 1991 and 2012. Child Geogr. 2016. https://doi.org/10.1080/14733285.2015.1082083.

16. Kytta M, Hirvonen J, Rudner J, Pirjola I, Laatikainen T. The last free-range children? Children's independent mobility in finland in the 1990s and 2010s. J Transp Health. 2015. https://doi.org/10.1016/j.jtrangeo.2015.07.004.

17. Fyhri A, Hjorthol R, Mackett RL, Fotel TN, Kytta M. Children's active travel and independent mobility in four countries: development, social contributing trends and measures. Transp Policy. 2011. https://doi.org/10.1016/j.tranpol.2011.01.005.

18. Shaw B, Bicket M, Elliott B, Fagan-Watson B, Mocca E, Hillmann M. Children's independent mobility. An international comparison and recommondation for action. London: Policy Studies Institute; 2015.

19. Sallis JF, Cervero RB, Ascher W, Henderson KA, Kraft MK, Kerr J. An ecological approach to creating active living communities. Annu Rev Public Health. 2006. https://doi.org/10.1146/annurev.publhealth.27.021405.102100

20. Giles-Corti B, Kelty SF, Zubrick SR, Villanueva KP. Encouraging walking for transport and physical activity in children and adolescents how important is the built environment? Sports Med. 2009. https://doi.org/10.2165/11319620-000000000-00000.

21. Schmidt W. Kindheit und sportzugang im wandel: Konsequenzen fuer die bewegungserziehung? [childhood and sport in transition: consequences for physical education?]. 1993; 42(1):24–32.

22. Hillman M, Adams J, Whitelegg J. One false move. London: Policy Studies Institute; 1990.

23. Cordovil R, Lopes F, Neto C. Children's (in)dependent mobility in Portugal. J Sci Med Sport. 2015. https://doi.org/10.1016/j.jsams.2014.04.013.

24. Mitra R, Faulkner GEJ, Buliung RN, Stone MR. Do parental perceptions of the neighbourhood environment influence children's independent mobility? Evidence from Toronto, Canada. Urban Stud. 2014. https://doi.org/10.1177/0042098013519140.

25. Alparone FR, Pacilli MG. On children's independent mobility: the interplay of demographic, environmental, and psychosocial factors. Child Geogr. 2012. https://doi.org/10.1080/14733285.2011.638173.

26. Mammen G, Faulkner G, Buliung R, Lay J. Understanding the drive to escort: a cross-sectional analysis examining parental attitudes towards children's school travel and independent mobility. BMC Public Health. 2012. https://doi.org/10.1186/1471-2458-12-862.

27. Christian H, Villanueva K, Klinker CD, Knuiman MW, Divitini M, Giles-Corti B. The effect of siblings and family dog ownership on children's independent mobility to neighbourhood destinations. Aust Nz J Publ Health. 2016. https://doi.org/10.1111/1753-6405.12528.

28. Ristvedt SL. The evolution of gender. JAMA Psychiatry. 2014. https://doi.org/10.1001/jamapsychiatry.2013.3199.

29. Kilvington J, Wood A. Gender, sex and children's play. London: Bloomsbury Publishing; 2016.

30. Slater A, Tiggemann M. Gender differences in adolescent sport participation, teasing, self-objectification and body image concerns. J Adolesc. 2011. https://doi.org/10.1016/j.adolescence.2010.06.007.

31. Vilhjalmsson R, Kristjansdottir G. Gender differences in physical activity in older children and adolescents: the central role of organized sport. Soc Sci Med. 2003. https://doi.org/10.1016/S0277-9536(02)00042-4.

32. Buliung RN, Larsen K, Faulkner G, Ross T. Children's independent mobility in the city of Toronto, Canada. Travel Behav Soc. 2017. https://doi.org/10.1016/j.tbs.2017.06.001.

33. Villanueva K, Giles-Corti B, Bulsara M, Trapp G, Timperio A, McCormack G, et al. Does the walkability of neighbourhoods affect children's independent mobility, independent of parental, socio-cultural and individual factors? Child Geogr. 2014. https://doi.org/10.1080/14733285.2013.812311.

34. Brown B, Mackett R, Gong Y, Kitazawa K, Paskins J. Gender differences in children's pathways to independent mobility. Child Geogr. 2008. https://doi.org/10.1080/14733280802338080.

35. Ghekiere A, Deforche B, Carver A, Mertens L, de Geus B, Clarys P, et al. Insights into children's independent mobility for transportation cycling which socio-ecological factors matter? J Sci Med Sport. 2017. https://doi.org/10.1016/j.jsams.2016.08.002.

36. Foster S, Villanueva K, Wood L, Christian H, Giles-Corti B. The impact of parents' fear of strangers and perceptions of informal social control on children's independent mobility. Health Place. 2014. https://doi.org/10.1016/j.healthplace.2013.11.006.

37. Golden SD, Earp JAL. Social ecological approaches to individuals and their contexts: twenty years of health education and behavior health promotion interventions. Health Educ Behav. 2012;39(3):364–72.

38. Kok G, Gottlieb NH, Commers M, Smerecnik C. The ecological approach in health promotion programs: a decade later. Am J Health Promot. 2008;22(6):437–41.

39. Panter JR, Jones AP, van Sluijs EM. Environmental determinants of active travel in youth: a review and framework for future research. Int J Behav Nutr Phys Act. 2008. https://doi.org/10.1186/1479-5868-5-34.

40. Sharmin S, Kamruzzaman M. Association between the built environment and children's independent mobility: a meta-analytic review. J Transp Health. 2017. https://doi.org/10.1016/j.jtrangeo.2017.04.004.

41. Qiu L, Zhu X. Impacts of housing and community environments on children's independent mobility: a systematic literature review. Int J Cont Archit. 2017. https://doi.org/10.14621/tna.20170205.

42. Moher D, Liberati A, Tetzlaff J, Altmann DG. The PRISMA Group. Preferred reporting items for systematic reviews and meta-analyses: the PRISMA Statement. PLoS Med. 2009. https://doi.org/10.1371/journal.pmed.1000097.

43. Ding D, Sallis JF, Kerr J, Lee S, Rosenberg DE. Neighborhood environment and physical activity among youth: a review. Am J Prev Med. 2011. https://doi.org/10.1016/j.amepre.2011.06.036.

44. Analytics Clarivate. Endnote X7. Philidelphia: Clarivate Analytics; 2013.

45. Downes MJ, Brennan ML, Williams HC, Dean RS. Development of a critical appraisal tool to assess the quality of cross-sectional studies (AXIS). BMJ Open. 2016. https://doi.org/10.1136/bmjopen-2016-011458.

46. Uijtdewilligen L, Nauta J, Singh AS, van Mechelen W, Twisk JWR, van der

Horst K, et al. Determinants of physical activity and sedentary behaviour in young people: a review and quality synthesis of prospective studies. Br J Sport Med. 2011. https://doi.org/10.1136/bjsports-2011-090197.

47. Sallis JF, Prochaska JJ, Taylor WC. A review of correlates of physical activity of children and adolescents. Med Sci Sports Exerc. 2000. https://doi.org/10.1097/00005768-200005000-00014.

48. Villanueva K, Giles-Corti B, Bulsara M, Timperio A, McCormack G, Beesley B, et al. Where do children travel to and what local opportunities are available? The relationship between neighborhood destinations and children's independent mobility. Environ Behav. 2012. https://doi.org/10.1177/0013916512440705.

49. Christian H, Klinker CD, Villanueva K, Knuiman MW, Foster SA, Zubrick SR, et al. The effect of the social and physical environment on children's independent mobility to neighborhood destinations. J Phys Act Health. 2015. https://doi.org/10.1123/jpah.2014-0271.

50. Lam WWY, Loo BPY. Determinants of children's independent mobility in Hong Kong. Asian Trans Stud. 2014. https://doi.org/10.11175/eastsats.3.250.

51. Broberg A, Salminen S, Kytta M. Physical environmental characteristics promoting independent and active transport to children's meaningful places. Appl Georgr. 2013. https://doi.org/10.1016/j.apgeog.2012.11.014.

52. Carver A, Panter JR, Jones AP, van Sluijs EMF. Independent mobility on the journey to school: a joint cross-sectional and prospective exploration of social and physical environmental influences. J Transp Health. 2014;1(1):25–32.

53. Carver A, Timperio AF, Crawford DA. Young and free? A study of independent mobility among urban and rural dwelling Australian children. J Sci Med Sport. 2012. https://doi.org/10.1016/j.jsams.2012.03.005.

54. Carver A, Watson B, Shaw B, Hillman M. A comparison study of children's independent mobility in England and Australia. Child Geogr. 2013. https://doi.org/10.1080/14733285.2013.812303.

55. Chaudhury M, Oliver M, Badland H, Garrett N, Witten K. Using the public open space attributable index tool to assess children's public open space use and access by independent mobility. Child Geogr. 2017. https://doi.org/10.1080/14733285.2016.1214684.

56. Johansson M. Environment and parental factors as determinants of mode for children's leisure travel. J Environ Psychol. 2006. https://doi.org/10.1016/j.jenvp.2006.05.005.

57. Lin E-Y, Witten K, Oliver M, Carroll P, Asiasiga L, Badland H, et al. Social and built-environment factors related to children's independent mobility: the importance of neighbourhood cohesion and connectedness. Health Place. 2017. https://doi.org/10.1016/j.healthplace.2017.05.002.

58. Lopes F, Cordovil R, Neto C. Children's independent mobility in Portugal: effects of urbanization degree and motorized modes of travel. J Transp Health. 2014. https://doi.org/10.1016/j.jtrangeo.2014.10.002.

59. Santos MP, Pizarro AN, Mota J, Marques EA. Parental physical activity, safety perceptions and children's independent mobility. BMC Public Health. 2013. https://doi.org/10.1186/1471-2458-13-584.

60. Veitch J, Carver A, Salmon J, Abbott G, Ball K, Crawford D, et al. What predicts children's active transport and independent mobility in disadvantaged neighborhoods? Health Place. 2017. https://doi.org/10.1016/j.healthplace.2017.02.003.

61. Wolfe MK, McDonald NC. Association between neighborhood social environment and children's independent mobility. J Phys Act Health. 2016. https://doi.org/10.1123/jpah.2015-0662.

62. Fyhri A, Hjorthol R. Children's independent mobility to school, friends and leisure activities. J Transp Health. 2009. https://doi.org/10.1016/j.jtrangeo.2008.10.010.

63. Janssen I, Ferrao T, King N. Individual, family, and neighborhood correlates of independent mobility among 7 to 11-year-olds. Prevent Med Rep. 2015. https://doi.org/10.1016/j.pmedr.2015.12.008.

64. Kytta M. The extent of children's independent mobility and the number of actualized affordances as criteria for child-friendly environments. J Environ Psychol. 2004. https://doi.org/10.1016/s0272-4944(03)00073-2.

65. Rothman L, Buliung R, Macarthur C, To T, Howard A. Walking and child pedestrian injury: a systematic review of built environment correlates of safe walking. Inj Prev. 2014. https://doi.org/10.1136/injuryprev-2012-040701.

66. Panter JR, Jones A. Attitudes and the environment as determinants of active travel in adults: What do and don't we know? J Phys Act Health. 2010. https://doi.org/10.1123/jpah.7.4.551.

67. Cerin E, Nathan A, van Cauwenberg J, Barnett DW, Barnett A, Council Environm Phys A. The neighbourhood physical environment and active travel in older adults: a systematic review and meta-analysis. Int J Behav Nutr Phys Act. 2017. https://doi.org/10.1186/s12966-017-0471-5.

68. Broberg A, Kytta M, Fagerholm N. Child-friendly urban structures: buller by revisited. J Environ Psychol. 2013. https://doi.org/10.1016/j.jenvp.2013.06.001.

69. Xu HL, Wen LM, Rissel C. Associations of parental influences with physical activity and screen time among young children: a systematic review. J Obes. 2015. https://doi.org/10.1155/2015/546925.

70. Hutchens A, Lee RE. Parenting practices and children's physical activity: an integrative review. J Sch Nurs. 2018. https://doi.org/10.1177/1059840517714852.

71. Mackett R, Brown B, Gong Y, Kitazawa K, Paskins J. Children's independent movement in the local environment. Built Environ. 2007. https://doi.org/10.2148/benv.33.4.454.

72. Reimers AK, Wagner M, Alvanides S, Steinmayr A, Reiner M, Schmidt S, et al. Proximity to sports facilities and sports participation for adolescents in Germany. PLoS ONE. 2014. https://doi.org/10.1371/journal.pone.0093059.

73. Cleland V, Dwyer T, Venn A. Which domains of childhood physical activity predict physical activity in adulthood? A 20-year prospective tracking study. Br J Sports Med. 2012. https://doi.org/10.1136/bjsports-2011-090508.

74. Malina RM. Tracking of physical activity and physical fitness across the lifespan. Res Q Exerc Sport. 1996;67(3 Suppl):S48–57.

75. Bhosale J, Duncan S, Stewart T, Chaix B, Kestens Y, Schofield G. Measuring children's independent mobility: comparing interactive mapping with destination access and licence to roam. Child Geogr. 2017. https://doi.org/10.1080/14733285.2017.1293232.

76. Bates B, Stone MR. Measures of outdoor play and independent mobility in children and youth: a methodological review. J Sci Med Sport. 2015. https://doi.org/10.1016/j.jsams.2014.07.006.

77. Bartholomew Eldredge LK, Markham CM, Ruiter RAC, Fernãndez ME, Kok G, Parcel GS. Planning health promotion programs: an intervention mapping approach. London: Wiley; 2016.

78. Bennetts SK, Cooklin AR, Crawford S, D'Esposito F, Hackworth NJ, Green J, et al. What influences parents' fear about children's independent mobility? Evidence from a state-wide survey of Australian parents. Am J Health Promot. 2017. https://doi.org/10.1177/0890117117740442.

Estimating the prevalence of 26 health-related indicators at neighbourhood level in the Netherlands using structured additive regression

Jan van de Kassteele[*], Laurens Zwakhals, Oscar Breugelmans, Caroline Ameling and Carolien van den Brink

Abstract

Background: Local policy makers increasingly need information on health-related indicators at smaller geographic levels like districts or neighbourhoods. Although more large data sources have become available, direct estimates of the prevalence of a health-related indicator cannot be produced for neighbourhoods for which only small samples or no samples are available. Small area estimation provides a solution, but unit-level models for binary-valued outcomes that can handle both non-linear effects of the predictors and spatially correlated random effects in a unified framework are rarely encountered.

Methods: We used data on 26 binary-valued health-related indicators collected on 387,195 persons in the Netherlands. We associated the health-related indicators at the individual level with a set of 12 predictors obtained from national registry data. We formulated a structured additive regression model for small area estimation. The model captured potential non-linear relations between the predictors and the outcome through additive terms in a functional form using penalized splines and included a term that accounted for spatially correlated heterogeneity between neighbourhoods. The registry data were used to predict individual outcomes which in turn are aggregated into higher geographical levels, i.e. neighbourhoods. We validated our method by comparing the estimated prevalences with observed prevalences at the individual level and by comparing the estimated prevalences with direct estimates obtained by weighting methods at municipality level.

Results: We estimated the prevalence of the 26 health-related indicators for 415 municipalities, 2599 districts and 11,432 neighbourhoods in the Netherlands. We illustrate our method on overweight data and show that there are distinct geographic patterns in the overweight prevalence. Calibration plots show that the estimated prevalences agree very well with observed prevalences at the individual level. The estimated prevalences agree reasonably well with the direct estimates at the municipal level.

Conclusions: Structured additive regression is a useful tool to provide small area estimates in a unified framework. We are able to produce valid nationwide small area estimates of 26 health-related indicators at neighbourhood level in the Netherlands. The results can be used for local policy makers to make appropriate health policy decisions.

Keywords: Small area estimation, Health-related indicators, Public health, Structured additive regression, Neighbourhoods

---

*Correspondence: Jan.van.de.Kassteele@rivm.nl

National Institute for Public Health and the Environment - RIVM, PO Box 1,
3720BA Bilthoven, The Netherlands

Background

From 2015 onwards, municipalities in the Netherlands were given more tasks and greater responsibilities that are of importance in the living environment of people: the so-called decentralizations of the social policy domain. As a consequence of the decentralizations, local policy makers and health care services increasingly require information on health-related indicators at smaller geographical scales, like districts or neighbourhoods.

In recent years more large data sources on health-related indicators have become available. One particular important new data source is the Dutch Public Health Monitor [1]. It is a national survey database containing figures on self-reported health, health perception, and health-related behaviours of persons aged 19 years and older. Currently, the prevalence of a large number of health-related indicators for nearly 80% of the Dutch municipalities can be provided by means of weighting methods, which are usually called 'direct estimates'.

However, direct estimates of the prevalence of such health-related indicators cannot be produced for neighbourhoods for which only small samples or no samples are available. This implies that monitoring and target-setting can only be done at a relatively crude geographical scale. This is an important constraint for decentralized public health activities. Oversampling could provide the required information, but this is very costly. An alternative strategy to produce local estimates is to use auxiliary data, or values of the variable of interest from related areas, or both. Even when local information is not directly available, estimations for small areas can be obtained in this way. This is called small area estimation (SAE) [2]. In this paper we focus on the so-called unit-level model with a binary-valued outcome. The unit-level model uses individual observations on both the response and auxiliary data.

In recent years the statistical methodology for producing small area estimates has greatly improved. In order to capture potential non-linearities, numerically-valued predictors can be put in a SAE model in a functional form using penalized splines, although the use of P-splines in SAE models is not very common. Examples are found in [3] and [4]. A random intercept term is usually added to the model to capture heterogeneity between neighbourhoods. For area level models with a Gaussian response, the well-known Fay–Herriot model, correlated random effects can be included to account for correlation between neighbourhoods. Examples can be found in [5, 6] and [7]. However, to our knowledge, the inclusion of spatially correlated effects in the unit-level model with binary-valued outcomes is hardly ever seen, mainly because of computational issues, while it can be expected that also for binary-valued regional health-related indicators, apart from individual effects, correlation exists between adjacent neighbourhoods.

The objective of this paper is therefore twofold. First, we extend the possibilities of the Public Health Monitor and produce nationwide small area estimates of the prevalence of 26 health-related indicators at neighbourhood level in the Netherlands. Second, we present a unit-level model for binary-valued outcomes that allows us to handle both P-splines and spatially correlated random effects.

We show that it is possible to estimate the prevalence of each health-related indicator using data at the individual level. We associate the outcome with a carefully selected set of predictor variables obtained from a large national registry database. In turn, the registry data are used to predict the prevalence in the entire population. We model the associations by structured additive regression (STAR) for small area estimation, which provides a unified framework for handling both P-splines and spatial effects in the presence of non-Gaussian outcomes. See [8] for an overview, and [9] and [10] for more details. Recent computational developments make it possible to use STAR models in combination with very large datasets [11].

We validate our method by using calibration plots, in which the estimated prevalences are compared with observed prevalences at the individual level. Additionally, we compare the estimated prevalences with already available direct estimates at municipality level. Eventually, the results can be used to make appropriate health policy decisions at the local level and to respond to local care needs.

Methods

Municipalities, districts and neighbourhoods

In the Netherlands a municipality is an urban administrative division having corporate status and powers of self-government or jurisdiction. Municipalities are the second-level administrative division in the Netherlands and are subdivisions of their respective provinces. Their duties are delegated to them by the central government. A Municipal Health Service (MHS) is the service which every municipality must have by law in the Netherlands to carry out a number of tasks in the field of public health. Municipal Health Services work through a common system for several municipalities in a given region, called a MHS region.

For administrative use by municipalities and data collection by Statistics Netherlands (CBS), all municipalities are subdivided into districts, which in turn are subdivided into neighbourhoods. Districts and neighbourhoods have no formal status. Districts and neighbourhoods are coherent regions that are based on several characteristics like age, geographical barriers such as busy roads, having similar urban and/or architectural features, or having similar functional, social or political characteristics. As of 2012, the reference year in this paper, the Netherlands consisted of 28 MHS regions and 415 municipalities that are subdivided into 2621 districts and 11,896 neighbourhoods.

Data sources
Public health monitor
The Dutch Public Health Monitor is a national survey database developed under collaboration of the National Institute for Public Health and the Environment (RIVM), the MHS's and CBS. The database contains information on health and health perception among the Dutch population aged 19 years and older. The data were collected in 2012 on 387,195 respondents (3.0% of the Dutch population, proportionally sampled) by a questionnaire survey. It is a combination of the local monitors of the 28 MHS regions, in which 376,384 (97.2%) persons were surveyed, and the National Health Survey of the CBS, in which 10,811 (2.8%) persons were surveyed. Questions in the questionnaires and instruments were harmonized as much as possible. A secured identification number was given to each participant. It was therefore possible to link the Public Health Monitor with registry data at individual level. Authorization for this linkage has been provided by the MHS's and CBS. Disclosure and tracing of individuals was not possible.

In this paper the following 26 health-related indicators will be considered: overweight, obesity, drinker, heavy drinker, excessive drinker, smoker, heavy smoker, diabetes, high blood pressure, asthma or COPD, joint degeneration of hips or knees, chronic arthritis, back problem, disease of the neck or shoulder, at least one chronic condition, hearing impairment, visual impairment, mobility impairment, at least one impairment, perceived good or very good health, adherence to the cardio-respiratory fitness guideline, adherence to the physical activity guideline, moderate or high risk of anxiety disorder or depression, loneliness, informal caregiver, and difficulty with making ends meet. All indicators were reported as binary-valued outcomes in the survey.

The Public Health Monitor takes place once every four years; the most recent Public Health Monitor, following the one in 2012, took place in 2016 and data will become available in 2017. More information on the Public Health Monitor, including definitions of the health-related indicators, can be found in [1].

Registry data
Characteristics of the Dutch population aged 19 years and older were obtained from registry data from CBS

with reference date September 1, 2012. Based on expert knowledge of the MHS's and the RIVM, 12 characteristics were chosen as possible health-related predictors. At the individual level we had age, sex, ethnicity and marital status. At household level we had household type, size, capital, income, income source and home ownership. At the neighbourhood level we had urbanization and neighbourhood code. Table 1 summarizes the population characteristics that were used as predictors in our model. Neighbourhood code was used in the model as a discrete location variable.

The registry data themselves had three sources. First, the municipal personal records database, which contains the characteristics of the individuals and the secured identification number, secured household identifier and secured living address identifier. Second, the household statistics database, which contains the characteristics of the households, including the secured household identifier. Third, the neighbourhood statistics database, which contains the characteristics of the neighbourhoods,

Table 1 Summary of population characteristics obtained from registry data that were used as predictors, with abbreviations that are used in the model between parentheses

Age (age)	Household size (hhsize)
Years	1, 2, …, 9, 10+
Sex (sex)	Household capital (hhcap)
Male	100 percentile classes
Female	Household income (hhinc)
Ethnicity (eth)	100 percentile classes
Autochthonous	Household income source (hhincsrc)
Morocco	Salaried
Turkey	Independent
Suriname	Capital
Netherlands Antilles	Unemployment benefit
Other non-western	Disability benefit
Other western	Old-age benefit
Marital status (mar)	Social welfare benefit
Unmarried	Other benefit
Married	Student loan
Divorced	Other
Widower	None
Household type (hhtype)	Home ownership (home)
Single person household	Homeowner
Unmarried without children	Renting with housing allowance
Married without children	Renting with no housing allowance
Unmarried with children	Neighbourhood urbanization (urb)
Married with children	100 percentile classes
Single parent family	Neighbourhood (neigh)
Other	Code

including the secured living address identifier. Subsequently, all records were linked through household identifier and address identifier, resulting in one large dataset of 13,073,969 records containing characteristics at the individual level, household level and neighbourhood level.

For 345 records (0.0026%) household type and household size were missing, and for 91,669 records (0.70%) household capital, household income, household income source and home ownership were missing. These records were imputed (single imputation) by using a multinomial logit model containing age (using a natural cubic spline with knots placed on age 22, 30, 50, and 80, chosen by visual inspection), sex, ethnicity and marital status as predictors. For this purpose, the number of categories for household capital and household income was reduced from 100 to five. Given the imputed category, we then uniformly sampled one integer-valued realisation for the corresponding capital or income.

Direct estimates

We compared our results with already available direct estimates, which were only available at municipality level. The direct estimates were based on the Public Health Monitor database. The following weighting scheme was applied, with the number of levels between parentheses: MHS (28) × Sex (2) × Age (13) + MHS (28) × Marital status (4) + MHS (28) × Urbanization (5) + MHS (28) × Household size (5) + MHS (28) × Sex (2) × Age (3) × Marital status (2) + MHS (28) × Ethnicity (3) + MHS (28) × Income(5) + Partially merged municipality (391) × Marital status (2) + Partially merged municipality (391) × Sex (2). More information can be found in [12, 13].

Structured additive regression model
Model formulation

We used a generalized structured additive regression (STAR) model to relate the predictors to the health-related indicators. Generalized STAR models provide a flexible framework for modelling (possible) nonlinear effects of the predictors on a, for example, binary-valued outcome, and allow for other effects, like spatial information. The well-established frameworks of generalized linear models and generalized additive models are considered special cases of STAR models [8].

Here, for individual i, $i = 1, ..., n$, the stochastic response variable Y_i has a Bernoulli distribution (0/1 health-related indicator outcome) with expectation $E(Y_i) = p_i$, the probability of having one as outcome:

$$Y_i \sim Bern(p_i).$$

The relationship between p_i and the linear predictor η_i is provided by the logit link function, which is the logarithm of the odds $p_i/(1 - p_i)$:

$$\log it(p_i) = \eta_i.$$

In STAR models, the linear predictor is a flexible, structured additive predictor:

$$\eta_i = \beta_0 + \beta_1 x_{i1} + \cdots + \beta_k x_{ik} + f_1(z_{i1}) + \cdots + f_q(z_{iq}),$$

where $x_{i1}, ..., x_{ik}$ are predictors associated with individual i whose effect on η_i can be modelled through a linear predictor with unknown regression coefficients β_1, ..., β_k. Typically, $x_{i1}, ..., x_{ik}$ are binary-coded characteristics of an individual, such as sex, where the reference category is absorbed in the intercept β_0. The functions $f_1(z_{i1}), ..., f_q(z_{iq})$ are nonlinear smooth effects of the predictors $z_{i1}, ..., z_{iq}$, which are typically numerically-valued characteristics, such as age, but they also may represent spatially correlated effects. Interactions may exist between predictors, such as $\beta_1 x_{i1} + f_1(z_{i1}) + f_{z1|x1}(z_{i1})x_{i1}$. To ensure identification of the model, it is necessary to centre the functions around zero, such that $\sum_{i=1}^{n} f_1(z_{i1}) = \cdots = \sum_{i=1}^{n} f_q(z_{iq}) = 0$ holds.

The functions $f_j(z_{ij})$, $j = 1, ..., q$, are specified by a basis function approach, in which the function $f_j(z_{ij})$ is written as a linear combination of d basis functions B_j:

$$f_j(z_{ij}) = \gamma_1 B_{j1}(z_{ij}) + \cdots + \gamma_d B_{jd}(z_{ij}).$$

For numerically-valued predictors typically B-spline basis functions are chosen. B-splines are piecewise polynomials of a given degree, usually cubic, which are fused smoothly in a pre-specified number of equidistant knots. The main advantage of the B-splines basis is its local definition, i.e. being zero everywhere, except on an interval around a knot.

To prevent overfitting as the number of knots, and therefore the number of coefficients, increases, the estimation of the unknown coefficients $\gamma_1, ..., \gamma_d$ is regularized through the introduction of a roughness penalty. These penalized B-splines are called P-splines [14]. For computational reasons, usually a quadratic penalty is assumed on the coefficients:

$$\lambda \sum_{l=r+1}^{d} (\Delta^r \gamma_l)^2,$$

where $\lambda \geq 0$ is an unknown smoothing parameter that controls the influence of the penalty. As $\lambda \to 0$, the effect of the penalty disappears. Δ^r denotes rth order differences on the adjacent coefficients $\gamma_1, ..., \gamma_d$. Usually $r = 2$

is chosen, as we did, which represents the discrete analogue of penalizing the second derivative of a continuous function, i.e. putting a penalty on large changes in the curvature. As $\lambda \to \infty$, the fit approaches a polynomial of degree $r - 1$, i.e. a straight line in our case. We can write

$$\Delta^2 \gamma_l = \gamma_l - 2\gamma_{l-1} + \gamma_{l-2},$$

which in matrix notation can be written as a $(d - 2) \times d$ difference matrix $\mathbf{D}$

$$\mathbf{D} = \begin{pmatrix} 1 & -2 & 1 & & \\ & 1 & -2 & 1 & \\ & & \ddots & \ddots & \ddots \\ & & & 1 & -2 & 1 \end{pmatrix},$$

where empty cells are equal to zero. This yields the penalty

$$\lambda \sum_{l=r+1}^{d} \left(\Delta^2 \gamma_l \right)^2 = \lambda \boldsymbol{\gamma}' \mathbf{D}' \mathbf{D} \boldsymbol{\gamma} = \lambda \boldsymbol{\gamma}' \mathbf{K} \boldsymbol{\gamma},$$

with a $d \times d$ penalty matrix

$$\mathbf{K} = \begin{pmatrix} 1 & -2 & 1 & & & \\ -2 & 5 & -4 & 1 & & \\ 1 & -4 & 6 & -4 & 1 & \\ & \ddots & \ddots & \ddots & \ddots & \ddots \\ & & 1 & -4 & 6 & -4 & 1 \\ & & & 1 & -4 & 5 & -2 \\ & & & & 1 & -2 & 1 \end{pmatrix}.$$

A similar principle of penalized basis functions applies to spatial data as well. For regional health-related indicators, it can be expected that, apart from individual and household effects, spatial heterogeneity may exist. In our case we had discrete spatial information in the form of neighbourhoods, where correlation may exist between adjacent neighbourhoods.

For data observed on a regular or irregular lattice, a common approach for the correlated spatial effect is based on Markov random fields [15]. Each individual i belongs to a particular neighbourhood s. A regression coefficient γ_s is assigned to each neighbourhood s, $s = 1, ..., d$. The corresponding basis function B_{is} is 1 if individual i belongs to neighbourhood s, and is 0 otherwise. Adjacent neighbourhoods are usually defined by common boundaries (Rook type contiguity). We use the notation $s \sim r$ to denote that neighbourhoods s and r are adjacent. The penalty again consists of squared differences and can compactly be written as $\lambda \boldsymbol{\gamma}' \mathbf{K} \boldsymbol{\gamma}$, where $\mathbf{K}$ is a $d \times d$ matrix with elements $\mathbf{K}_{sr} = -1$ if $s \neq r$, $s \sim r$, $\mathbf{K}_{sr} = 0$ if $s \neq r$, $s \nsim r$, and $\mathbf{K}_{sr} = |N(s)|$ if $s = r$, and where $|N(s)|$ is the number of adjacent neighbourhoods of s. In other words, large first order differences between adjacent neighbourhoods are penalised. For example, for $d = 9$ neighbourhoods in a regular 3×3 lattice, numbered from left to right and from top to bottom, the penalty matrix $\mathbf{K}$ is given by

$$\mathbf{K} = \begin{pmatrix} 2 & -1 & & -1 & & & & & \\ -1 & 3 & -1 & & -1 & & & & \\ & -1 & 2 & & & -1 & & & \\ -1 & & & 3 & -1 & & -1 & & \\ & -1 & & -1 & 4 & -1 & & -1 & \\ & & -1 & & -1 & 3 & & & -1 \\ & & & -1 & & & 2 & -1 & \\ & & & & -1 & & -1 & 3 & -1 \\ & & & & & -1 & & -1 & 2 \end{pmatrix}.$$

The linear predictor can now be written as follows:

$$\begin{aligned} \eta_i =\ & \beta_0 + \beta_{sex}\, sex_i + f_{age}(age_i) + f_{age|sex}(age_i) \\ & + \sum_{j=1}^{6} \beta_{eth,j}\, eth_{ij} + \sum_{j=1}^{3} \beta_{mar,j}\, mar_{ij} \\ & + \sum_{j=1}^{6} \beta_{hhtype,j}\, hhtype_{ij} + f_{hhsize}(hhsize_i) \\ & + f_{hhcap}(hhcap_i) + f_{hhinc}(hhinc_i) \\ & + \sum_{j=1}^{10} \beta_{hhincsrc,j}\, hhincscr_{ij} + \sum_{j=1}^{2} \beta_{home,j}\, home_{ij} \\ & + f_{urb}(urb_i) + f_{neigh}(neigh_i) \end{aligned}$$

The non-linear functions of all numerically-valued predictors were modelled by cubic B-splines basis functions with 10 knots and a penalty on the second order differences of the coefficients, except for household size, which had five knots. These numbers were based on preliminary analyses. The choice of the number of knots was not critical, but it was important not to make it restrictively small, nor very large and computationally costly. Furthermore, the spatial correlation between neighbourhoods was taken into account. Although the number of regression coefficients was large, the effective number of coefficients was usually much lower because of the smoothing penalties. The amount of smoothing was selected automatically as will be explained in the next section.

Parameter estimation

All data preparations and analyses were carried out in R [16], using the data.table package for handling the large datasets [17] and the sp and maptools packages for handling the spatial data [18, 19]. Estimation of parameters was carried out via restricted maximum likelihood (REML) in the R package mgcv [10, 20].

Because of the large dataset in combination with the model's complexity, it was impossible to fit the model to the whole dataset. Therefore the dataset was split by

MHS region, and for each combination of MHS region (28) and health-related indicator (26) a model was run. We combined MHS regions *GGD Drenthe* and *GGD Groningen*, located in the north-east of the Netherlands, because the number of respondents in *GGD Drenthe* appeared too low for a proper estimation of the regression coefficients for those regions separately. So, in total there were $27 \times 26 = 702$ model runs. For each run, the same model formulation was used. The fitted models differed only in their sets of estimated regression coefficients and smoothing parameters.

To avoid boundary effects, first a 10 km buffer was created around each MHS region using the rgeos package [21]. Neighbourhoods (and all individuals within) with their centroid located within the buffer were included in the estimation procedure. Next, a neighbourhood adjacency list (graph) was created, based on neighbourhoods with contiguous boundaries, using the spdep package [22]. The creation of the 10 km buffer sometimes resulted in artificial islands that were disconnected with the considered region, i.e. subgraphs. Besides, natural islands are also a common feature in the Netherlands. To avoid a disconnected graph, neighbourhoods in two

unconnected subgraphs that were located the closest to each other were connected, using the RANN package [23]. The Euclidian distance between centroids was taken as distance measure. This was repeated until there was only one connected graph left.

The construction of the 10 km buffer and the adjacency list is illustrated in Fig. 1. The region corresponds to the Dutch province of Utrecht (for illustrative purpose the MHS regions '*GGD Midden Nederland*' and '*GG en GD Utrecht*' were combined here) and is indicated by the dark blue colour. The thick black line indicates the 10 km buffer and the additional neighbourhoods that were included in the estimation procedure are indicated by a light blue colour. Adjacent neighbourhoods are connected by a black line. In the east, indicated by an orange circle, an artificial island can be seen, now connected with the rest of the region.

Although the splitting of the dataset by MHS region reduced the number of records considerably, the introduction of the 10 km buffer and inclusion of the spatial and heterogeneity terms in the model still resulted in very large numbers to handle. The following numbers are averages for each model run: 34,782 individuals and 975

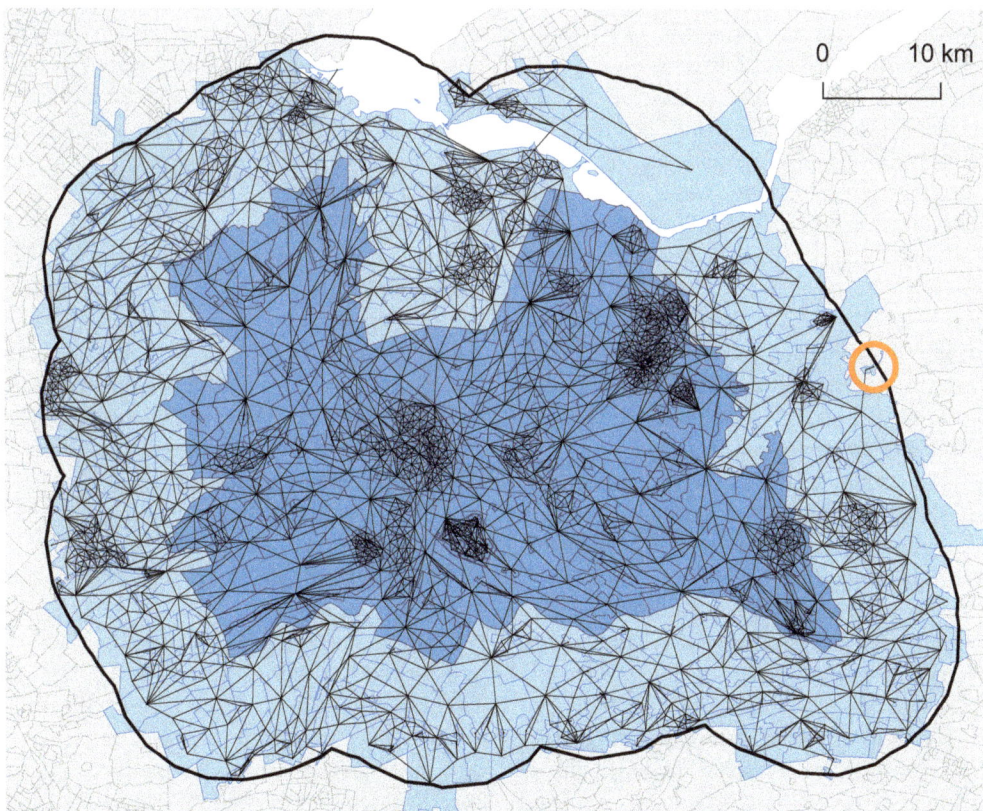

Fig. 1 Illustration of the construction of the 10 km buffer (*light blue area*) and adjacency list (*thin black lines*) for the MHS regions 'GGD Midden Nederland' and 'GG en GD Utrecht' (*dark blue area*). An artificial island is marked by the *orange circle*. North is up

neighbourhoods were used for estimation, 1052 regression coefficients were estimated and 484,221 individuals and 441 neighbourhoods were predicted. For this reason, we used the bam function in mgcv, which is much like the standard gam function in mgcv, except that the numerical methods are designed for very large datasets. The advantage of bam is a much lower memory footprint than gam, but it can also be much faster and can be run in parallel [11].

Prediction

Once the regression coefficients for a combination of a MHS region and health-related indicator were estimated, the formula for the linear predictor was applied to all individuals in the registry data for that region. This resulted in a log-odds of having one as an outcome for each individual. The log-odds were subsequently transformed into probabilities. Because on average the outcome was actually known for 3.0% of the individuals, the probabilities for these individuals were replaced by their observed binary-valued outcome, as is the common procedure in small area estimation [2]. The individual outcomes were aggregated to neighbourhood (11,432), district (2599) and municipality level (415) to obtain prevalence estimates. To prevent disclosure or privacy issues, results for regions with fewer than 10 inhabitants aged 19+ were sanitised (i.e. not reported). This was the case for 464 neighbourhoods and 22 districts.

Each estimation and prediction step took on average 3 m 19 s to run on an Intel® Xeon® X5560 2.80 GHz CPU with four sockets running a 64-bit Windows 7 operating system. One health-related indicator took 1 h 30 m to run. The whole exercise took 1 day 14 h 51 m to run.

Validation
Calibration plots

The model's validity was checked using calibration plots. Calibration refers to the agreement between estimated outcomes and observations. In a calibration plot the estimated prevalences is compared with the observed prevalence [24]. For example, if the model predicts that a respondent has a 20% probability of having overweight, the observed frequency of overweight should be approximately 20 out of 100 respondents with such a prediction.

Here, the 387,195 respondents were randomly split in 2/3 training individuals and 1/3 validation individuals. Next, for each health-related indicator, the model was fitted to the training dataset as described in the previous section (i.e. same model formulation and estimation procedure, and stratification by MHS region). Subsequently, the estimated regression coefficients were used to make predictions for all individuals in the validation dataset. Because it is impossible to compare a predicted

probability with a binary response at the individual level, the predicted probabilities in the validation dataset were divided into 200 equally sized intervals according to their quantiles. Then for each interval, the predicted probabilities and corresponding observed binary responses were averaged, resulting in an averaged predicted prevalence and an observed prevalence for that interval, which can be compared in a scatterplot [24]. The points in the scatter-plot should lie near the 1:1 line. It is assumed that if the model can accurately predict the indicator of an individual, then at neighbourhood, district or municipality level the estimated prevalence will be close to the true prevalence.

Comparison between small area estimates and direct estimates

At municipality level we compared the small area estimates with the already available direct estimates, obtained by weighted estimation. Since the true prevalence is unknown, this is not an actual validation, but it can give an impression of how well the small area estimates agree with the direct estimates.

Results

We illustrate the small area estimation procedure for overweight. First we consider the province of Utrecht, represented in Fig. 1, for which we show the estimated regression coefficients. Other regions are alike. Next, we show the overweight prevalence for all 11,896 neighbourhoods in the Netherlands. We end with assessing the model's performance.

Estimated effect sizes

Figure 2 shows the estimated regression coefficients corresponding to the categorical predictors (top six panels) and the smooth terms corresponding to the numerically-valued predictors (bottom six panel), corresponding to the terms in the formula for the linear predictor. The values can be interpreted as differences in log-odds. Similar patterns for overweight are visible in other MHS regions (figures not shown) and similar graphs can be made for the other health-related indicators (figures not shown). Note that it is not the goal of this paper to explain effect sizes and differences. Here, they are solely used to make the predictions.

Compared to males, females have lower overweight prevalence, but there is also a strong interaction with age. Compared to the autochthonous population, most ethnicities have higher prevalence, especially people with a Turkish background. Compared to (un)married people, divorced or widowed people have higher prevalence. Compared to single-person households, other household types have a higher prevalence. Compared to households

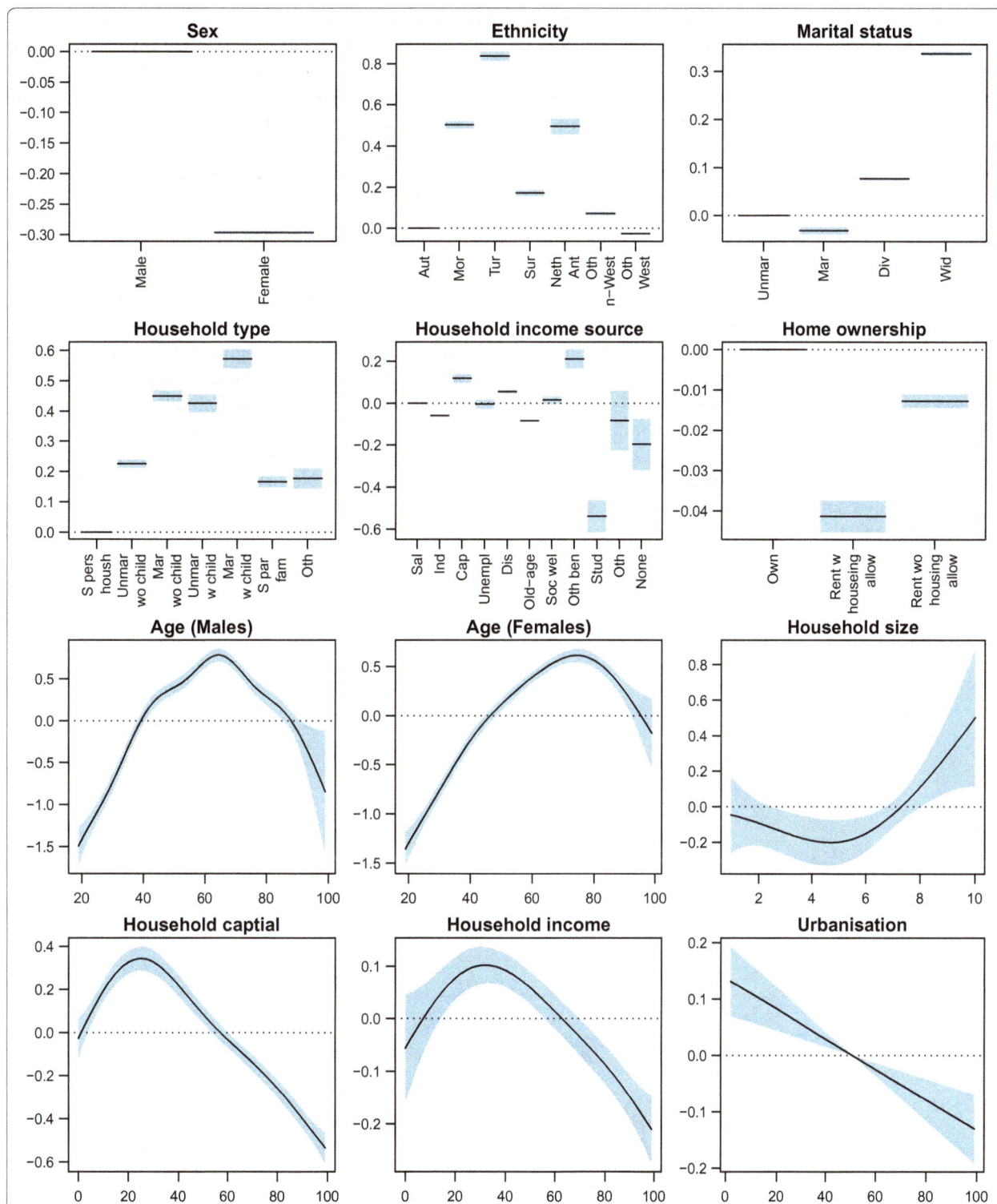

Fig. 2 Estimated regression coefficients for the overweight model for the province of Utrecht (MHS regions 'GGD Midden Nederland' and 'GG en GD Utrecht'). Levels or values of each predictor are given on the x-axis. The estimated effect size, in terms of differences in log-odds compared to the reference category or value, is given on the y-axis. The *shaded areas* represent the 95% confidence intervals. The reference category is always on the *horizontal dotted line* at zero

having a salaried income, households having their income from capital and other benefits have higher prevalence. On the other hand, student households have lower prevalence. Home ownership is not an important predictor for overweight, as can be seen from the small differences between the three categories. Age is an important predictor for overweight. Younger people have a lower prevalence, whereas the prevalence increases with age, reaching a maximum around 65 years for men and 75 years for women. For the elderly, especially men, the prevalence decreases again. The prevalence increases with household size. Households with a lower capital or income have higher prevalence, whereas the prevalence decreases with increasing capital and income. Finally, the prevalence decreases with increasing urbanisation (note: although the effect of urbanisation is modelled with a P-spline, the relation is estimated to be a straight line. The disappearing of the 95% confidence interval near the mean is a result of the sum-to-zero identifiability constraints).

Figure 3 shows for the province of Utrecht the estimated spatial effect, corresponding to the last term in the formula for the linear predictor. The term represents the estimated spatial heterogeneity, apart from individual,

household and urbanisation effects. Blue colours indicate lower overweight prevalence than expected. Orange colours indicate higher overweight prevalence than expected. Clear geographic patterns are visible. In the large cities Utrecht and Amersfoort, respectively located in the centre and in the north east, the prevalence is lower than expected. In the rural areas in the south, the prevalence is higher than expected. Note that it is not the goal of this paper to explain these patterns.

Prevalence map

Figure 4 shows a map of the estimated overweight prevalence (%) at neighbourhood level in the Netherlands. The darker the colour, the higher the prevalence. Neighbourhoods with fewer than 10 inhabitants aged 19+ are indicated with "No data". Although differences are small, there are distinct geographic patterns visible. High prevalences are especially seen in the north-eastern and south-western part of the Netherlands. Other clusters of high prevalence are seen at the 'Veluwe', a forested area just east of the country's centre, and in the south-east, around the so-called 'Parkstad', a former mining colony. Lower overweight prevalences are found elsewhere.

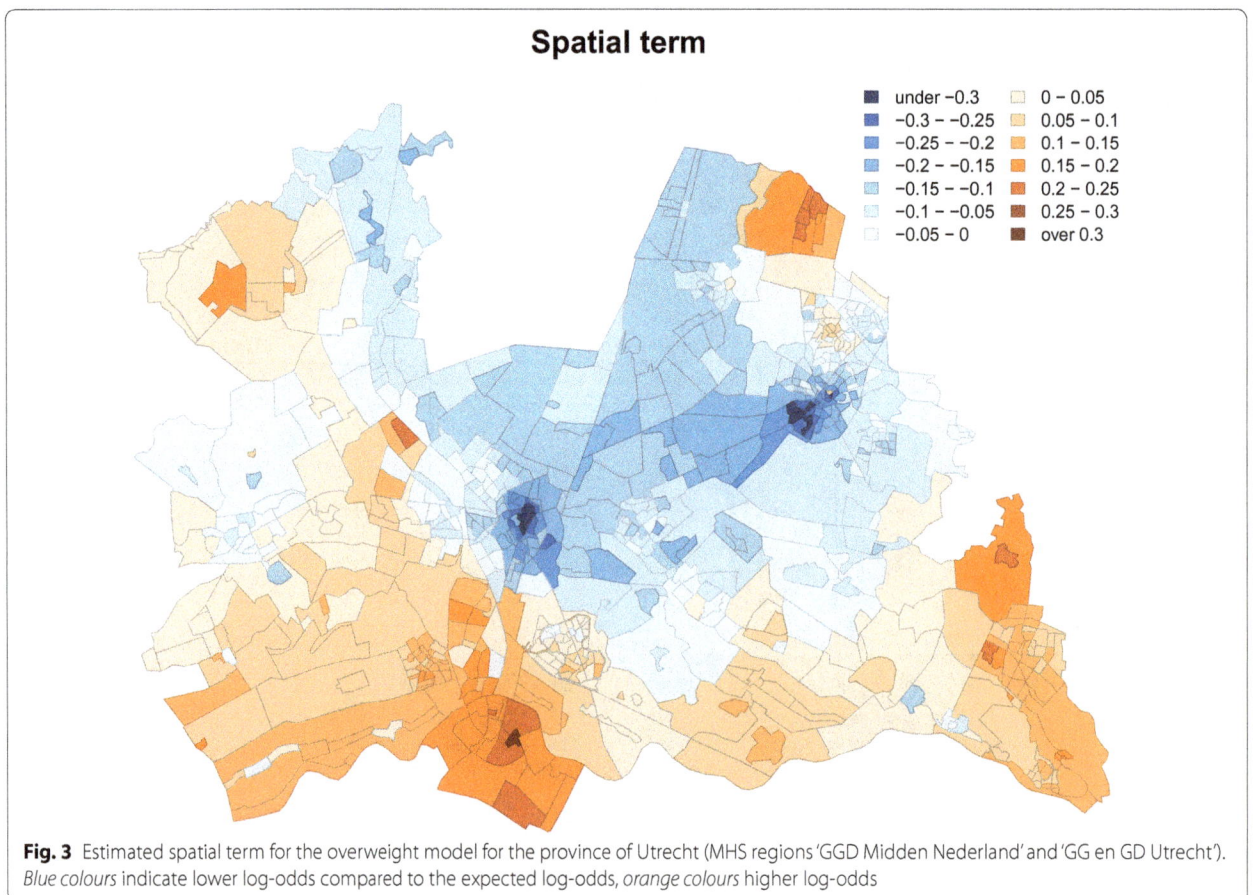

Fig. 3 Estimated spatial term for the overweight model for the province of Utrecht (MHS regions 'GGD Midden Nederland' and 'GG en GD Utrecht'). *Blue colours* indicate lower log-odds compared to the expected log-odds, *orange colours* higher log-odds

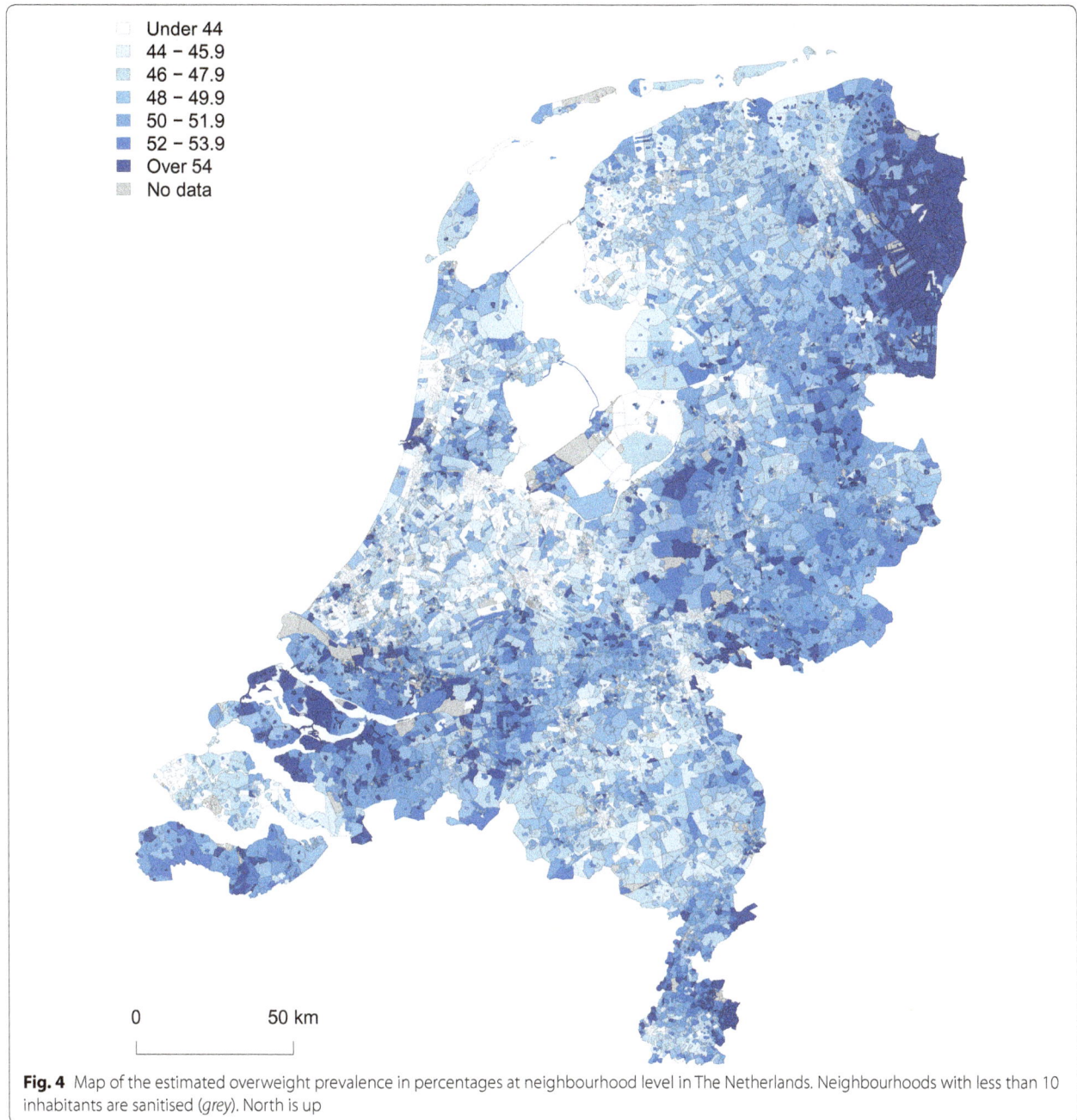

Fig. 4 Map of the estimated overweight prevalence in percentages at neighbourhood level in The Netherlands. Neighbourhoods with less than 10 inhabitants are sanitised (*grey*). North is up

Assessing the model's performance

Figure 5 shows calibration plots to see how well the model is able to predict the prevalence of the 26 health-related indicators at the individual level. Each dot represents the average of about 645 respondents. On the x-axis the predicted prevalence is shown, on the y-axis the corresponding observed prevalence. The diagonal line is the 1:1 line. All dots are close to the 1:1 line over the whole prevalence range for almost

all health-related indicators. This indicates that the model is very capable of predicting the prevalence at the individual level.

Figure 6 shows the small area estimates on the y-axis compared to the direct estimates on the x-axis. Each dot represents a municipality. For the health-related indicator 'Making ends meet' no direct estimates were available. There exists a moderate correlation between the two estimates. There seems to be a tendency for the small

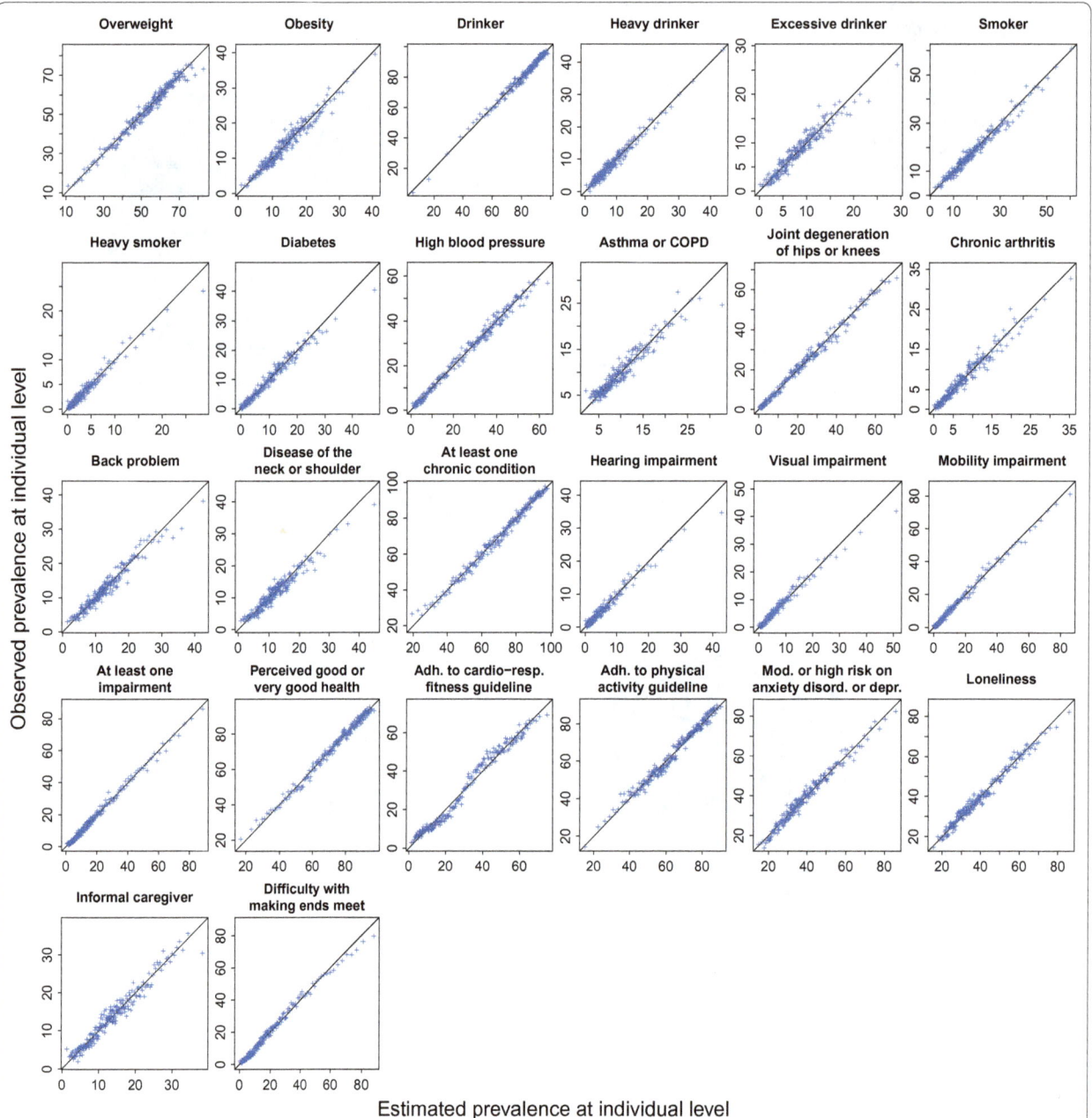

Fig. 5 Calibration plots of the 26 health-related indicators. Estimated prevalence is given on the *x*-axis, observed prevalence on the *y*-axis. Each *dot* is the average of 645 individuals

area estimates being both somewhat higher and less extreme than the direct estimates.

Discussion
STAR models in small area estimation
We have shown that it is possible to extrapolate the data from the Public Health Monitor by providing estimates of the prevalence of 26 health-related indicators for 11,896 neighbourhoods, 2621 districts and 415 municipalities in

the Netherlands. This was done by relating each indicator to a given set of predictors at the individual, household and neighbourhood level, obtained from registry data. We have used a generalized structured additive regression model, which is, to our knowledge, a relatively new concept in SAE. Another application of STAR models in SAE can be found in [25].

STAR models allow modelling of non-linear relationships using P-splines and modelling spatially correlated

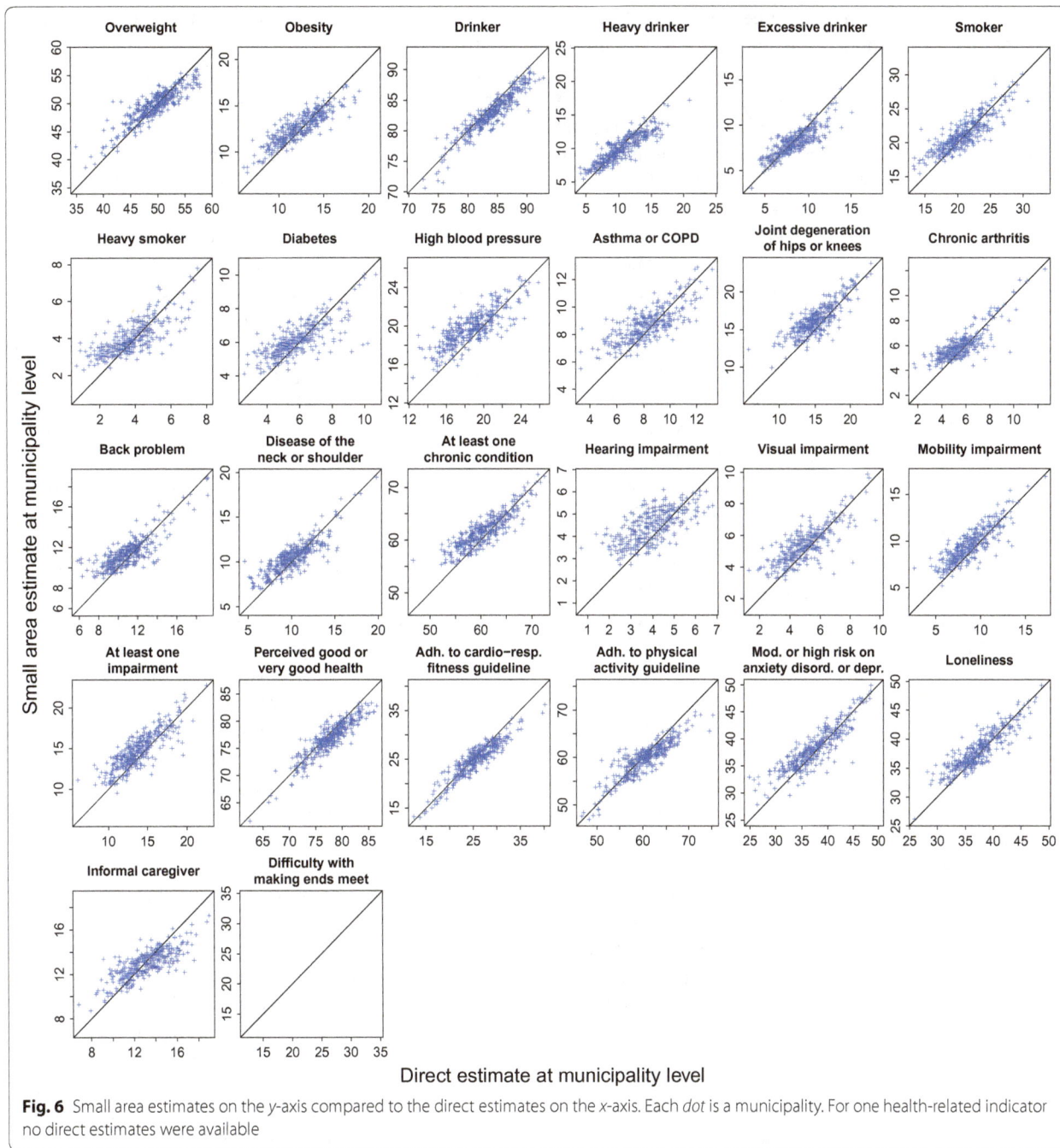

Fig. 6 Small area estimates on the *y*-axis compared to the direct estimates on the *x*-axis. Each *dot* is a municipality. For one health-related indicator no direct estimates were available

data in a unified way. This is accomplished by using basis functions, of which the corresponding regression coefficients are automatically regularized through a roughness penalty to prevent overfitting. We have seen that, for the numerically-valued predictors, effects can be non-linear. There was usually enough information in the data to pick up such signals, as on average 34,782 individuals and 975 neighbourhoods were used for estimation. If for some reason no relationship exists, the roughness penalty becomes so high that the result is a (non-significant) straight line, as we have seen for the relation between household size and overweight.

We have seen that the individuals' characteristics alone are not able to explain the outcome entirely. Still (spatial) patterns exist that are unaccounted for, which should be included as additional random effects in the model. This is often encountered in hierarchical Bayes SAE models (e.g. [2]). The STAR modelling approach treats these random effects in a similar way as the numerically-valued predictors. The amount of smoothing is automatically determined by the amount of information in the data. A spatially correlated random effect has the additional advantage that it interpolates to neighbourhoods where no individuals are sampled. It borrows information from adjacent neighbourhoods in a similar way the P-splines do for numerically-valued predictors. However there still may exist additional heterogeneity between neighbourhoods that cannot be described by individual or spatial effects. This effect is usually modelled by a random intercept, and in the STAR framework it can be similarly modelled as a spatial random effect, except that the penalty matrix $\mathbf{K}$ simplifies to a $d \times d$ identity matrix, which is the classical ridge penalty [8]. We investigated whether a random intercept should be included in the model, but no effect was found.

The creation of a 10 km buffer around each MHS region seemed necessary. Without the buffer, unrealistic clear-cut boundaries between MHS regions appeared in the results. Although the buffer considerably diminished boundary effects, still some regional effects could be recognized because of the stratification by MHS region, even though the data collection and cleaning were harmonized between MHS regions.

Accuracy of the model

The accuracy of the model's estimate has been checked by calibration plots and by comparing the small area estimates with the direct estimates. The binary-valued survey data at the individual level are the best we have to compare the estimates with. The model tries to follow the survey data as well as possible. The calibration plots showed that the model is very capable of estimating the prevalence of the 26 health-related indicators at the individual level. Although not guaranteed, since the true prevalence at neighbourhood level cannot be observed, this suggests that the prevalence at neighbourhood level (or at district or municipality level) may be very close to the true prevalence.

The small area estimates agree reasonably well with the direct estimates already available at municipality level. Although the set of predictors that were accounted for in the weighting scheme showed many similarities with our selected set, we should realise that two totally different estimation procedures are compared here. We additionally included household type, household capital, household income source, and home ownership as predictors in our model and the numerically-valued predictors have not been categorized into an arbitrary number of classes.

Plausibility of the estimates

Plausibility of the estimates was checked in two ways: first, by identifying and explaining extreme estimates, and second, by asking feedback from the Municipal Health Services.

For each health-related indicator we identified the most extreme estimates, i.e. identified the healthiest and unhealthiest neighbourhoods. We located the neighbourhoods on a map and investigated the properties of these neighbourhoods and the residents within. First we noticed that the extremes are not caused by a low number of residents in the neighbourhood; almost all identified outlying neighbourhoods consisted of around 30–300 residents. Instead, extremes were caused by homogeneous groups of individuals sharing the same characteristics that are associated with high or low prevalences, for example, elderly, or people of a certain ethnicity. There was often some institution present in the neighbourhood, e.g. a nursing home, an institute for the mentally disabled, a university campus or an asylum centre. Note that the associations are based on all sampled individuals in a MHS region. A neighbourhood with a homogeneous group of typical individuals then subsequently results in an extreme prevalence. We think it is a good sign that the model is able to pick up such signals.

The feedback from the MHS's, whether the estimates make sense based on their familiarity with the local situation, was mostly positive. Note that this was a qualitative assessment. The estimates did agree with what was expected, although it was noticed, that the small area estimates were less extreme than the direct estimates (when available). The expected differences between neighbourhoods were noticeable and logical. Deprived neighbourhoods, often associated with an unhealthy lifestyle, were in the top rank as expected.

Some results, however, were remarkable. For example, for one neighbourhood that mainly consisted of students the model estimated the prevalence of smokers to be 44%, heavy smokers 12%, and risk of anxiety disorder or depression 49%. This was doubted by the MHS. After further investigation we found that most residents were 19–25 years old, were of an 'other Western' background, were mostly unmarried, and living in single person households. The household capital and income was mainly (very) low, and if any income was generated, it was by employment or a student benefit. Home ownership was mainly rent without housing allowance. By looking at the associations between smoking behaviour and the predictors (as described by Fig. 2), we saw that smoking was associated with young age, small households, low household capital and income, and rent without housing allowance. These associations are based on all participants in the corresponding MHS. It is therefore not surprising that the model subsequently produced such a high smoking prevalence for this neighbourhood.

What is missing is educational level, which is usually considered as a strong predictor for health-related indicators. Household capital, income, income source and home ownership were used as a proxy, but for this specific neighbourhood this seemed to be insufficient. Furthermore, the estimate is the product of an expected value based on the individual's characteristics and a spatial random effect at neighbourhood level. The latter can be estimated better if more people would have participated in the Public Health Monitor in that neighbourhood (currently only two). With less information, the estimate is shrunken towards the expected value based on individual's characteristics and the random effect borrows more information from of the surrounding neighbourhoods. In other words, if the information was there, then we would have gotten a better estimate for this specific neighbourhood.

Limitations and possible extensions

This brings us to the limitations and possible extensions of the model. First, sufficient data should be available; registry data as well as survey data. In the Netherlands, high-resolution registry data is available (in a secured environment). Such data may not be available in other countries. We have also noticed that educational level should have been included as a predictor. However this predictor is only partly available in the registry data and therefore cannot be included. This may improve in the future as more data on educational level becomes available. Next to appropriate registry data, still sufficient survey data are needed to be able to associate the health-related indicators with the predictors. Here, conveniently, 387,195 participants were incorporated that were proportionally sampled throughout the Netherlands. We have not investigated what the minimum number of respondents would be in relation to the number of predictors and neighbourhoods, but this may be a topic for further research.

The availability of appropriate registry data is related to the selection of predictors. Here selection was done by expert knowledge. We have not considered applying any variable selection methods, e.g. [26], but this may be also a topic for further research. As there is no information on the non-responders, we had to assume that the predictors were evenly distributed across responder and non-responders. However, we realize that survey research frequently involves some selection bias.

One must bear in mind that inappropriate modelling choices may produce incorrect results. For instance, our methodology could be applied to other indicators, e.g. experienced noise annoyance, which could be associated with local environmental exposure to noise. However, if local exposure to noise is not included as a predictor in the model and an association is found with e.g. low household capital, this does not automatically mean that all individuals with low household capital experience noise annoyance.

Although recent computational developments make it possible to use STAR models in combination with very large datasets [11], it is currently unfeasible to provide estimates of prediction uncertainties. The model does provide uncertainty estimates at the individual level, but aggregation to neighbourhood, district or municipality level causes difficulties. In theory Monte Carlo simulation could be a solution: (1) Draw a large number, say 1000, realisations of the estimated regression coefficients from a multivariate Normal distribution, which takes care of the covariances. (2) For a given set of coefficients, predict the prevalences at the individual level. (3) For each given prevalence, draw a realisation of the outcome from a Bernoulli distribution. Replace the realisation by the observed response for individuals whose outcome is actually known. (4) For each neighbourhood, add up the individuals' outcome and divide by the total number of individuals in that neighbourhood. (5) Calculate the desired summary statistics, e.g. mean or standard deviation. The main problem is that these steps have to be carried out for 13,073,969 individuals. In combination with, on average, 1052 regression coefficients, this results in a huge linear predictor matrix. This is computationally infeasible at the moment and may be a topic for further research.

Conclusions

The possibilities of Public Health Monitor can be extended to produce nationwide small area estimates of 26 health-related indicators at neighbourhood level in the Netherlands. Registry data is needed to make predictions. Structured additive regression is a useful tool to provide small area estimates in a unified framework. The model can handle both non-linear relations and spatial effects in the presence of binary-valued outcomes.

The model tries to follow the survey data as well as possible. The estimated prevalences agree very well with observed prevalences at the individual level. The estimated prevalences agree reasonably well with the direct estimates at the municipal level. The estimates seem plausible. The results can be used by local and policy makers to make appropriate health policy decisions at the local level and by health care services to respond to local care needs.

Abbreviations

CBS: Centraal Bureau voor de Statistiek (Statistics Netherlands); COPD: chronic obstructive pulmonary disease; GGD: Gemeentelijke Gezondheidsdienst (Municipal Health Service); MHS: Municipal Health Service; REML: restricted maximum likelihood; RIVM: Rijksinstituut voor de Volksgezondheid en Milieu (National Institute for Public Health and the Environment); SAE: small area estimation; STAR: structured additive regression.

Authors' contributions

JvdK prepared the datasets, carried out the analyses, prepared the manuscript and joined the discussions with the Municipal Health Services. LZ added the geographical view to the project. He co-supervised the project, joined the discussions with the Municipal Health Services and other stakeholders, and discussed the manuscript. OB discussed the manuscript. CA prepared the datasets. CvdB coordinated the data collection of the Public Health Monitor and supervised the project of the small area estimates. She consulted the Municipal Health Services and discussed the manuscript. All authors read and approved the final manuscript.

Acknowledgements

We thank Suzan van Dijken of the MHS *GGD Flevoland* for her expert knowledge with regard to the selection of the predictors. We also thank Daan Uitenbroek of MHS *GGD Amsterdam* for his input and support. We thank the MHS Working Group on Small Area Estimation for their input, suggestions, comments and plausibility checks.

Competing interests

The authors declare that they have no competing interests.

Availability of data and materials

Results are based on calculations by the National Institute for Public Health and the Environment, based on non-publicly accessible microdata from Statistics Netherlands on the Public Health Monitor 2012, which originate from the Municipal Health Services, Statistics Netherlands and the National Institute for Public Health and the Environment. The datasets analysed during the current study are not publicly available due to restricted access. Only authorised institutions have access to the microdata of Statistics Netherlands. Microdata are linkable data at the level of individuals, companies and addresses, which can only be made available to researchers under strict conditions for statistical research. The datasets generated during the current study are not publicly available, but data are however available from the authors upon reasonable request.

Funding

This research was carried out in the framework of the Strategic Program RIVM (SPR), in which expertise and innovative projects prepare RIVM to respond to future issues in health and sustainability.

References

1. Centraal Bureau voor de Statistiek. Opbouw en instructie totaalbestand Gezondheidsmonitor Volwassenen 2012 [Internet]. Centraal Bureau voor de Statistiek; 2015. https://www.cbs.nl/nl-nl/onze-diensten/methoden/onderzoeksomschrijvingen/korte-onderzoeksbeschrijvingen/gezondheidsmonitor.
2. Pfeffermann D. New important developments in small area estimation. Stat Sci. 2013;28:40–68.
3. Opsomer JD, Claeskens G, Ranalli MG, Kauermann G, Breidt FJ. Non-parametric small area estimation using penalized spline regression. J R Stat Soc Ser B Stat Methodol. 2008;70:265–86.
4. Ugarte MD, Goicoa T, Militino AF, Durbán M. Spline smoothing in small area trend estimation and forecasting. Comput Stat Data Anal. 2009;53:3616–29.
5. Pratesi M, Salvati N. Small area estimation in the presence of correlated random area effects. J Off Stat. 2009;25:37–53.
6. You Y, Zhou QM. Hierarchical bayes small area estimation under a spatial model with application to health survey data. Surv Methodol. 2011;37:25–37.
7. Porter AT, Holan SH, Wikle CK, Cressie N. Spatial Fay–Herriot models for small area estimation with functional covariates. Spat Stat. 2014;10:27–42.
8. Fahrmeir L, Kneib T, Lang S, Marx B. Regression: models, methods and applications. Berlin: Springer; 2013.
9. Brezger A, Lang S. Generalized structured additive regression based on Bayesian P-splines. Comput Stat Data Anal. 2006;50:967–91.
10. Wood S. Generalized additive models: an introduction with R. Boca Raton: Chapman and Hall/CRC; 2006.
11. Wood SN, Goude Y, Shaw S. Generalized additive models for large data sets. J R Stat Soc Ser C Appl Stat. 2015;64:139–55.
12. Buelens B, Meijers R, Tennekes M. Weging gezondheidsmonitor 2012. Centraal Bureau voor de Statistiek; 2013.
13. Nieuwenbroek N, Boonstra HJ. Bascula 4.0 for weighting sample survey data with estimation of variances. Surv Stat. 2002;46:6–11.
14. Eilers PHC, Marx BD. Flexible smoothing with B-splines and penalties. Stat Sci. 1996;11:89–121.
15. Besag J, York J, Mollié A. Bayesian image restoration, with two applications in spatial statistics. Ann Inst Stat Math. 1991;43:1–20.
16. R Development Core Team. R: A language and environment for statistical computing [Internet]. Vienna: R Foundation for Statistical Computing; 2016. https://www.R-project.org/.
17. Dowle M, Srinivasan A, Short T, Saporta SL with contributions from R, Antonyan E. data.table: Extension of data.frame [Internet]; 2015. https://cran.r-project.org/web/packages/data.table/index.html.
18. Bivand RS, Pebesma E, Gómez-Rubio V. Applied spatial data analysis with R. New York: Springer; 2013.
19. Bivand R, Lewin-Koh N, Pebesma E, Archer E, Baddeley A, Bearman N, et al. Maptools: tools for reading and handling spatial objects [Internet]; 2016. https://cran.r-project.org/web/packages/maptools/index.html.
20. Wood SN. Fast stable restricted maximum likelihood and marginal likelihood estimation of semiparametric generalized linear models. J R Stat Soc Ser B Stat Methodol. 2011;73:3–36.
21. Bivand R, Rundel C, Pebesma E, Stuetz R, Hufthammer KO. rgeos: Interface to Geometry Engine-Open Source (GEOS) [Internet]; 2016. https://cran.r-project.org/web/packages/rgeos/index.html.
22. Bivand R, Piras G. Comparing implementations of estimation methods for spatial econometrics. J Stat Softw. [Internet]; 2015;63. https://www.jstatsoft.org/article/view/v063i18.
23. Arya S, Mount D, Kemp SE, Jefferis G. RANN: Fast nearest neighbour search (Wraps Arya and Mount's ANN Library) [Internet]; 2015. https://cran.r-project.org/web/packages/RANN/index.html.
24. Steyerberg EW. Clinical prediction models; A practical approach to development, validation, and updating [Internet]. New York: Springer; 2009. http://link.springer.com/10.1007/978-0-387-77244-8.
25. Brunauer W, Lang S, Umlauf N. Modelling house prices using multilevel structured additive regression. Stat Model. 2013;13:95–123.
26. Scheipl F, Fahrmeir L, Kneib T. Spike-and-slab priors for function selection in structured additive regression models. J Am Stat Assoc. 2012;107:1518–32.

Determining the spatial heterogeneity underlying racial and ethnic differences in timely mammography screening

Joseph Gibbons[1]*[iD] and Melody K. Schiaffino[2]

Abstract

Background: The leading cause of cancer death for women worldwide continues to be breast cancer. Early detection through timely mammography has been recognized to increase the probability of survival. While mammography rates have risen for many women in recent years, disparities in screening along racial/ethnic lines persist across nations. In this paper, we argue that the role of local context, as identified through spatial heterogeneity, is an unexplored dynamic which explains some of the gaps in mammography utilization by race/ethnicity.

Methods: We apply geographically weighted regression methods to responses from the 2008 Public Health Corporations' Southeastern Household Health Survey, to examine the spatial heterogeneity in mammograms in the Philadelphia metropolitan area.

Results: We find first aspatially that minority identity, in fact, increases the odds of a timely mammogram: 74% for non-Hispanic Blacks and 80% for Hispanic/Latinas. However, the geographically weighted regression confirms the relation of race/ethnicity to mammograms varies by space. Notably, the coefficients for Hispanic/Latinas are only significant in portions of the region. In other words, the increased odds of a timely mammography we found are not constant spatially. Other key variables that are known to influence timely screening, such as the source of healthcare and social capital, measured as community connection, also vary by space.

Conclusions: These results have ramifications globally, demonstrating that the influence of individual characteristics which motivate, or inhibit, cancer screening may not be constant across space. This inconsistency calls for healthcare practitioners and outreach services to be mindful of the local context in their planning and resource allocation efforts.

Keywords: Timely mammograms, Geographically weighted regression, Spatial heterogeneity, Race/ethnicity, Community connection

Background

Breast cancer persists as a leading cause of cancer death in women worldwide [1]. Early detection of breast cancer, defined as timely or guideline-concordant screening mammography and diagnosis contribute to survivorship. Specifically, stage 0–1 detection results in nearly 100% 5-year survival while stage IV detection only has a 22% survival rate according to a recent American Cancer Society estimate [2, 3]. Screening rates have risen among women, in particular for women in countries where screening was not previously available [3, 4]. However, disparities along the continuum of breast cancer persist among underserved women, a situation that reflects the experiences of underserved women everywhere. In particular, Non-Hispanic Black (henceforth, Black) women in the U.S. experience later stage diagnosis at much higher rates compared to White women [3, 4]. In addition, Hispanic/Latina women continue to experience lower comparable rates of timely screening mammography than both White and Black women as well as late-stage diagnoses comparable to Black women [4]. Recently, screening recommendations have also

*Correspondence: jgibbons@mail.sdsu.edu
[1] Department of Sociology Health, San Diego State University, 5500 Campanile Dr., San Diego, CA 92182-4493, USA
Full list of author information is available at the end of the article

experienced variation with technological advances in screening modalities, changes in recommended ages for screening initiation contingent on genetics, familial history, and other nuanced risk factors have lead to the flattening of disparities [2, 5]. However, largely overlooked in this discussion is the role of spatial variation, or heterogeneity, in local screening rates. We argue that the spatial heterogeneity of mammograms by race/ethnicity helps to understand the disparities in rates overall, underlining the subtle role of local context on cancer screening.

While differences in outcomes across socially and racially/ethnically diverse populations are known, the role of local variation in breast cancer screening behaviors among underserved minority populations is not as well understood. Studies of geographic access to mammograms demonstrate disparities in screening rates by race/ethnicity, but often stop short of examining other contextual influences [6–9]. More subtle social, cultural, and other local factors are also found to shape timely cancer screenings [10–13]. We highlight for this study one's community connection, group membership, and perceived medical discrimination as these factors are associated with healthy minority behaviors and vary at a local level [14–17], thus contributing to the risk of disease for minorities in a community [18, 19].

Community connection has been framed through a number of different terms, including social capital [14, 20] and collective efficacy [17]. It is derived from several measures including interpersonal trust with neighbors, a feeling of belongingness to the place, and the sense that residents share mutual interests [21]. Strong community connection within a group may facilitate leverage for treatment and survival by promoting timely screening. The protective effects of local ties can assist the spread of local health information such as where health services can be accessed, securing assistance in transportation to services, or the encouragement from peers to seek them out [17, 22, 23]. Membership in local community groups, ranging from churches to local nonprofits, provides another avenue to encourage service usage as it often puts members in contact with others outside of their proximate friend and family circle [23–25]. Group membership can be a facilitator to mobilize individuals toward healthy behaviors effectively [26, 27]. Put simply, the ability of friends or one's pastor to inform and encourage one to seek out services like mammograms is more viable when these exchanges take place in a local day to day setting, such as a neighborhood.

The impact of community connection and group membership on health outcomes is noted to vary between racial/ethnic groups [14, 20, 26]. For example, community connection has been found to have a stronger positive effect on health outcomes among Latino populations,

ceteris paribus, compared to the health outcomes of Black populations [28]. Sampson shows, in his study of collective efficacy, that the strength of community connection and group membership is not equal across space, being deeply stratified by local disparities such as racial segregation [17]. How these matter locally for mammograms for minority women is unclear. Dean and colleagues found that while local social capital influenced the relationship of Black women to mammography utilization, postulating a relationship with collective efficacy, they could not establish the direction of the relationship [14].

Another factor which may influence the use of health services by underserved minorities related to local context is discrimination from medical practitioners or medical discrimination. Medical discrimination as a barrier to health outcomes was widely described in the IOM report *Unequal Treatment* when it was one of the first empirical reports on the validated effect of medical discrimination on health outcomes [29]. Evidence regarding continued medical discrimination in health services experienced by women suggests this is a persistent issue that remains unaddressed [30, 31]. Jacobs et al. [32] found that medical discrimination related inversely to receiving screening mammography, they also found that more Black women compared to other groups reported health services discrimination.

While medical discrimination is a form of institutional racial discrimination, thus taking place within the larger context of the health service system, there is evidence that the perception of this discrimination for minority patients is not consistent across space. Studies on businesses and nonprofits, for example, have both found the institutional environment of professional settings is subject to local context [33, 34]. What's more, Hunt et al. [15] found through a health survey on minority women that the perception of discrimination was lower in segregated communities. This evidence suggests medical discrimination may not be homogenous across communities and may be subject to spatial heterogeneity that warrants further study.

Examining the influence of local context on timely mammography requires an estimation strategy which accounts for granular variations of effects within a place. To this end, geographically weighted regression (GWR) is a novel way to examine the spatial heterogeneity in rates of timely mammography by race/ethnicity. Past studies have shown that GWR is an effective way to not only document local variations in health outcomes, [35] but also service usage [36]. While multi-level modeling strategies, commonly used in urban health research [37–40], can examine the interrelation between individual and neighborhood characteristics, they are limited in that they treat local effects as stationary and mutually independent across neighborhoods [41]. Multi-level strategies overlook the underlying spatial structures that would influence timely mammography rates within and between neighborhood boundaries.

To our knowledge, this is the first study to use GWR to understand the role of spatial heterogeneity to explore within race and social category variation in the utilization of timely screening mammography. The expected contributions of these findings relate to the potential of GWR as a tool for healthcare professionals better understand nuance *within* places to improve patient- and community-centered responses to the need for timely mammography that may not always be easily answered by broader designations. Further, our results suggest other factors such as social and spatial determinants also need to be considered or re-configured. The objectives of this analysis are to assess the spatial factors associated with timely mammography utilization in a cohort of women. With GWR, we can compare the local variation in our predictors localized population parameters at the census tract level. Through this comparison, we can begin to contextualize the spatial relationship of population factors to timely mammographies among women in the study sample, isolating potential neighborhood impacts on the local spatial structure.

Timely mammography theoretical and conceptual foundations

Variation in the utilization of timely mammography outcomes is multi-dimensional and complex. The *Andersen Model of Health Services Utilization* is a valuable model that takes into account this complexity and offers a framework that allows us to adapt, conceptualize, and study these dimensions for our present analysis [42]. Broadly, Andersen describes multi-level factors that operationalize the complexity of access to care and utilization as a product of how multiple social, contextual, and perceived factors can influence our utilization or lack thereof. As Fig. 1 shows, these factors are operationalized as *predisposing*, or background characteristics which shape a person's inclination to seek out healthcare and are not mutable. For example, African–Americans are less likely to find care due to historical systemic racism within the health system [43, 44]. Next, *enabling* factors include those which facilitate or hinder, if absent, one's efforts to find healthcare. For example, lacking insurance makes it nearly impossible for one to obtain timely and affordable healthcare. Finally, *need* factors reflect ailments a person might be experiencing that would require healthcare in the first place, these are subject to a perceived and evaluated need that can be influenced by discrimination when they do visit a doctor. The Andersen Model has been adapted successfully in multiple cases,

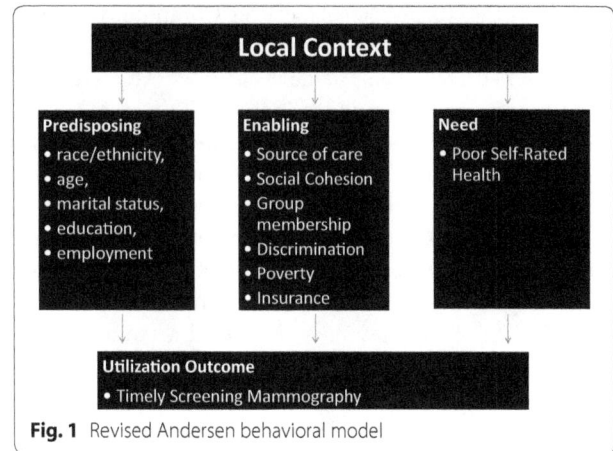

Fig. 1 Revised Andersen behavioral model

and part of the strength of this model is its adaptability to study context and outcomes related to health utilization behavior [45]. With the present analysis, we adapted the Andersen Model to include *local* context as it relates to spatial heterogeneity across all levels of need from predisposing to outcome.

Hypotheses

To address the potential effect of local context on cancer screening disparities, our study explores the spatial heterogeneity in factors associated with timely mammography within racial and ethnic minority populations. To this end, we propose the following hypotheses:

1. Utilization of timely screening mammography by Latina/Hispanic women will be negatively associated versus non-Hispanic women, and will not vary significantly between Black women versus White women.

    (a) Utilization of timely mammography will vary significantly by geography among Black women.
    (b) Utilization of timely mammography will vary significantly by geography among Hispanic women.

2. Utilization of timely screening mammography will be positively associated with community connection.

    (a) Utilization of timely screening mammography will vary significantly by geography among respondents reporting community connection.

Data and methods
Data source

To empirically examine our hypotheses, we used a sample of female respondents from the 2008 Public Health Management Corporation (PHMC) Southeastern Pennsylvania Household Survey (N = 3261) with geocodes to link to the 2005–2009 American Community Survey (ACS) geographic dataset consisting of approximately N = 998 census tracts. The goal of the PHMC is to collect the information on individual's health status, behaviors, attitudes, and access to healthcare in the following five counties of the Philadelphia metropolitan area [46]. PHMC respondents used in this study are those eligible to receive guideline concordant recommendations appropriate for the data collection time period of 2008, specifically women aged 40 and over [47]. While the U.S. Preventive Services Task Force has since suggested a reduced marginal benefit in the range of participants to include in population-based screening mammography [48], for the purposes of the present analysis we included the population appropriate to the time period. On the reliability and validity of the PHMC surveys, a recent study [21] reported that several health and socioeconomic indicators (e.g., obesity rate and poverty) drawn from PHMC data were comparable with those estimated by the Centers for Diseases Control and Prevention.

Measurements

The dependent variable is the self-reported use of timely *Breast Cancer Screening Mammography*. Participants were asked if they had received a screening mammography within the guideline concordant time frame recommended by their medical practitioner for the time period in which data were collected. Following the common practice, we dichotomized the answers into no (coded 0, reference group) and yes (coded 1). Our predictors were determined based on Andersen's Behavioral Model [42, 49], including Predisposing, Enabling and Need factors which would compel one to seek out medical services like a mammography. Starting with Predisposing factors, our focal predictors are *race/ethnicity*; the PHMC classified respondents into non-Hispanic White (reference group, hence just White), Black, Hispanic/Latinas, and non-Hispanic other minorities. Three race/ethnicity dummy variables were included in the analysis. Other predisposing covariates include age, poverty, race/ethnicity, marital status, employment status, and education attainment. Respondents reported their ages in years, and we treated *age* as a continuous variable. In keeping with the screening guidelines circa 200 [8, 48] we restrict our sample to age 40 and above. *Marital status* was categorized into four groups: single (reference group), married or living with a partner, widowed/divorced/separated (WDS), and another marital status. Gender was not included as a predictor given the surveys focus on female breast cancer screening.

Turning to Enabling factors, we add as focal variables community connection and medical discrimination given their strong association with race. First, we include a measure of *Medical discrimination*; the respondents

were asked if they have ever experienced discrimination when getting medical care because of their race, ethnicity, or color. Those who perceived medical discrimination were coded 1, otherwise 0. Next, we include a measure of *community connection*, a composite score based on the principal components analysis (PCA) of respondents' answers to the following three questions: (1) *Willingness*, "Would you say that most people in your neighborhood are always, often, sometimes, rarely, or never willing to help their neighbors?" From *always* to *never*, we coded from 5 to 1. (2) *Belonging*, "Do you strongly agree, agree, disagree, or strongly disagree that you feel that you belong and are part of your neighborhood?" We coded the answers with a four-level Likert-type scale where 4 means *strongly agree*, and 1 indicates *strongly disagree*. (3) *Trust*, "Do you strongly agree, agree, disagree, or strongly disagree with the statement that most people in your neighborhood can be trusted?" The coding scheme is also a four-level Likert-type scale (4 = *strongly agree*, and 1 = *strongly disagree*). The PCA results suggested that one factor is sufficient to capture over 60% of the variance among these three questions. We used the regression method to obtain the factor score as our dependent variable (with a mean of 0 and a standard deviation of 1). A higher score indicates stronger community connection.

Also, we include enabling factors more commonly found in behavioral models [49], consisting of those who lived under the federal poverty line as a measure of the financial situation, coding 1 as in *poverty* and 0 otherwise. For *employment status*, we classified those will full-time employment status as employed. Next, we include a measure of *insurance status*; a respondent coded 1 when a respondent reported that she had health insurance, otherwise 0. Next, we included variables for *Source of Health Care*, where an individual goes to get medical services, as a way to understand healthcare access. We categorized the answers into four groups: private doctor's office, community health center or public clinic, outpatient clinic, and other places (e.g., hospital emergency room). To test our hypotheses, the "other places" category was used as the reference group, and three dummy variables were considered in the analysis. We also include a measure of *Local group participation*, the total number of local groups that a respondent participates in such as social, political, religious, school-related, and athletic groups. Finally, we include a measure of residence in the city and county of Philadelphia, *City*.

Finally, for factors of *Need*, we use a measure of *self-rated health*. The respondents were asked to evaluate their health as poor, fair, good, very good or excellent. Their answers were further dichotomized into poor/fair (coded 1) and good/very good/excellent (coded 0), which is a conventional practice. While it is common in GWR studies using administrative units like census tracts to utilize the geographic centroids of the unit as a proxy of the individual level, this approach has been criticized for underestimating the spatial variation across research area [41]. To address this issue, and following the precedent established by previous studies, we used ArcGIS to generate coordinates for each respondent that fall at random within their respective census tract [41, 50]. To ensure the reliability of this approach, multiple coordinates were generated for each observation and sensitivity analysis were conducted (results available on request). This approach of spatial randomization has been found to be a useful method to preserve spatial variation [41].

Analytic methods and strategy

To explore the spatial variation between timely mammograms and other covariates across the Philadelphia metropolitan area, we employed logistic GWR to handle the binary dependent variable [51]. As we randomly created the coordinates for each individual, the model below can be applied to our data:

$$\log\left(\frac{y_i}{1-y_i}\right) = \beta_{0i}(u_i, v_i) + \sum_{n=1}^{k} \beta_{ni}(u_i, v_i) * x_{ni}$$

where y_i is the probability of reporting timely mammograms for an individual i, (u_i, v_i) denotes the coordinates of individual i, x_{ni} represents the explanatory variables ($n = 1, ..., k$) discussed above for individual i, and β_{ni} represents the estimated association of variable n with mammograms for individual i. We used the software program developed by Fotheringham et al. [51] to implement the analysis. The estimation method is the iteratively reweighted least squares and the kernel density function is the bi-square weighting function, which is a commonly used weighting scheme [51]. When the data points are dense in a study area, the choice of kernel density function may not affect the results greatly.

One advantage of GWR is that it is an extension of generalized regression models, and thus the interpretations of regression coefficients remain unchanged [52–54]. Explicitly, the regression coefficient of a specific variable at a specific location, (u_i, v_i), in the model above indicates the change in the log-odds of having a timely mammograms given a one-unit change in this variable. Similar to the conventional logistic regression, exponentiating the coefficient yields the odds ratio associated with this variable at a particular location. As the model above generates results for each individual in our data, it is ineffective to show all local estimates. Following previous studies [41, 53, 55], we reported the estimates of conventional logistic results, presented the five-number summary (i.e., minimum, three quartiles, and maximum) of local

estimates, and visualized the GWR results with thematic maps using a recently developed method [50]. The corrected Akaike Information Criterion (AIC) was used to understand whether the logistic GWR fits the data better than the conventional logistic model [51]. As a rule of thumb, when the difference in AICs between two models is larger than 4, the model with the smaller AIC is strongly preferred [56].

Results

Aspatial results

Table 1 presents the descriptive statistics for this study. Overall, 74.03% of the PHMC respondents received timely screening mammographies. As for racial composition, the 2008 PHMC survey included 70.84% of White, 22.85% of Black, 3.93% of Hispanic/Latinas, and roughly 2.39% of non-Hispanic other minority groups. These figures closely matched to those reported by the 2005–2009 ACS. Most of those surveyed, 95.95%, had some insurance. Only 6.10% reported experiencing medical discrimination. As for healthcare access, most respondents went to a private practice for regular care, 88.87%, compared to a community health center, which amounted to only 5.24% of those surveyed. Regarding other individual characteristics, 6.69% of the interviewees did not complete high school, while more than 40.08% of the individuals had a college degree or greater. As for group membership, most respondents reported membership in at least one group. Community connection was not reported in Table 1 as it is a means-centered variable.

Table 2 presents the global, or conventional logistic findings. The results for predisposing factors are somewhat surprising, given the previous literature. Both Black and Hispanic/Latina women reported greater odds of getting timely screening mammograms. Being Black increases the odds of a timely mammogram by 74% ($1.738 - 1 = 0.738$; $p < 0.01$) while being Hispanic/Latina increases the odds by 80% ($p < 0.0501$). The other predisposing factors are more in line with the past literature. A college education (or greater) and being married both increase the likelihood one will get a mammogram. Turning to enabling factors, employment and having insurance both increase the odds one will get a timely mammogram. Also, where one goes for healthcare consistently has an important role in screening. Based on our findings, any place other than a center like a hospital will increase odds of a timely mammogram. Access to a community health center appears to matter the most in encouraging a mammogram. Meanwhile, experiencing medical discrimination was inversely related to reporting receipt of a timely mammogram though this association was not significant (AOR 0.784). What is more, community connection was not significant in the global models

Table 1 Descriptive statistics

Outcome variable	Count[a]	(%)
Received timely screening		
Yes	2414	74.03
No (ref)	847	25.97
Predisposing variables		
Age (average)	56.68	–
Race/ethnicity		
White (ref)	2310	70.84
Black	745	22.85
Hispanic/Latina	128	3.93
Other race	78	2.39
Educational attainment		
No high school diploma (ref)	218	6.69
High school	1077	33.03
Some college	659	20.21
College or greater	1307	40.08
Marital status		
Married	1761	54.00
Not married (ref)	1500	46.00
Enabling		
Poverty status		
Lives below 100% FPL	260	7.97
Above 100% federal poverty level (ref)	3001	92.03
Fulltime employment status		
Yes	1918	58.82
No (ref)	1343	41.18
Insurance status		
Yes	3129	95.95
No (ref)	132	4.05
Source of healthcare		
Other center (ref)	65	1.99
Community health center	171	5.24
Private practice	2898	88.87
Outpatient clinic	127	3.89
Experienced medical discrimination		
Yes	199	6.10
No (ref)	3062	93.90
Respondent Residence		
Urban (Philadelphia Residence)	1377	42.23
Suburban (ref)	1884	57.77
Group participation (average)	1.224	–
Need		
Self-rated health status		
Poor or fair	732	22.45
Good, very good or excellent (ref)	2529	77.55
N	3261	

[a] Numbers are total counts unless otherwise noted

and membership in groups only had a marginally significant effect. Turning lastly to need, women with poor/fair self-rated health reported 30% lower odds of receiving a mammogram in a timely manner by 30% ($p < 0.01$).

GWR results

GWR logistic regression generated a set of coefficient estimates for each individual, which makes it difficult, if not impossible, to present all results. Following Fotheringham et al. [51], we reported the five-number summary in Table 3 and visualized the GWR findings into thematic maps. The goal of this table is to present the spatial range in magnitude of the variable coefficients. Local statistical significance for select GWR coefficients is mapped out in Figs. 2 and 3. While several methods have been proposed to examine spatial heterogeneity of significance and coefficients [57, 58], these methods are not applicable to the logistic GWR model and visualization remains an appropriate way to explore this spatial heterogeneity.

On the question of whether the GWR logistic model fit our data better than the global logistic model, we compared the corrected AICs in Tables 2 and 3. Because the GWR AIC is smaller than the global AIC by 4, it indicates the GWR provides superior fit for our predictors. As Table 3 shows, the GWR estimates range quite dramatically, suggesting that the relationships between our independent variables and receipt of timely mammograms may depend on where an individual resides. This offers support to the importance of geographically weighted results over the global results. Starting with our focal predisposing predictors, the maximum size of the coefficient for being Hispanic/Latina is nearly 4 times as large as its minimum, suggesting substantial variation in how being Hispanic/Latina impacts timely mammograms. The coefficients for Blacks also increase, albeit not as dramatically. These results mean that the impact of race on mammograms is not consistent across the region. Turning to our focal enabling variables, community connection, group membership, and medical discrimination also vary, although most notably there are some local coefficients for which community connection relates negatively to mammograms.

To better contextualize our GWR estimates, we make use of a series of maps of the region to unpack the local spatial relations for Black and Hispanic/Latina coefficients, presented in Fig. 2. To help with the easy interpretation, we first created the spatially smoothed local estimates and local t-values with the GWR results. We then overlaid local estimates with t-values in the geographic information systems and showed the local

Table 2 Global logistic regression results of breast cancer screening (1 = yes; 0 = no)

Variable	Odds ratio	95% confidence interval		Coefficient	S.E.	Significance
Predisposing						
Race/ethnicity (ref. = non-Hispanic White)						
Black	1.738	1.371	2.203	0.552	0.120	***
Hispanic/Latina	1.799	1.126	2.875	0.587	0.239	**
Other race	0.726	0.444	1.187	−0.319	0.250	
Age	1.000	0.992	1.009	0.001	0.004	
Educational attainment (ref. = no high school diploma)						
High school	1.092	0.781	1.529	0.088	0.171	
Some college	1.068	0.743	1.535	0.065	0.185	
College or greater	1.349	0.941	1.935	0.299	0.184	
Married	1.304	1.094	1.554	0.265	0.089	**
Enabling						
Poverty status (1 = poor, 0 = non-poor)	0.979	0.714	1.341	−0.021	0.160	
Employment status (1 = employed, others = 0)	1.206	0.994	1.463	0.186	0.098	*
Insured (1 = having health insurance, 0 = no health insurance)	3.857	2.616	5.687	1.349	0.198	***
Source of healthcare						
Community health center	2.728	1.449	5.138	1.003	0.322	**
Private practice	2.053	1.228	3.432	0.719	0.262	**
Outpatient clinic	1.671	0.882	3.166	0.513	0.326	
Experienced medical discrimination	0.784	0.563	1.092	−0.243	0.168	
Community connection	1.056	0.988	1.130	0.054	0.034	
Group membership	1.060	0.996	1.128	0.058	0.031	*
Respondent residence—city (ref = suburban)	1.026	0.849	1.240	0.025	0.096	
Need						
Poor or fair self-rated health	0.700	0.570	0.861	−0.356	0.105	***
Constant				−1.475	0.462	***
N	3261					
Akaike Inf. Crit.	3613.910					

* *p* < 0.1; ** *p* < 0.05; *** *p* < 0.01

estimates with a t-value that is greater than 1.96 (*p* value <0.05). That is, the colored areas were estimated to have statistically significant associations of covariates with receipt of timely mammograms. We used the red–orange gradient scheme to show different magnitudes of the local estimates, red signifying strong effects and orange indicating weak associations. Second, in a separate set of maps we then overlaid the areas with insignificant coefficients (with t-values between −1.96 and 1.96) on top of census tract data displaying ACS estimates. While one should proceed with caution in interpreting these visuals without multi-level models, given the risk of ecological fallacy, they do provide some indication of the context as to why the significant coefficients are located where they are.

The localized coefficients for Hispanic/Latinas present an interesting find. These results show that the higher odds of receiving timely mammography among Hispanic/Latina is only significant in roughly half of the region, especially in the suburban Bucks County, not across all

respondents in that ethnic category as regression results suggest in Table 1. This is unexpected for one as this area only has a few large Hispanic populations, suggesting that 'being Hispanic/Latina' matters for reasons other than being in a mostly Hispanic area. Spatial heterogeneity for Black coefficients, in contrast, are significant across the region, growing in strength as one moves east. The lowest coefficients are generally found in Delaware County. It is not clear, based on where the mostly Black populations are found, why this variation exists as all counties have areas with large Black populations, although Philadelphia has the strongest concentrations. One possible explanation why Delaware County has the lowest coefficients is that it is only of the region that does not directly share a border with Philadelphia or inner ring suburban communities, and thereby is the furthest from the largest Black populations.

Turning to our enabling variables of community connection and medical discrimination we find spatial

Table 3 Five-number summary of the GWR logistic regression results; bandwidth 3000

Variable	Min	Q1	Median	Q3	Max
Predisposing					
Race/ethnicity (ref. = non-Hispanic White)					
Black	0.434	0.516	0.561	0.602	0.666
Hispanic/Latina	0.270	0.485	0.601	0.683	1.054
Other race	−0.734	−0.368	−0.214	−0.148	−0.091
Age	−0.007	−0.002	0.001	0.003	0.004
Educational attainment (ref. = no high school diploma)					
High school	−0.261	−0.104	−0.065	−0.021	0.338
Some college	−0.170	−0.156	−0.145	−0.061	0.622
College or greater	−0.056	−0.019	0.012	0.070	0.818
Married	0.209	0.248	0.270	0.298	0.388
Enabling					
Poverty status (1 = poor, 0 = non-poor)	−0.214	−0.184	−0.172	−0.123	0.285
Employment status (1 = employed, others = 0)	0.063	0.131	0.191	0.214	0.241
Insured (1 = having health insurance, 0 = no health insurance)	1.147	1.438	1.476	1.502	1.755
Source of healthcare					
Community health center	0.818	0.846	0.857	0.900	1.352
Private practice	0.464	0.502	0.528	0.609	1.060
Outpatient clinic	0.289	0.302	0.348	0.505	1.031
Experienced medical discrimination	−0.494	−0.191	−0.144	−0.126	−0.106
Community connection	−0.004	0.065	0.076	0.079	0.080
Group membership	−0.033	0.036	0.062	0.075	0.099
Respondent residence—city (ref = suburban)	−0.022	0.015	0.041	0.053	0.092
Need					
Poor of fair self-rated health	−0.575	−0.404	−0.368	−0.353	−0.259
Intercept	−2.354	−1.457	−1.344	−1.174	−0.759
Akaike Inf. Crit.	3609.497				

Min minimum, *Q1* first quartile, *Q3* third quartile, *max* maximum

findings of interest. First, Fig. 3 reveals the coefficients for community connection were significant in select parts of the region, encompassing most of the city of Philadelphia and its immediate surrounding areas. This is notable as community connection was not significant in the global model. Comparing this map to the ACS data in Fig. 2 shows that the significant coefficients appear to co-occur in the areas where the highest concentrations of Black and Hispanic populations are found. These results do not mean that no other area of the region lacked community connection, but our findings do suggest that there is a significant relationship between community connection and women seeking out mammograms that is confined spatially to the area presented in the figure.

Conclusion

Broadly, our results report greater odds of timely screening mammography among racial and ethnic minority populations that appear to be better for this well-insured cohort study sample. However, our primary study purpose, the study of spatial heterogeneity, illustrates a salient point. Geographically weighted regression results support our hypotheses that spatial heterogeneity exists in timely mammograms among Black and Hispanic/Latina women as they compare to white women, and what appear to be greater odds of timely mammography among the whole racial/ethnic group may in fact be limited. In addition, we found that other predisposing and enabling factors like community connection also vary substantially over space. This presents an important innovation to our understanding of health service provision, demonstrating the overlooked role local context carries when considering Andersen's Behavioral Model of utilization. While racial/ethnic groups are typically considered homogenous, our findings show that unaccounted variation across space and place exist within these groups, even when accounting for standard controls like socio-economic and demographic variables. This illustrates that social factors persist even among the insured as we saw that health status persisted as a barrier to timely care.

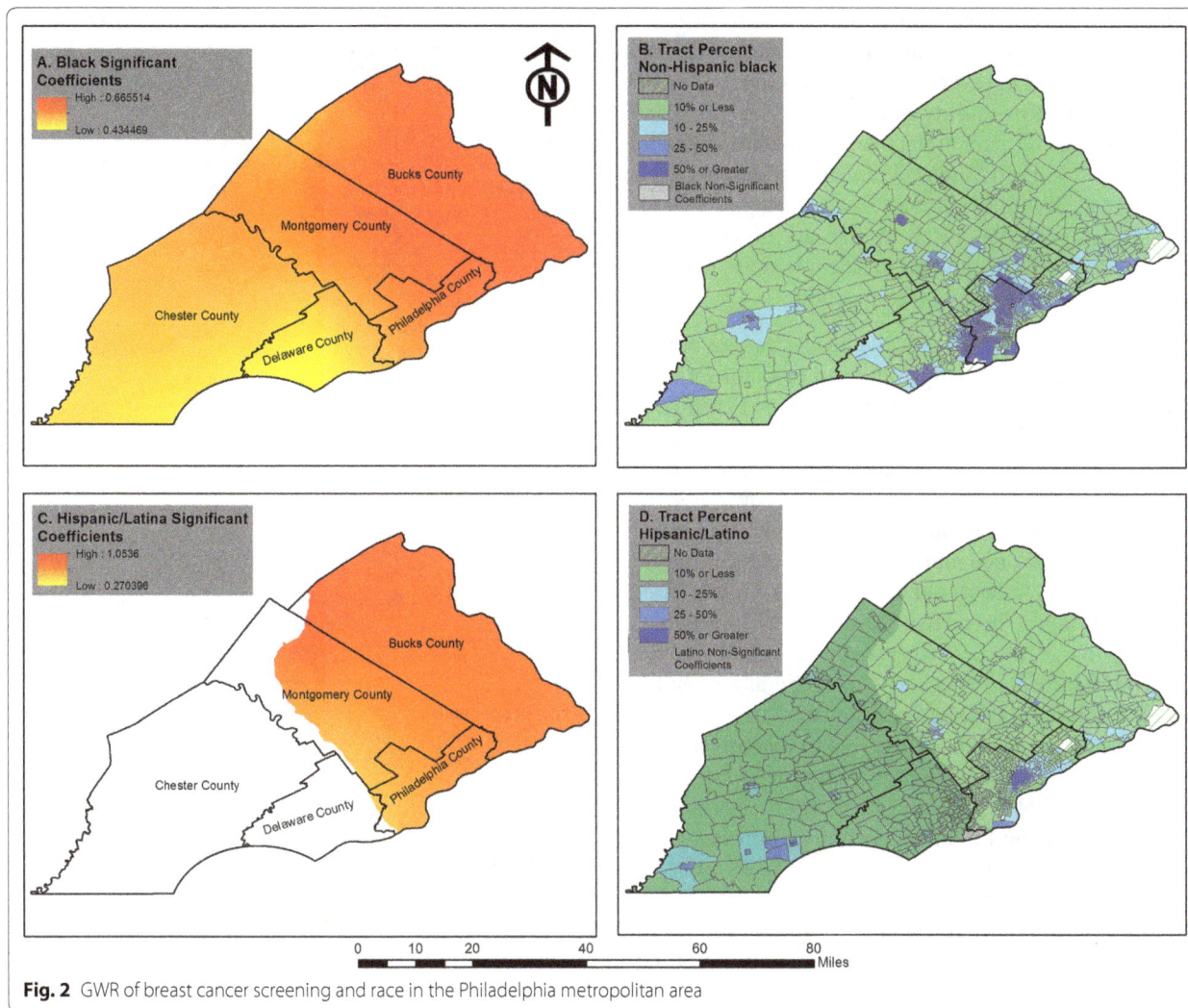

Fig. 2 GWR of breast cancer screening and race in the Philadelphia metropolitan area

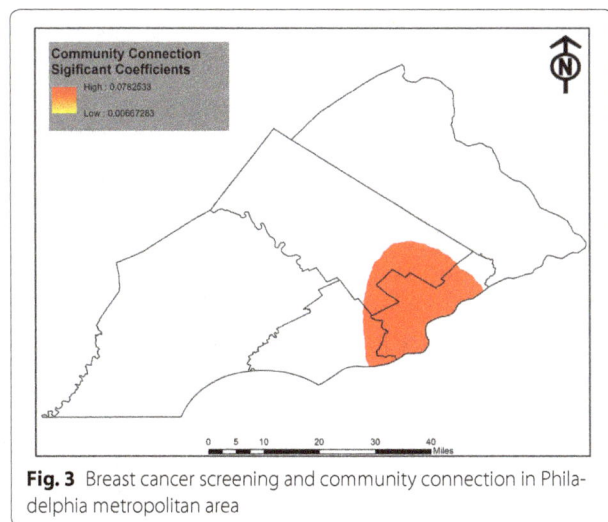

Fig. 3 Breast cancer screening and community connection in Philadelphia metropolitan area

While GWR is an exploratory tool, comparing the GWR maps to one another, as well as to the neighborhood census tract data, reveals patterns allowing informed speculation as for the role race/ethnicity has on mammography. First, significant Hispanic/Latina coefficients are mainly found in the suburban counties of Bucks and Montgomery. One's Hispanic/Latina identity thus appears to matter in encouraging mammographies in these suburban areas. This may reflect recent patterns of immigration in the United States as Hispanic migrants have increasingly dispersed into suburban and rural 'new destinations' as opposed to concentrating in cities [59]. Future research should investigate screening practices for suburban Hispanic/Latinas to understand this trend better. Second, while the coefficients for Black respondents are significant and positive across the region, a close analysis of the other GWR results suggests a more localized dynamic is taking place. Community connection's effect in encouraging mammograms is localized to a mostly

Black and Hispanic area. This could be a reflection of a phenomenon known as 'ethnic density'. Ethnic density a process identified in several countries wherein minorities residing in mostly minority communities, such as places racially segregated, gain protective health effects from the close connections and reduced discrimination enjoyed in these places [38, 60, 61]. Indeed, it would support Dean's et al. [14] theory that Black women are more likely to pursue mammograms in their local context based on the presence of local community connection.

There are a number of possible considerations for the high overall mammography utilization rates for minority women, including income and insurance status. Indeed, insurance was one of the most salient predictors in our models, which is not surprising given our highly insured study population. On the other hand, high overall mammography utilization among minorities could be a reflection of high levels of community health centers in the city of Philadelphia. Indeed, our results show these centers had the strongest predictive power on mammograms. Laiteerapong et al. [62] suggested that Black women visit community health centers like Federally Qualified Health Centers (FQHCs) at rates greater than White or Hispanic/Latina women and that mammograms are also more likely to occur among FQHC attendees, suggesting a positive effect of FQHC utilization. These results could also be affected by the disproportionate representation in the PHMC of respondents with high levels of socioeconomic status or some other unmolded factors unique to Philadelphia. Future research should seek to replicate this analysis in other regions to determine the singularity of our study. While the exact spatial character of race/ethnicity's relation to screening is likely to vary based on location, the bottom line is that the impact of local context on mammography matters differently for racial/ethnic groups across space, a finding likely to be applicable globally.

Timely mammography screening is the first step in understanding and acting to mitigate the devastating impact of breast cancer. There is substantial literature supporting the need for better access to timely screening and care; we lack an understanding of the localized racial/ethnic, cultural and economic factors that continue to make these barriers persist. It is not sufficient to aspatially examine the predisposing and enabling factors that facilitate or bar access to timely screening mammograms among racial/ethnic minorities. Indeed, as our results show, the impact of one's race/ethnicity on pursuing mammograms, as well as other intervening variables, changes from one area to another. Thus, efforts to ensure equitable screening rates among groups must investigate local potential variations in their instances, seeking to determine why these disparities exist and, when necessary, how to manage them.

Abbreviations
GWR: geographically weighted regression; PHMC: Public Health Management Corporation; ACS: American Community Survey; AIC: Akaike Information Criterion; FQHC: Federally Qualified Health Centers.

Authors' contributions
JG contributed to the design of the study, carried out all analyses, contributed to the drafting of the manuscript, and led the interpretation of research results. MS contributed to the design of the study, participated in the interpretation of the research results, and contributed to the drafting of the manuscript. Both authors read and approved the final manuscript.

Author details
[1] Department of Sociology Health, San Diego State University, 5500 Campanile Dr., San Diego, CA 92182-4493, USA. [2] Graduate School of Public Health, San Diego State University, 5500 Campanile Dr., San Diego, CA 92182-4493, USA.

Acknowledgements
The authors would like to thank Tse-Chuan Yang for his advice and input towards the development of the study design and interpretation of results.

Competing interests
The authors declare that they have no competing interests.

References
1. Torre LA, Bray F, Siegel RL, Ferlay J, Lortet-Tieulent J, Jemal A. Global cancer statistics, 2012: global cancer statistics, 2012. CA Cancer J Clin. 2015;65(2):87–108. doi:10.3322/caac.21262.
2. ACS. Breast cancer survival rates by stage. http://www.cancer.org/cancer/breastcancer/detailedguide/breast-cancer-survival-by-stage. Published 2014.
3. ACS. Breast cancer facts and figures for Hispanics/Latinos 2015–2017. http://www.cancer.org/acs/groups/content/@research/documents/document/acspc-046405.pdf. Published 2016.
4. ACS. Cancer facts and figures for African Americans 2013–2014. Am Cancer Soc. 2013. http://www.cancer.org/acs/groups/content/@epidemiologysurveilance/documents/document/acspc-036921.pdf.
5. Siu AL. Screening for breast cancer: U.S. preventive services task force recommendation statement. Ann Intern Med. 2016;164(4):279–96. doi:10.7326/m15-2886.
6. Alford-Teaster J, Lange JM, Hubbard RA, et al. Is the closest facility the one actually used? An assessment of travel time estimation based on mammography facilities. Int J Health Geogr. 2016;15(8):1–10. doi:10.1186/s12942-016-0039-7.
7. Khan-Gates JA, Ersek JL, Eberth JM, Adams SA, Pruitt SL. Geographic access to mammography and its relationship to breast cancer screening and stage at diagnosis: a systematic review. Womens Health Issues. 2015;25(5):482–93. doi:10.1016/j.whi.2015.05.010.
8. Onega T, Cook A, Kirlin B, et al. The influence of travel time on breast cancer characteristics, receipt of primary therapy, and surveillance mammography. Breast Cancer Res Treat. 2011;129(1):269–75. doi:10.1007/s10549-011-1549-4.

9. Huang B, Dignan M, Han D, Johnson O. Does distance matter? Distance to mammography facilities and stage at diagnosis of breast cancer in Kentucky. J Rural Health. 2009;25(4):366–71.

10. Iqbal J, Ginsburg O, Rochon PA, Sun P, Narod SA. Differences in breast cancer stage at diagnosis and cancer-specific survival by race and ethnicity in the United States. JAMA. 2015;313(2):165–73. doi:10.1001/jama.2014.17322.

11. Mejia de Grubb MC, Kilbourne B, Kihlberg C, Levine RS. Demographic and geographic variations in breast cancer mortality among U.S. Hispanics. J Health Care Poor Underserved. 2013;24(Suppl 1):140–52. doi:10.1353/hpu.2013.0043.

12. Tian N, Gaines Wilson J, Benjamin Zhan F. Female breast cancer mortality clusters within racial groups in the United States. Health Place. 2010;16(2):209–18. doi:10.1016/j.healthplace.2009.09.012.

13. Wang F, McLafferty S, Escamilla V, Luo L. Late-stage breast cancer diagnosis and health care access in Illinois. Prof Geogr. 2008;60(1):54–69. doi:10.1080/00330120701724087.

14. Dean L, Subramanian SV, Williams DR, Armstrong K, Charles CZ, Kawachi I. The role of social capital in African-American women's use of mammography. Soc Sci Med. 2014;104:148–56. doi:10.1016/j.socscimed.2013.11.057.

15. Hunt MO, Wise LA, Jipguep M-C, Cozier YC, Rosenberg L. Neighborhood racial composition and perceptions of racial discrimination: evidence from the Black Women's Health Study. Soc Psychol Q. 2007;70(3):272–89.

16. Chen D, Yang T-C. The pathways from perceived discrimination to self-rated health: an investigation of the roles of distrust, social capital, and health behaviors. Soc Sci Med. 2014;104:64–73. doi:10.1016/j.socscimed.2013.12.021.

17. Sampson RJ. Great American City: Chicago and the enduring neighborhood effect. 1st ed. Chicago: University of Chicago Press; 2012.

18. Clark WAV, Burt JE. The impact of workplace on residential relocation. Ann Assoc Am Geogr. 1980;70(1):59–66. doi:10.1111/j.1467-8306.1980.tb01297.x.

19. Cromley E, McLafferty S. GIS and public health. 2nd ed. New York: The Guilford Press; 2012.

20. Kawachi I, Kennedy BP, Glass R. Social capital and self-rated health: a contextual analysis. Am J Public Health. 1998;89(8):1187–93.

21. Gibbons J, Yang T-C. Connecting across the divides of race/ethnicity: how does segregation matter? Urban Aff Rev. 2015;Online First:1–28. doi:10.1177/1078087415589193.

22. Putnam RD. Bowling alone: the collapse and revival of American Community. New York: Simon and Schuster; 2000.

23. Small ML. Unanticipated gains: origins of network inequality in everyday life. New York: Oxford University Press; 2009.

24. Benjamins MR. Religious influences on trust in physicians and the health care system. Int J Psychiatry Med. 2006;36(1):69–83.

25. Ahern MM, Hendryx MS. Social capital and trust in providers. Soc Sci Med. 2003;57(7):1195–203. doi:10.1016/S0277-9536(02)00494-X.

26. Kim D. Bonding versus bridging social capital and their associations with self rated health: a multilevel analysis of 40 US communities. J Epidemiol Community Health. 2006;60(2):116–22. doi:10.1136/jech.2005.038281.

27. Hutchinson RN, Putt MA, Dean LT, Long JA, Montagnet CA, Armstrong K. Neighborhood racial composition, social capital and black all-cause mortality in Philadelphia. Soc Sci Med. 2009;68(10):1859–65. doi:10.1016/j.socscimed.2009.02.005.

28. Klinenberg E. Heat wave: a social autopsy of disaster in Chicago. Chicago: University of Chicago Press; 2003.

29. Smedley B, Stith A, Nelson A, editors. Unequal treatment: confronting racial and ethnic disparities in health care. Washington: The National Academies Press; 2002.

30. Hausmann LR, Jeong K, Bost JE, Ibrahim SA. Perceived discrimination in health care and use of preventive health services. J Gen Intern Med. 2008;23(10):1679–84. doi:10.1007/s11606-008-0730-x.

31. Abramson CM, Hashemi M, Sanchez-Jankowski M. Perceived discrimination in US healthcare: charting the effects of key social characteristics within and across racial groups. Prev Med Rep. 2015;2:615–21. doi:10.1016/j.pmedr.2015.07.006.

32. Jacobs EA, Rathouz PJ, Karavolos K, et al. Perceived discrimination is associated with reduced breast and cervical cancer screening: the Study of Women's Health Across the Nation (SWAN). J Womens Health Larchmt. 2014;23(2):138–45. doi:10.1089/jwh.2013.4328.

33. Gibbons J. Does racial segregation make community-based organizations more territorial? Evidence from Newark, NJ, and Jersey City, NJ: does racial segregation make community-based organizations more territorial? J Urban Aff. 2015;37(5):600–19. doi:10.1111/juaf.12170.

34. Marquis C, Battilana J. Acting globally but thinking locally? The enduring influence of local communities on organizations. Res Organ Behav. 2009;29:283–302. doi:10.1016/j.riob.2009.06.001.

35. Black NC. An ecological approach to understanding adult obesity prevalence in the United States: a county-level analysis using geographically weighted regression. Appl Spat Anal Policy. 2014;7(3):283–99. doi:10.1007/s12061-014-9108-0.

36. Comber AJ, Brunsdon C, Phillips M. The varying impact of geographic distance as a predictor of dissatisfaction over facility access. Appl Spat Anal Policy. 2012;5(4):333–52. doi:10.1007/s12061-011-9074-8.

37. Acevedo-Garcia D, Lochner KA, Osypuk TL, Subramanian SV. Future directions in residential segregation and health research: a multilevel approach. Am J Public Health. 2003;93(2):215–21.

38. Gibbons J, Yang T-C. Self-rated health and residential segregation: how does race/ethnicity matter? J Urban Health. 2014;91(4):648–60. doi:10.1007/s11524-013-9863-2.

39. Kramer MR, Hogue CR. Is segregation bad for your health? Epidemiol Rev. 2009;31(1):178–94. doi:10.1093/epirev/mxp001.

40. Subramanian SV. Racial residential segregation and geographic heterogeneity in black/white disparity in poor self-rated health in the US: a multilevel statistical analysis. Soc Sci Med. 2005;60(8):1667–79. doi:10.1016/j.socscimed.2004.08.040.

41. Yang T-C, Matthews SA. Understanding the non-stationary associations between distrust of the health care system, health conditions, and self-rated health in the elderly: a geographically weighted regression approach. Health Place. 2012;18(3):576–85. doi:10.1016/j.healthplace.2012.01.007.

42. Andersen RM. Revisiting the behavioral model and access to medical care: does it matter? J Health Soc Behav. 1995;36(1):1. doi:10.2307/2137284.

43. Armstrong K, McMurphy S, Dean LT, et al. Differences in the patterns of health care system distrust between Blacks and Whites. J Gen Intern Med. 2008;23(6):827–33. doi:10.1007/s11606-008-0561-9.

44. Yang T-C, Matthews SA, Hillemeier MM. Effect of health care system distrust on breast and cervical cancer screening in Philadelphia, Pennsylvania. Am J Public Health. 2011;101(7):1297.

45. Gelberg L, Andersen RM, Leake BD. The behavioral model for vulnerable populations: application to medical care use and outcomes for homeless people. Health Serv Res. 2000;34(6):1273–302.

46. PHMC. Household health survey documentation. Philadelphia: Public Health Management Corporation; 2008.

47. Final Recommendation Statement Breast Cancer: Screening. Rockville, MD: U.S. Preventative Task Force; 2002. https://www.uspreventiveservicestaskforce.org/Page/Document/RecommendationStatementFinal/breast-cancer-screening-2002.

48. Final Recommendation Statement Breast Cancer: Screening. Rockville, MD: U.S. Preventative Task Force; 2016. http://www.uspreventiveservicestaskforce.org/Page/Document/UpdateSummaryFinal/breast-cancer-screening1.

49. Babitsch B, Gohl D, von Lengerke T. Re-revisiting Andersen's behavioral model of health services use: a systematic review of studies from 1998–2011. GMS Psycho-Soc-Med. 2012;9. http://www.ncbi.nlm.nih.gov/pmc/articles/PMC3488807/. Accessed 16 Dec 2015.

50. Matthews SA, Yang T-C. Mapping the results of local statistics: using geographically weighted regression. Demogr Res. 2012;26:151–66. doi:10.4054/DemRes.2012.26.6.

51. Fotheringham S, Brunsdon C, Charlton M. Geographically weighted regression: the analysis of spatially varying relationships. New York: Wiley; 2003.

52. Brunsdon C, Fotheringham AS, Charlton M. Geographically weighted regression: a method for exploring spatial nonstationarity. In: Kemp K, editor. Encyclopedia of geographic information science. California: Sage; 2008. p. 558.

53. Brunsdon C, Fotheringham S, Charlton M. Geographically weighted regression. J R Stat Soc Ser Stat. 1998;47(3):431–43.

54. Chen VY-J, Yang T-C. SAS macro programs for geographically weighted generalized linear modeling with spatial point data: applications to

health research. Comput Methods Prog Biomed. 2012;107(2):262–73. doi:10.1016/j.cmpb.2011.10.006.

55. Shoff C, Yang T-C. Untangling the associations among distrust, race, and neighborhood social environment: a social disorganization perspective. Soc Sci Med. 2012;74(9):1342–52. doi:10.1016/j.socscimed.2012.01.012.

56. Burnham K, Anderson D. Model selection and multimodel inference: a practical information-theoretic approach. New York: Springer; 2002.

57. Brunsdon C, Fotheringham AS, Charlton M. Spatial nonstationarity and autoregressive models. Environ Plan A. 1998;30(6):957–73. doi:10.1068/a300957.

58. Leung Y, Mei C-L, Zhang W-X. Statistical tests for spatial nonstationarity based on the geographically weighted regression model. Environ Plan A. 2000;32(1):9–32. doi:10.1068/a3162.

59. Massey DS. New faces in new places: the changing geography of American immigration. New York: Russell Sage Foundation; 2008.

60. Bécares L, Cormack D, Harris R. Ethnic density and area deprivation: Neighbourhood effects on Māori health and racial discrimination in Aotearoa/New Zealand. Soc Sci Med. 2013;88:76–82. doi:10.1016/j.socscimed.2013.04.007.

61. Bécares L, Nazroo J, Stafford M. The buffering effects of ethnic density on experienced racism and health. Health Place. 2009;15(3):700–8. doi:10.1016/j.healthplace.2008.10.008.

62. Laiteerapong N, Kirby J, Gao Y, et al. Health care utilization and receipt of preventive care for patients seen at federally funded health centers compared to other sites of primary care. Health Serv Res. 2014;49(5):1498–518. doi:10.1111/1475-6773.12178.

Evaluation of geoimputation strategies in a large case study

Naci Dilekli[1,3]* , Amanda E. Janitz[2], Janis E. Campbell[2] and Kirsten M. de Beurs[3]

Abstract

Background: Health data usually has missing or incomplete location information, which impacts the quality of research. Geoimputation methods are used by health professionals to increase the spatial resolution of address information for more accurate analyses. The objective of this study was to evaluate geo-imputation methods with respect to the demographic and spatial characteristics of the data.

Methods: We evaluated four geoimputation methods for increasing spatial resolution of records with known locational information at a coarse level. In order to test and rigorously evaluate two stochastic and two deterministic strategies, we used the Texas Sex Offender registry database with over 50,000 records with known demographic and coordinate information. We reduced the spatial resolution of each record to a census block group and attempted to recover coordinate information using the four strategies. We rigorously evaluated the results in terms of the error distance between the original coordinates and recovered coordinates by studying the results by demographic sub groups and the characteristics of the underlying geography.

Results: We observed that in estimating the actual location of a case, the weighted mean method is the most superior for each demographic group followed by the maximum imputation centroid, the random point in matching sub-geographies and the random point in all sub-geographies methods. Higher accuracies were observed for minority populations because minorities tend to cluster in certain neighborhoods, which makes it easier to impute their location. Results are greatly affected by the population density of the underlying geographies. We observed high accuracies in high population density areas, which often exist within smaller census blocks, which makes the search space smaller. Similarly, mapping geoimputation accuracies in a spatially explicit manner reveals that metropolitan areas yield higher accuracy results.

Conclusions: Based on gains in standard error, reduction in mean error and validation results, we conclude that characteristics of the estimated records such as the demographic profile and population density information provide a measure of certainty of geographic imputation.

Keywords: Geo-imputation, Address data, Coarse resolution, Census data, Demographics

Background

Spatial epidemiology is the study of geographic variation of diseases. Locational accuracy is essential in geographical studies including epidemiological studies where the locational characteristics and behaviors of the patient are key to understand the underlying risk factors to inform policymaking. For example, underlying spatial factors such as environmental exposures have been linked to cancer including, asbestos exposure and mesothelioma, polychlorinated biphenyls (PCBs) and melanoma, aflatoxin and liver cancer, benzene and acute myeloid leukemia, tobacco and multiple cancers, and air pollution and lung cancer [1–8]. Besides cancer, environmental exposures are also associated with other diseases, for example, air pollution has been linked with respiratory disease, cardiovascular disease, and reproductive health [9–12]. Spatial epidemiology and geographic information systems (GIS) have also been applied to non-environmental

*Correspondence: ndilekli@ou.edu
[1] Center for Spatial Analysis, University of Oklahoma, 3100 Monitor Ave. Suite 180, Norman, OK, USA
Full list of author information is available at the end of the article

health issues, including understanding the built environment [13], health planning [14], and crime data [15].

While high quality scholarly research requires reliable locational information of exposures and outcomes, the level of spatial detail available to health researchers is often not sufficiently fine resolution. This is for two main reasons: (a) while health information is exceedingly valuable, it is protected by federal law and thus it is imperative to protect the privacy of individuals; and (b) information is often only collected or made available at a lower resolution, such as the zip code or county level. For health data, the exact geographic coordinates of participants are often not available without a data request and several levels of approval to ensure the confidentiality of participants is maintained. Failure to accurately and precisely capture geographic information may lead to incorrect findings and conclusions, including an overestimation of the true association [16] or imprecise estimates [17, 18]. Researchers often work with data with coarse resolution (e.g. when the complete street address is missing and only the ZIP code is available), resulting in omitted records and potentially creating biases due to misclassification [19]. Geocoding to ZIP code area centroids, a common practice in health research, often falsely indicates clustering at the centroid [20, 21], especially so in rural communities [22].

In order to rectify issues associated with imprecise spatial data, several spatially informed geo-imputation methods have been developed to increase the spatial resolution. They are similar to disaggregation methods [15], which interpolate data at smaller units using the spatial distribution of ancillary data.

Geo-imputation strategies can generally be divided into stochastic and deterministic methods. One method for stochastic geo-imputation is the use of the cumulative distribution function to randomly assign a case to a locale [23–25]. A variety of this method uses a variable such as population to construct the probability of a locale being chosen [24]. Deterministic methods assign cases to locales deterministically, based on a set of rules, such as the geographically weighted mean of locales, or the centroid of the locale [26] that is the best fit. A mixture of the two can be used as well by selecting a random point within a deterministically chosen locale. Although the literature on the use of imputation for missing address information is sparse, authors have used both stochastic and deterministic methods, including alone and in combination [23, 27–32]. For example, Curriero et al. [23] found that misclassification in assignment of correct census tract was reduced most using deterministic geo-imputation weighted by specific ethnicity/age population in comparison to a stochastic method and other types of deterministic methods. Walter and Rose [30] devised

a stochastic method called random property allocation, which randomly assigns each case with incomplete address information to an address that was previously geocoded within the corresponding geographical unit, where each address has equal probability. They compared this method to one stochastic and three deterministic geo-imputation methods, which assign incomplete addresses to geographic centroids, population weighed centroids, areal proportion using random function and areal proportion using deterministic function, similar to the methods mentioned before. The authors observed that while all geo-imputation methods performed well, the random allocation method was the least prone to bias, as centroid based methods can create artificial clustering and bias.

The accuracy of geographic imputation methods is typically assessed by comparing the results from several methods. The results can be assessed based on: (a) the ratio of correct estimates, e.g. the number of times a case was assigned to the correct geographical unit; or (b) based on the distance between the predicted and known coordinates. Theoretically, when ground truth data is not available, it is not possible to evaluate the accuracy of the results. In this study, we are not focused on missing spatial data but rather our focus is on the application of geo-imputation methods to improve the spatial accuracy of spatial data by estimating higher resolution locations of events or persons based on known lower resolution spatial information (such as ZIP code) and supporting information (such as demographic characteristics). In this study, we apply four geo-imputation methods, including both stochastic and deterministic, to impute coordinate level information followed by an evaluation of the performance of the geo-imputation methods using the demographic sub groups and the characteristics of the underlying geography.

Methods

Data

As discussed in the introduction, the development and discussion of geo-imputation methods is most relevant for the analysis of spatial interactions in disease patterns. However, since most of the actual hospital records are justifiably protected by privacy laws, we instead have selected a subset of the Texas Sex Offender Registry as the population to include in our case study. This dataset provides address, age, gender and race information on all convicted sex offenders in Texas [33]. Of the 88,552 records that were acquired at the access date (August 28, 2017), 52,260 had known Texas address information that were previously geocoded to X,Y coordinates. Of these records, 52,229 had a known race, and only this subset of the data with

Table 1 Demographic summary of the Texas Sex Offender Registry 2017 used in the study

	White			Asian			Black			Hispanic			Native American			All		
	Male	Female	Total	Male	Female	Total	Male	Female	Total	Male	Female	Total	Male	Female	Total	Male	Female	Total
Age<20	814	39	853	16	1	17	389	12	401	769	12	781	2	–	2	1990	64	2054
20≤Age<50	14,948	695	15,643	168	3	171	7653	160	7813	9538	229	9767	21	–	21	32,328	1087	33,415
50≤Age<65	7729	139	7868	50	–	50	3103	22	3125	2775	20	2795	6	–	6	13,663	181	13,844
65≤Age<85	1960	11	1971	8	–	8	355	1	356	553	–	553	2	–	2	2878	12	2890
Age≥85	13	–	13	–	–	–	5	–	5	6	–	6	–	–	–	24	–	24
All	25,464	884	26,348	242	4	246	11,505	195	11,700	13,641	261	13,902	31	–	31	50,883	1344	52,227

known address and race information was used in the subsequent analyses. A breakdown of the data by race, age and gender is provided in Table 1, which shows the existing race groups in the registry and summarizes records into five age groups. These records were spatially joined to the Texas Census Block layer to add the census block information. Here are the characteristics of this data that are relevant to this project [33]:

- The sex offender registration laws in Texas went into effect on September 1, 1991. Among other information, The Texas Sex Offender Registration Program requires offenders to submit full name, date of birth, sex, race, height, weight, eye color, hair color, social security number, driver's license number, shoe size, home address or a detailed description of each geographical location at which the person resides or intends to reside.
- Adult sex offenders must register either for life or for 10 years depending on certain conditions.
- Registered offenders must report address changes.
- Sex offenders may be prohibited from living in child safety zones defined by laws and city ordinances, as well as campuses of higher education.

This information means the data is not collected at specified, regular intervals, but whenever there is a new entry and as soon as possible after an address change. Demographic data for the population includes age, gender and ethnicity information from 2010 Census Summary File 1 (SF1) [34] at census block level, which is the target resolution to assign our data. The SF1 data includes nine ethnic groups and 23 population ranges for both males and females, resulting in 414 possible demographic combinations. Additional file 1: Tables S1 and S2 list the complete list of race and age groups in the Census data.

This demographic data was merged and joined to the census block shapefile with NAD 1983 Texas Centric Mapping System Albers projection. There are 914,231 census blocks in the State of Texas.

Study design

For all records with existing X, Y coordinates, we carry out the following steps:

(a) Obtain census block information using GIS.
(b) Obtain census block group (to reduce data quality for the purposes of validating imputation).
(c) Impute X, Y coordinates based on census blocks with census information for each method.
(d) Calculate error distance for each strategy.

Thus, we first reduce the data quality of each X, Y record by selecting its block group in order to make the data comparable to the more coarse spatial data quality (steps a and b). In the next step (c), we attempt to improve the spatial data quality by correctly assigning each X, Y record to the correct census block. In the last step (d) we evaluate our results by calculating the distance between the point assigned to the census block, and the original X, Y record.

Geo-imputation strategies

The chosen geo-imputation methods were derived from the literature, in order to assign a non-geocoded record with census block group information to (a) a random point within the entire census block group; (b) a random point within the extents of matching blocks; (c) the centroid of census block with the highest weight; and (d) the weighted centroid of the matching census blocks. We chose the following methods which are either stochastic or deterministic methods identified from the literature [23, 28–30].

Imputation Strategy #1 and #2

The following two imputation methods generate geoimputed results based on a complete random spatial function. These methods provide a basis to test the relative usefulness of the deterministic methods (3 and 4) that rely on the underlying demographic characteristics.

Strategy #1, random in Block Group, assigns the record to a random point within the entire block group as used in Henry and Boscoe [28]. Strategy #2, random in Matching blocks, randomly assigns a random point only within blocks that have matching demographic population to the individual record.

Imputation Strategy #3

This method assigns the record to the centroid of the geographical unit with the highest calculated weight. The weight is determined as in Eq. 1 [23]. For example, in the case of a 71-year-old white female person, the weight of a particular block would be calculated as the following:

$$Block\ Weight = \frac{No.\ of\ White\ Female\ 70-74\ in\ Block}{Total\ of\ White\ Female\ 70-74\ in\ Block\ Group} \tag{1}$$

This method can be prone to generating artificial clusters [29], as all imputed coordinates from a particular geographical unit (which is chosen as it has the highest weight) will be identical.

Imputation Strategy #4

This strategy assigns the record to the weighted centroid of the matching census blocks using the mean center of the available population similar to the approach used by Walter and Rose [30]. However, we matched demographics to target smaller population (as in Eq. 1) rather than the general population only. This strategy requires first calculating the centroid of each census block, and then calculating one final centroid based on their imputation weights calculated according to Eq. 1. In this approach, the weight of each block is calculated using one of the 414 combinations based on the case's gender, age, and race within the block group to which it belongs. This method can be compared to the previous imputation strategy, as both methods make use of the block weights. The difference is that this method results in an estimation built by the entire set of candidate geographies based on how likely they are to contain a specific case. Also, unlike the previous imputation strategy, this strategy is not prone to artificial clustering since it is nearly impossible to generate the same weighted mean center. Two imputations would overlap only if they are in the same census block group with identical demographic characteristics.

Evaluation of the accuracy of the imputation strategies

We evaluate the imputation strategies described above by comparing the original coordinates with geo-imputed coordinates using all records. We calculated the distance between the imputed location and the actual location (accuracy), stratified by age groups and ethnicities since certain demographic groups may cluster spatially, while others distribute more uniformly. Thus, high accuracy location data can be deduced when the target demographics are very particular and only exist in one or a few candidate geographies. We also evaluated the results by population density, as we expected the results to be more accurate when the underlying geographical unit is smaller.

We developed box and whisker plots to display the accuracy of each geo-imputation method and underlying factors, validated the stochastic methods using multiple imputation, assess the sensitivity of results based on the administrative boundary type, and map the geographic inaccuracy. We expected to observe differences in geographical patterns of imputation accuracy across space (e.g. particular neighborhoods, rural areas, etc.).

Results

We geoimputed 96.7% of records (n = 50,494) by all four strategies; the other 1734 records could not be geoimputed by Strategies #3 and #4 as they did not have any matching population in the searched census block group. This is potentially due to the difference in dates of data collection (Texas Sexual Offender Registry date of offense vs. US Census data restricted to 2010, the date census data was collected) combined with addresses change, or inaccuracies in data collection. In addition, many factors could account for this small number of records that could not be imputed including known racial misclassification issues [35, 36].

Accuracy by imputation strategy and demographic group

Figure 1 displays the range of error distances (minimum, maximum, median, first quartile and third quartile) between each geoimputed location and the actual location in meters for the four imputation methods. We observed that the weighted mean method (Strategy #4) had the lowest error distance, followed by maximum imputation centroid (Strategy #3), random point in matching sub-geographies (Strategy #2) and random point in all sub-geographies (Strategy #1) methods. This indicates there is less uncertainty around the estimate of the mean measurement of the weighted mean method (Strategy #4), compared to random methods. In addition, the weighted mean method has a median error of 522 m, providing an almost 40% more accurate estimate than the complete random estimate method which revealed

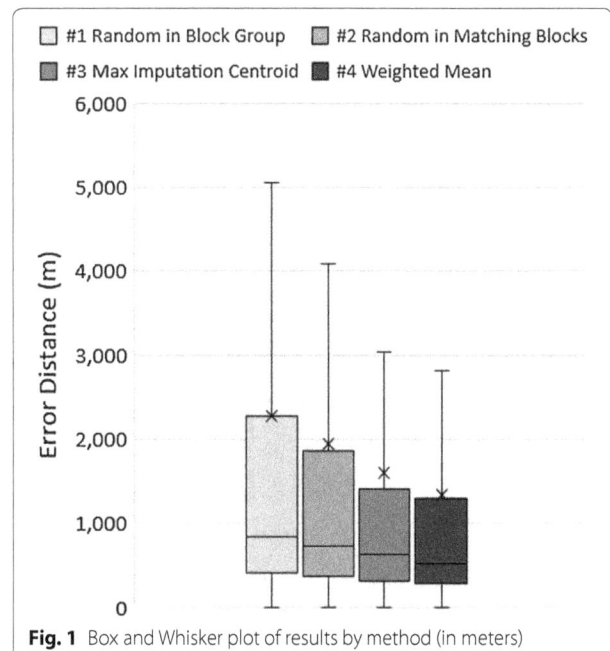

Fig. 1 Box and Whisker plot of results by method (in meters)

a median error of 845 m. Although the weighted mean method consistently reveals superior results, we observed differences among the demographic groups (Additional file 1: Table S3).

Accuracies were higher for minority populations because minorities tend to cluster in certain neighborhoods which makes it easier to impute their location (Fig. 2). However, the geoimputation accuracy appears to decline for older populations. This might be particularly due to elderly people living in rural areas (Fig. 3).

Figure 3 provides the mean error distance between the imputed points and the actual points broken down by age group and geo-imputation method (see Additional file 1: Table S3 for information on gender). These results also indicate that in estimating the actual location of a case, the weighted mean method (Strategy #4) is almost always

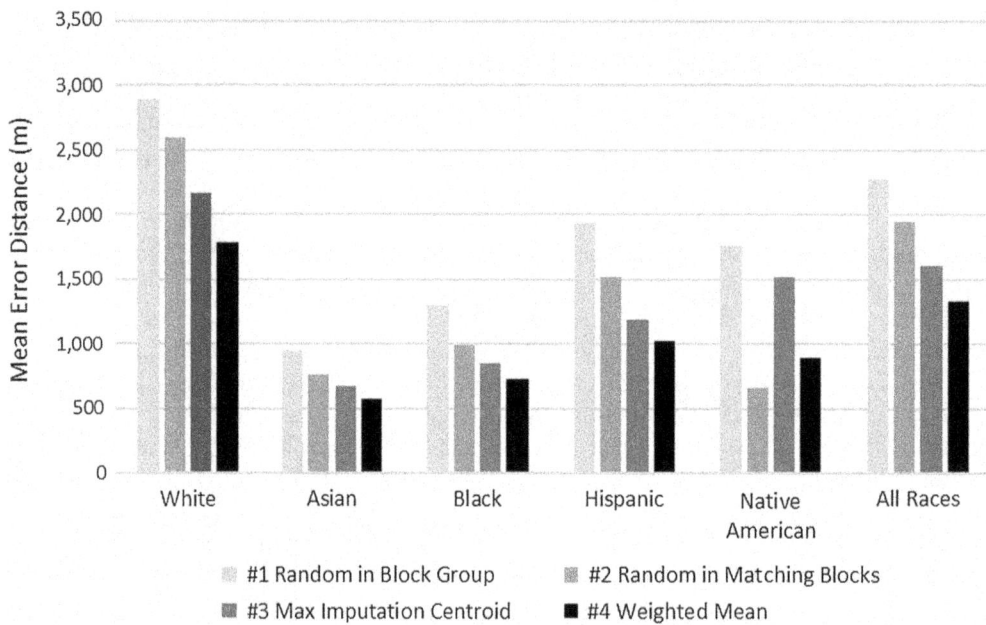

Fig. 2 Mean error distance by race and method

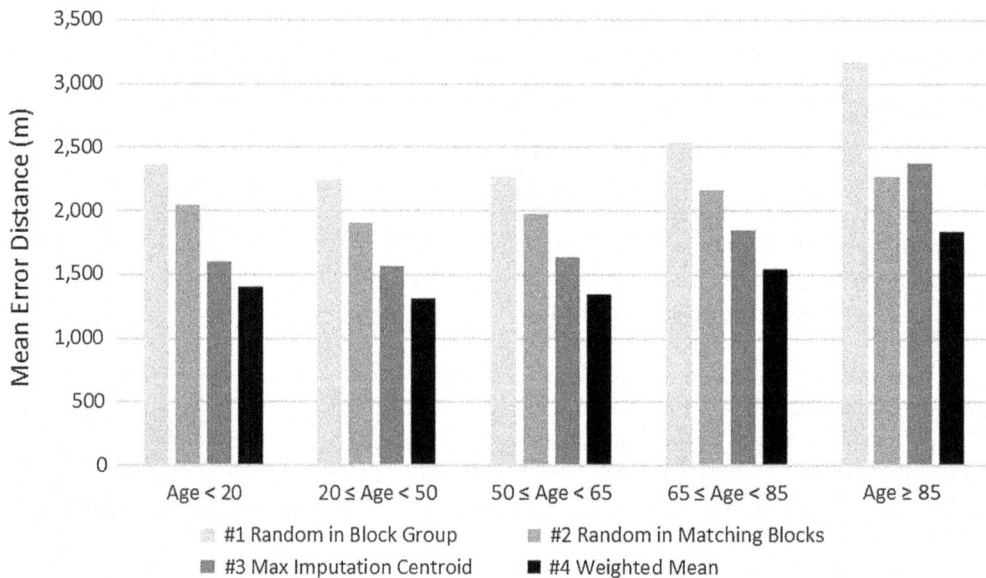

Fig. 3 Mean error distance by age group and method

the most superior for each demographic group followed by the maximum imputation centroid (Strategy #3), the random point in matching sub-geographies (Strategy #2) and the random point in all sub-geographies methods (Strategy #1). The only exception is the 65–85-year-old Asian subgroup, which has only 5 cases, as well as the American Indian/Alaska Native (AI/AN) group as a whole.

Accuracy by imputation strategy and population density

The population density varies greatly in the study area, from 0.08 people to 30,142 people per km^2; thus, we applied a logarithmic scale to the x-axis to allow for the large differences in population densities. Figure 4 shows mean error distances as well as standard errors based on population densities. As is expected, all methods reveal a steep drop-off for increasing population densities with error distances and standard errors much larger in areas with very low population densities and lower error distances and standard errors for areas with higher population densities (for detailed information: Additional file 1: Table S4). For this reason, error bars are not visible at high density ranges. The weighted mean method reveals the lowest error distances for all population densities, which are indicative of the size of the geographical units. Figure 5 provides an enhanced view for areas with relatively high population densities (>100 people/km^2) only

and indicates that the weighted mean method performs the best.

Certainly, it makes sense to expect high accuracies in areas with high population density, these areas are typically identified by smaller census blocks and decreasing the search space. Error results range from 48,300 m by a random estimate to only 58 m by the weighted mean estimate in our population density analysis. We observed that at the low end of the population density (0.01–0.1 people/km^2), the performance of methods #1, #2, and #3 were not significantly different while method #4 performs significantly better than the first three methods. At the high end of the population density (10,000–35,000 people/km^2) the methods fall into two groups with methods #3 and #4 performing better than methods #1 and #2 (Fig. 5).

Multiple imputation

We conducted multiple imputation using a sample size of 4864 records to further validate the results. We imputed each record 10 times and computed the error distance for each imputation for the methods #1 and #2, which are stochastic. We did not conduct multiple imputation for methods #3 and #4 since they are deterministic methods resulting in the same point estimate no matter how many times the method is run. We observed that the average

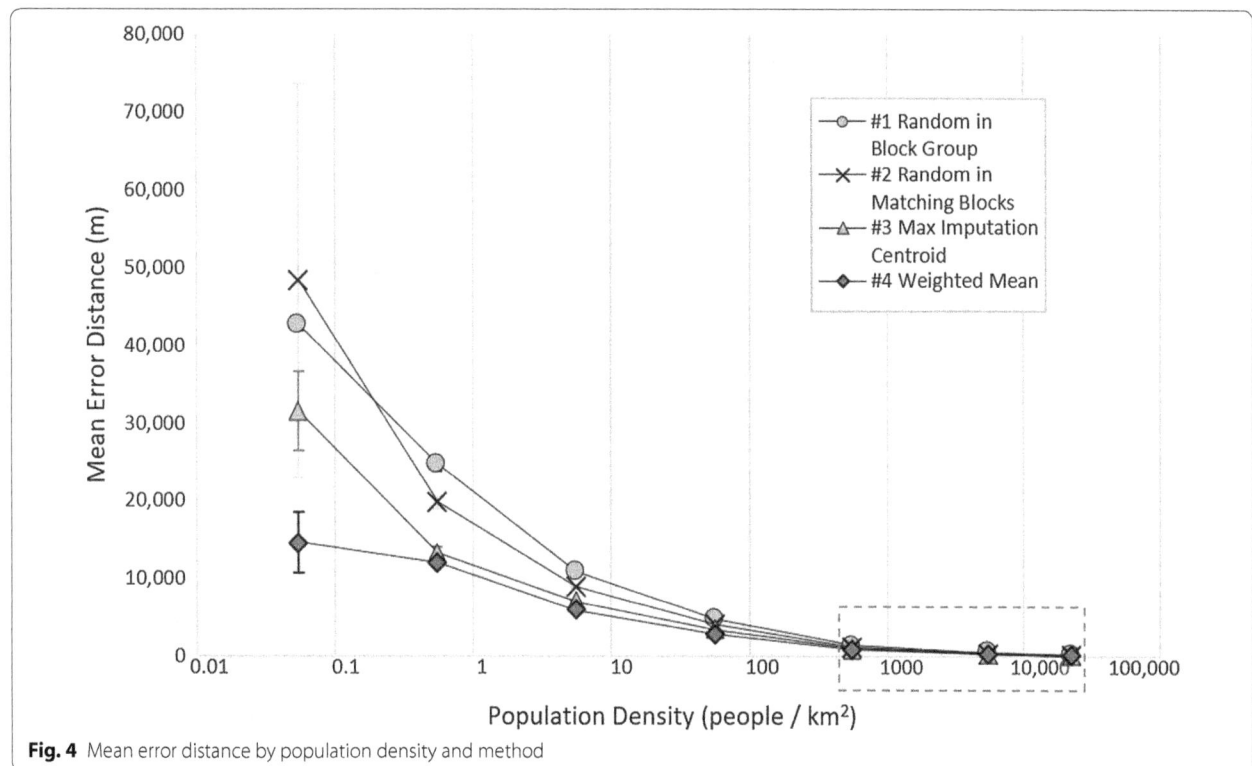

Fig. 4 Mean error distance by population density and method

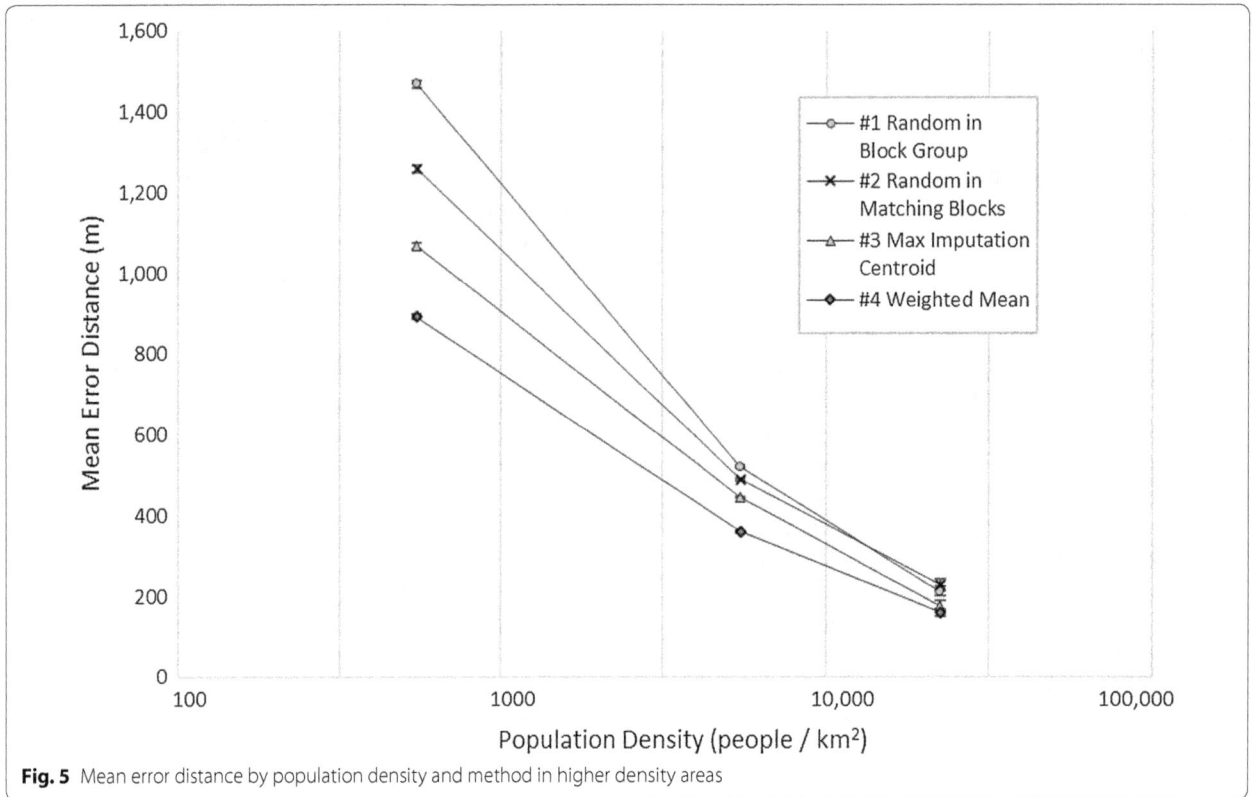

Fig. 5 Mean error distance by population density and method in higher density areas

error values from multiple imputation experience are comparable to the original results (Fig. 6).

Sensitivity analysis

To evaluate the sensitivity with respect to different spatial units, we used the smaller sample set and reduced the spatial resolution first to census tracts and then to counties. We then conducted the identical analyses with all four strategies using these spatial units.

Figures 7 and 8 reveal that the difference between impacts of the census tract and county level information, respectively, depends on the underlying population density. There are only two imputations at the lowest density bin, which is the reason for the unexpected result for the first method. Overall, rural census tracts and counties have poorer performance compared to urban census tracts and counties.

Accuracy across geography

We plotted each of the 50,494 results on the map and performed an inverse distance weighted interpolation using weighted mean results (Fig. 9). Results, ranging from 52.8 to 47,992 m, reveal how the accuracy changes across the study area. As expected, Dallas, Houston, Austin and San Antonio metropolitan areas yield higher accuracy results. We aggregated the results to census tract level presenting

the highest error distance and removed census tracts with < 0.001 imputed records per km^2 to avoid reporting unreliable interpolation results.

Discussions

We developed a methodological approach to evaluate various geoimputation methods with a large data set with complete, known, addresses and demographic information. Through rigorously evaluating the results stratified by demographic sub groups, population density, and geography, we have contributed additional knowledge to the field [23–25, 30].

This approach can be applied in contexts with missing addresses to increase the spatial resolution of the existing information. In such application, limitations and potential uncertainties of the geoimputation can be deduced from the size and population density of the underlying geography, as well as particular characteristics of the demographical profile of the particular record. We found that strategy #4, the Weighted Mean method, performed the best overall as in Curriero et al. [23], and in almost all sub evaluation criteria. This also supports Henry and Boscoe's [24] stochastic method weighted by race and ethnicity population as opposed to a random point or a geographic centroid. As in Henry and Boscoe's [24] study, we presented results by ethnicity, age and population

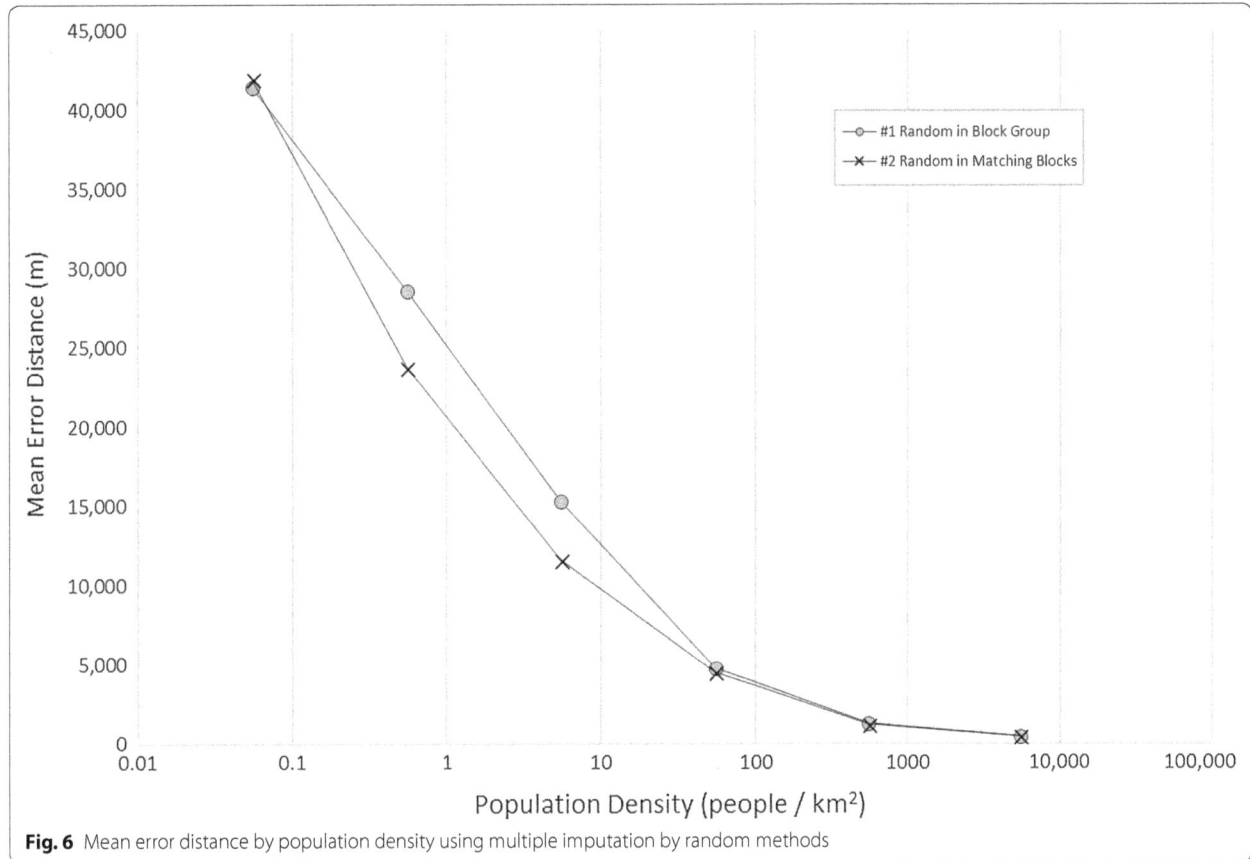

Fig. 6 Mean error distance by population density using multiple imputation by random methods

density (also as in Walter and Rose [30] who evaluated them based on Metropolitan vs. Non-Metropolitan areas), but with further detail. Similar to Hibbert et al. [25], which report results by geography (i.e. four states), we report the results across the space. As in JD Hibbert et al. [36] and FC Curriero et al. [34], we also conducted multiple imputation of a sample set to validate our results. In addition, we conducted sensitivity analyses using two coarser spatial units of census tracts and counties. All the reviewed studies evaluated results based on assignment to correct unit, while we reported the results based on distance between predicted point and the actual point. We argue that correct assignment probability depends on the number of high resolution units in the search space, and therefore reporting the error distance can be viewed as an alternative way to evaluate different methods.

The range of error based on the demographic char acteristics and population density is instructive for researchers working with limited locational information. For example, for some exposures of interest, sub kilometer gains in accuracy in urban core areas may not be very significant on epidemiological associations.

On the other hand, the accuracy gains based on certain demographic groups or population densities (such as rural areas) may provide required level of accuracy to establish such associations.

There are a few potential issues in the evaluation of the results:

(a) We use demographic data from the Census Bureau from 2010. If the demographics of the case's location changed from the time of the decennial census, our error estimates would be impacted. Similarly, the individuals on the sex offender registry could have moved, and would report a different address to the registry than the address reported at the census. This might explain some of the 1734 records that could not be geoimputed by Strategies #3 and #4.

(b) Potential data collection inaccuracies could also result in misclassification of race/ethnicity. For example, there are 13,336 records reporting a white race with unknown ethnicity, which we corresponded as white race in the Census data. We also corresponded the 26,135 records with white race with Hispanic ethnicity to the Hispanic or Latino race category in the Census data (Additional file 1:

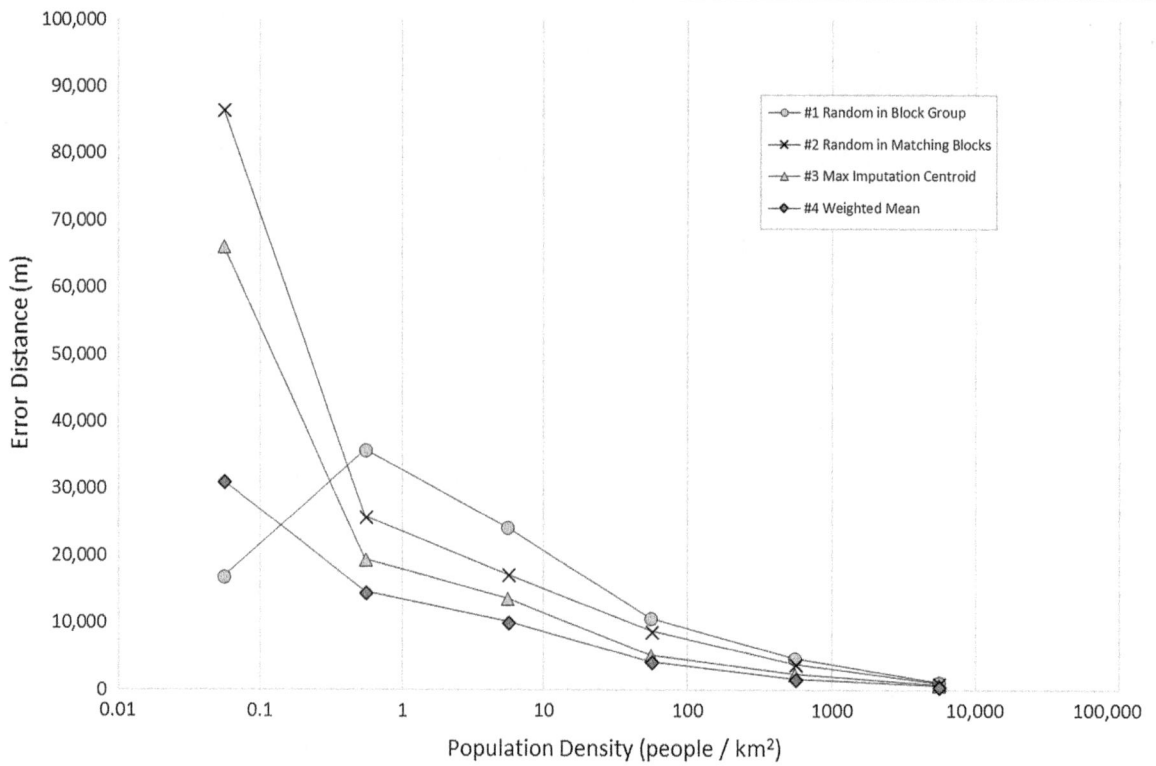

Fig. 7 Mean error distance by population density using census tract level information

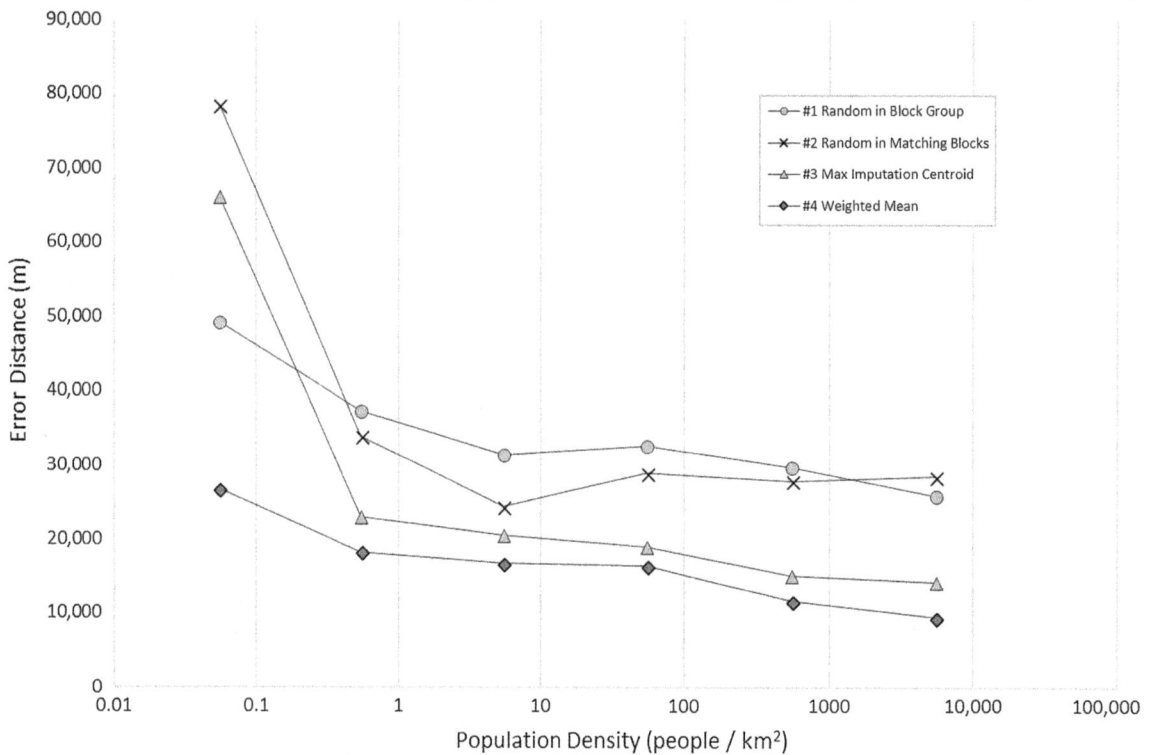

Fig. 8 Mean error distance by population density using county level information

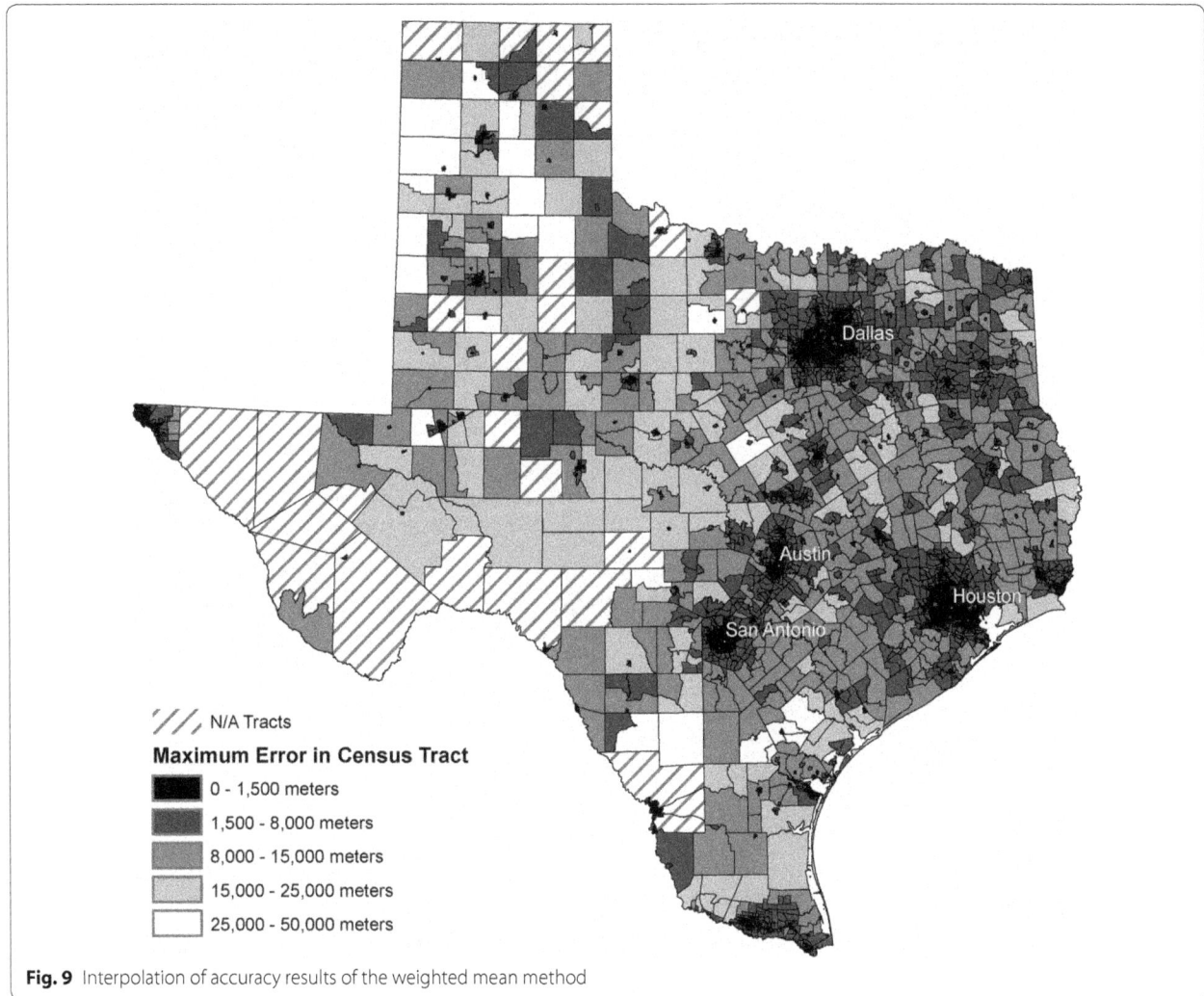

Fig. 9 Interpolation of accuracy results of the weighted mean method

Legend:
- N/A Tracts
- **Maximum Error in Census Tract**
- 0 - 1,500 meters
- 1,500 - 8,000 meters
- 8,000 - 15,000 meters
- 15,000 - 25,000 meters
- 25,000 - 50,000 meters

Map labels: Dallas, Austin, Houston, San Antonio

Table S1). While we assumed that other attributes are collected correctly, while there is no feasible way to validate them.

(c) While the sexual offender dataset is very large, it may still not be representative of the general population in terms of demographics as well as living preferences/limitations. For example, only 2.5% of the records belong to females. This is not comparable to many other health outcomes where these methods may be applied, including cancer rates among men and women, which ranges between 7:4 and 3:2 [37]. Additionally, we assume that the individuals in this database are randomly dispersed throughout the community, which is unlikely because of their status as a sexual offender.

Many publicly-available datasets, including state-level cancer incidence and mortality data and the Surveillance Epidemiology and End Results program data are generally available at the county level, prohibiting detailed analysis with complete address information due to privacy and confidentiality concerns. Although additional validation in other datasets that include both genders are needed, these methods are generalizable to other publicly-available datasets. Future studies may apply these methods to other types of health data with missing complete address information and to data sources that lack certain demographic information, at the expense of generating additional uncertainty.

Future studies should consider conducting geoimputation at other geographic levels, including ZIP code level information or applying a method based on cumulative random function, which would assign cases to finer spatial units randomly based on weights. Theoretically the deterministic imputation methods used in this study can be further improved by utilizing additional data, such as income, education etc., if available. These methods can be further enhanced by additional GIS or Remote Sensing data to exclude areas that do not contain residences. For example, we could eliminate areas without any residential buildings with a combination of GIS (zoning) and RS (impervious surface) data and methods.

Conclusions

Based on gains in standard error, reduction in mean error and validation results, we conclude that methods #3 and #4, Maximum Imputation and Weighted Mean methods were preferable in this study when no fine level spatial information is available, though this should be replicated in a population that is more randomly dispersed. We conclude that characteristics of the estimated records such as the demographic profile and population density information impact accuracy of results. In the absence of ground truthing information, such variables can provide accuracy information using the error ranges provided in this study.

Authors' contributions
ND obtained the registry data, collected census and geographical data, developed and ran the code for geo-imputation, conducted the statistical analyses and wrote the first draft. AEJ, JEB and KMB provided guidance in interpretation of results. All authors helped to draft the manuscript. All authors read and approved the final manuscript.

Author details
[1] Center for Spatial Analysis, University of Oklahoma, 3100 Monitor Ave. Suite 180, Norman, OK, USA. [2] The University of Oklahoma Health Sciences Center, 801 NE 13th Street, Oklahoma City, OK, USA. [3] Department of Geography and Environmental Sustainability, University of Oklahoma, 100 East Boyd Street, Norman, OK, USA.

Competing interests
The authors declare that they have no competing interests.

Funding
This work was supported by The Oklahoma Center for the Advancement of Science and Technology, Grant No. HR16-048.

References
1. Berwick M, Buller DB, Cust A, Gallagher R, Lee TK, Meyskens F, Pandey S, Thomas NE, Veierød MB, Ward S. Melanoma epidemiology and prevention. In: Kaufman LH, Mehnert MJ, editors. Melanoma. Cham: Springer; 2016. p. 17–49.
2. Saracci R, Wild CP. International Agency for Research on Cancer: the first 50 years, 1965–2015. Lyon: International Agency for Research on Cancer; 2015 **(distributed by World Health Organization Press)**.
3. Steenland K, Hein MJ, Cassinelli RT, Prince MM, Nilsen NB, Whelan EA, Waters MA, Ruder AM, Schnorr TM. Polychlorinated biphenyls and neurodegenerative disease mortality in an occupational cohort. Epidemiology. 2006;17(1):8–13.
4. Straif K, Cohen A. International Agency for Research on Cancer: air pollution and cancer. Lyon: International Agency for Research on Cancer; 2013 **(distributed by World Health Organization Press)**.
5. IARC Working Group on the Evaluation of Carcinogenic Risks to Humans. Arsenic, metals, fibres and dusts: a review of human carcinogens. In: IARC monographs on the evaluation of carcinogenic risks to humans, vol. 100C. Lyon: International Agency on Cancer, World Health Organization; 2012.
6. International Agency for Research and Cancer. IARC monographs on the evaluation of carcinogenic risks to humans: preamble. Lyon: International Agency for Research and Cancer; 2015.
7. Grosse Y, Loomis D, Guyton KZ, El Ghissassi F, Bouvard V, Benbrahim-Tallaa L, Mattock H, Straif K. Carcinogenicity of some industrial chemicals. Lancet Oncol. 2016;17:419–20.
8. Benbrahim-Tallaa L, Baan RA, Grosse Y, Lauby-Secretan B, El Ghissassi F, Bouvard V, Guha N, Loomis D, Straif K. Carcinogenicity of diesel-engine and gasoline-engine exhausts and some nitroarenes. Lancet Oncology. 2012;13(7):663–4.
9. Nardone A, Neophytou AM, Balmes J, Thakur N. Ambient air pollution and asthma-related outcomes in children of color of the USA: a scoping review of literature published between 2013 and 2017. Current Allergy and Asthma Reports. 2018;18(5):29.
10. Vidale S, Campana C. Ambient air pollution and cardiovascular diseases: from bench to bedside. European Journal of Preventive Cardiology. 2018;25(8):818–25.
11. Carre J, Gatimel N, Moreau J, Parinaud J, Leandri R. Does air pollution play a role in infertility? A systematic review. Environ Health. 2017;16(1):82.
12. Checa Vizcaino MA, Gonzalez-Comadran M, Jacquemin B. Outdoor air pollution and human infertility: a systematic review. Fertil Steril. 2016;106(4):897–904.e891.
13. Wang X, Khattak A, Chen J. Accuracy of geoimputation. Transportation Research Record: Journal of the Transportation Research Board. 2013;2382:10–9.
14. Nykiforuk CIJ, Flaman LM. Geographic information systems (GIS) for health promotion and public health: a review. Health Promotion Practice. 2009;12(1):63–73.
15. Kounadi O, Ristea A, Leitner M, Langford C. Population at risk: using areal interpolation and Twitter messages to create population models for burglaries and robberies. Cartography and Geographic Information Science. 2018;45(3):205–20.
16. Jacquemin B, Lepeule J, Boudier A, Arnould C. Impact of the geocoding technique on the associations between long-term exposure to urban air pollution and lung function. Environ Health Perspect. 2013;1054:1–93.
17. Mazumdar S, Rushton G, Smith BJ, Zimmerman DL, Donham KJ. Geocoding accuracy and the recovery of relationships between environmental exposures and health. International Journal of Health Geographics. 2008;7:13.
18. Zandbergen PA, Green JW. Error and bias in determining exposure potential of children at school locations using proximity-based GIS techniques. Environ Health Perspect. 2007;115:1363–70.
19. Hurley SE, Saunders TM, Nivas R, Hertz A, Reynolds P. Post office box addresses: a challenge for geographic information system-based studies. Epidemiology. 2003;14(4):386–91.
20. Zimmerman DL, Fang X, Mazumdar S. Spatial clustering of the failure to geocode and its implications for the detection of disease clustering. Stat Med. 2008;27:4254–66.
21. Krieger N, Waterman P, Chen JT, Soobader MJ, Subramanian SV, Carson R. Zip code caveat: bias due to spatiotemporal mismatches between zip codes and US census-defined geographic areas—the public health disparities geocoding project. Am J Public Health. 2002;92(7):1100–2.
22. Kravets N, Hadden WC. The accuracy of address coding and the effects of coding errors. Health and Place. 2007;13:293–8.
23. Curriero FC, Kulldorff M, Boscoe FP, Klassen AC. Using imputation to provide location information for nongeocoded addresses. PLoS ONE. 2010;5(2):e8998.
24. Henry KA, Boscoe FP. Estimating the accuracy of geographical imputation. Int J Health Geogr. 2008;7:3.
25. Hibbert JD, Liese AD, Lawson A, Porter DE, Puett RC, Standiford D, Liu L, Dabelea D. Evaluating geographic imputation approaches for zip code level data: an application to a study of pediatric diabetes. Int J Health Geogr. 2009;8:54.

26. Jones SG, Ashby AJ, Momin SR, Naidoo A. Spatial implications associated with using Euclidean distance measurements and geographic centroid imputation in health care research. Health Serv Res. 2010;45(1):316–27.

27. Baker J, White N, Mengersen K. Missing in space: an evaluation of imputation methods for missing data in spatial analysis of risk factors for type II diabetes. International Journal of Health Geographics. 2014;13(1):47.

28. Henry KA, Boscoe FP. Estimating the accuracy of geographical imputation. International Journal of Health Geographics. 2008;7:3.

29. Hibbert JD, Liese AD, Lawson A, Porter DE, Puett RC, Standiford D, Liu L, Dabelea D. Evaluating geographic imputation approaches for zip code level data: an application to a study of pediatric diabetes. International Journal of Health Geographics. 2009;8:54.

30. Walter SR, Rose N. Random property allocation: a novel geographic imputation procedure based on a complete geocoded address file. Spatial and spatio-temporal epidemiology. 2013;6:7–16.

31. Seon-Ju Y, Shon C. How can we assess the effects of urban environment on obesity using aggregated data? [abstract]. Paper presented at international society for disease surveillance annual conference proceedings 2018. Orlando, FL. https://doi.org/10.5210/ojphi.v10i1.8329.

32. Wang X, Khattak A, Chen J. Accuracy of geoimputation: an approach to capture microenvironment. Transp Res Rec. 2013;2382(1):10–9.

33. Texas Public Sex Offender Registry. https://records.txdps.state.tx.us/sexoffender/. Accessed 28 Aug 2017.

34. U.S. Census Bureau. 2010 Census Summary File 1 Texas. 2011.

35. Strmic-Pawl HV, Jackson BA, Garner S. Race counts: racial and ethnic data on the US census and the implications for tracking inequality. Sociology of Race and Ethnicity. 2018;4(1):1–13.

36. Terry RL, Schwede L, King R, Martinez M, Childs JH. Exploring inconsistent counts of racial/ethnic minorities in a 2010 census ethnographic evaluation. Bulletin of Sociological Methodology. 2017;135(1):32–49.

37. Cancer Rates by Race/Ethnicity and Sex. https://www.cdc.gov/cancer/dcpc/data/race.htm. Accessed 22 Mar 2018.

Relative risk estimation of dengue disease at small spatial scale

Daniel Adyro Martínez-Bello[1]* [iD], Antonio López-Quílez[1] and Alexander Torres Prieto[2]

Abstract

Background: Dengue is a high incidence arboviral disease in tropical countries around the world. Colombia is an endemic country due to the favourable environmental conditions for vector survival and spread. Dengue surveillance in Colombia is based in passive notification of cases, supporting monitoring, prediction, risk factor identification and intervention measures. Even though the surveillance network works adequately, disease mapping techniques currently developed and employed for many health problems are not widely applied. We select the Colombian city of Bucaramanga to apply Bayesian areal disease mapping models, testing the challenges and difficulties of the approach.

Methods: We estimated the relative risk of dengue disease by census section (a geographical unit composed approximately by 1–20 city blocks) for the period January 2008 to December 2015. We included the covariates normalized difference vegetation index (NDVI) and land surface temperature (LST), obtained by satellite images. We fitted Bayesian areal models at the complete period and annual aggregation time scales for 2008–2015, with fixed and space-varying coefficients for the covariates, using Markov Chain Monte Carlo simulations. In addition, we used Cohen's Kappa agreement measures to compare the risk from year to year, and from every year to the complete period aggregation.

Results: We found the NDVI providing more information than LST for estimating relative risk of dengue, although their effects were small. NDVI was directly associated to high relative risk of dengue. Risk maps of dengue were produced from the estimates obtained by the modeling process. The year to year risk agreement by census section was sligth to fair.

Conclusion: The study provides an example of implementation of relative risk estimation using Bayesian models for disease mapping at small spatial scale with covariates. We relate satellite data to dengue disease, using an areal data approach, which is not commonly found in the literature. The main difficulty of the study was to find quality data for generating expected values as input for the models. We remark the importance of creating population registry at small spatial scale, which is not only relevant for the risk estimation of dengue but also important to the surveillance of all notifiable diseases.

Keywords: Disease mapping, Satellite images, Bayesian modeling, Cohen's Kappa

Background

Dengue is an arboviral disease characterized by fever and vascular complications and is endemic in many tropical and subtropical regions of the world [1]. Within the global efforts to control the disease, representation of the problem in space and time is key to supporting disease surveillance systems [2]. Spatial and spatio-temporal models are useful for generating risk maps for dengue disease, supporting early warning systems and intervention programs [2, 3].

Disease mapping tools correlated dengue incidence with socioeconomic, demographic and environmental variables using the Moran index in Brazil [4], while its

---
*Correspondence: danieladyro@gmail.com
[1] Departament d'Estadística i Investigació Operativa, Facultat de Matemàtiques, Universitat de València, C/Dr Moliner 50, 46100 Burjassot, Valencia, Spain
Full list of author information is available at the end of the article

geographical distribution has been characterized using spatial statistics and geographical information system (GIS) analysis in Ecuador [5]. Dengue disease mapping has also been combined with surveillance and monitoring of the *Aedes aegypti* vector in the Middle East [6], and in Peru, investigators have explored the association between dengue and clinical, meteorological, climatic, and sociopolitical variables through fuzzy association rule mining in a spatial setting [7]. At a micro-regional scale, Lowe et al. [8] included temperature, rainfall, the El Niño Southern Oscillation index, and other relevant socioeconomic and environmental variables in a spatio-temporal Bayesian hierarchical model implemented with Markov Chain Monte Carlo (MCMC), generating predictions at spatial and temporal levels and supporting a dengue alert system. Honorato et al. [9] studied the relationship between risk of dengue and sociodemographic variables using Bayesian spatial regression models in the municipalities of Espírito Santo, Brazil, while Ferreira and Smith [10] modeled the number of cases of dengue fever in Rio de Janeiro, Brazil, considering the cases as a Poisson random variable, with conditional autoregressive (CAR) priors in the spatial random effects, testing different neighborhood structures and covariates with fixed coefficients.

Colombia is highly endemic for dengue disease. From 2000 to 2011, the country experienced a stable annual incidence of dengue, with major outbreaks in 2001–2003 and 2010, followed by a considerable decrease of incidence in 2011, with cases mainly occurring in children (<15 years of age) and the highest incidence in 2009 in infants (<1 year of age) [11]. Small scale studies using dengue reports have investigated the spatial autocorrelation of dengue cases [12] and the association between dengue and satellite environmental data using spatially stratified tests of ecological niche models [13]. Hagenlocher et al. [14] performed a spatial assessment of current socioeconomic vulnerabilities to dengue fever in 340 neighborhoods of a Colombian city through a spatial approach that included expert-based and purely statistical-based modeling of current vulnerability levels using a GIS.

At national level, Quintero et al. [15] used epidemiological surveillance data (weekly cases) and Poisson regression models to assess the influence of the El Niño Southern Oscillation index and pluviometry on dengue incidence, adjusting by year and week. At a regional scale, Cadavid-Restrepo et al. [16] explored the variation in spatial distribution of notified dengue cases in Colombia from 2007 to 2010, exploring associations between the disease and selected environmental risk factors through a Bayesian spatio-temporal conditional autoregressive model. The results elucidate the role of environmental risk factors in the spatial distribution of dengue disease, explaining how these factors can be used to develop and refine preventive approaches for dengue in Colombia. All these studies are strategic to the research of surveillance and control of dengue disease, demonstrating the importance of representation of the disease in space and time.

In Colombia, dengue epidemiological surveillance is based in passive notification of cases, coordinated by the 'Instituto Nacional de Salud' (Colombia National Institute of Health) [17], and supports monitoring, prediction, risk factor identification and intervention measures. Even though the surveillance network works adequately, and provides information to all the national institutions involved in dengue control, we appreciate that disease mapping techniques currently developed and employed for many health problems are not widely applied.

We selected the Colombian city of Bucaramanga to use Bayesian areal disease mapping models, testing the challenges and difficulties of the approach to dengue disease mapping. Bucaramanga was one of the cities with the highest dengue incidence in Colombia by year during the period 2008–2015. We estimated the relative risk of dengue disease, applying Bayesian spatial areal models to dengue case counts and satellite covariates (normalized difference vegetation index (NDVI) and land surface temperature (LST)) with fixed and space-varying coefficients, at a small spatial scale and with global and annual aggregation time scales, for the 2008–2015 period. Ideally, we would use data on the vector presence, distribution and ecology, but that kind of data does not exist for the city of Bucaramanga at the aggregation level of the study. We relied on satellite images to search associations between dengue incidence and environmental data. In addition, we provided a Bayesian model to estimate the Cohen's Kappa measure of agreement for the interpretation of the change in relative risk of dengue between the global and annual time scales.

Methods

Cases of dengue disease from Bucaramanga, Colombia

The city of Bucaramanga, Colombia is located at coordinates 7°7'07"N–73°06'58" W, at 959 m above sea level. It covers an urban area of 27 km^2 and it has a population of 527,913 people in 2016, living in 220 neighborhoods nested in 17 communes. While Colombia presented an incidence rate of 436 cases per 100,000 persons in 2010, Bucaramanga reported an incidence rate of 1359.1 per 100,000 persons. We obtained data on incident cases of dengue disease (dengue and severe dengue) from the SIVIGILA (public health surveillance system) for the urban area of Bucaramanga for the period from January 2008 to December 2015.

We geocoded and allocated every case of dengue disease to one of 293 Bucaramanga census sections (geographical unit composed by approximately 20 closed city blocks) according to the cartography of the 2005 census from the national geostatistical framework of the 'Departamento Nacional de Estadística' (Colombia national statistics office) [18]. For geocoding purposes, we started with a database of 30,063 cases corresponding to the notified dengue cases from health institutions in Bucaramanga to the surveillance system. The cases were obtained from the database checked for duplicates reported to the surveillance system. The dengue cases data included address, sex, age and an identification code which anonymized the name and personal identification of the case to the geocoder. From this database, we selected the cases with address of residence belonging to Bucaramanga. We discarded cases without address, cases with rural address and wrong addresses. Then, an R [19] script sent batches of addresses to the web geocoding service of ArcGIS server. The returned geocoding were checked and accepted, or revised for a new geocoding cycle. At the end of the process, we succesfully geocoded to the urban area of Bucaramanga a total of 27,301 cases, which were aggregated to the spatial scale defined above, therefore our data does not relate to an identifiable natural person thus the data subject is not identifiable.

The cases aggregated by census section were aggregated along two time scales: a global scale, running for the entire study period (2008–2015); and an annual scale, resulting in eight respective datasets for each included year.

We obtained disaggregated data by census section, sex and five-years age groups from the 2005 census and calculated annual and global crude incidence rates according to these variables. We calculated expected values for dengue case counts by multiplying the global and annual crude incidence of dengue times the population by sex and age at census section level.

Satellite images for normalized difference vegetation index

We used satellite raster images obtained from Landsat Surface Reflectance (SR) Enhanced Thematic Mapper (ETM) 7, bands 3 and 4 (60 m resolution) for the years 2008, 2009, 2010, 2011; and from Landsat SR Operational Land Imager (OLI) and Thermal Infrared Sensor (TIRS) 8, bands 4 and 5 (30 m resolution) for years 2013, 2014, and 2015 (Landsat Surface Reflectance products courtesy of the U.S. Geological Survey). We selected Landsat multispectral images based on those with the least cloud cover. Images covered the city of Bucaramanga and were taken from row 55, path 8 or path 7, with Universal Transversal Mercator (UTM) projection, zone 18

North and datum WGS-84. From Landsat SR ETM 7, we selected images from January 2, 2008; January 27, 2009; January, 14 2010; and February 2, 2011. From Landsat SR OLI-TIRS 8, we chose images from June 16, 2013; January 10, 2014; and January 4, 2015. We did not find any suitable Landsat images for the year 2012.

Satellite images for land surface temperature

We use Moderate Resolution Imaging Spectroradiometer (MODIS) satellite raster images from the MOD11A2 version 6 product [20] to obtain mean 8-day, per-pixel land surface temperature (LST), in a 1200 km × 1200 km grid. Each pixel value in the MOD11A2 is a simple average of all the corresponding MOD11A1 LST pixels collected within that 8-day period, with a pixel size of 1000 m × 1000 m. We selected the 'day time surface temperature' band.

Image processing

For the Landsat SR 7 ETM raster images, we calculated a composite NDVI raster image for the annual satellite images using band 4 [near infra red (NIR)] and band 3 (red). For the Landsat SR 8 OLI-TIRS raster images, we calculated a composite NDVI raster image for the annual satellite images using band 5 NIR and band 4 (red). We applied the formula NDVI = (NIR band − red band)/ (NIR band + red band), following Yuan et al. [21]. Due to the absence of good quality images for 2012, we created a composite NDVI image for 2012 by pixel averaging of the composite NDVI images for 2011 and 2013.

To obtain an NDVI value by census section, we superimposed a mask comprised by the polygons (census sections) from the shape file of the city of Bucaramanga, onto the composite NDVI raster image, calculating the NDVI pixel mean by census section to the composite NDVI annual satellite images. We also produced a composite NDVI image at global aggregation scale (2008–2015 period) by pixel averaging by census section of all the composite NDVI images per year. For the composite NDVI image at global scale, we followed the same masking procedure to produce NDVI pixel mean by census section applied to the composite NDVI images by year.

For the MODIS LST raster images, we first reprojected the images from sinusoidal projection to UTM 18N projection, datum WGS84, and resampled to 30 m using the Modis reprojection tool (MRT) software [22]. We then created composite LST raster images per epidemiological period by pixel averaging all the reprojected and resampled images available in every epidemiological period. We generated composite LST images per year by pixel averaging all the composite LST raster images per epidemiological period. For every composite LST raster image per year, we applied a mask comprised by the polygons (census sections) from the shape file of the city of Bucaramanga, and calculated the average LST by polygon (census section).

Finally, we created a composite LST image at global aggregation scale (2008–2015 period) by pixel averaging all the composite LST images per year. We produced LST average by census section in the composite LST image at global scale, following the same masking process to obtain LST average by census section per year. Raster image processing was done using the R software version 3.3 [19] with the `raster` package version 2.5-8 [23].

Statistical models

Disease mapping is the area of epidemiology that estimates the spatial pattern in disease risk over an extended geographical region in order to identify areas at high risk [24]. Besag et al. [25] developed a Bayesian hierarchical model for spatial analysis of areal data. Let θ_i be the log relative risk of a contagious disease with low transmission, O_i the observed number of cases and E_i the expected number of cases in area i. Assuming O_i are independent Poisson variables with mean $E_i \exp(\theta_i)$, where $\exp(\theta_i)$ is the relative risk of the disease and the linear predictor $\theta = t + u + v$ is adopted, where t is a term associated with measured covariates; and u and v are surrogates for unknown observed covariates. The u_i's represent variables with spatial structure and the v_i's represent spatially unstructured variables. In the hierarchical framework, prior probability distributions are assigned to u and v. For v, Normal prior with zero mean and variance λ, and for u,

$$p(u) \propto \left\{ -\sum_{i<j} \zeta_{ij} \phi(u_i - u_j) \right\}, \quad u \in \mathcal{R} \tag{1}$$

where ϕ is a function of pairwise differences among u's, and ζ_{ij} are weights equal to zero for i non-contiguous to j. Besag et al. [25] consider two options for ϕ: $\phi(z) = z^2/2\kappa$ or $\phi(z) = |z|/\kappa$, where κ is an unknown constant. Choosing the first options for ϕ, the conditional structure of u follows

$$p(u|\kappa) \propto \frac{1}{\kappa^{n/2}} \left\{ -\frac{1}{2\kappa} \sum_{i \sim j} \zeta_{ij}(u_i - u_j)^2 \right\} \tag{2}$$

where $i \sim j$ represent neighbor areas, and the model is referred to as the 'Normal intrinsic autoregression.' For the non-zero ζ_{ij} several options are available, such as 1 for zones sharing a border and 0 otherwise, or the length of the boundary between contiguous zones [10]. The model with independent normal priors for v_i and Normal intrinsic priors for u_i is known as the 'convolution model'.

We fitted Poisson log normal models for relative risk, following Besag et al. [25], to the aggregated data at annual and global scale, with observation equation,

$$O_i \sim \text{Poisson}(E_i e^{\theta_i}) \tag{3}$$

where O_i, E_i and $\exp(\theta_i)$ are the observed count, the expected count, and the relative risk of dengue disease, respectively, in census section i ($i = 1, \ldots, m, m = 293$). For the linear predictor, we explored the following structures:

$$\theta_i = \begin{cases} \alpha + u_i + v_i \\ \alpha + u_i + v_i + \beta_1 \text{ NDVI}_i \\ \alpha + u_i + v_i + \beta_2 \text{ LST}_i \\ \alpha + u_i + v_i + \beta_1 \text{ NDVI}_i + \beta_2 \text{ LST}_i \end{cases} \tag{4}$$

where the u_i are spatially correlated effects with Normal intrinsic conditional autoregressive (ICAR) priors distribution with precision parameter τ_u, and the v_i are the spatially uncorrelated effects with Normal prior distribution with zero mean and precision parameter τ_v. β_j ($j = 1, 2$) are normally distributed fixed coefficients for NDVI and LST, with zero mean and precision 100. Uniform (0,1) hyperpriors were assigned to $\tau_u^{-1/2}$ and $\tau_v^{-1/2}$.

Next, we fitted models with spatially correlated effects with Leroux [26] Normal conditional autorregressive (CAR) prior distribution and fixed coefficients for the covariates,

$$\theta_i = \begin{cases} \alpha + w_i \\ \alpha + w_i + \beta_1 \text{ NDVI}_i \\ \alpha + w_i + \beta_2 \text{ LST}_i \\ \alpha + w_i + \beta_1 \text{ NDVI}_i + \beta_2 \text{ LST}_i \end{cases} \tag{5}$$

The w_i are the spatially correlated effects with Leroux Normal CAR prior distributions, with precision matrix τ_w with Gamma(1, 0.001) hyperpriors. Finally, models were fitted with fixed and spatially varying coefficients for the covariates with Leroux CAR priors as follow:

$$\theta_i = \begin{cases} \alpha + (\beta_1 + b_{i,1}) \text{ NDVI}_i + (\beta_2 + b_{i,2}) \text{ LST}_i \\ \alpha + (\beta_1 + b_{i,1}) \text{ NDVI}_i \\ \alpha + (\beta_2 + b_{i,2}) \text{ LST}_i \end{cases} \tag{6}$$

where the $b_{i,j}$ are spatially varying coefficients for NDVI ($j = 1$) and LST ($j = 2$). For the linear predictor including two spatially varying coefficients $b_{i,j}$, these coefficients are modelled multivariate Normal with Leroux conditional mean vector $\mu_{i,j}$ ($j = 1, 2$) and precision matrix $\xi_{2\times2}$ following Congdon (2014) [27], where $\mu_{i,j}|\mu_{k\in\partial_{i,j}} = (\rho/(1 - \rho + \rho d_i)) \sum_{k\in\partial_i} \mu_{k,j}$ and $\xi_{2\times2} = (1 - \rho + \rho d_i)\Xi_{2\times2}$, where the precision matrix $\Xi_{2\times2}$ is Wishart distributed with symmetric matrix S and 2 degrees of freedom.

The coefficient ρ establishes the degree of spatial structure of the spatial effects $\mu_{i,j}$. When $\rho = 1$, the Leroux prior for the spatial effects implies an Normal ICAR prior, while, $\rho = 0$, we have an independent model [28].

For the models with linear predictor including spatially varying coefficients for only one covariate, the $b_{i,1}$ or $b_{i,2}$ space-varying coefficients for NDVI or LST are modelled with Leroux conditional mean vector $\mu_{i,j}$ ($j = 1, 2$) and precision τ_{b_j} ($j = 1$ for NDVI or $j = 2$ for LST), with Gamma(1,0.001) hyperpriors. All models included an intercept α with a diffuse improper prior .

From the Poisson log Normal models, we obtain the relative risk $\exp(\theta_i)$ of dengue disease by census section and calculate point-wise mean estimates and 95% credible intervals (CI). Choropleth maps were produced using the logarithm of the mean relative risk (θ_i) and the mean spatially correlated effects u_i by census section.

Additionally, the relative risk of dengue disease by census section was discretized as *low* or *high* risk, based on the lower bound of the 95% CI, where a value of 1 or less for the lower bound of the relative risk of dengue disease by census section indicates a *low* risk, and values exceeding 1 signify a *high* risk. Choropleth maps of the discretized relative risk (DRR) of dengue disease are produced at global and annual aggregation scale.

Using the DRR of dengue disease, we calculated the Cohen's Kappa [29] coefficients for global-to-annual or annual-to-annual agreement of *low-high* risk by census section, using the following Bayesian model adapted from Lee and Wagenmakers [30]:

$$\kappa = (\delta - \psi)/(1 - \psi)$$
$$\delta = \pi_1 + \pi_4$$
$$\psi = (\pi_1 + \pi_2)(\pi_1 + \pi_3) + (\pi_3 + \pi_4)(\pi_2 + \pi_4) \quad (7)$$
$$\mathbf{y} \sim \text{Multinomial}\ ([\pi_1, \pi_2, \pi_3, \pi_4], n)$$
$$\pi_i \sim \text{Dirichlet}\ (1, 1, 1, 1)$$

where κ is the Kappa coefficient and $\mathbf{y}$ is the vector of counts in categories from the cross tabulation of *low* and *high* risk from global-to-annual or annual-to-annual agreement. Let $year_a$ be one the eight study years and $year_b$ other year not equal to $year_a$, the categories are as follows: $y_1 = low$ risk in global scale or $year_a$ and *low* risk in $year_b$; $y_2 = low$ risk in global scale or $year_a$ and *high* risk in $year_b$; $y_3 = high$ risk in global scale or $year_a$ and *low* risk in $year_b$; and $y_4 = high$ risk in global scale or $year_a$ and *low* risk in $year_b$.

We first calculated the global-to-annual agreement of DRR, between the pairs of DRR from model by global

aggregation scale and the models for the data at annual aggregation scale. Second, we calculated the annual-to-annual agreement of DRR between all pairs of models fitted at annual aggregation scale. For the interpretation of the Kappa coefficients, we used the categories in Table 1, from Broemeling [31].

Models were fitted with Markov Chain Monte Carlo (MCMC) using the WinBUGS software version 1.4 [32]. We utilize three chains with a burn-in period of 30,000 iterations, a final run of 10,000 iterations and thinning rate of 10, deriving a final sample of 1000 iterations by chain for the inference. To evaluate convergence, we check trace and density plots as well as the Gelman, Brooks and Rubin and Geweke tests [19]. Model selection was accomplished using the deviance, the deviance information criterion (DIC) and the number of effective parameters (p_D) [33].

Results
Summary statistics

Table 2 presents summary statistics for the dengue case counts, the standardized morbidity rate (SMR, the observed dengue cases divided by the expected dengue cases by census section), the NDVI, the LST and, the correlations between these variables, for the data aggregated at global and annual scales.

For the global scale, a total of 27,301 cases (range by census section: 1–433) were reported and geocoded. The mean SMR for all census section was 1.098, with a minimum of 0.225 and a maximum of 4.05. The mean value of NDVI was 0.368, with a minimum of 0.135 and a maximum of 0.792. Mean LST for the aggregated data was 32.1 °C, with a minimum of 28.8 °C and a maximum of 34 °C. Linear correlations between counts of cases of Dengue and NDVI (r $= -0.071$) and LST (r $= 0.127$) was weak, while, correlation between the NDVI and LST was moderate and negative (r $= -0.629$).

For the summary statistics at annual scale, 2010 was the year with the highest number of cases (n = 6932) followed by 2014 (n = 4956) and 2013 (n = 4839), with 2011 showing the lowest number of cases (896). The maximum number of cases in a census section ocurred in 2013 (n = 115), followed by 2010 (109) and 2014 (84). For the annual SMR, the year 2011 presented the highest average SMR (1.193) followed by 2010 (SMR = 1.143) and 2015 (SMR = 1.165).

Table 1 Degree of agreement for Kappa

Degree of agreement	Poor	Slight	Fair	Moderate	Substantial	Perfect
Kappa	<0	0–0.20	0.21–0.40	0.41–0.60	0.61–0.80	0.81–1.00

Table 2 Summary statistics for counts of dengue disease, NDVI and LST, by Bucaramanga census section, for globally and annually aggregated data, 2008–2015

Statistic	Global (2008–2015)	2008	2009	2010	2011	2012	2013	2014	2015
Dengue disease case counts									
Total	27,301	1936	3131	6932	896	1546	4839	4956	3065
Min.	1	0	0	0	0	0	0	0	0
Max.	433	31	56	109	17	39	115	84	58
Mean	93.2	6.6	10.7	23.7	3.0	5.3	16.5	16.9	10.5
Standardized morbidity rate									
Min.	0.225	0.000	0.000	0.000	0.000	0.000	0.000	0.000	0.000
Max.	4.052	8.409	6.346	5.401	12.294	5.979	4.683	5.129	5.502
Mean	1.098	1.125	1.082	1.143	1.193	1.089	1.096	1.101	1.165
NDVI									
Min.	0.135	0.091	0.130	0.096	0.134	0.144	0.142	0.146	0.129
Max.	0.792	0.767	0.813	0.757	0.803	0.850	0.896	0.784	0.779
Mean	0.368	0.346	0.394	0.355	0.368	0.379	0.390	0.367	0.346
LST									
Min.	28.8	29.3	28.8	27.6	28.4	29.1	29.3	28.9	28.5
Max.	34.0	34.2	34.9	32.9	34.2	34.5	34.6	34.8	32.8
Mean	32.1	32.3	32.5	30.7	31.8	32.4	32.2	32.9	31.7
Linear correlation									
Dengue-NDVI	−0.071	0.062	0.170	0.108	0.080	0.061	0.198	−0.014	0.086
Dengue-LST	0.127	0.016	−0.038	0.056	−0.063	−0.039	−0.126	0.017	−0.043
NDVI-LST	−0.629	−0.533	−0.640	−0.546	−0.583	−0.629	−0.568	−0.543	−0.522

The lowest maximum NDVI by census section corresponded to the year 2010 (NDVI = 0.757) followed, in order, by 2008 (NDVI = 0.767) and 2014 (NDVI = 0.784), while the lowest mean NDVI were for years 2008 and 2015 (mean NDVI = 0.346) followed by 2010 (mean NDVI = 0.355).

With respect to the LST, the year 2010 displayed the lowest mean temperature (30.7 °C), followed by 2015 (31.7 °C) and 2011 (31.8 °C), while for the rest of the years, the LST mean was close to 32 °C.

The linear correlations between dengue case counts and NDVI or LST were low, whereas the most pronounced correlation was for 2013: between dengue and NDVI, r = 0.198; and between dengue and LST, r = −0.126. At an annual scale, the correlation between NDVI and LST was moderate and inverse for all years, with the strongest correlations for 2009 (r = −0.640) and 2012 (r = −0.629).

Model selection

Table 3 shows the selection statistics deviance, number of effective parameters (p_D) and DIC, for the models fitted at global and annual aggregation scales in Bucaramanga.

In general, the convolution models with CAR priors fitted the data better than the models with Leroux CAR priors, evidenced by the smallest deviance in the convolution models. For the data at global aggregation scale,

the model with spatially correlated and uncorrelated effects with fixed coefficient for NDVI ($u_i + v_i + \beta_1$) presented the smallest DIC (DIC = 2364.6). For the year 2008, the smallest DIC was for the model with spatial effects with Leroux CAR priors and fixed coefficient for NDVI ($\beta_1 + w_i$) (DIC = 1457.8). For the years 2009, 2010, and 2014, we selected the models with correlated and uncorrelated spatial effects plus a fixed coefficient for NDVI ($u_i + v_i + \beta_1$), which presented the smallest DIC values of 1618.4, 1916.5, and 1798.3, respectively. For the years 2011, 2012, 2013, and 2015, the selected models contained space-varying coefficients for NDVI with Leroux CAR priors and a fixed coefficient for NDVI ($\beta_1 + b_{i,1}$), displaying the smallest DIC values of 1178.4, 1361.8, 1772.2, and 1629.1 respectively.

Parameter estimates of the selected model at global aggregation scale, 2008–2015

The selected model at global scale was the convolution model with fixed coefficient for NDVI ($u_i + v_i + \beta_1$). Figure 1 shows the map of the SMR logarithm, the map of the logarithm of the mean relative risk of dengue disease θ_i, the DRR of dengue disease, and the spatially correlated effects (u_i) from the model at global scale. The log mean relative risk of dengue disease shows high risk clusters in the south and north-west census sections of the city.

Table 3 Information criterion statistics, for relative risk models of dengue disease, 2008–2015

Model	Deviance	p_D	DIC	Deviance	p_D	DIC	Deviance	p_D	DIC
	Global scale 2008–2015			2008			2008		
$u_i + v_i$	2098.0	268.3	2366.3	1290.5	168.5	1459.0	1428.0	191.9	1619.9
$u_i + v_i + \beta_1$	*2097.2*	*267.4*	*2364.6*	1291.3	168.7	1460.0	*1427.7*	*190.7*	*1618.4*
$u_i + v_i + \beta_2$	2097.3	267.4	2364.7	1289.8	168.2	1458.0	1427.0	192.2	1619.2
$u_i + v_i + \beta_1 + \beta_2$	2097.8	267.9	2365.8	1289.5	168.7	1458.2	1427.9	191.7	1619.6
w_i	2098.1	268.9	2367.1	1296.2	163.3	1459.5	1428.8	196.0	1624.8
$w_i + \beta_1 + \beta_2$	2098.1	268.6	2366.7	1295.7	163.5	1459.1	1429.0	194.5	1623.5
$w_i + \beta_1$	2098.3	268.9	2367.2	*1294.5*	*163.3*	*1457.8*	1429.1	194.5	1623.6
$w_i + \beta_2$	2098.0	269.0	2367.0	1296.2	163.7	1459.9	1428.7	196.0	1624.6
$\beta_1 + b_{i,1} + \beta_2 + b_{i,2}$	2108.4	261.8	2370.2	1323.6	157.2	1480.8	1443.5	186.9	1630.5
$\beta_1 + b_{i,1}$	2113.8	257.0	2370.8	1346.2	140.6	1486.9	1465.5	175.7	1641.3
$\beta_2 + b_{i,2}$	2279.2	267.1	2546.3	1423.8	133.7	1557.5	1616.1	158.7	1774.8
	2010			2011			2012		
$u_i + v_i$	1684.3	233.5	1917.7	1063.3	120.5	1183.8	1198.4	164.8	1363.2
$u_i + v_i + \beta_1$	*1683.9*	*232.6*	*1916.5*	1063.5	120.6	1184.1	1199.6	165.6	1365.2
$u_i + v_i + \beta_2$	1684.4	233.8	1918.2	1063.0	119.9	1182.9	1198.2	165.6	1363.8
$u_i + v_i + \beta_1 + \beta_2$	1683.7	232.8	1916.5	1063.6	121.4	1185.0	1198.5	165.9	1364.5
w_i	1685.6	236.9	1922.5	1072.2	115.1	1187.3	1208.2	163.3	1371.4
$w_i + \beta_1 + \beta_2$	1686.0	236.0	1922.0	1071.0	117.4	1188.4	1207.7	163.6	1371.3
$w_i + \beta_1$	1686.0	236.5	1922.6	1072.2	115.9	1188.2	1208.4	163.3	1371.7
$w_i + \beta_2$	1684.0	236.2	1920.2	1071.8	115.9	1187.7	1207.8	163.8	1371.7
$\beta_1 + b_{i,1} + \beta_2 + b_{i,2}$	1694.3	227.6	1921.8	1065.9	121.0	1186.9	1206.8	156.6	1363.4
$\beta_1 + b_{i,1}$	1699.1	220.5	1919.6	*1077.6*	*100.7*	*1178.4*	*1214.9*	*146.8*	*1361.8*
$\beta_2 + b_{i,2}$	1823.0	228.0	2051.0	1168.5	69.3	1237.8	1332.8	119.6	1452.4
	2013			2014			2015		
$u_i + v_i$	1556.9	216.5	1773.4	1582.5	216.7	1799.2	1443.9	193.5	1637.4
$u_i + v_i + \beta_1$	1557.8	215.3	1773.1	*1581.9*	*216.4*	*1798.3*	1443.2	193.3	1636.5
$u_i + v_i + \beta_2$	1557.4	216.2	1773.6	1582.5	216.6	1799.2	1443.4	193.4	1636.8
$u_i + v_i + \beta_1 + \beta_2$	1557.7	215.4	1773.1	1581.8	217.3	1799.1	1443.4	193.8	1637.2
w_i	1560.0	216.5	1776.5	1586.4	220.0	1806.4	1447.1	197.5	1644.6
$w_i + \beta_1 + \beta_2$	1559.9	215.4	1775.3	1584.6	219.3	1803.9	1447.1	197.2	1644.3
$w_i + \beta_1$	1560.0	215.0	1775.0	1585.2	219.4	1804.7	1446.8	196.9	1643.7
$w_i + \beta_2$	1560.4	216.8	1777.2	1584.8	219.4	1804.2	1447.1	197.2	1644.3
$\beta_1 + b_{i,1} + \beta_2 + b_{i,2}$	1570.4	202.8	1773.1	1589.6	209.7	1799.3	1452.5	179.6	1632.1
$\beta_1 + b_{i,1}$	*1579.3*	*192.9*	*1772.2*	1597.2	202.3	1799.5	*1452.9*	*176.2*	*1629.1*
$\beta_2 + b_{i,2}$	1912.6	178.8	2091.4	1764.9	200.9	1965.8	1635.3	160.2	1795.5

p_D is defined as number of effective parameters

The DRR map presents the areas where the 95% CIs for the relative risk do not include 1, and the map of spatial effects displays spatial correlation at the south of the city.

Parameter estimates from models at annual aggregation scale, 2008–2015

Table 4 presents the mean point-wise parameters estimates and 95% CI from the selected models fitted at the annual aggregation scale.

The selected model for 2008 was the model with spatially correlated effects with Leroux CAR priors plus fixed coefficient for NDVI ($w_i + \beta_1$). The point-wise mean estimate for the NDVI fixed coefficient is positive (0.294), and the 95% CI include zero (−0.214, 0.814), suggesting a weak association between dengue and NDVI by census section, at the same time, the point mean estimate of ρ is 0.486, which denotes moderate spatially correlated effects w_i in the relative risk of dengue disease.

The convolution model plus fixed coefficient for NDVI was the selected model for the years 2009, 2010, and 2014 ($u_i + v_i + \beta_1$). The point-wise mean and 95% CI estimates of the fixed coefficients for NDVI for years 2009, 2010,

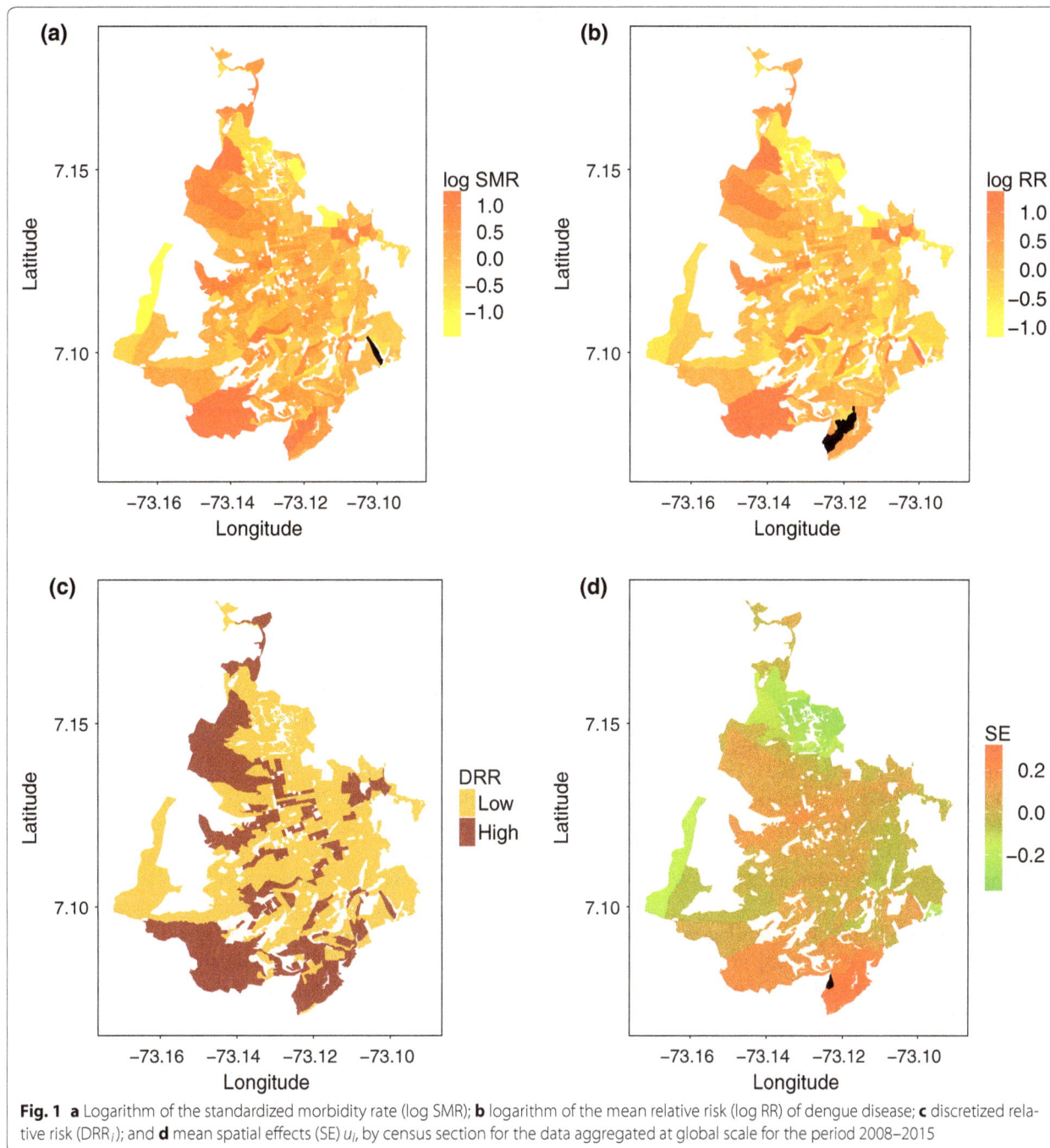

Fig. 1 **a** Logarithm of the standardized morbidity rate (log SMR); **b** logarithm of the mean relative risk (log RR) of dengue disease; **c** discretized relative risk (DRR$_i$); and **d** mean spatial effects (SE) u_i, by census section for the data aggregated at global scale for the period 2008–2015

and 2014 show a strong, positive association between Dengue and NDVI for 2009 (0.589; 95% C.I: 0.168, 1.024), but not for 2010 and 2014. The mean of the spatially correlated effects w_i (2008) and u_i (2009, 2010 and 2014) are presented in Fig. 2a. We observe the highest values of the mean spatial effects for the south of the city in 2008, but a scattered pattern of the mean of the spatially correlated effects for the rest of the years.

The model with fixed coefficient and space-varying coefficients for NDVI was selected for years 2011, 2012, 2013, and 2014 ($\beta_1 + b_{i,1}$). The fixed coefficients for NDVI have to be accompanied by the space-varying coefficients, to be fully interpreted. The mean estimates for the fixed coefficient plus the space-varying coefficients for NDVI ($\beta_1 + b_{i,1}$) are presented in the Fig. 2b. We discretized the space-varying coefficients in a similar way

Table 4 Parameter estimates (point-wise mean and 95% CI) from the selected model at annual scale, 2008–2015 period

Parameter	Year			
	2008	2009	2010	2011
α	−0.173 (−0.399, 0.059)	−0.305 (−0.494, −0.115)	−0.19 (−0.363, −0.007)	0.108 (−0.12, 0.332)
σ_u	0.811 (0.658, 1.008)	0.323 (0.153, 0.512)	0.342 (0.199, 0.494)	
σ_v		0.457 (0.372, 0.543)	0.45 (0.386, 0.518)	
β_1	0.294 (−0.214, 0.814)	0.589 (0.168, 1.024)	0.43 (−0.041, 0.885)	−0.398 (−1.042, 0.249)
$\sigma_{b_{i,1}}$				1.399 (1.063, 1.835)
ρ	0.486 (0.217, 0.868)			0.062 (0.002, 0.236)
Parameter	**2012**	**2013**	**2014**	**2015**
α	0.116 (−0.11, 0.346)	−0.08 (−0.224, 0.071)	−0.093 (−0.28, 0.083)	0.049 (−0.138, 0.223)
σ_u			0.5 (0.346, 0.684)	
σ_v			0.404 (0.322, 0.483)	
β_1	−0.635 (−1.367, 0.12)	0.002 (−0.496, 0.502)	0.058 (−0.39, 0.536)	−0.222 (−0.867, 0.456)
$\sigma_{b_{i,1}}$	2.068 (1.601, 2.711)	1.785 (1.469, 2.188)		2.034 (1.666, 2.506)
ρ	0.279 (0.081, 0.592)	0.314 (0.146, 0.567)		0.316 (0.141, 0.575)

as the discretized relative risk (DRR). We considered the association between the NDVI and dengue by census section to be *weak* when the lower bound of the 95% CI was 1 or less and, to be *strong* otherwise (Fig. 2c). The discretized space-varying (DSV) NDVI coefficients enabled us to identify census sections where there was strong association between dengue incidence and NDVI. For 2012, 2013, and 2015, we observe a strong association in 4 to 8 census sections, while for 2011, the discretized effect was so low that there were no census sections showing an association between the covariate and dengue disease.

Mapping of relative risk of dengue disease, from models by annual scale

In this section, we begin by presenting the maps for the logarithm of the mean relative risk of dengue disease, and then we display the maps of the DRR of dengue, from the models selected by year 2008–2015.

Figure 3a presents the logarithm of the mean relative risk (Log RR) by year, for the period 2008–2015. The smoothed estimates of the Log RR let us discern patterns of the disease distribution in Bucaramanga. We observe similar patterns for 2009, 2010, and 2011, with clusters of high relative risk in the southern and northwestern census sections. For 2008, 2012, 2013 and 2015, we observe slightly fewer zones with high relative risk. Estimates of relative risk of dengue for 2014 presented a great number of high-risk census sections in the northwestern, southern and central zones of the city.

The maps of DRR of dengue disease help us to identify rapidly those census sections presenting the highest risk for each year (Fig. 3b). The areas along the southern and northwestern edges of the city show a consistent tendency towards high relative risk, while the center generally presents a low risk, with some exceptions.

Kappa coefficient for the global-toa-annual and annual-to-annual agreement of DRR of dengue disease

We present estimates for the Kappa coefficient (point-wise mean and 95% CI) for global-to-annual and annual-to-annual agreement of DRR of dengue disease in Table 5. We interpreted the Kappa coefficient for agreement based on the coverage of the 95% CI over the categories of 'degree of agreement' from Table 1. Firstly, we established the global-to-annual agreement of DRRs of dengue disease. Secondly, we determined the annual-to-annual agreement of the DRR of dengue disease.

From Table 5, we interpreted the global-to-annual agreement in DRR at years 2008, 2009, 2012, and 2015 to be *poor to fair*, while the agreement was *poor to slight* for 2011. Agreement of DRR of dengue disease was *slight to moderate* between the model at global scale and models for 2013 and 2014, and, *substantial to moderate* for the global scale model and the model for 2010.

For the annual-to-annual agreement of DRR, from 2009 to 2010, there was *poor to fair* agreement of DRR. From years 2011 to 2012 and 2012 to 2013, the agreement of DRR for dengue disease was *slight to moderate*. Additionally, the agreement was *slight to fair* from 2010 to 2011, 2013 to 2014, and 2014 to 2015. Finally, annual-to-annual agreement of DRR between other year pairs was almost always *poor to slight*.

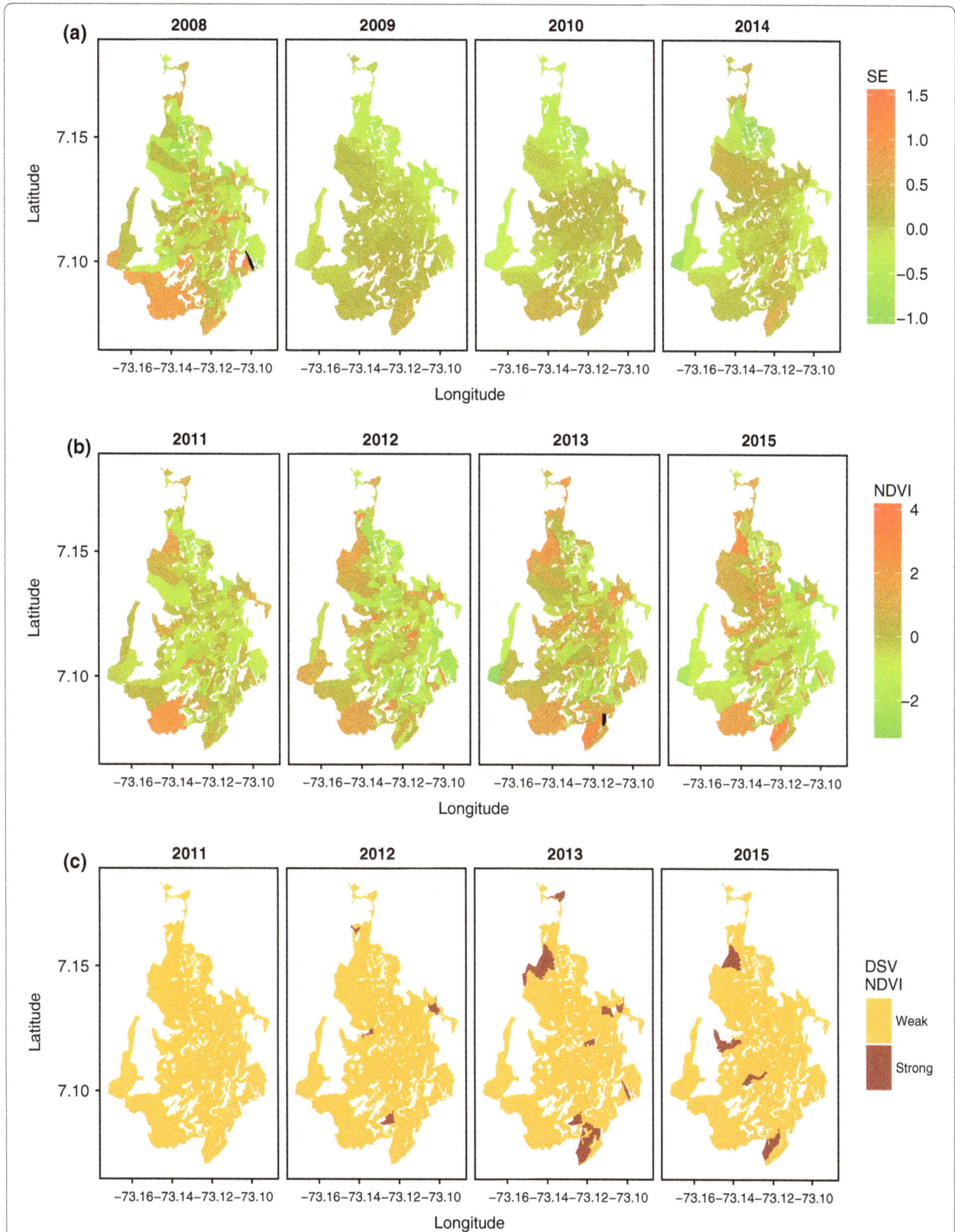

Fig. 2 **a** Mean spatial effects (SE) w_i (2008) and u_i (2009, 2010, and 2014) from the selected models at annual aggregation scale; **b** mean space-varying NDVI coefficients ($\beta_1 + b_{i,1}$); and **c** discretized space-varying (DSV) NDVI coefficients ($\beta_1 + b_{i,1}$) for years 2011, 2012, 2013, 2015, from models at annual aggregation scale

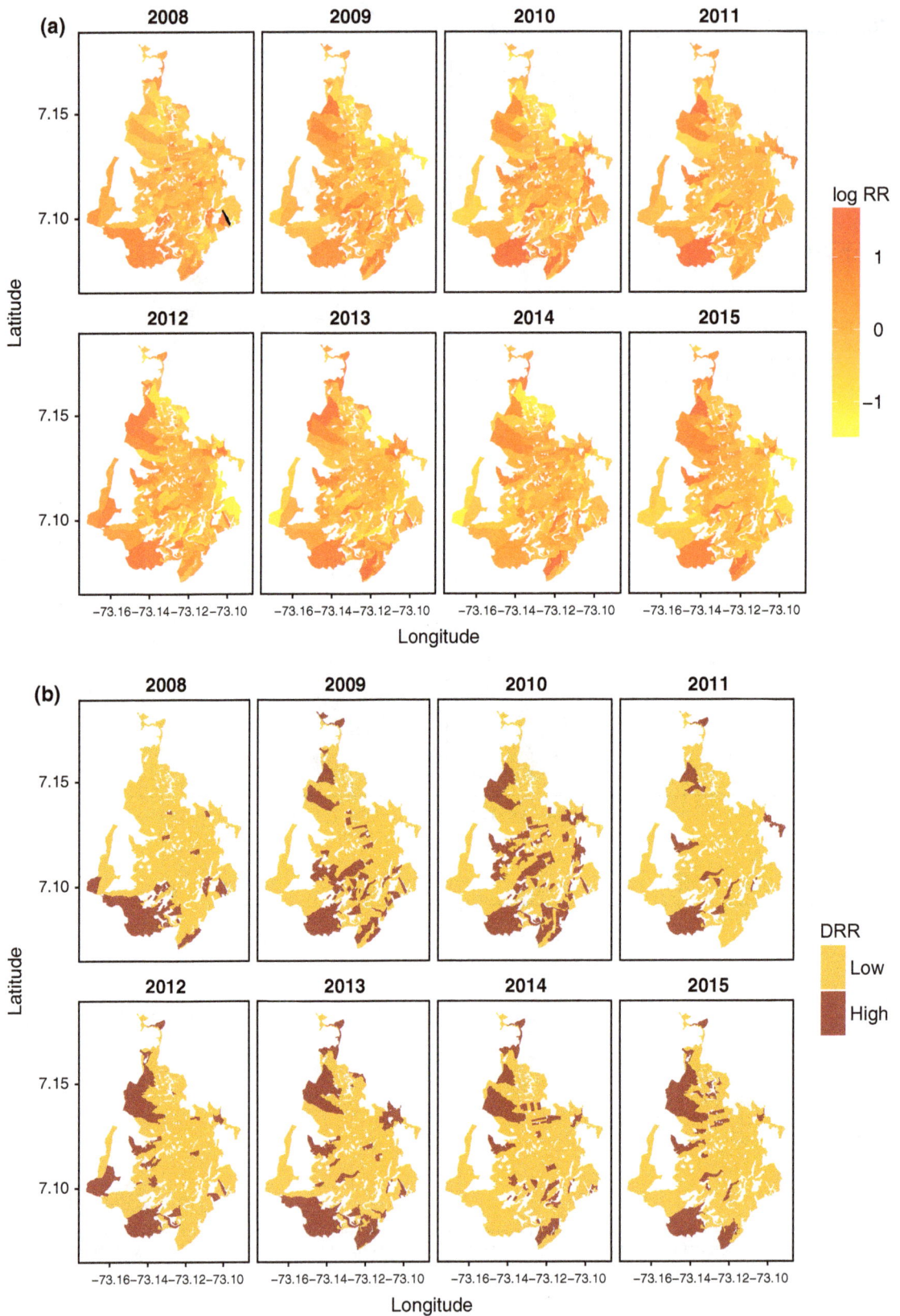

Fig. 3 a Logarithm of the mean relative risk (log RR) of dengue disease , from models at annual aggregation scale 2008–2015; **b** discretized relative risk (DRR) of dengue disease, 2008–2015

Table 5 Kappa coefficient (point-wise mean and 95% CI) for global-to-annual and annual-to-annual agreement of discretized relative risk (DRR) of dengue by census sections, from models at global and annual aggregation scales in Bucaramanga, 2008–2015

Year	Global scale	Annual scale						
		2009	2010	2011	2012	2013	2014	2015
2008	0.231	0.146	0.107	0.087	0.142	0.115	0.003	0.042
	(0.124, 0.347)	(0.021, 0.288)	(0, 0.235)	(−0.027, 0.251)	(0.007, 0.303)	(−0.003, 0.255)	(−0.087, 0.126)	(−0.059, 0.173)
2009	0.327		0.271	0.207	0.207	0.226	0.141	0.097
	(0.207, 0.448)		(0.144, 0.402)	(0.078, 0.36)	(0.072, 0.355)	(0.094, 0.366)	(0.012, 0.281)	(−0.02, 0.234)
2010	0.513			0.143	0.158	0.294	0.134	0.075
	(0.397, 0.621)			(0.043, 0.261)	(0.046, 0.284)	(0.162, 0.425)	(0.013, 0.264)	(−0.035, 0.202)
2011	0.166				0.293	0.279	0.185	0.196
	(0.079, 0.271)				(0.116, 0.486)	(0.14, 0.431)	(0.054, 0.341)	(0.062, 0.357)
2012	0.254					0.363	0.225	0.269
	(0.144, 0.369)					(0.212, 0.513)	(0.085, 0.378)	(0.121, 0.424)
2013	0.466						0.219	0.231
	(0.352, 0.577)						(0.089, 0.361)	(0.1, 0.375)
2014	0.307							0.25
	(0.188, 0.428)							(0.112, 0.393)
2015	0.22							
	(0.099, 0.34)							

Discussion

In this study we applied Bayesian hierarchical models for spatial analysis of areal data to the estimation of relative risk of dengue disease in a Colombian city. We chose this particular city for its high incidence of dengue disease, in 2008–2015. We fitted models at global and annual scales for the study period. The hierarchical models included covariates (NDVI and LST) obtained from satellite raster images.

From the descriptive statistics, we found low correlation between the covariates and the dengue case counts by census section. NDVI and LST were moderately correlated by census sections at global and annual scales. Two main models were fitted: first the convolution model (spatially correlated effects with Normal ICAR priors, and uncorrelated spatial effects with Normal zero mean priors and precision τ_v); and second, spatially correlated effects model with Leroux Normal CAR priors. We used those structures with or without covariates. The covariates effects were modeled as fixed coefficients with Normal prior distributions with zero mean and high precision, or space-varying coefficients with Leroux Normal CAR priors.

We used MCMC to fit the models, and selected the models for inference, applying DIC measures. All the selected models (at global and annual scale) included NDVI fixed coefficients (2008, 2009, 2010, and 2015), and NDVI space-varying coefficients (2011, 2012, 2013, and 2014).

The convolution model was selected at global and annual scale for 2009, 2010, and 2014. The models with spatially correlated effects with Leroux Normal CAR priors were selected for 2008, 2011, 2012, 2013, and 2015. We illustrated the relative risk of dengue disease using two types of maps. First, we produced maps of the logarithm of the mean relative risk, containing smoothed estimates of relative risk, allowing us to distinguish clusters of high relative risk at global and annual scales. Second, we created maps of DRR of dengue disease, allowing us to identify zones where the risk is higher than in zones with 95% CIs including 1.

We employed satellite images from two sources (Landsat and MODIS) to calculate NDVI and LST data at areal level (census section). We were interested in establishing association between the information from raster images and dengue incidence at global and annual scale according to census section. The selected models for inferences did include NDVI but not LST. Parameter estimates (point-wise mean and 95% CI) for the association of the NDVI and dengue disease are mainly positive; however, they only reveal a strong association between dengue and NDVI, in 2009 (95% CI not including zero). Our results were different from some results in the literature. In Costa Rica, Troyo et al. [34] found negative coefficients for NDVI suggesting an inverse association with relative risk of dengue disease. They reported NDVI from satellite images at different resolutions, finding an association between high NDVI and low incidence of dengue. Meza-Ballesta et al. [35] reported the association between dengue incidence and high air temperature, high rainfall, and vegetation deterioration. Araujo et al. [36] analyzed dengue incidence in São Paulo, Brazil. They associated thermal remote sensing images, census data, and dengue incidence, and their findings point to low dengue incidence in areas with high vegetation cover, and high incidence in areas with low vegetation coverage and land surface temperatures above 29 °C; however Nazri et al. [37] did not find NDVI to be a major factor influencing dengue incidence in Malaysia. Qi et al. [38] found that the associations between cases of Dengue disease and population density, GDP per capita, road density, and NDVI were nonlinear, and the risk of dengue disease declined gradually with rising NDVI.

These reports involving NDVI as a covariate did not use areal data, or the aggregation resolution was higher than the resolution used in our study. Additionally, at high spatial scale, the link between NDVI and rainfall variability in zones with epidemiological reports of dengue or malaria has been reported across South America [39], contributing to a better understanding of climate, environment, and epidemics facilitating the implementation of local and regional health early warning systems. In this context, our study contributes to understand the relationship between NDVI and incidence of dengue disease at a finer resolution.

As limitations of the satellite data employed in our study, we noted that for the period 2008–2011, we had to impute the NDVI in some census sections because of known issues with the sensor from Landsat ETM 7. We employed a convolution model to make the imputation of the missing NDVI values. For the NDVI data, the pixel resolution was 30 m, while the pixel resolution of the MODIS LST data was 1000 m, resampled to 30 meters, which makes some census section highly associated with respect to the LST. Additionally, for LST, we used single raster image per year, which is a composite of around 48 MODIS images. Moreover, finding high-quality Landsat images for the period was difficult, mainly because of cloud cover. In addition, we used a non-conventional method to treat information from satellite images, as compared to the literature, because we employed continuous variables such as NDVI and LST in space obtaining areal inputs as covariates, using the mean value for every census section.

With respect to the data quality on dengue, we employed official data, aggregating the cases into census sections acknowledging factors such as age or sex by means of internal standardization. We consider our dengue case counts to be high-quality data given that the

surveillance system is based on compulsory reporting physicians in Colombia at all service levels, but keeping in mind critic considerations regarding possible underreporting as shown by Romero-Vega et al. [40].

For the spatial aggregation level and census data, we based our population estimates on the 2005 census, with the assumption that city's population has been fairly stable throughout the study period. We recognize the possible bias produced by the use of 2005 data for estimation of the expected values for the study period. This is one of the challenges of the study, but it is not only for the disease under study. At the time of the realization of this study, there were not updated data for population living in Bucaramanga, at census section level. The Colombian government updates its census every ten years. It was programmed a census for 2016, but was not developed. We consider this finding extremely important, if public health authorities are interested to provide information, not only for temporal analysis (as is currently done) but also for spatial analysis at finer resolution scales (census block, section or sector). This study provides the space to recommend to the Colombian authorities, to build real-time registries of population, which support evaluation, decision making and intervention, not only for dengue disease, but for all the notifiable diseases. Additionally, we are aware that the spatial aggregation scale changes the conclusion from areal data as shown by Khormi and Kumar [41], as does the choice of neighborhood structure [10]. The spatial aggregation scale used in this study corresponds to the spatial scale supplied by the official cartography from the 2005 census.

Together with the generation of relative risk maps and the evaluation of satellite data associated with incidence of dengue disease, we determined whether there was an association in the DRR of dengue disease by census section from year to year, and from the risk at global scale and annual scale. To this end, we employed the Kappa coefficients to define the global-to-annual agreement of risk when the relative risk is discretized as *low* or *high* risk, estimating the Kappa coefficients, using a Bayesian model. We have found substantial to moderate agreeement between the DRR at global scale and the year 2010, and moderate to fair agreeement for 2013 and 2014. For the rest of the global-to-annual agreement or all the annual-to-annual agreement of the DRR for consecutive years, we found slight to fair agreement, reflecting a volatile pattern of dengue risk by census section from year to year. The main results for the annual-to-annual agreement of the discretized relative risk for non consecutive year, point to low agreeement between census sections in terms of risk level between years.

Conclusions

We applied disease mapping models at small spatial scale in a Colombian city with fixed and space-varying coefficients for covariates derived of satellite images. We found the NDVI associated to high dengue risk by census section. The modeling process produced relative risk maps of dengue disease, allowing us to identify areas with high risk in the city. We compared the concordance of high risk by census section between the global aggregated model and the annual aggregated models, and between years in the 2008–2015 period. We found in general, slight to fair agreement in high risk. The information obtained by the use of disease mapping models is not currently available to public health authorities in Colombia. We highlight the importance of transforming raw spatial data into relative risk maps of dengue disease for planning and implementation of public health strategies. The map quality depends on high-quality population data at the selected spatial aggregation scale, which are sometimes difficult to obtain; and the geocoding process to allocate every case to a correct spatial coordinate. Information from satellite images improves the output of the spatial modeling, by associating environmental variables to the dengue incidence. For future research we are interested to apply disease mapping models in similar datasets from municipalities in Colombia. The main limitation is the cost of geocoding the data from the official records in terms of work-time and accurate geocoding. However, after the geocoding task is finished, the data will be available not only to spatial analysis, but also to temporal and spatiotemporal analysis, including the covariates with constant or time-varying coefficients[42]. We would like to present the method to the public health authorities from diverse surveillance offices in Colombia, and test the field applicability of the disease mapping models discussed in our study. Finally, we also are interested to apply disease mapping methods based on hierarchical Bayesian models to map the relative risk not only for dengue disease, but also for arboviral diseases like Chykungunya and Zika at small spatial scale in Colombia, to support public health authorities in disease surveillance and control strategies.

Abbreviations
CAR: conditional autorregressive; CI: credible interval; DANE: Departamento Nacional de Estadística; DIC: deviance information criterion; DRR: discretized relative risk; DSV: discretized space-varying; ICAR: intrinsic conditional autoregressive; GIS: geographic information system; LST: land surface temperature; MODIS: moderate resolution imaging spectroradiometer; NDVI: normalized difference vegetation index; SIVIGILA: Sistema de Vigilancia en Salud Pública; SMR: standardized morbidity rate.

Authors' contributions
DMB and ALQ conceived and designed the modeling process, performed the modeling process and analyzed the data; ATP contributed materials; DMB, ALQ and ATP wrote the paper. All authors read and approved the final manuscript.

Author details
[1] Departament d'Estadística i Investigació Operativa, Facultat de Matemátiques, Universitat de València, C/Dr Moliner 50, 46100 Burjassot, Valencia, Spain. [2] Epidemiological Surveillance, Health Office of Department of Santander, Cl. 45 11-52, Bucaramanga 680001, Colombia.

Competing interests
The founding sponsors had no role in the design of the study; in the collection, analyses, or interpretation of data; in the writing of the manuscript, and in the decision to publish the results. The authors declare that they have no competing interests.

Funding
DMB acknowledges the support of the Colombian Administrative Department of Science and Technology (COLCIENCIAS) by the Grant 646-2014 for doctoral studies abroad. ALQ would like to thank the "Ministerio de Economía y Competitividad" for its support in the form of the research Grant MTM2016-77501-P (jointly financed with the European Regional Development Fund).

References
1. Whitehorn J, Simmons CP. The pathogenesis of dengue. Vaccine. 2011;29(42):7221–8.
2. Louis VR, Phalkey R, Horstick O, Ratanawong P, Wilder-Smith A, Tozan Y, Dambach P. Modeling tools for dengue risk mapping—a systematic review. Int J Health Geogr. 2014;13(1):50.
3. Racloz V, Ramsey R, Tong S, Hu W. Surveillance of dengue fever virus: a review of epidemiological models and early warning systems. PLoS Negl Trop Dis. 2012;6(5):1648.
4. Mondini A, Chiaravalloti-Neto F. Spatial correlation of incidence of dengue with socioeconomic, demographic and environmental variables in a Brazilian city. Sci Total Environ. 2008;393(2):241–8.
5. Castillo KC, Körbl B, Stewart A, Gonzalez JF, Ponce F. Application of spatial analysis to the examination of dengue fever in Guayaquil, Ecuador. Procedia Environ Sci. 2011;7:188–93.
6. Khormi HM, Kumar L, Elzahrany RA. Modeling spatio-temporal risk changes in the incidence of dengue fever in Saudi Arabia: a geographical information system case study. Geospat Health. 2011;6(1):77–84.
7. Buczak AL, Koshute PT, Babin SM, Feighner BH, Lewis SH. A data-driven epidemiological prediction method for dengue outbreaks using local and remote sensing data. BMC Med Inform Decis Mak. 2012;12:124.
8. Lowe R, Bailey TC, Stephenson DB, Graham RJ, Coelho CA, Carvalho MS, Barcellos C. Spatio-temporal modelling of climate-sensitive disease risk: towards an early warning system for dengue in Brazil. Comput Geosci. 2011;37(3):371–81.
9. Honorato T, Lapa PPDA, Sales CMM, Reis-Santos B, Tristão-Sá R, Bertolde AI, Maciel ELN. Spatial analysis of distribution of dengue cases in Espírito Santo, Brazil, in 2010: use of Bayesian model. Revista Bras Epidemiol. 2014;17(Suppl D.S.S.):150–9.
10. Ferreira G, Schmidt A. Spatial modelling of the relative risk of dengue fever in Rio de Janeiro for the epidemic period between 2001 and 2002. Braz J Probab Stat. 2006;20:29–47.
11. Villar LA, Rojas DP, Besada-Lombana S, Sarti E. Epidemiological trends of dengue disease in Colombia (2000–2011): a systematic review. PLoS Negl Trop Dis. 2015;9(3):1–16.
12. Londoño CLA, Restrepo CE, Marulanda EO, Distribución ME. Spatial distribution of dengue based on Geographic Information Systems tools, Aburra Valley. Revista Fac Nac Salud Pública. 2014;32(1):7–15.

13. Arboleda S, Jaramillo ON, Peterson AT. Mapping environmental dimensions of dengue fever transmission risk in the Aburrá Valley, Colombia. Int J Environ Res Public Health. 2009;6(12):3040–55.

14. Hagenlocher M, Delmelle E, Casas I, Kienberger S. Assessing socioeconomic vulnerability to dengue fever in Cali, Colombia: statistical vs expert-based modeling. Int J Health Geogr. 2013;12(1):36.

15. Quintero-Herrera LL, Ramírez-Jaramillo V, Bernal-Gutiérrez S, Cárdenas-Giraldo EV, Guerrero-Matituy EA, Molina-Delgado AH, Montoya-Arias CP, Rico-Gallego JA, Herrera-Giraldo AC, Botero-Franco S, Rodríguez-Morales AJ. Potential impact of climatic variability on the epidemiology of dengue in Risaralda, Colombia, 2010–2011. J Infect Public Health. 2015;8(3):291–7.

16. Cadavid-Restrepo A, Baker P, Clements ACA. National spatial and temporal patterns of notified dengue cases, Colombia 2007–2010. Trop Med Int Health. 2014;19(7):863–71.

17. Zambrano P. Protocolo de Vigilancia en Salud Pública, Dengue (Surveillance Protocol in Public Health, Dengue). Instituto Nacional de Salud (National Institute of Health), Santafé de Bogota, Colombia. Instituto Nacional de Salud (National Institute of Health). 2014. http://www.ins.gov.co/lineas-de-accion/Subdireccion-Vigilancia/sivigila/Paginas/protocolos.aspx.

18. Departamento Administrativo Nacional de Estadística, g.o. Dirección de Geoestadística (National Administrative Department of Statistics: Capa del Nivel de Sector Urbano (urban Sector Level Layer). Marco geoestadístico nacional (national geostatistical framework). 2005. http://www.dane.gov.co/.

19. R Core Team: R: A language and environment for statistical computing. R foundation for statistical computing, Vienna, Austria. R Foundation for Statistical Computing. 2016. https://www.R-project.org/.

20. Wan Z, Hook, S, Hulley G. MOD11A2 MODIS/Terra Land Surface Temperature/Emissivity 8-Day L3 Global 1km SIN Grid V006. NASA EOSDIS Land Processes DAAC, 2015. NASA EOSDIS Land Processes DAAC. 2015. https://doi.org/10.5067/MODIS/MOD11A2.006.

21. Yuan F, Bauer ME. Comparison of impervious surface area and normalized difference vegetation index as indicators of surface urban heat island effects in Landsat imagery. Remote Sens Environ. 2007;106(3):375–86.

22. United States Geological Service: Modis Reprojection Tool User's Manual. Release 4.1 April 2011. Land Processes DAAC. USGS Earth Resources Observation and Science. Land Processes DAAC. USGS Earth Resources Observation and Science. 2011.

23. Hijmans RJ, van Etten JR. Geographic analysis and modeling with raster data. R package version 2.5-8. 2016. http://CRAN.R-project.org/package=raster.

24. Lee D. A comparison of conditional autoregressive models used in Bayesian disease mapping. Spat Spatio Temporal Epidemiol. 2011;2(2):79–89.

25. Besag J, York J, Mollie A. Bayesian image restoration with two applications in spatial statistics. Ann Inst Stat Math. 1991;43(1):1–59.

26. Leroux BG, Lei X, Breslow N. Estimation of disease rates in small areas: a new mixed model for spatial dependence. In: Halloran ME, Berry D, editors. Statistical models in epidemiology, the environment and clinical trials. New York: Springer; 1999. p. 179–91.

27. Congdon P. Applied Bayesian modelling. 2nd ed. West Sussex: Wiley; 2014.

28. Banerjee S, Carlin B, Gelfand A. Hierarchical modeling and analyisis for spatial data. Boca Raton: Chapman & Hall/CRC Biostatistics Series; 2015.

29. Cohen J. A coefficient of agreement for nominal scales. Educ Psychol Meas. 1960;20:37–46.

30. Lee MD, Wagenmakers EJ. Bayesian cognitive modeling: a practical course. Cambridge: Cambridge University Press; 2014.

31. Broemeling LD. Bayesian methods for measures of agreement. Boca Raton: Chapman & Hall/CRC Biostatistics Series; 2009.

32. Lunn D, Spiegelhalter D, Thomas A, Best N. The BUGS project: evolution, critique, and future directions. Stat Med. 2009;28:3049–67.

33. Spiegelhalter DJ, Best NG, Carlin BP. Bayesian measures of model complexity and fit. J R Stat Soc Ser B (Stat Methodol). 2002;64(4):583–639.

34. Troyo A, Fuller DO, Calderón-Arguedas O, Solano ME, Beier JC. Urban structure and dengue fever in Puntarenas, Costa Rica. Singap J Trop Geogr. 2009;30(2):265–82.

35. Meza-Ballesta A, Gónima L. Influencia Del Clima Y De La Cobertura Vegetal En La Ocurrencia Del Dengue (2001–2010). Revista Salud Pública. 2004;16(2):293–306.

36. Araujo RV, Albertini MR, Costa-da-Silva AL, Suesdek L, Franceschi NCS, Bastos NM, Katz G, Cardoso VA, Castro BC, Capurro ML, Allegro VLAC. São Paulo urban heat islands have a higher incidence of dengue than other urban areas. Braz J Infect Dis. 2015;19(2):146–55.

37. Nazri C, Hashim A, Rodziah I. Distribution pattern of a dengue fever outbreak using GIS. J Environ Health Res. 2009;9(2002):1–10.

38. Qi X, Wang Y, Li Y, Meng Y, Chen Q, Ma J, Gao G. The effects of socioeconomic and environmental factors on the incidence of dengue fever in the Pearl River Delta, China, 2013. PLoS Negl Trop Dis. 2015;10:0004159.

39. Tourre YM, Jarlan L, Lacaux JP, Rotela CH, Lafaye M. Spatio-temporal variability of NDVI-precipitation over southernmost South America: possible linkages between climate signals and epidemics. Environ Res Lett. 2008;3:044008.

40. Romero-Vega L, Pacheco O, de la Hoz-Restrepo F, Díaz-Quijano FA. Evaluation of dengue fever reports during an epidemic, Colombia. Revista de Saude Publica. 2014;48(6):899–905.

41. Khormi HM, Kumar L. The importance of appropriate temporal and spatial scales for dengue fever control and management. Sci Total Environ. 2012;430:144–9.

42. Martínez-Bello D, López-Quílez A, Torres-Prieto A. Bayesian dynamic modeling of time series of dengue disease case counts. PLoS Negl Trop Dis. 2017;11(7):0005696.

Influence of Pokémon Go on physical activity levels of university players

Fiona Y. Wong[*]

Abstract

Background: The prevalence of overweight is increasing and the effectiveness of various weight management and exercise programs varied. An augmented reality smartphone game, Pokémon Go, appears to increase activity levels of players. This study assessed the players and ex-players' frequencies and durations of staying outdoors, and walking/jogging before and during the time they played Pokémon Go, evaluated the physical activity levels of players, ex-players and non-players, and investigated the potential factors which determined their play statuses.

Methods: Students in a university answered an online-questionnaire survey. The IPAQ-short form was incorporated to measure vigorous-intensity activities, moderate-intensity activities and walking. Chi square tests were used to compare frequencies and durations of staying outdoors and walking/jogging, health discomforts and physical activity levels between players, ex-players and non-players. Wilcoxon signed ranks tests were performed to assess the changes prior to and during the time when the players and ex-players played Pokémon Go. Logistic regression analyses were performed to assess factors contributing to playing, quitting or not playing Pokémon Go.

Results: 644 university students answered the questionnaire. Compared with the ex-players, the players were significantly more frequent to stay outdoors when playing Pokémon Go (P < 0.001), walk/jog to a location to catch Pokémon, to Pokéstops or Gyms (P < 0.005), as well as walking/jogging to hatch eggs (P < 0.001). Players who never or rarely walked/jogged before spent a mean of 108.19 ± 158.21 min/week to walk/jog in order to play the game which is equivalent to burning 357 kcal/week for a 60-kg person walking a moderate pace. Compared with the non-players, players were more likely to be aged 18–25 years [OR (95% CI) 3.28 (1.28–8.40), P = 0.013], never [OR (95% CI) 10.51 (1.12–98.57), P = 0.039] or rarely [OR (95% CI) 4.00 (1.95–8.23), P < 0.001] stayed outdoors and rarely walked/jogged prior to playing the game [OR (95% CI) 3.88 (1.86–8.05), P < 0.001]. However, there was no significant difference in physical activity levels between the three groups (P = 0.573).

Conclusions: Players who used to be sedentary benefited the most from Pokémon Go. The game can be used as a starting point for sedentary people to begin an active lifestyle. The impact of Pokémon Go on physical activity can provide insights to public health workers in using novel strategies in health promotion.

Keywords: Physical activity levels, Pokémon Go, Active lifestyle, Augmented reality games

Background

Sedentary lifestyle and physical inactivity are associated with obesity and chronic illness. According to WHO, 60–85% of people in the world lead a sedentary lifestyle.

A sedentary lifestyle doubles the risk of cardiovascular diseases, diabetes and obesity, and increases the risks of colon cancer, high blood pressure, lipid disorders and depression [1]. Similar to populations in many countries, people in Hong Kong tend to have less physical activities. According to the statistics of the Centre for Health Protection collected in April 2014, 20.3% of the Hong Kong people had low physical activity level [2]. Compared with

*Correspondence: fiona.y.wong@polyu.edu.hk
Faculty of Health and Social Sciences, The Hong Kong Polytechnic University, Kowloon, Hong Kong, China

the same survey conducted in Oct 2005 in which 19.7% were categorized as having low physical activity, this indicates that there has been no significant improvement in people's physical activity level regardless of the exercise promotion programs delivered in the past 10 years [3]. WHO recommends adults aged 18–64 to have at least 150 min of moderate-intensity aerobic physical activity throughout the week, or at least 75 min of vigorous intensity physical activity a week, or an equivalent combination of moderate and vigorous physical activity [4]. However, in Hong Kong only 37.4% of the people surveyed met the WHO recommendation in 2014 [5].

In the past few decades, weight management programs primarily using dietary and exercise interventions had been developed and delivered to help people to achieve desirable anthropometric and metabolic outcomes. However, the effects of these programs varied [1, 6]. The prevalence of overweight and obesity is increasing regardless of the hard work of the health workers. In the US, the prevalence of overweight of people aged 18 years or above increased from 70.3% in 2010 to 72.1% in 2014 while in China, the prevalence rate increased from 31.1 to 36.2% [7]. As smartphones and mobile games are becoming more popular, and it seems that there are limitations in the traditional approaches in promoting exercises and physical activities, mobile exergames (mobile games which combine exercising with game play) could be another option to increase physical activity levels in daily life [8]. The potential for smartphone applications to facilitate health behavioral change has been supported [9, 10]. Some mobile phone games for health behaviors have been tested for their short-term effectiveness in promoting physical activity and healthy eating [11, 12]. The most popular smartphone applications are found to be those incorporated with virtual avatars, gaming and social media [12]. The self-determination theory (SDT), a motivational theory, has been used in examining participation in digital games [13–15]. SDT explains the relationships between motives, psychological needs, motivations and outcomes [16]. The three basic psychological needs—competence (capable and challenged), autonomy (volitional and controllable) and relatedness (sense of belongingness) are essential for people's well-being and psychological growth. Games with virtual avatars are generally higher in autonomy satisfaction as they allow players to develop their own in-game characters and engage in any activities they want. Gaining points, rewards and prestige in games increase motivations as the players feel more competent. Interactions between players can facilitate relatedness needs. The latest augmented reality (AR) smartphone game, Pokémon Go, which has been downloaded by millions of people since its launch, seems to be able to satisfy the psychological needs in SDT.

Pokémon Go is an AR game combining real-world and virtual elements. The mission is to capture all Pokémon creatures appear on the screen [17]. First the player needs to create his on-screen avatar, the trainer. Using the global positioning system (GPS), the smartphone will vibrate to inform the player that a Pokémon is nearby as he moves around. The player then needs to throw a Pokéball to catch it. The game uses a real-world map of the streets and landmarks to help players to locate Pokémon, Pokéstops (for collecting Pokéballs and other special items) and Gyms (for putting the Pokémon in a battle with other players' Pokémon). Players can play Pokémon Go indoors if they come close to a Pokéstop. However, if players want to level up quickly and collect as many Pokémon as possible, especially those rare ones, they need to be active. They need to move around outdoors in real life to look for Pokémon, go to different Pokéstops and Gyms, as well as walking/jogging for a certain distance in order to hatch eggs. Some studies have found that Pokémon Go has the potential to increase short-term activity [18–21], and provide emotional benefits to players [22, 23].

Since the launch of Pokémon Go, it has become one of popular game applications around the world [24, 25]. The game was released in Hong Kong on 25 July 2016. It is easy to find people, especially young adults, playing Pokémon Go on the streets. Unlike most of the computer and video games which require players to play indoors, Pokémon trainers need to be physically active. Well-designed games played on mobile phones have the potential to encourage voluntary physical activity. The aim of this study is to investigate the impact of Pokémon Go on physical activity of student players in a local university. The objectives are (1) to compare the players and ex-players' frequencies and durations of staying outdoors, and walking/jogging before and during the time they played Pokémon Go; (2) to assess and compare the physical activity levels, including vigorous activities, moderate activities and walking, of players, ex-players and non-players of Pokémon Go; and (3) to investigate the potential factors which determine play statuses of the university students.

Methods

Setting and target group

This is a cross-sectional study using an online-questionnaire survey approach. An invitation email was sent to all students in a local university. Those who refused to receive commercial electronic messages (CEM) were excluded. According to the email system of the university, a total of 21,935 students were willing to receive CEM from the university. A sample of 378 students would provide a margin of error of 5% from the true values at 95% confidence level.

The survey was conducted 28 days after the game was released in Hong Kong. An invitation email explaining the purpose of the survey was sent to all students who agreed to receive CEM on 22 Aug 2016. Two hyperlinks, one for accessing the Chinese online questionnaire and another one for accessing the English online questionnaire, were enclosed in the email. The online-questionnaire survey ended on 5 Sep 2016.

Measuring instrument

The questionnaire consisted of 31 closed-ended questions in the format of multiple choice and Likert-scale. Depending on the play statuses of the participants, the questions they needed to answer varied. The questions measured time spent in playing Pokémon Go, frequencies and time spent in staying outdoors, walking and/or jogging intentionally when playing the game and before started playing the game, and health discomforts experienced. Characteristics of the respondents including sex, age, academic program attending and employment status were also studied.

The International Physical Activity Questionnaire (IPAQ)—short form has been validated and translated into different languages, including Chinese, was used to measure three specific types of activity, including vigorous-intensity activities, moderate-intensity activities and walking, in the past seven days [26]. Metabolic Equivalent of Task (MET) is the energy cost of physical activities. The three activities have different MET values [vigorous physical activity (PA) = 8.0 METs; moderate PA = 4.0 METs and walking = 3.3 METs]. The separate scores on vigorous-intensity activities, moderate-intensity activities and walking, and a combined total PA score were calculated and expressed in MET-min/week [27]. Physical activity levels were categorized as low, moderate and high based on the total PA and the criteria listed in the scoring protocol.

The questionnaire was pilot-tested online with 16 subjects aged 18–40 years. Eleven were players, three were ex-players and two were non-players. Among the players, six (54.5%) spent 60 min or less a day to play Pokémon Go, eight (72.7%) reported that they stayed outdoors sometimes or most of the time and four (36.4%) claimed that they stayed outdoors at least an hour a day intentionally to play the game. Regarding walking/jogging when playing Pokémon Go, seven (63.6%) of them would walk/jog to specific locations to catch Pokémon, to reach Pokéstops or Gyms sometimes or most of the time, and five (45.5%) would walk/jog for 10–30 min a day. Six players (54.5%) claimed that that would walk/jog sometimes or most of the time in order to hatch eggs. The questionnaire was appropriately adjusted before implementation of the main study. The response choices of those questions regarding frequencies and durations in staying

outdoors, walking/jogging were revised. To facilitate the respondents in completing the questionnaire online, the wordings and formats of some of the questions were also revised.

Statistical analysis

Statistical analysis was performed using SPSS (version 21). Descriptive statistics were reported by mean ± standard deviation or percentage, as appropriate. Chi square tests were used to compare frequencies and durations of staying outdoors and walking/jogging, health discomforts and physical activity levels between players, ex-players and non-players. Wilcoxon signed ranks tests were performed to assess the changes in frequencies in staying outdoors and walking/jogging prior to and during the time they played Pokémon Go. Univariate analyses, followed by logistic regression analyses were performed to assess socio-demographic factors and play behaviors which determined play statuses. A P value of <0.05 was considered as statistically significant.

Results

Characteristics of the subjects

A total of 784 students responded to the online questionnaire. Among these 784 subjects, 644 completed the questionnaire. 39.5% claimed that they were players (still playing Pokémon Go at the time of the survey), 30.9% claimed that they were ex-players (played before but had not played for at least 7 consecutive days), and the remaining 29.6% were non-players (never played the game) (Table 1). 48.2% of these respondents were male, and the majority were 18–25 years old (72.5%) and currently enrolling in the full-time bachelor's degree programs (70.1%) in the University. Approximately half of them were not employed (49.1%).

Play behaviors of players and ex-players

Play behaviors of players and ex-players were compared. For players, questions focused on their behaviors in the past seven days. For ex-players, questions focused on the period they were still playing Pokémon Go. Players played 4.79 days (SD = 2.11) a week which was significantly longer compared with the ex-players who played 3.57 days (SD = 2.26) a week (P < 0.001) but there was no significant difference in their time spent on the game each day (Table 2). Approximately 60 and 62% of the players and ex-players, respectively, spent less than one hour a day on the game (P = 0.274).

Compared with the ex-players group, the players group was significantly more frequent to stay outdoors when playing Pokémon Go, walk/jog to locations to catch Pokémon, to Pokéstops or Gyms, as well as walking/jogging in order to hatch eggs (Table 2). Around half of

Table 1 Play status and socio-demographics of subjects

	N = 644 N (%)
Play status	
Players	243 (37.7%)
Ex-players	178 (27.6%)
Non-players	223 (34.6%)
Sex	
Male	275 (48.2%)
Female	296 (51.8%)
Missing/reject	73
Age (years)	
Under 18	75 (13.1%)
18–25	416 (72.5%)
26–30	46 (8.0%)
31–40	29 (5.1%)
41–50	6 (1.0%)
51–60	2 (0.3%)
Missing/reject	70
Academic program attending	
Full-time bachelor's degree	387 (70.1%)
Full-time postgraduate degree	85 (15.4%)
Part-time postgraduate degree	44 (8.0%)
Higher diploma	36 (6.5%)
Missing/reject	92
Employment status	
Not working	277 (49.1%)
Working full-time	95 (16.8%)
Working part-time	192 (34.0%)
Missing/reject	80

the respondents in the players group (51.1%) stayed outdoors sometimes or most of the time to play the game but only 29.2% in the ex-players group would do the same (P < 0.001). Compared with the players group, more ex-players (28.7 vs 20.6%) claimed that they never stayed outdoors to play Pokémon Go but less ex-players (43.8 vs 53.9%) claimed that they spent at least 60 min a day in outdoor to play the game, however, the differences were insignificant (P = 0.096). On the other hand, 42.8% of the players group reported that they walked/jogged to specific locations to catch Pokémon, to Pokéstops or Gyms sometimes or most of the time but only 26.9% of the ex-players group would do the same (P = 0.005). 31.3% of the players walked/jogged for more than 20 min a day to catch Pokémon, to Pokéstops or Gyms, which was also significantly more than the ex-players (21.3%) (P = 0.046). In order to hatch eggs, 30.9% of the players would walk/jog sometimes or most of the time, but 87.1% of the ex-players claimed that they never or rarely walked/jogged to hatch eggs (P < 0.001).

We also estimated the time the players and ex-players spent in a week to walk/jog intentionally to play Pokémon Go by multiplying the reported number of days they played the game in a week and the length of time they walked/jogged to catch Pokémon. The players spent a mean of 98.43 ± 151.21 min/week to walk/jog intentionally which was significantly longer than the ex-players (68.23 ± 141.82 min/week) (P = 0.038) (Table 2). According to their frequencies of walking/jogging prior to playing the game, the players and ex-players were separated into two groups. One group was those who claimed that they never or rarely walked/jogged before playing Pokémon Go and another group was those who used to walk/jog sometimes or most of the time. Among the players, those who claimed that they never or rarely walked/jogged before spent a longer time each week in walking/jogging when playing the game (108.19 ± 158.21 min/week) compared with those players who used to walk/jog sometimes or most of the time (89.88 ± 145.43 min/week), however the difference was insignificant (P = 0.351). Insignificant difference was also found among the ex-players (P = 0.838).

Regarding health discomforts, the players (12.3%) reported significantly more leg pain or tiredness than the ex-players (3.9%) ($X^2 = 9.07$, P = 0.003) (Table 2). A significantly higher proportion of respondents in the ex-players group (76.4 vs 67.5%) reported that they did not have any health discomforts associated with playing Pokémon Go ($X^2 = 3.99$, P = 0.05). When the players were asked to estimate how long they would continue playing the game, 12.0% stated that they would continue playing the game for more than a year, however, 47% had no idea how long they would play (Table 2). The non-players were asked why they did not play the game, the majority stated that they were not interested or did not have time.

Compare frequencies of staying outdoors and walking/jogging prior to and during playing Pokémon Go

To understand whether Pokémon Go can encourage players to increase physical activity levels, changes in frequencies of staying outdoors and walking/jogging prior to and during the time playing Pokémon Go were assessed using Wilcoxon signed ranks tests. No significant change was found in both the players group and the ex-players groups. However, if only those who claimed that they never or rarely stayed outdoors or walked/jogged prior to playing Pokémon Go were selected for the analyses, positive changes were found.

Regarding staying outdoors, positive ranks indicated that the respondents "stayed outdoors more often to play Pokémon Go" and negative ranks indicated that they "stayed outdoors less often to play Pokémon Go", compared with the frequencies before playing the game. A

Table 2 Play behaviors and health discomforts between players and ex-players

	Players group N (%)	Ex-players Group N (%)	Chi-square χ^2	P
Time spent each day in playing Pokémon Go				
≤15 min	37 (15.2%)	40 (22.5%)	7.54	0.274
16–30 min	48 (19.8%)	40 (22.5%)		
31–60 min	61 (25.2%)	30 (16.9%)		
>60 min to 2 h	46 (18.9%)	30 (16.9%)		
2–3 h	26 (10.7%)	16 (9.0%)		
3–4 h	14 (5.8%)	13 (7.3%)		
≥4 h	11 (4.5%)	9 (5.1%)		
Frequency in staying outdoors to play Pokémon Go				
Never	50 (20.6%)	51 (28.7%)	20.43	<0.001
Rarely	69 (28.4%)	75 (42.1%)		
Sometimes	100 (41.2%)	40 (22.5%)		
Most of the time	24 (9.9%)	12 (6.7%)		
Time spent each day in staying outdoors to play Pokémon Go				
0 min	50 (20.6%)	51 (28.7%)	9.34	0.096
≤15 min	37 (15.2%)	24 (13.5%)		
16–30 min	42 (17.3%)	33 (18.5%)		
31 – 60 min	52 (21.4%)	21 (11.8%)		
>60 min – 2 hr	35 (14.4%)	24 (13.5%)		
≥2 h	27 (11.1%)	25 (14.0%)		
Frequency in walking/ jogging to catch Pokémon, go to Pokéstops or Gyms				
Never	67 (27.6%)	70 (39.3%)	13.06	0.005
Rarely	72 (29.6%)	60 (33.75)		
Sometimes	80 (32.9%)	33 (18.5%)		
Most of the time	24 (9.9%)	15 (8.4%)		
Time spent each day in walking/ jogging to catch Pokémon, go to Pokéstops or Gyms				
0 min	67 (27.6%)	70 (39.3%)	11.26	0.046
<10 min	52 (21.4%)	36 (20.2%)		
10–20 min	48 (19.8%)	34 (19.1%)		
21–30 min	37 (15.2%)	13 (7.3%)		
31–60 min	24 (9.9%)	12 (6.7%)		
≥1 h	15 (6.2%)	13 (7.3%)		
Frequency in walking/jogging to hatch eggs				
Never	92 (37.9%)	99 (55.6%)	22.09	<0.001
Rarely	76 (31.3%)	56 (31.5%)		
Sometimes	58 (23.9%)	20 (11.2%)		
Most of the time	17 (7.0%)	3 (1.7%)		
Health discomforts				
Eye strain	28 (11.5%)	22 (12.4%)	0.07	0.879
Neck pain	22 (9.1%)	11 (6.2%)	1.17	0.360
Shoulder pain	18 (7.4%)	13 (7.3%)	0.002	1.000
Wrist pain	10 (4.1%)	2 (1.1%)	3.32	0.080
Finger fatigue	18 (7.4%)	7 (3.9%)	2.22	0.150
Leg pain/tiredness	30 (12.3%)	7 (3.9%)	9.07	0.003
Mental tiredness/weariness	15 (6.2%)	15 (8.4%)	0.79	0.444
None	164 (67.5%)	136 (76.4%)	3.99	0.050

Table 2 continued

	Players group N (%)	Ex-players Group N (%)	Chi-square χ^2	P
Game continuation[a]				
Few days—a week	18 (7.7%)	NA		
2–3 weeks	19 (8.1%)			
1 month	20 (8.5%)			
2–3 months	23 (9.9%)			
4–12 months	16 (6.8%)			
>l year	28 (12.0%)			
Don't know	110 (47.0%)			
Missing	9			

	T-test		P	
	Players Group Mean ± SD	Ex-players group Mean ± SD		
Estimated time spent in walking/ jogging to catch Pokémon, go to Pokéstops or Gyms (min/week) All respondents in the group	98.43 ± 151.21	68.23 ± 141.82	0.038	

	Players Group		Ex-players group	
	Mean ± SD	P	Mean ± SD	P
Prior walking/jogging frequencies				
Never/rarely	108.19 ± 158.21	0.351	70.39 ± 148.25	0.838
Sometimes/most of the time	89.88 ± 145.43		66.02 ± 135.73	

Refers to play behaviors of players in the last 7 days, and play behaviors of ex-players when they were still playing Pokémon Go

[a] The question on game continuation is for players only

positive sum of ranks of 3457.50 and a negative sum of ranks of 637.50 showed that players who never or rarely stayed outdoors prior to playing Pokémon Go, had significantly changed to stay outdoors more often to play the game (Z = −6.11, P < 0.001) (Table 3). Similarly, those who claimed that they never or rarely walked/jogged before playing Pokémon Go, had significantly changed to walk/jog more often to catch Pokémon, to reach Pokéstops or Gyms (Z = −4.34, P < 0.001), and had significantly changed to walk/jog more often in order to hatch eggs (Z = −2.72, P = 0.007).

For ex-players who never or rarely stayed outdoors prior to playing the game, had significant changed to stay outdoors more often to play Pokémon Go (Z = −3.02, P = 0.003). A significant negative change was found in hatching eggs which indicated that those ex-players who never or rarely walked/jogged before, significantly walked/jogged less often to hatch eggs (Z = −3.31, P = 0.001). No positive change was found in both players and ex-players who claimed that they used to stay outdoors or walk/jog sometimes or most of the time prior to playing the game.

Factors determine playing or not playing Pokémon Go
Chi square analyses were performed to assess the relationships between play statuses and demographic characteristics, physical activity levels determined by IPAQ and frequencies of staying outdoors and walking/jogging prior to playing Pokémon Go. The three different play statuses were found to have significant relationships with age, employment status and frequencies of staying outdoors and walking/jogging prior to playing the game.

A multinomial logistic regression was used to further assess factors which determined the play statuses (Table 4). Compared with the non-players, players were more likely to be aged 18–25 years [OR (95% CI) 3.28 (1.28–8.40), P = 0.013], never [OR (95% CI) 10.51 (1.12–98.57), P = 0.039] or rarely [OR (95% CI) 4.00 (1.95–8.23), P < 0.001] stayed outdoors and rarely walked/jogged prior to the game [OR (95% CI) 3.88 (1.86–8.05), P < 0.001]. Similarly, compared with the non-players, the ex-players were more likely to be aged <18 [OR (95% CI) 4.05 (1.13–14.56), P = 0.032] or 18–25 [OR (95% CI) 3.17 (1.03–9.72), P = 0.044], never [OR (95% CI) 17.57 (1.81–170.64), P = 0.013] or rarely [OR (95% CI)

Table 3 Compare the change of frequency of players and ex-players who *never or rarely* staying outdoors and walking/jogging before playing Pokémon Go

	N	Mean rank	Sum of ranks	Z	P
Players group					
Frequency in staying outdoors when playing Pokémon Go (–) Before playing Pokémon Go					
Negative ranks	17	37.50	637.50	−6.11	<0.001
Positive ranks	73	47.36	3457.50		
Ties	37				
Frequency in walking/jogging to catch Pokémon, to reach Pokéstops/Gyms (–) Before playing Pokémon Go					
Negative ranks	26	36.00	936.00	−4.34	<0.001
Positive ranks	60	46.75	2805.00		
Ties	31				
Frequency in walking/jogging to hatch eggs (–) Before playing Pokémon Go					
Negative ranks	34	37.00	1258.00	−2.72	0.007
Positive ranks	51	47.00	2397.00		
Ties	32				
Ex-players group					
Frequency in staying outdoors when playing Pokémon Go (–) Before playing Pokémon Go					
Negative ranks	12	18.00	216.00	−3.02	0.003
Positive ranks	29	22.24	645.00		
Ties	45				
Frequency in walking/jogging to catch Pokémon, to reach Pokéstops/Gyms (–) Before playing Pokémon Go					
Negative ranks	30	24.00	720.00	−0.69	0.491
Positive ranks	26	33.69	876.00		
Ties	34				
Frequency in walking/jogging to hatch eggs (–) Before playing Pokémon Go					
Negative ranks	40	27.00	1080.00	−3.31	0.001
Positive ranks	14	28.93	405.00		
Ties	36				

3.34 (1.53–7.28), P = 0.002] stayed outdoors and rarely walked/jogged prior to the game [OR (95% CI) 3.62 (1.67–7.87), P = 0.001].

To study game enjoyment factors which determined the students continued playing or quitted the game for at least seven consecutive days, Chi square tests were performed to assess the relationships between play statuses (players and ex-players) and number of days played in a week, frequencies of and time spent in staying outdoors and walking/jogging when playing Pokémon Go, and health discomforts. Significant relationships were found in number of days played in a week, frequencies of staying outdoors, walking/jogging to catch Pokémon, to reach Pokéstops/Gyms and walking/jogging to hatch eggs, time spent in walking/jogging to catch Pokémon, to reach Pokéstops/Gyms, and leg pain/tiredness.

A binary logistic regression was used to further assess factors which determined the students continued playing (players) or quitted the game (ex-players) (Table 5). Those who played at least 4 days a week [OR (95% CI) 1.87 (1.21–2.90), P = 0.005] and walked/jogged sometimes [OR (95% CI) 2.25 (1.05–4.83), P = 0.038] or most of the time [OR (95% CI) 6.62 (1.54–28.53), P = 0.011] in order to hatch eggs, were likely to continue playing Pokémon Go (Table 5).

Table 4 Factors determine play statuses of Pokémon Go using multinomial logistic regression

	Players OR (95% CI)	P	Ex-players OR (95% CI)	P
Age (years)				
<18	2.94 (0.95–9.14)	0.062	4.05 (1.13–14.56)	0.032
18–25	3.28 (1.28–8.40)	0.013	3.17 (1.03–9.72)	0.044
26–30	2.34 (0.79–6.94)	0.125	1.43 (0.37–5.58)	0.604
≥31	1.00		1.00	
Employment status				
Not working	0.97 (0.59–1.59)	0.902	1.16 (0.70–1.95)	0.565
Working full-time	0.78 (0.39–1.57)	0.483	0.51 (0.22–1.17)	0.114
Working part-time	1.00		1.00	
Staying outdoors prior to playing Pokémon Go				
Never	10.51 (1.12–98.57)	0.039	17.57 (1.81–170.64)	0.013
Rarely	4.00 (1.95–8.23)	<0.001	3.34 (1.53–7.28)	0.002
Sometimes	1.56 (0.83–2.91)	0.164	1.57 (0.80–3.09)	0.188
Most of the time	1.00		1.00	
Walking/jogging prior to playing Pokémon Go				
Never	3.64 (0.84–15.80)	0.085	1.93 (0.39–9.56)	0.420
Rarely	3.88 (1.86–8.05)	<0.001	3.62 (1.67–7.87)	0.001
Sometimes	1.72 (0.93–3.19)	0.084	1.34 (0.69–2.61)	0.394
Most of the time	1.00		1.00	

Reference category: non-players

Table 5 Factors determine whether respondents continued playing Pokémon Go using binary logistic regression

	Players OR (95% CI)	P
Nos of days played/week (days)		
1–3	1.00	
4–7	1.87 (1.21–2.90)	0.005
Frequency in staying outdoors to play Pokémon Go in the last 7 days		
Never	1.00	
Rarely	0.74 (0.40–1.39)	0.350
Sometimes	1.57 (0.70–3.55)	0.277
Most of the time	1.48 (0.44–4.98)	0.530
Frequency in walking/jogging to catch Pokémon, go to a Pokéstop or a Gym		
Never	1.00	
Rarely	0.11 (0.01–1.94)	0.132
Sometimes	0.12 (0.01–2.17)	0.152
Most of the time	0.08 (0.004–1.47)	0.088
Time spent each day in walking/jogging to catch Pokémon, go to a Pokéstop or a Gym		
0 min	1.00	
<10 min	10.30 (0.60–175.79)	0.107
10–20 min	5.95 (0.36–98.36)	0.212
21–30 min	8.95 (0.52–153.15)	0.130
31–60 min	5.35 (0.31–92.09)	0.248
1–2 h	3.19 (0.19–53.93)	0.421
Frequency in walking/jogging to hatch eggs		
Never	1.00	
Rarely	1.53 (0.87–2.67)	0.140
Sometimes	2.25 (1.05–4.83)	0.038
Most of the time	6.62 (1.54–28.53)	0.011
Leg pain/tiredness		
Yes	1.00	
No	0.43 (0.17–1.08)	0.071

Physical activity levels

In addition to play behaviors, physical activity levels in the past seven days were also assessed using IPAQ. A total of 420 subjects, including 166 players, 107 ex-players and 147 non-players, completed this assessment. There was no significant difference in physical activity levels between the three groups (P = 0.573) (Table 6). Around 40–48% of these student respondents were having moderate physical activity level while 31–38% was having high physical activity level (Fig. 1).

Since the ex-players had not played the game for at least seven consecutive days at the time of the survey, they were combined with the non-players to compare walking, moderate, vigorous and total PA with the players using T-tests. The players were found to have higher walking and moderate PA, however, these were not statistically significant (Table 7).

Discussion

This is the first study assessing the play behaviors of Pokémon Go and the physical activity levels of university students in Hong Kong. Our results showed that players who were used to being sedentary benefited the most

Table 6 Physical activity levels of players, ex-players and non-players using Chi square

	Players	Ex-players	Non-players	X^2	P
Physical activity levels					
Low	41 (24.7%)	23 (21.5%)	29 (19.7%)	2.91	0.573
Moderate	73 (44.0%)	43 (40.2%)	71 (48.3%)		
High	52 (31.3%)	41 (38.3%)	47 (32.0%)		

from Pokémon Go. Players who never or rarely stayed outdoors or walked/jogged before would significantly stay outdoors more frequently as well as walking/jogging more often in order to play Pokémon Go. The players group walked/jogged 98.43 min a week intentionally for playing Pokémon Go. Since walking a moderate pace of 4.8 km/h is estimated to burn 3.3 kcal/kg/h [28], walking

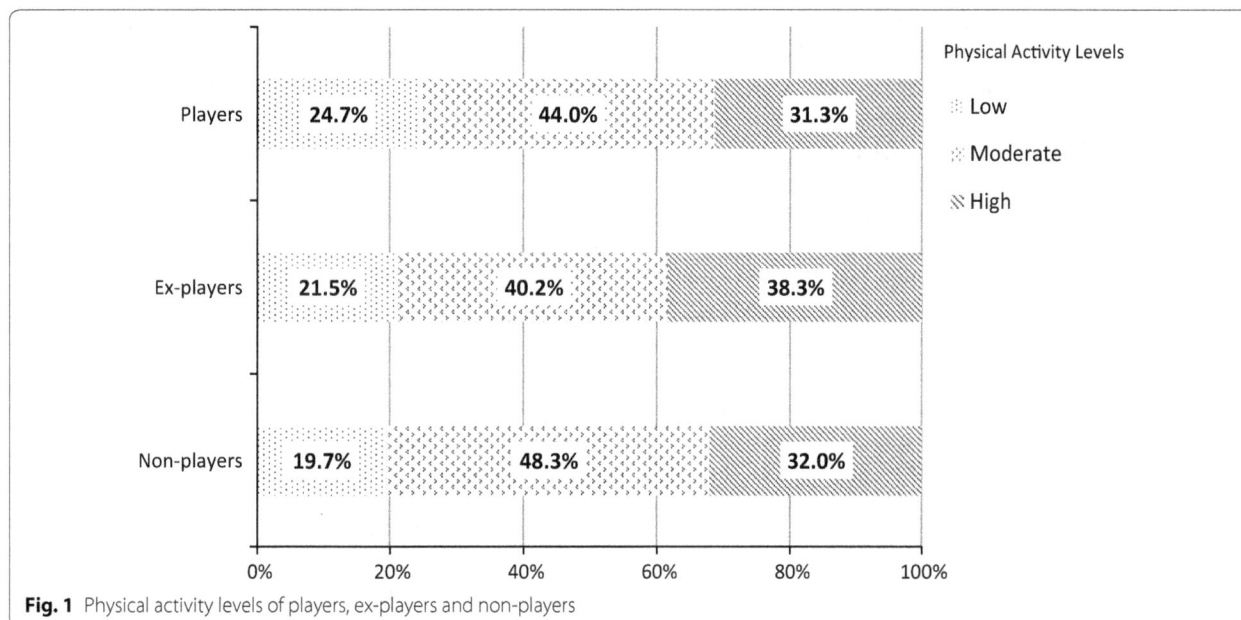

Fig. 1 Physical activity levels of players, ex-players and non-players

98.43 min/week is equivalent to burning 325 kcal a week for a 60-kg person walking a moderate pace. Most importantly, those players who used to be more sedentary (i.e. never or rarely walked/jogged prior to playing Pokémon Go), walked/jogged 108.19 min a week just for playing Pokémon Go, about 10 min more than the mean of the whole players group. Walking 108.19 min/week is equivalent to burning 357 kcal a week. However, the length of time in walking/jogging prior to playing the game was not studied because of the possibility of recall bias, therefore, the changes in walking time and calorie expenditure were uncertain. A recent study showed that Pokémon Go players walked 1473 steps more a day in average, a 25% increase compared to prior activity level [18]. Another study also found that Pokémon Go users increased their daily average steps by 955 additional steps during the first week of installation although the number of daily steps

had gone back to pre-installation levels by the sixth week [19]. From the IPAQ assessment, our players were found to have higher mean walking PA compared with the ex-players and non-players although the difference was insignificant. The higher walking PA in the players group could be attributed to the playing of Pokémon Go.

Players did not spend more time each day to play Pokémon Go compared with the ex-players, but they were more willing to play the game outdoor. The players were also more eager and active when playing. They were more frequent and spent longer period of time to walk or jog to catch Pokémon, to Pokéstops to get more Pokéballs and special items, to Gyms to fight battles, and to hatch eggs in order to get new Pokémon. Although there was no significant difference in the overall physical activity levels and total PA between players, ex-players and non-players, the impact of Pokémon Go on walking or jogging was important, especially to those players who never or rarely walked or jogged before playing the game. Pokémon Go could motivate players who were previously sedentary to become more physically active. As previously discussed, if they did not play Pokémon Go, they were likely to walk 108.19 min less a week. This finding was in line with Althoff's study of which they found that Pokémon Go players who used to be very inactive exhibited large activity increases [18]. Getting inactive people to do a little bit of physical activity is believed to provide greater population health gains even the goal of 150 min a week cannot be achieved [29]. Participation in leisure time activity, even below the recommended level, is associated with a reduced risk of mortality and longer life expectancy [30], as well as decreasing lifetime medical expenditure [31].

Table 7 Walking PA, Moderate PA, Vigorous PA and Total PA of Players and Ex-players/Non-players Using T-tests

	Players Mean ± SD	Ex-players/non-players Mean ± SD	P
Walking PA (MET-min/week)	1437.02 ± 1959.75	1346.61 ± 1740.48	0.579
Moderate PA (MET-min/week)	443.66 ± 1184.71	433.52 ± 1178.05	0.928
Vigorous PA (MET-min/week)	678.04 ± 1313.33	866.95 ± 1750.31	0.187
Total PA (MET-min/week)	2508.83 ± 2947.37	2549.72 ± 3097.30	0.893

Significant positive increases in frequencies of staying outdoors and walking/jogging could not be observed in players who were relatively more active prior to playing Pokémon Go. Outdoor activities, walking or jogging could be already part of the regular daily activities of these players, therefore, they did not need to spend extra time to walk or jog outdoors intentionally as the players who used to be less active. Ex-players who never or rarely stayed outdoors before were found to stay outdoors more often to play the game, however, they did not walk or jog more often in order to catch Pokémon, to go to Pokéstops or Gyms, or to hatch eggs. Ex-players could be less interested in or enthusiastic about playing Pokémon Go, so they put less effort and quit finally. This was consistent with their significantly lower frequencies in walking/jogging when playing Pokémon Go, compared with the players.

In addition, we found that university students aged 18–25 years, who never or rarely stayed outdoors before and rarely walked/jogged before were more likely to play Pokémon Go, compared with students who were non-players. When we asked the non-players why they did not play the game, the majority stated that they were not interested or did not have time. The overall physical activity levels were determined by the total PA obtained from IPAQ which assessed a combination of walking, moderate and vigorous PA in the past seven days. In this study, there was no significant difference in the overall physical activity levels and total PA between players, ex-players and non-players. The non-players had the highest proportion of people (48.3%) having a moderate physical activity level and the lowest proportion of people having a low physical activity level (19.7%). The reasons behind were uncertain but it seemed that many non-players might participate in regular moderate exercise and they were not interested in Pokémon Go. Sometimes self-reported physical activity could be unreliable because of the possibility of recall bias and reporting bias by social desirability [12]. Some non-players could over-report their activity levels as they did not want to leave the impression that they did not play Pokémon Go because they were lazy to move. Further in-depth assessment is needed to collect more objective data on the types and durations of their exercise. The players group was found to have a higher walking PA than the ex-players/non-players group although there was no significant difference. Part of the walking PA could be attributed to the playing of Pokémon Go. In this study, walking, moderate and vigorous PA prior to playing Pokémon Go were not measured, however, a previous study found that playing Pokémon GO increased moderate to vigorous physical activity by about 50 min per week and reduced sedentary behavior by about 30 min per day [21].

According to the self-determination theory (SDT), autonomy, competence and relatedness were positively associated with enjoyment and preference for future play [15]. In Pokémon Go, an individual can take full control of the movement of his avatar. Collecting different Pokémon may provide people with optimal challenges and a feeling of success. Players can earn rewards every time they catch a Pokémon, put in effort to walk to a Pokéstop, as well as walking or jogging for a certain distance. With regard to relatedness needs, they can fight a battle with other players' Pokémon, and there are social media groups for sharing play strategies and locations where the rare Pokémon appear. It seems that Pokémon Go can satisfy the three psychological needs in SDT which are responsible for motivating people to continue playing the game; but 47% of the players had no idea how long they would continue playing the game.

One of the challenges of using computer and mobile games to promote health behaviors is that the game enthusiasm usually decreases with time [12]. Pokémon Go is still one of the most downloaded game apps in Apple's free downloads category three months after its release. However, it is possible that players will stop playing or play less often a few months later if they have collected all the Pokémon. A study found that instant enjoyment, exploration intention (exploration of the game environment) and attention demand (focus on the game) were predictors of interest of game players [32]. Enjoyment of the game was found to increase Pokémon Go players' physical activities outdoors [33]. Games with an internal social network which allows users to interact, post updates, spread content and comments on others' posts can help users to remain active and less likely to drop out of the games [34]. The study of the influence of social networks on user behavior in a physical activity tracking application found that the social network increased user offline real-world physical activity by 7% [34]. Researchers need to further explore motivators and appealing features and characteristics of mobile games for sustaining people to continue playing the game or at least for a longer period of time. Although an increase in physical activity could be found in some exergame players but many were short-term impact and there was no strong evidence to support that exergaming was a gateway to behavior change [35]. Identifying significant enjoyment predictors, game features and under what conditions mobile games can enhance behavior change are necessary.

There are some tricks and barriers that may limit the effects of Pokémon Go on players' physical activity. Players may cheat by taking slow-moving transportations like buses and trams to earn distances. Instead of walking, those who own a car can drive to Pokéstops. Other issues such as battery drain, running out of mobile data, GPS problems with inaccurate location, and body discomforts like leg tiredness, eye strain and neck pain, etc., can limit people's playing time. A common limitation in using smartphone games in health promotion, especially to the economically disadvantaged people, is the availabilities of a smartphone and mobile data. Elderly people and those with poor vision may also have difficulties in operating smartphones. Choosing budget smartphones with a large screen and a bigger keypad, and using economic data plans with slower data speed may help minimizing the problems.

The study population was limited to students in a local university and they are not representative to the general population. The time spent in walking/jogging activities and physical activity levels prior to playing the game was not studied because of the possibility of recall bias. The frequencies of and length of time in staying outdoors, walking and jogging, and other moderate and vigorous physical activities were self-reported by the respondents. There might be recall bias and the activity levels could also be over-reported because of social desirability effects. In future studies, the walking distances of players, ex-players and non-players need to be measured using distance measuring applications or pedometers while physical activity patterns can be recorded using accelerometers to obtain more precise data. Prior physical activities of players have to be recorded for comparison. Changes in BMI or body weight, and the extent of users replacing indoor activities with outdoor activities can also be studied to investigate the potential of incorporating Pokémon Go or similar AR games into exercise and weight management programs. The long-term impact of Pokémon Go on physical activity levels of the general population and motivators to sustain an active lifestyle can also be further explored.

Conclusions

This study showed that players who were used to being sedentary benefited the most from Pokémon Go. Players who never or rarely stayed outdoors or walked/jogged before significantly stay outdoors more frequently as well as walking/jogging more often in order to play Pokémon Go. However, substantial impact on physical activity levels of players could not be identified. A possible alternative to promote physical activity is to engage people in using tools and technology they currently possess and are familiar with, such as mobile devices and games [12]. Developing a mobile health app is costly and the testing usually takes a long time. As user satisfaction and interest on new exergames are uncertain, using existing popular apps is another option. A well-rounded physical activity should include aerobic exercise and

resistance training. Although Pokémon Go cannot be used to replace ordinary exercise as its benefits on cardio health are limited unless the players jog and walk briskly, it can be used as a starting point for sedentary people to begin an active lifestyle. The influence of Pokémon Go and other exergames on people's health can provide insights to public health workers in using novel strategies in health promotion.

Acknowledgements
The author would like to thank the students who participated in this study.

Competing interests
The authors declare that they have no competing interests.

References
1. WHO: Physical inactivity a leading cause of disease and disability, warns WHO. http://www.who.int/mediacentre/news/releases/release23/en/ (2002). Accessed 30 Oct 2016.
2. Centre for Health Protection: Statistics on behavioral risk factors, level of physical activity. Centre for Health Protection, HKSAR. http://www.chp.gov.hk/en/data/1/10/280/3998.html (2014). Accessed 30 Oct 2016.
3. Centre for Health Protection: Statistics on behavioral risk factors, level of physical activity. Centre for Health Protection, HKSAR. http://www.chp.gov.hk/en/data/4/10/280/246.html (2005). Accessed 30 Oct 2016.
4. WHO: Global recommendations on physical activity for health. WHO. http://www.who.int/dietphysicalactivity/physical-activity-recommendations-18-64years.pdf (2011). Accessed 30 Oct 2016.
5. Centre for Health Protection: Statistics on behavioral risk factors, television watching. Centre for Health Protection, HKSAR. http://www.chp.gov.hk/en/data/4/10/280/355.html (2008). Accessed 30 Oct 2016.
6. Ho M, Garnett SP, Baur LA, Burrows T, Stewart L, Neve M, et al. Impact of dietary and exercise interventions on weight change and metabolic outcomes in obese children and adolescents: a systematic review and meta-analysis of randomized trials. JAMA Pediatr. 2013;167:759–68.
7. WHO: Global Health Observatory (GHO) data. Overweight and obesity. http://www.who.int/gho/ncd/risk_factors/overweight/en/. Accessed 30 Oct 2016.
8. Monroe CM, Thompson DL, Bassett DR, Fitzhugh EC, Raynor HA. Usability of mobile phones in physical activity—related research: a systematic review. Am J Health Educ. 2015;46(4):196–206.
9. Patrick K, Raab F, Adams MA, Dillon L, Zabinski M, Rock CL, et al. A text message-based intervention for weight loss: randomized controlled trial. J Med Internet Res. 2009;11:e1.
10. Morak J, Schindler K, Goerzer E, Kastner P, Toplak H, Ludvik B, et al. A pilot study of mobile phone-based therapy for obese patients. J Telemed Telecare. 2008;14:147–9.
11. Garde A, Umedaly A, Abulnaga M, Robertson L, Junker A, Chanoine JP, et al. Assessment of a mobile game ("MobileKids Monster Manor") to promote physical activity among children. Games Health J. 2015;4:149–58.
12. Hswen Y, Murti V, Vormawor AA, Bhattacharjee R, Naslund JA. Virtual avatars, gaming, and social media: designing a mobile health app to help children choose healthier food options. J Mob Technol Med. 2013;2:8–14.
13. Li F. The exercise motivation scale: its multifaceted structure and construct validity. J Appl Sport Psychol. 1999;11:97–115.
14. Vallerand RJ, Losier GF. An integrative analysis of intrinsic and extrinsic motivation in sport. J Appl Sport Psychol. 1999;11:142–69.
15. Uysal A, Yildirim IG. Self-determination theory in digital games. In: Bostan B, editor. Gamer psychology and behavior, international series on computer entertainment and media technology. Basel: Springer; 2016. p. 123–35.

16. Deci EL, Ryan RM. Motivation, personality, and development within embedded social contexts: an overview of self-determination theory. In: Ryan RM, editor. The Oxford handbook of human motivation. New York: Oxford University Press; 2012. p. 85–107.

17. Pokemon Go: Nintendo. http://www.pokemon.com/us/pokemon-video-games/pokemon-go/ (2017). Accessed 3 Feb 2017.

18. Althoff T, White RW, Horvitz E. Influence of Pokémon Go on physical activity: study and implications. J Med Internet Res. 2016;18(12):e315.

19. Howe KB, Suharlim C, Ueda P, Howe D, Kawachi I, Rimm EB. Gotta catch'em all! Pokémon Go and physical activity among young adults: difference in differences study. BMJ. 2016;355:i6270.

20. LeBlanc AG, Chaput JP. Pokémon Go: a game changer for the physical inactivity crisis? Prev Med. 2016. doi:10.1016/j.ypmed.2016.11.012.

21. Nigg CR, Mateo DJ, An J. Pokémon Go may increase physical activity and decrease sedentary behaviors. Am J Public Health. 2017;107(1):37–8.

22. McCartney M. Game on for Pokémon Go. BMJ. 2016;354:i4306. doi:10.1136/bmj.i4306.

23. Serino M, Corfrey K, McLaughlin L, Milanaik RL. Pokémon Go and augmented virtual reality games: a cautionary commentary for parents and pediatricians. Curr Opin Pediatr. 2016;28(5):673–7.

24. Tunes Chart, Free Apps: Apple Inc. http://www.apple.com/itunes/charts/free-apps/ (2016). Accessed 30 Oct 2016.

25. Google Play Chart, Game Category: Google. https://play.google.com/store/apps/category/GAME/collection/topgrossing (2016). Accessed 30 Oct 2016.

26. Craig CL, Marshall AL, Sjöström M, Bauman AE, Booth ML, Ainsworth BE, et al. International physical activity questionnaire: 12-country reliability and validity. Med Sci Sports Exerc. 2003;35:1381–95.

27. Guidelines for data processing and analysis of the International Physical Activity Questionnaire (IPAQ)—Short and long forms. The IPAQ Group. https://sites.google.com/site/theipaq/scoring-protocol (2005). Accessed 3 Feb 2017.

28. Ainsworth BE, Haskell WL, Whitt MC, Irwin ML, Swarta AM, Strath SJ, et al. Compendium of physical activities: an update of activity codes and MET intensities. Med Sci Sports Exerc. 2000;32(Suppl):S498–516.

29. de Souto Barreto P. Global health agenda on non-communicable diseases: has WHO set a smart goal for physical activity? BMJ. 2015;350:h23.

30. Moore SC, Patel AV, Matthews CE, de Gonzalez AB, Park Y, Katki HA, et al. Leisure time physical activity of moderate to vigorous intensity and mortality: a large pooled cohort analysis. PLoS Med. 2012;9:e1001335.

31. Nagai M, Kuriyama S, Kakizaki M, Ohmori-Matsuda K, Sone T, Hozawa A, et al. Impact of walking on life expectancy and lifetime medical expenditure: the Ohsaki Cohort Study. BMJ Open. 2011;1:e000240.

32. Pasco D, Roure C, Kermarrec G, Pope Z, Gao Z. The effects of a bike active video game on players' physical activity and motivation. J Sport Health Sci. 2016. doi:10.1016/j.jshs.2016.11.007.

33. Zach FJ, Tussyadiah IP. To catch them all—the (un)intended consequences of Pokémon GO on mobility, consumption, and wellbeing. In: Information and communication technologies in tourism 2017. Proceedings of the international conference in Rome, Italy, January 24–36; 2017. p. 217–27. doi:10.1007/978-3-319-51168-9_16.

34. Althoff T, Jindal P, Leskovec J. Online actions with offline impact: how online social networks influence online and offline user behavior. In: WSDM' 17. Cambridge, UK—Feb 06–10; 2017. Proceedings of the Tenth ACM international conference on web search and data mining. p 537–46. doi:10.1145/3018661.3018672. Accessed 3 Feb 2017.

35. Baranowski T. Exergaming: hope for future physical activity? Or blight on mankind? J Sport Health Sci. 2016. doi:10.1016/j.jshs.2016.11.006.

Current and future distribution of *Aedes aegypti* and *Aedes albopictus* (Diptera: Culicidae) in WHO Eastern Mediterranean Region

Els Ducheyne[1*] , Nhu Nguyen Tran Minh[2], Nabil Haddad[3], Ward Bryssinckx[1], Evans Buliva[2], Frédéric Simard[4], Mamunur Rahman Malik[2], Johannes Charlier[1], Valérie De Waele[1], Osama Mahmoud[5], Muhammad Mukhtar[6], Ali Bouattour[7], Abdulhafid Hussain[8], Guy Hendrickx[1] and David Roiz[2,4]

Abstract

Background: *Aedes*-borne diseases as dengue, zika, chikungunya and yellow fever are an emerging problem worldwide, being transmitted by *Aedes aegypti* and *Aedes albopictus*. Lack of up to date information about the distribution of *Aedes* species hampers surveillance and control. Global databases have been compiled but these did not capture data in the WHO Eastern Mediterranean Region (EMR), and any models built using these datasets fail to identify highly suitable areas where one or both species may occur. The first objective of this study was therefore to update the existing *Ae. aegypti* (Linnaeus, 1762) and *Ae. albopictus* (Skuse, 1895) compendia and the second objective was to generate species distribution models targeted to the EMR. A final objective was to engage the WHO points of contacts within the region to provide feedback and hence validate all model outputs.

Methods: The *Ae. aegypti* and *Ae. albopictus* compendia provided by Kraemer et al. (Sci Data 2:150035, 2015; Dryad Digit Repos, 2015) were used as starting points. These datasets were extended with more recent species and disease data. In the next step, these sets were filtered using the Köppen–Geiger classification and the Mahalanobis distance. The occurrence data were supplemented with pseudo-absence data as input to Random Forests. The resulting suitability and maximum risk of establishment maps were combined into hard-classified maps per country for expert validation.

Results: The EMR datasets consisted of 1995 presence locations for *Ae. aegypti* and 2868 presence locations for *Ae. albopictus*. The resulting suitability maps indicated that there exist areas with high suitability and/or maximum risk of establishment for these disease vectors in contrast with previous model output. Precipitation and host availability, expressed as population density and night-time lights, were the most important variables for *Ae. aegypti*. Host availability was the most important predictor in case of *Ae. albopictus*. Internal validation was assessed geographically. External validation showed high agreement between the predicted maps and the experts' extensive knowledge of the terrain.

Conclusion: Maps of distribution and maximum risk of establishment were created for *Ae. aegypti* and *Ae. albopictus* for the WHO EMR. These region-specific maps highlighted data gaps and these gaps will be filled using targeted monitoring and surveillance. This will increase the awareness and preparedness of the different countries for *Aedes* borne diseases.

Keywords: *Aedes*, *Aedes aegypti*, *Aedes albopictus*, Distribution, Chikungunya, Dengue, Spatial model, Surveillance, Yellow fever, Zika

*Correspondence: educheyne@avia-gis.com
[1] Avia-GIS, Zoersel, Belgium
Full list of author information is available at the end of the article

Background

Aedes-borne diseases (dengue, chikungunya, yellow fever and zika) are an emerging problem worldwide, escalating overall risk and burden of disease worldwide [3]. Lack of up to date and more precise *Aedes* distributional data and potential distributional modelling hampers effective vector surveillance and control. This is particularly true in the WHO Eastern Mediterranean Region (EMR), a region which includes Afghanistan, Bahrain, Djibouti, Egypt, Iraq, Iran, Jordan, Kuwait, Lebanon, Libya, Morocco, Oman, Pakistan, Palestine, Qatar, Saudi Arabia, Somalia, Sudan, Syria, Tunisia, United Arab Emirates and Yemen (Fig. 1). Detailed information about disease burden and the current and potential spatial distribution of *Aedes* vectors in the EMR is scarce. Humphrey et al. [4] listed the available information about dengue incidence and country scale vector distribution in the region.

Therefore, there is a clear need to focus on this area, especially in the light of the recent zika virus (ZIKV) pandemic. Even though none of the EMR countries had any reported ZIKV transmission, the risk of autochthonous zika transmission in the EMR, especially on the Red Sea rim and Pakistan, following introduction from endemic countries, cannot be overlooked.

Given the wide spread distribution and the abundance of *Aedes aegypti* and the reported cases of dengue, chikungunya and yellow fever, Tran Minh et al. [5] assumed that the potential risk of disease outbreaks is high in at least eight of the EMR countries: Djibouti, Egypt, Oman, Pakistan, Saudi Arabia, Somalia, Sudan and Yemen. Furthermore, in recent years the invasive vector *Aedes*

albopictus has spread in some countries, such as Lebanon [6] and Morocco [7], but the available occurrence database is not updated. The first objective of this study is therefore to build an up to date comprehensive dataset of observed presences of both *Aedes aegypti* (Linnaeus, 1762) and *Aedes albopictus* (Skuse, 1895) for the EMR.

Existing spatial distribution models for the two *Aedes* species can currently only be extracted from global modelling outputs [8–10]. In these models, observed presence data are strongly biased in favour of the Americas, the Indian subcontinent, South-East Asia and Europe, and the predicted probability for the EMR may therefore not reflect the actual situation. This bias is supported by the case of the TigerMaps models [11]. These models were based only on Mediterranean data, indicating a higher risk of occurrence of *Ae. albopictus* in Northern Africa as compared to any of the previously-mentioned global models. The second objective in this study is therefore to produce a new set of habitat suitability maps for *Ae. aegypti* and *Ae. albopictus* focused on the EMR. These maps will depict areas of potential introduction and maximum risk of establishment. Kraemer et al. [1, 2] compiled a global database of observed occurrences of *Ae. aegypti* and *Ae. albopictus*. These models improve our knowledge of the species' distribution globally and provide insight into environmental dependencies. On the other hand, model output can be biased when target area environmental conditions are not properly captured in the training set. Given that in Kraemer's data less than 1% of the observed points fall geographically within the EMR, a similarity mask was created to include

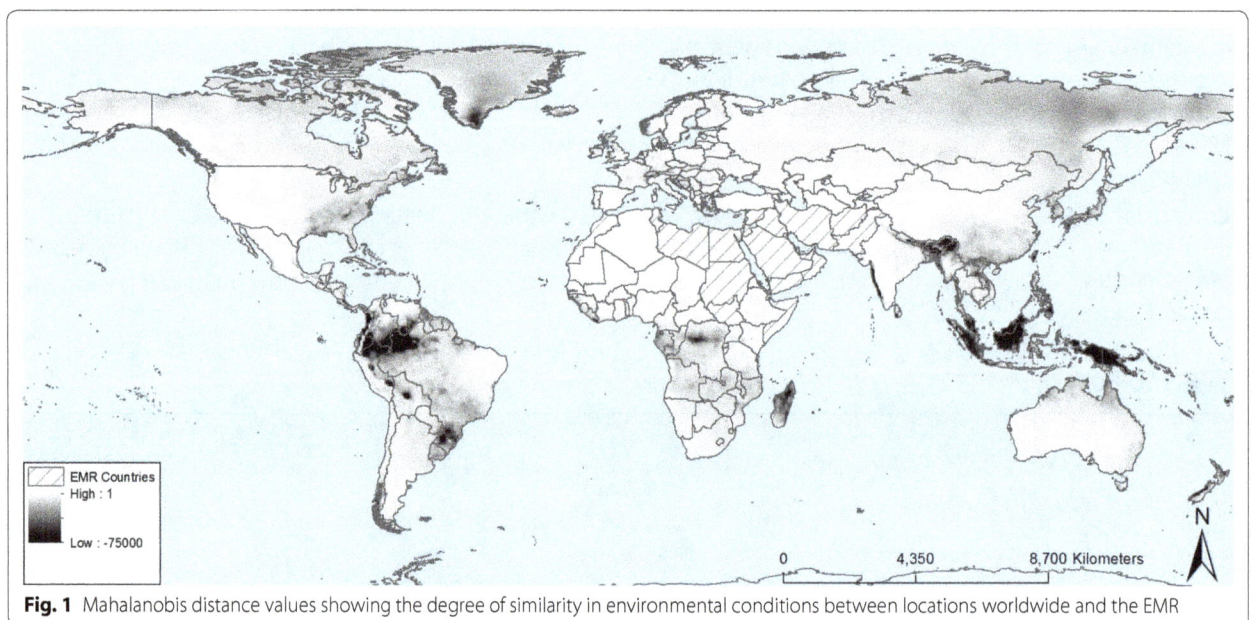

Fig. 1 Mahalanobis distance values showing the degree of similarity in environmental conditions between locations worldwide and the EMR

occurrence data only from areas similar in environmental conditions to the EMR.

Methods

Study area

The EMR has 22 member states/territories: Afghanistan, Bahrain, Djibouti, Egypt, Iraq, Iran, Jordan, Kuwait, Lebanon, Libya, Morocco, Oman, Pakistan, Palestine, Qatar, Saudi Arabia, Somalia, Sudan, Syria, Tunisia, United Arab Emirates and Yemen (Fig. 1). Many countries in the EMR are particularly vulnerable to communicable disease epidemics, because they are experiencing numerous environmental and social stresses, including armed conflicts, water scarcity, food insecurity, rapid population growth

and urbanization. Therefore, these countries often have weak governing institutions and health systems [12], although there does exist a large variability in the EMR.

Training data

First, the Köppen–Geiger classes [13] per EMR country were determined. A binary classification resulted in a mask where value 1 represents all areas globally with one of the classes found in the EMR countries and value 0 where the condition was not met. Secondly, the Mahalanobis distance was calculated using the set of environmental predictors listed in Table 1. The Mahalanobis distance is a unit-less and scale invariant similarity measure. Its value will increase when the

Table 1 Overview of the environmental and eco-climatic predictor variables used in spatial distribution modelling of *Ae. aegypti* and *Ae. albopictus* in the EMR

Data layer	Description	Resolution (km)	Units	Origin
Altitude	Elevation above sea level	5 × 5	m	WorldClim[a]
BIO1	Annual mean temperature	5 × 5	°C	WorldClim
BIO2	Mean diurnal range (mean of monthly (max temp − min temp))	5 × 5	°C	WorldClim
BIO3	Isothermality (BIO2/BIO7) (× 100)	5 × 5	%	WorldClim
BIO4	Temperature seasonality (standard deviation × 100)	5 × 5	%	WorldClim
BIO5	Max temperature of warmest month	5 × 5	°C	WorldClim
BIO6	Min temperature of coldest month	5 × 5	°C	WorldClim
BIO7	Temperature annual range (BIO5−BIO6)	5 × 5 km	°C	WorldClim
BIO8	Mean temperature of wettest quarter	5 × 5	°C	WorldClim
BIO9	Mean temperature of driest quarter	5 × 5	°C	WorldClim
BIO10	Mean temperature of warmest quarter	5 × 5	°C	WorldClim
BIO11	Mean temperature of coldest quarter	5 × 5	°C	WorldClim
BIO12	Annual precipitation	5 × 5	mm	WorldClim
BIO13	Precipitation of wettest month	5 × 5	mm	WorldClim
BIO14	Precipitation of driest month	5 × 5	mm	WorldClim
BIO15	Precipitation seasonality (coefficient of variation)	5 × 5	%	WorldClim
BIO16	Precipitation of wettest quarter	5 × 5	mm	WorldClim
BIO17	Precipitation of driest quarter	5 × 5	mm	WorldClim
BIO18	Precipitation of warmest quarter	5 × 5	mm	WorldClim
BIO19	Precipitation of coldest quarter	5 × 5	mm	WorldClim
Fourier transforms of T_{max}, T_{mean} and T_{min}	Amplitudes 1, 2, and 3	50 × 50	°C	EDENext[b]
	Phases 1, 2, and 3	50 × 50	Day of year	EDENext
Fourier transforms of precipitation	Amplitudes 1, 2 and 3	50 × 50	mm	EDENext
	Phases 1, 2, and 3	50 × 50	Day of year	EDENext
Night-time light	Night-time light	5 × 5	Unit-less	DMSP—NASA[c]
Average NDVI	Global annual sum NDVI	5 × 5	Unit-less	LADA[d]
Human population	Population density grid	5 × 5	Persons/pixel	SEDAC[e]

[a] http://www.worldclim.org/bioclim

[b] http://www.edenextdata.com

[c] http://ngdc.noaa.gov/eog/dmsp/downloadV4composites.html

[d] http://www.fao.org/geonetwork

[e] http://sedac.ciesin.columbia.edu/data/set/grump-v1-population-density/data-download

environmental conditions become more and more different than those observed in the target area.

The cut off for similarity pixels was set to the 99% percentile of the Mahalanobis distance within the Köppen–Geiger EMR mask. This procedure retained 1351 out of 17,280 entries for *Ae. albopictus* and 1938 out of 13,991 for *Ae. aegypti* (Additional file 2: Fig. S1).

To extend the dataset with data collected specifically in the EMR, additional *Ae. albopictus* presence/absence data from Lebanon were provided by one of the co-authors (N.H.): 186 locations were sampled during summer 2015 for *Ae. albopictus* presence in Lebanon, and the mosquito was found at 73 of them (unpublished data).

In addition, a literature review and personal communications with entomologists and environmental health officers in the EMR provided further presence locations for both *Ae. aegypti* and *Ae. albopictus* and for *Aedes*-borne disease outbreaks (we excluded seroprevalence studies) in the region of interest. This data set is provided as Additional file 1.

The current compiled data sources contain only observed occurrence data of *Ae. aegypti* and *Ae. albopictus*, except for Lebanon where absence data for *Ae. albopictus* was collected. Many modelling techniques require both occurrence and absence data as input data, except for presence-only modelling techniques such as MaxEnt [14]. While these occurrence-only models have proven their value for species distribution modelling in general [15] and *Aedes* modelling more specifically [16, 17], we feel that including simulated absence data, also called pseudo-absence data, would strengthen the model output. This is not only because extra information is added to the training set but also because the range of modelling techniques that can be used is much wider.

A surface range envelope (SRE) presence-only model was used to define the area suitable for both species together. Pseudo-absences were then generated randomly outside this area within the Köppen–Geiger/Mahalanobis EMR mask as a point shapefile without a minimum distance criterion [18]. SRE models were based on the presence training data included in the Mahalanobis distance mask using the BIOMOD package in R [19]. The suitable area was restricted by removing 1.25, 2.5 and 5% of the outer values in each of the environmental predictor variable envelopes. This yielded three different training datasets per species. The number of pseudo-absences that was generated was set equal to the number of presence data to obtain a balanced training dataset and avoid bias towards predicting presence or absence. No pseudo-absences were generated for Lebanon since absence locations were already available. The final absence dataset consisted of the generated pseudo-absences and the balanced subset of absence locations in Lebanon.

Environmental predictor data

From literature, temperature is a crucial factor limiting the distribution of *Ae. aegypti* and *Ae. albopictus*. Other listed variables include altitude, rainfall as well as land-use and anthropogenic factors. The predictor variable dataset was collated from a variety of sources and included both ground-measured and remotely-sensed data (Table 1).

All variables, except the Fourier transforms, were available at a spatial resolution of 5 × 5 km. The Fourier MODIS images were processed according to Scharlemann et al. [20] over the period of 2001–2012 and were available from the EDENext data archive (http://www.edenextdata.com/). These Fourier variables were downscaled using spatial inverse distance weighted interpolation. The interpolation results were assigned to 5 × 5 km pixels based on the average of the 12 nearest locations in the grid. A 5 × 5 km resolution land mask was then applied to obtain a fine-resolution border between land and water bodies (Additional file 3: Fig. S2).

Species distribution modelling

The suitability models were generated using Random Forests (RF) [21]. RF is a powerful data mining tool that can model complex interactions between different predictor variables and determine variable importance with great classification accuracy [22]. RF is a mixture of tree predictors that are randomly constructed by bootstrapping from the complete dataset with replacement but having the same distribution as the full dataset. Random forests of 1000 trees were trained using the VECMAP software (http://www.vecmap.com). Six predictor variables were randomly selected at each node to split it into two new branches. Given that the input data sets were balanced, the cut-off value to differentiate between suitable and unsuitable habitats is 0.5.

Variable importance was assessed using the Gini impurity criterion. The smaller the Gini impurity index, the more accurate the classification of the pixel. The Gini impurity index may therefore be very low when nodes are split by variables that are highly correlated with the species' probability of occurrence. During the training process, random subsets of predictor variables were considered for each split and each time the variable with the lowest Gini impurity index was chosen. To assess variable importance, the mean decrease in the Gini impurity index in each variable as compared the other variables in the model was calculated.

Although individual classification trees in a RF model are grown based on random subsets of training data, all available data was fed into the training process of our random forest model. The estimated habitat suitability for *Ae. aegypti* and *Ae. albopictus* therefore represents overall agreement by the training dataset to classify an area as suitable or unsuitable for the species. Subsets of the training data can, however, reveal extreme cases, i.e., areas where only a part of the training data would classify the area as suitable. These areas are characterized by environmental and anthropogenic conditions that are not ideal for the species but may be deemed sufficient for them to survive. To consider these extreme areas, 100 subsets of the random forest model, each containing 10 trees, were assessed and the maximum value of each pixel was retained.

Internal and external validation

The standard deviation per pixel of these 100 subsets of the random forest model, each containing 10 trees, was assessed to evaluate model uncertainty, permitting a more geographically based assessment of model uncertainty instead of using overall performance indices. A high pixel value represents large variability in the modelled probabilities of occurrence and therefore greater uncertainty. Pixels with small values indicate that many model repetitions estimated a similar probability of occurrence and therefore represent locations for which the model outcome is more robust.

To externally validate the model outputs, we contacted the WHO EMR point of contacts for every country in the region. To facilitate the interpretation, the four maps per country (current and maximum risk of establishment for *Ae. aegypti* and *Ae. albopictus* respectively) were combined into a single map. This map was obtained by hard classifying the suitable and maximum risk of

establishment maps with a threshold of 0.5. This means that if the probability is higher than 0.5 a value of 1 (current) and 2 (maximum risk of establishment) respectively was attributed. In the next step, the maps were combined and the maximum value of each map was retained in the final output.

The experts were asked to assess the model output by indicating areas that are of interest either because they confirm what was found during surveillance activities that were not yet reported or conversely because they show a mismatch between the predicted suitability and the observed suitability. The areas of agreement and disagreement where annotated on the maps and digitized. This was used as input for a confusion matrix with a random sample of 2000 pixels were used to quantify the experts' opinions, and the following accuracy indices were calculated: Percent Correctly Classified (PCC), Cohen's index of agreement κ and the sensitivity and specificity per class.

Results

Training data

Following the literature review and the expertise of entomologists in the region, the presence of *Aedes aegypti* was confirmed in several countries of the EMR: Djibouti, Egypt, Oman, Pakistan, Saudi Arabia, Somalia, Sudan, and Yemen (Fig. 2). The presence of *Ae. albopictus* was confirmed in Iran, Jordan, Lebanon, Morocco, Pakistan and Syria (Fig. 3). The two species were detected in nearby regions that are not part of the EMR, such as *Ae. aegypti* in Israel and Turkey and *Ae. albopictus* in

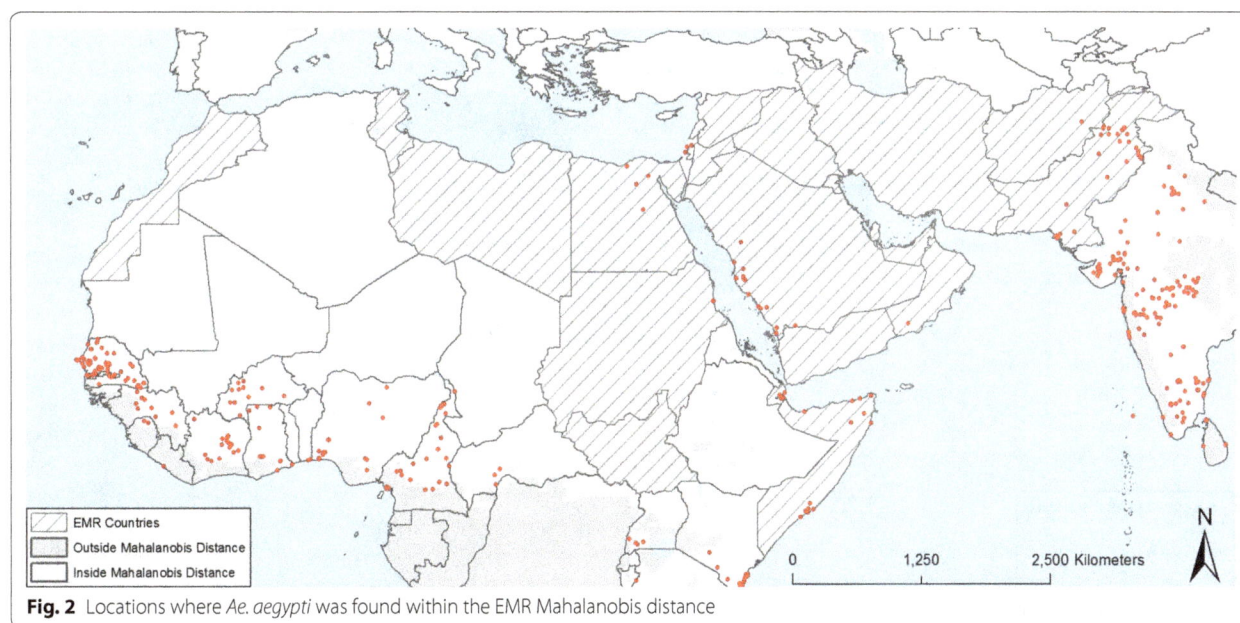

Fig. 2 Locations where *Ae. aegypti* was found within the EMR Mahalanobis distance

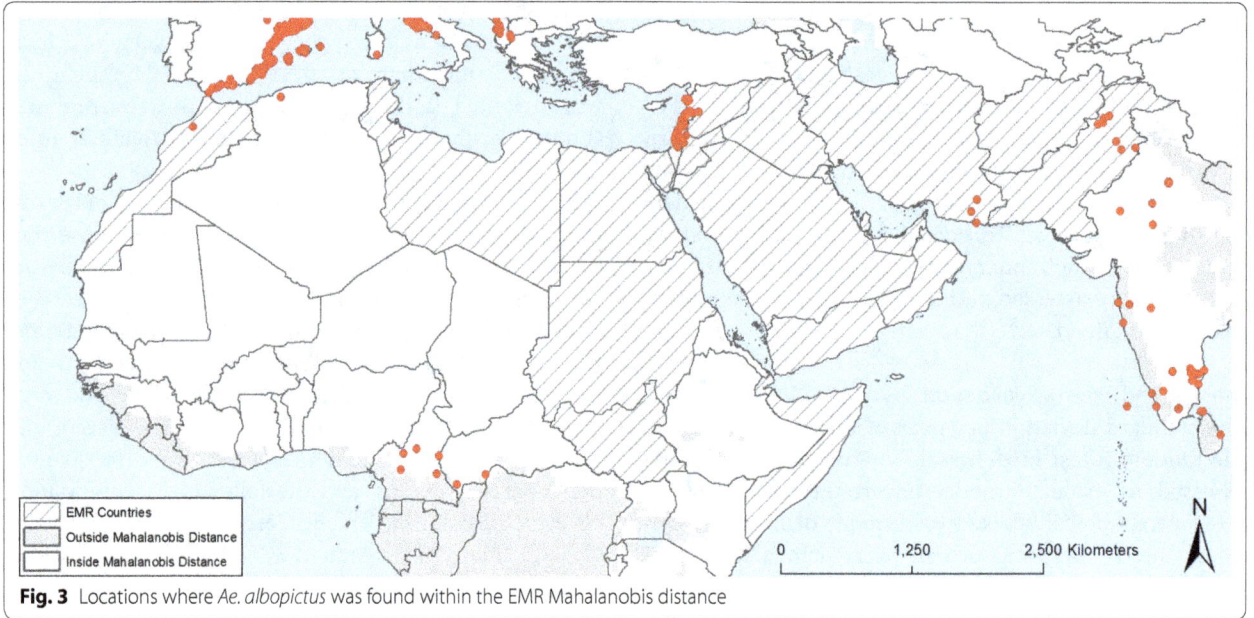

Fig. 3 Locations where *Ae. albopictus* was found within the EMR Mahalanobis distance

Algeria, Israel and Turkey. Dengue was reported in Djibouti, Egypt, Pakistan, Saudi Arabia, Somalia, Sudan and Yemen. Imported dengue cases were reported in Oman and Iran. Chikungunya was reported in Djibouti, Pakistan, Saudi Arabia, Somalia and Yemen, and yellow fever in Sudan. So far, no zika infection was reported in the EMR [3].

Based on this information, the resulting dataset included 1995 locations for *Ae. aegypti* and 2868 presence

locations for *Ae. albopictus* within the boundaries of the Mahalanobis distance mask.

Species distribution modelling

The distribution model and maximum risk of establishments are shown in Figs. 4, 5, 6, 7, 8 and 9.

The predicted probabilities of establishment and spread of *Ae. aegypti* in the EMR are displayed in Figs. 4 and 5, respectively. The first map shows areas of high probability

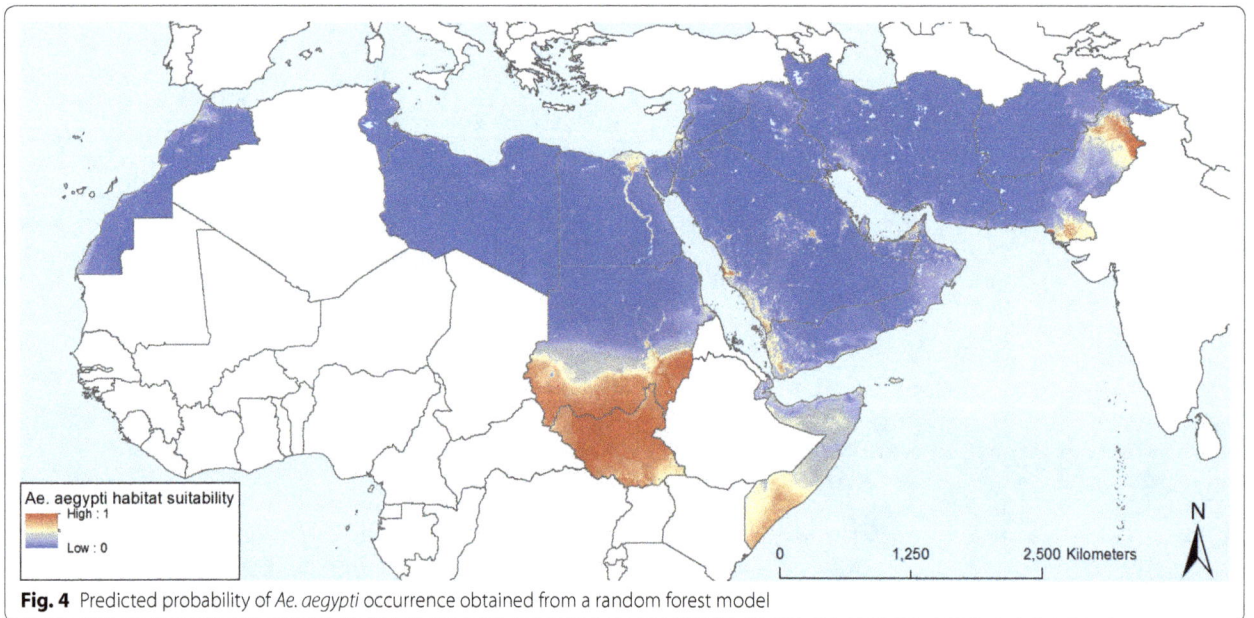

Fig. 4 Predicted probability of *Ae. aegypti* occurrence obtained from a random forest model

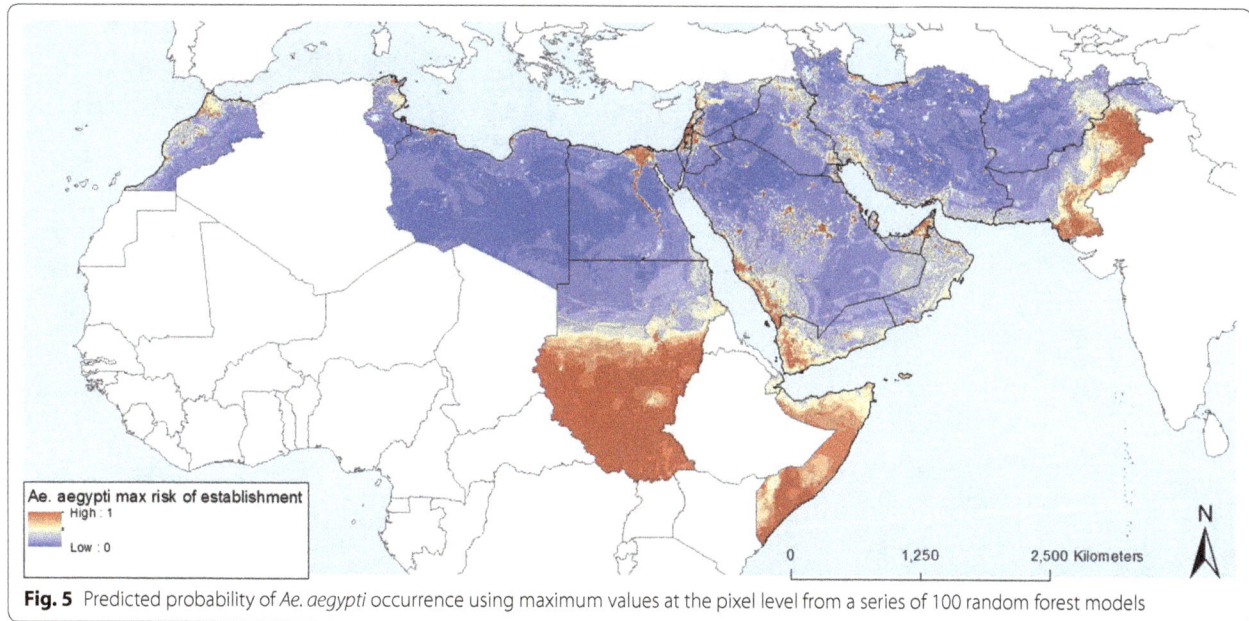

Fig. 5 Predicted probability of *Ae. aegypti* occurrence using maximum values at the pixel level from a series of 100 random forest models

of occurrence, these being the southern areas of Somalia and Sudan, South Sudan (not part of EMR), the Nile delta in Egypt, the Red Sea border of Saudi Arabia and Yemen, and Pakistan. Areas suitable for maximum risk of establishment are highlighted in Fig. 5. These areas are Morocco, the Mediterranean Sea border of Tunisia, Libya and Egypt, Palestine, Lebanon, Syria and countries around the Red Sea rim and the Persian Gulf. This highlights that all EMR countries are suitable for *Ae. aegypti* establishment. The uncertainty map in Fig. 6a shows areas with a high standard deviation of model predictions. Among these are areas in Morocco and Oman and a band between Iraq and Iran that was not identified as being suitable in the distribution model. The signal to noise map (Fig. 6b) indicates that the noise is highest in the south of Sudan, which could be attributed to forested areas.

The predicted probabilities of *Ae. albopictus* occurrence in the EMR are shown in Figs. 7 and 8, which map areas of suitability and maximum risk of establishment, respectively. The maps highlight the fact that all EMR countries have areas suitable for the *Ae. albopictus*. They also confirm field observations in Morocco, Palestine, Jordan, Lebanon, Syria and Pakistan. Both maps show patchy zones of higher probability, corresponding to urbanized areas. Suitable regions with a high probability of establishment were also found in countries that, so far have not reported any occurrence such as Tunisia, Libya, Egypt, Iraq, United Arab Emirates, Saudi Arabia (southwestern region), and Yemen. Figure 8 indicates where the maximum risk of establishment of *Ae. albopictus* could

be found. This includes the Nile delta in Egypt, the southern zones of South Sudan (outside EMR) and Somalia, and eastern Afghanistan. A map of uncertainty associated with the predictions for *Ae. albopictus* is presented in Fig. 9a. In the case of *Ae. albopictus* the noise is highest at the Mediterranean coast.

The random forest models show that the distributions of both *Aedes* species are highly influenced by demographic and climatic factors. Their relative importance is illustrated in Figs. 10 and 11 for *Ae. aegypti* and *Ae. albopictus*, respectively.

The five most important variables for *Ae. aegypti* were all related to precipitation and host availability, expressed as population density and night-time lights. The temperature variables scored less and ranked between rank five and rank ten. In case of *Aedes albopictus*, urbanisation was the most important factor, determined by population density and night-time lights. This is followed by temperature and precipitation.

Internal and external validation

We received feedback from Tunisia, Oman, Pakistan and Somalia. Feedback from Somalia could not be quantified, as the points of contacts generally confirmed the findings but did not indicate any regions or disagreement. The accuracy indices of Tunisia, Oman and Pakistan are listed in Table 2. The accuracy expressed as Percent Correctly Classified is very high in all cases. Similarly, Cohen's index of agreement κ can be classified as near perfect according to the benchmark categories defined by Landis and Koch [23]. The sensitivity and specificity

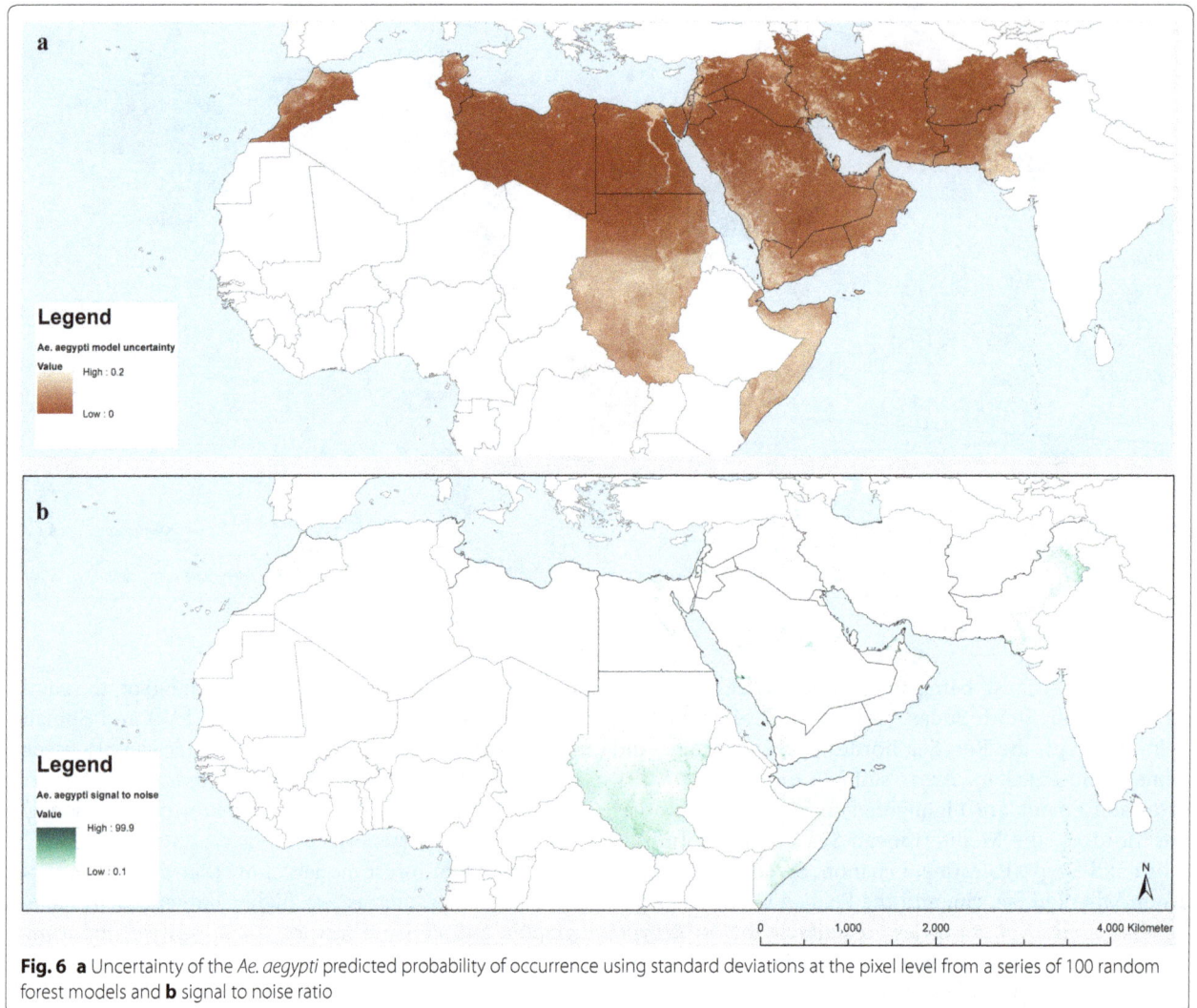

Fig. 6 a Uncertainty of the *Ae. aegypti* predicted probability of occurrence using standard deviations at the pixel level from a series of 100 random forest models and **b** signal to noise ratio

measures indicate that there exists a good discrimination between the classes 0 (not suitable) on the one hand and the classes 1 and 2 (current suitability and maximum risk of establishment) on the other hand. Between the two classes there is confusion, mostly pixels that are considered maximum risk of establishment whereas they are currently suitable.

Discussion

The distributions of *Ae. aegypti* and *Ae. albopictus* are, as expected, highly influenced by precipitation, demographic factors and temperature [24, 25]. Night-time light and human population density are among the most

important predictor variables for both *Aedes* species. Night-time light indicate urbanisation and both species are container-breeders within an urban environment [26]. Additionally, as both species are anthropophilic, with *Ae. albopictus* being the most opportunistic [27], human population indicates host availability.

The relative importance of precipitation is highly pronounced for *Ae. aegypti*, for which the importance of precipitation amplitude 3 and the precipitation of the wettest month is comparable to that of demographic factors. In comparison to other studies [16, 17], the variable importance of precipitation variables seems higher. We must bear in mind that the EMR is an arid area with shortages

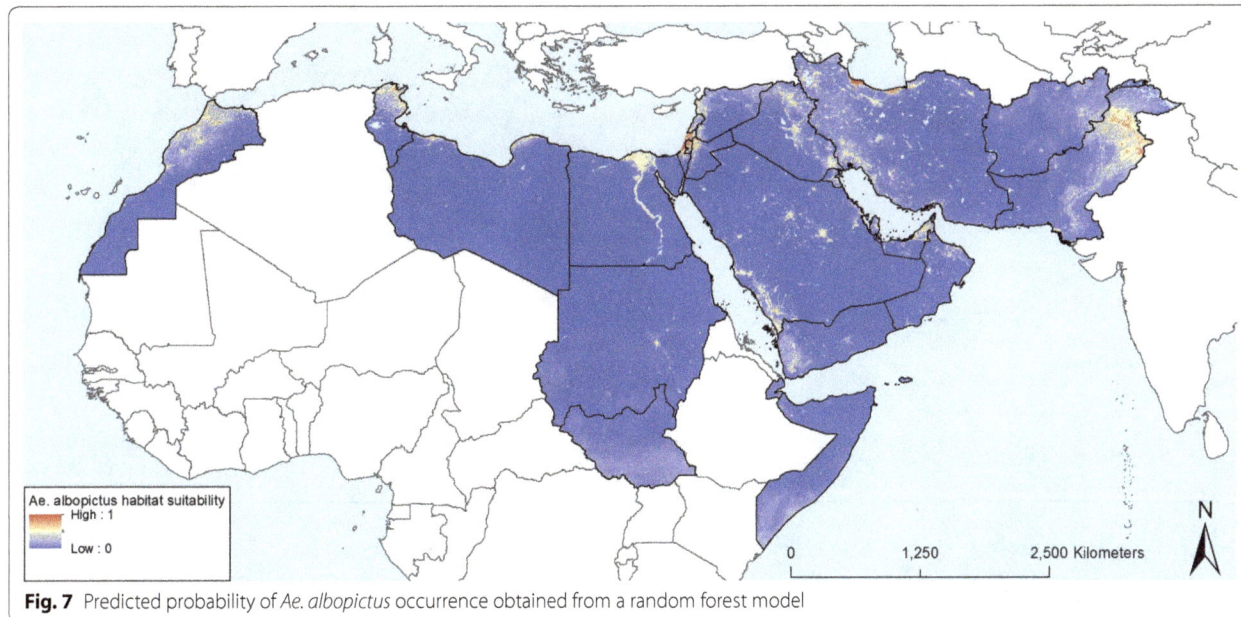

Fig. 7 Predicted probability of *Ae. albopictus* occurrence obtained from a random forest model

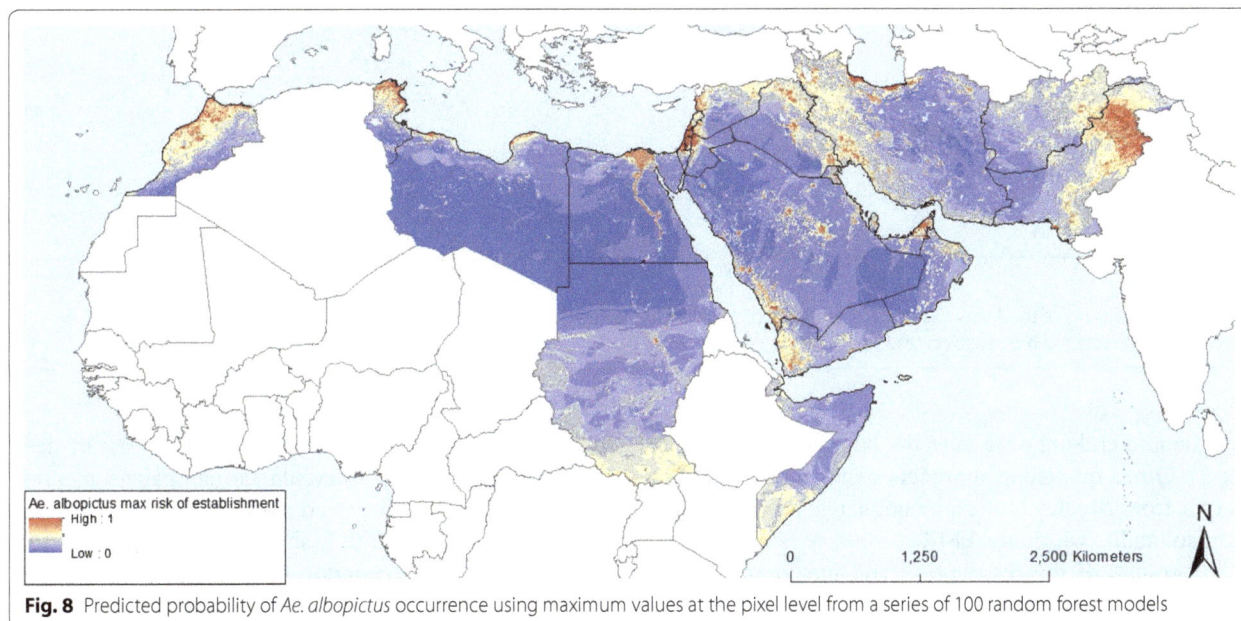

Fig. 8 Predicted probability of *Ae. albopictus* occurrence using maximum values at the pixel level from a series of 100 random forest models

in water supply. Therefore, precipitation may be more important than in other areas. These results highlight the fact that different key limit factors must be more relevant in different geographical areas, as suggested by Cunze et al. [28]. Altitude is included in the model in contrast to the study by Rochlin et al. [29] where this was irrelevant.

When the EMR specific model output is contrasted to the model output generated by Kraemer et al. [1]

(Figs. 12, 13) it is clear that the models differ especially in urban areas within the EMR. Whilst this might be considered a small spatial difference, it has serious implications in terms of vector-borne disease management. Indeed, these areas are where the highest population density can be found so if vectors and/or pathogens are introduced within these high probability areas this might lead to outbreaks, as confirmed by the reported cases of

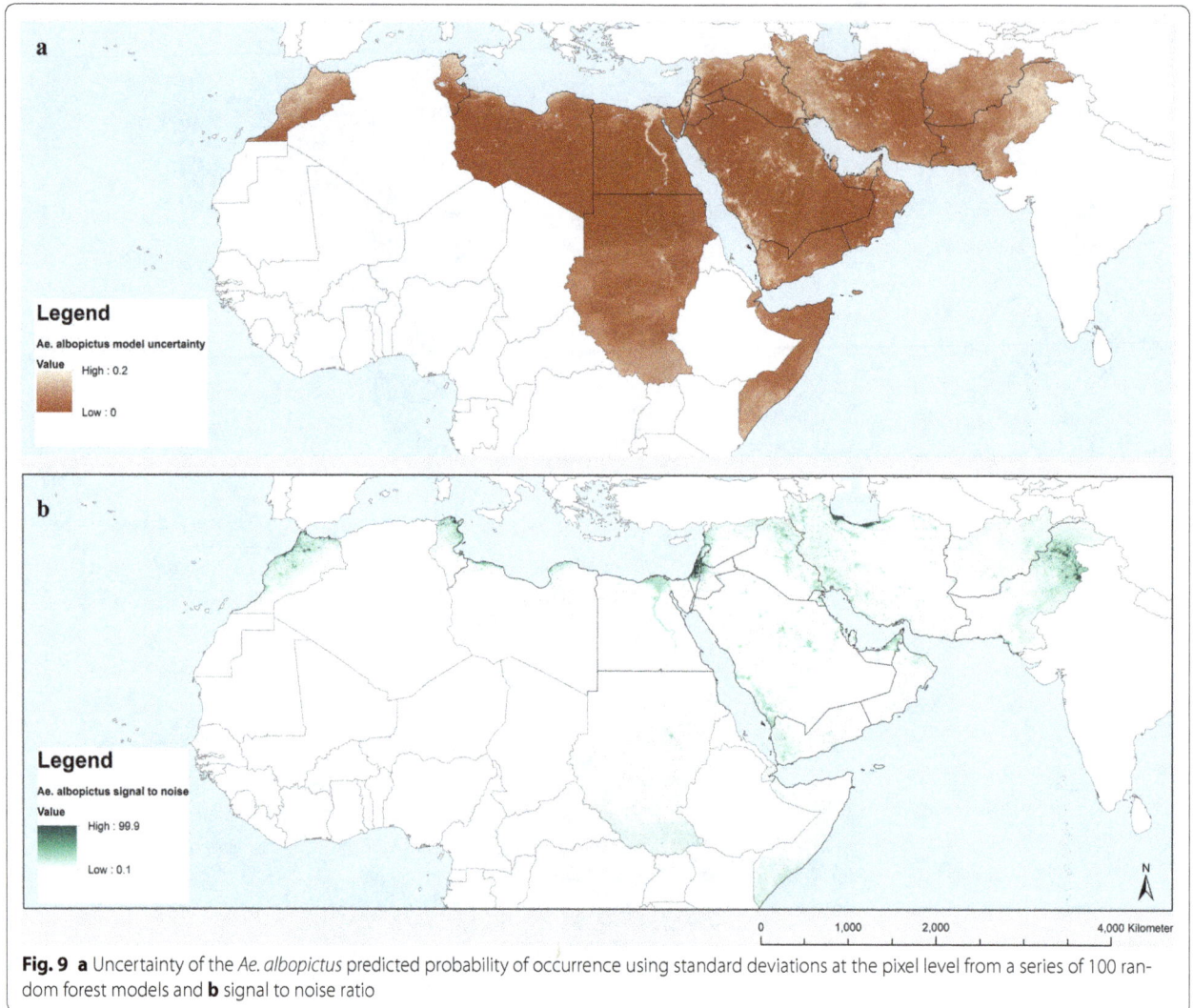

Fig. 9 a Uncertainty of the *Ae. albopictus* predicted probability of occurrence using standard deviations at the pixel level from a series of 100 random forest models and **b** signal to noise ratio

dengue and chikungunya over the last years (Additional file 1). Other modelling approaches such as the MaxEnt output from Medley [16] even completely failed to highlight suitability within the EMR.

The results of the distribution and maximum risk of establishment models show that there are numerous areas with suitable habitats for *Ae. aegypti* and *Ae. albopictus* throughout the EMR, although few field data are available for the region. Monitoring these areas will help detecting introduction of the species in areas that are generally regarded as less suitable for the species. This also includes reintroduction, as *Ae. aegypti* was widely distributed in the Mediterranean during the last century [30].

We cannot exclude that these other areas within the EMR have already been invaded, as there is little information available on *Ae. aegypti* and *Ae. albopictus* in the EMR. Therefore, increasing *Aedes* and *Aedes*-borne disease entomological and epidemiological surveillance

in the area is a priority. While there is an urgent need to undertake periodic surveillance campaigns in areas that are currently considered suitable for maximum risk of establishment, attention should also be paid to surveillance at larger population centres, at Points of Entry (PoE) for *Aedes*, such as harbours, roads and ground-crossings, and for *Aedes*-borne diseases and viruses, at airports and ports and larger urban areas.

As a first step towards capacity building for entomological surveillance in the area, training courses and guidelines for improving *Aedes* and *Aedes*-borne disease surveillance and control have been developed by the WHO Regional Office for the Eastern Mediterranean. However, it is also important to raise awareness of the key elements that affect habitat suitability for mosquitoes, especially in urban areas, such as unprotected storage of drinking water.

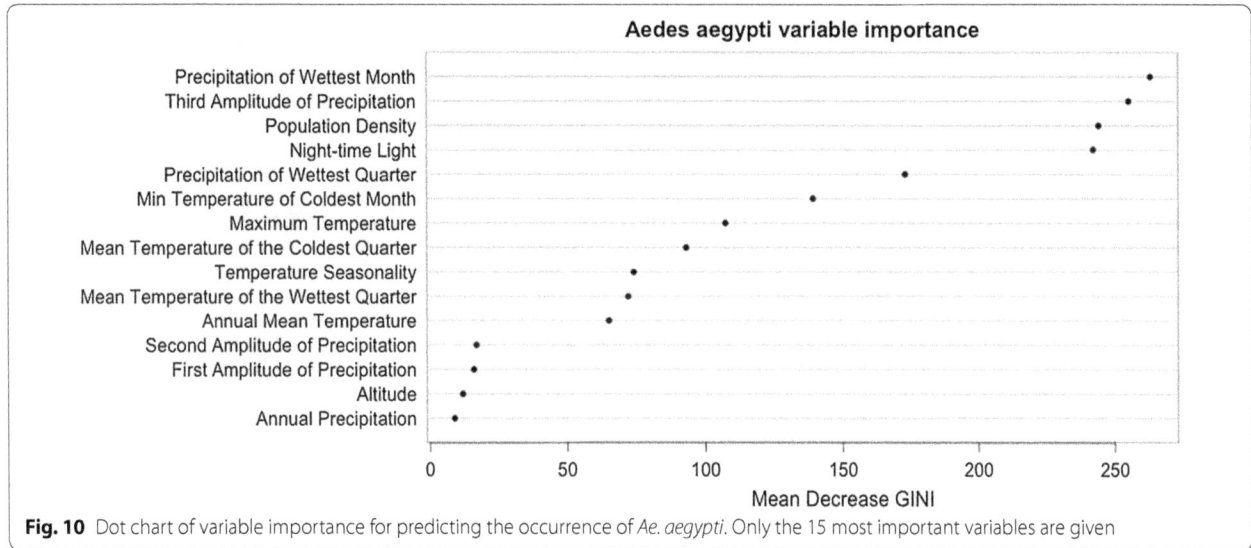

Fig. 10 Dot chart of variable importance for predicting the occurrence of *Ae. aegypti*. Only the 15 most important variables are given

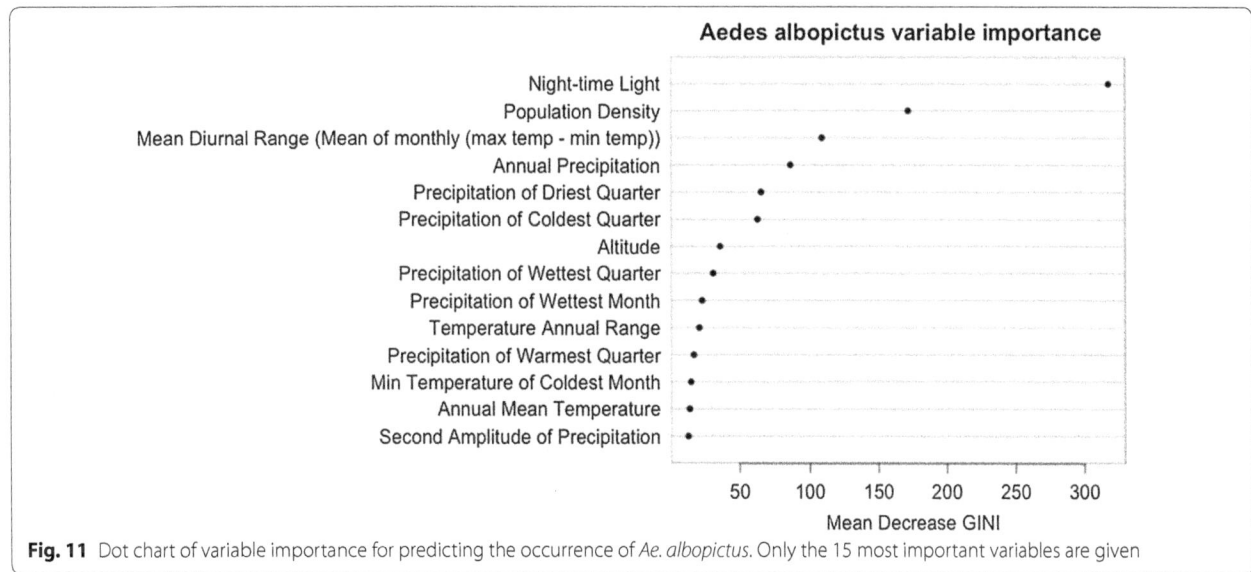

Fig. 11 Dot chart of variable importance for predicting the occurrence of *Ae. albopictus*. Only the 15 most important variables are given

Table 2 Results of the country-based expert validation

Country	Accuracy (CI)	Kappa	Sensitivity			Specificity		
			0	1	2	0	1	2
Tunisia	0.989 (0.985, 0.994)	0.976	0.98	1	0.99	0.992	0.998	0.991
Oman	0.987 (0.982, 0.992)	0.968	1	0.561	1	1	1	0.936
Pakistan	0.928 (0.916, 0.939)	0.879	1	0.75	0.93	0.85	1	0.994

Conclusion

This paper presented tailored distribution and maximum risk of establishment maps for the two major vectors of disease: *Aedes aegypti* and *Ae. albopictus* for the WHO EMR. Previous maps were highly biased towards data from the Americas and Asia and failed to identify risk areas in the target region. The obtained maps were provided to the points of contacts within the countries and their expertise was used to validate the outcome. Urban environment and host availability are among the most

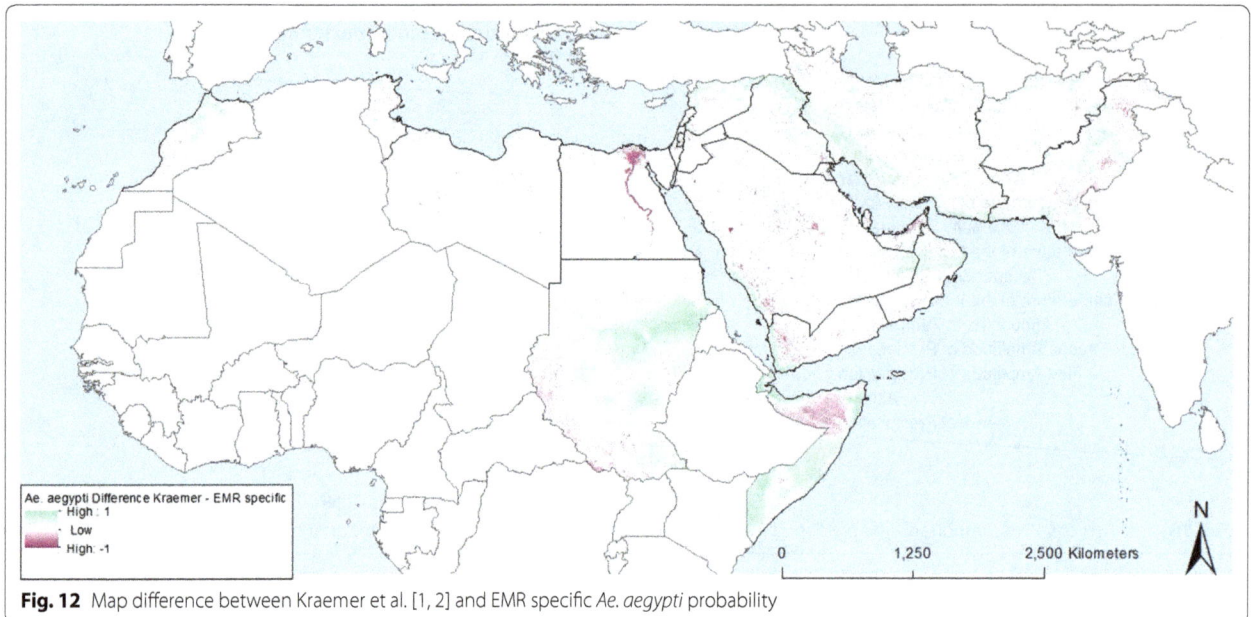

Fig. 12 Map difference between Kraemer et al. [1, 2] and EMR specific *Ae. aegypti* probability

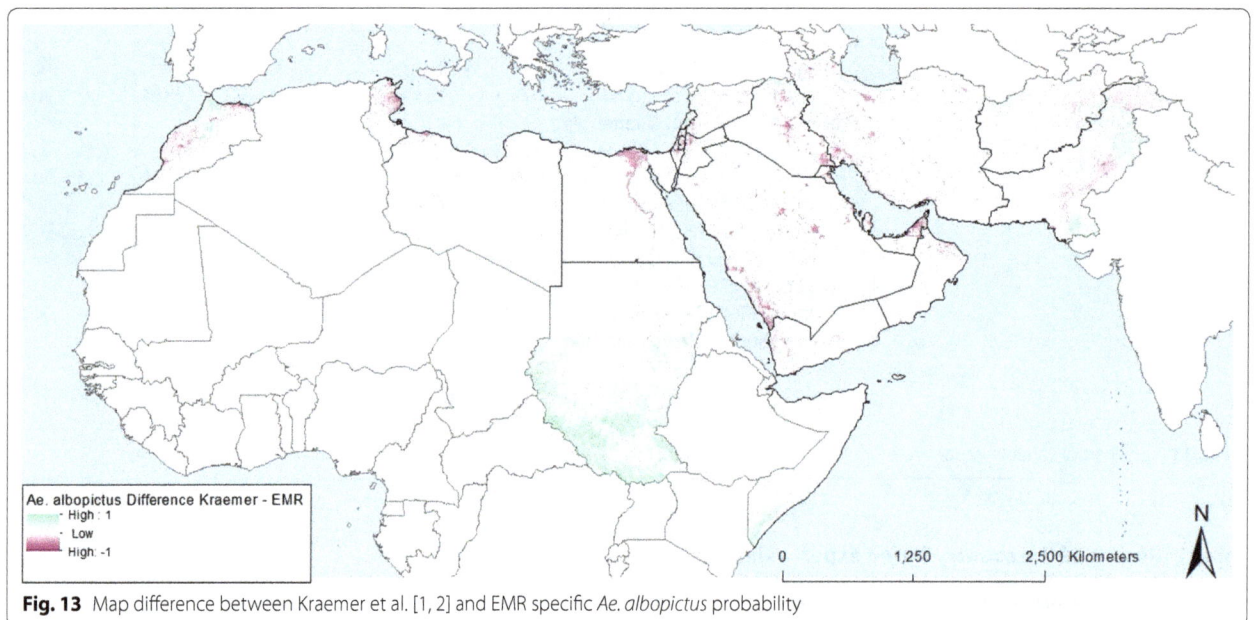

Fig. 13 Map difference between Kraemer et al. [1, 2] and EMR specific *Ae. albopictus* probability

important predictor variables for both *Aedes* species. The relative importance of precipitation is especially pronounced for *Ae. aegypti* which reflects the aridity of the region with shortages in water supply.

The maps generated specifically for the EMR highlighted data gaps and these gaps will be filled using targeted monitoring and surveillance. This will increase the awareness and preparedness of the different countries for *Aedes* borne diseases.

Additional files

Additional file 1. Presence of *Aedes aegypti* and *Aedes albopictus* and case data of Dengue, chikungunya and yellow fever in the EMR.

Additional file 2: Fig. S1. Presence data (*Ae. aegypti* and *Ae. albopictus*) taken from locations in areas with a Mahalanobis distance greater than 280 that were excluded from the model training data.

Additional file 3: Fig. S2. TFA processed precipitation data before (top) and after (bottom) spatial interpolation.

Authors' contributions
DR and GH conceptualize and supervise. NNTM, ED, WB, VDW, EB, ED, MM, GH, DR performed the data curation, analysis and investigation. NH performed active data collection in Lebanon. NH, OM, MM, AB, AH provided expert validation on the output. NNTM, EB, MM, GH, FS, DR obtained resources and funding. WB, GH, MM, FS administrated the project. WB, VDW, JC, DR, ED write the original draft. All authors read and approved the final manuscript.

Author details
[1] Avia-GIS, Zoersel, Belgium. [2] Regional Office for the Eastern Mediterranean, World Health Organisation, Cairo, Egypt. [3] Laboratory of Immunology and Vector-Borne Diseases, Faculty of Public Health, Lebanese University, Fanar, Lebanon. [4] MIVEGEC Lab, IRD/CNRS/UM, Montpellier, France. [5] Directorate General for Disease Surveillance and Control, Ministry of Health, Muscat, Sultanate of Oman. [6] Directorate of Malaria Control, Islamabad, Pakistan. [7] Institut Pasteur Tunis, Tunis, Tunisia. [8] Vector Control Focal Point, Ministry of Health, Puntland, Somalia.

Acknowledgements
We thank the numerous entomologists and health officers of the EMR who shared data with the WHO Regional Office for the Eastern Mediterranean. Ms. Barwa and Dr. Zayed are gratefully acknowledged for their technical assistance. We gratefully acknowledge the valuable input of the anonymous reviewers on the first version of this paper.

Competing interests
The authors declare that they have no competing interests.

Funding
This work was supported by the WHO Regional Office for the Eastern Mediterranean. The work was supported partially by the project InvaCosts (ANR-14-CE02-0021-01). Field work in Lebanon was supported by the WHO National Bureau (LEB1409860).

References
1. Kraemer MUG, Sinka ME, Duda KA, Mylne A, Shearer FM, Brady OJ, Messina JP, Barker CM, Moore CG, Carvalho RG, et al. The global compendium of Aedes aegypti and Ae. albopictus occurrence. Sci Data. 2015;2:150035.
2. Kraemer MUG, Sinka ME, Duda KA, Mylne A, Shearer FM, Brady OJ, Messina JP, Barker CM, Moore CG, Carvalho RG, Coelho GE, Van Bortel W, Hendrickx G, Schaffner F, Wint GRW, Elyazar IRF, Teng H, Hay SI. Data from: The global compendium of Aedes aegypti and Ae. albopictus occurrence. Dryad Digit Repos. 2015. https://doi.org/10.5061/dryad.47v3c.2.
3. Wilder-Smith A, Gubler DJ, Weaver SC, Monath TP, Heymann DL, Scott TW. Epidemic arboviral diseases: priorities for research and public health. Lancet Infect Dis. 2017;17:e101–6.
4. Humphrey JM, Cleton NB, Reusken CBEM, Glesby MJ, Koopmans MPG, Abu-Raddad LJ. Dengue in the Middle East and North Africa: a systematic review. PLOS Negl Trop Dis. 2016;10:e0005194.
5. Tran Minh N, Huda Q, Asghar H, Samhouri D, Abubakar A, Barwa C, Shaikh I, Buliva E, Mala P, Malik M. Zika virus: no cases in the Eastern Mediterranean Region but concerns remain. East Mediterr Health J. 2016;22:350–5.
6. Haddad N, Mousson L, Vazeille M, Chamat S, Tayeh J, Osta MA, Failloux A-B. Aedes albopictus in Lebanon, a potential risk of arboviruses outbreak. BMC Infect Dis. 2012;12:300. https://doi.org/10.1186/1471-2334-12-300.
7. Bennouna A, Balenghien T, El Rhaffouli H, Schaffner F, Garros C, GardÈS L, Lhor Y, Hammoumi S, Chlyeh G, Fassi Fihri O. First record of Stegomyia albopicta (= Aedes albopictus) in Morocco: a major threat to public health in North Africa? Med Vet Entomol. 2016;31:102–6.
8. Benedict MQ, Levine RS, Hawley WA, Lounibos LP. Spread of the tiger: global risk of invasion by the mosquito Aedes albopictus. Vector Borne Zoonotic Dis. 2007;7:76–85.
9. European Centre for Disease Control. Environmental risk mapping: Aedes albopictus in Europe. Stockholm: European Centre for Disease Control; 2013.
10. Khormi HM, Kumar L. Climate change and the potential global distribution of Aedes aegypti: spatial modelling using geographical information system and CLIMEX. Geospat Health. 2014;8:405.
11. European Centre for Disease Control. Development of Aedes albopictus risk maps. Stockholm: European Centre for Disease Control; 2009.
12. Habib RR, Zein KE, Ghanawi J. Climate change and health research in the Eastern Mediterranean Region. EcoHealth. 2010;7:156–75.
13. Rubel F, Brugger K, Haslinger K, Auer I. The climate of the European Alps: shift of very high resolution Köppen–Geiger climate zones 1800–2100. Meteorol Z. 2017;26:115–25.
14. Elith J, Graham CH, Anderson RP, Dudík M, Ferrier S, Guisan A, Hijmans RJ, Huettmann F, Leathwick JR, Lehmann A, et al. Novel methods improve prediction of species' distributions from occurrence data. Ecography. 2006;29:129–51.
15. Sallam MF, Xue R-D, Pereira RM, Koehler PG. Ecological niche modeling of mosquito vectors of West Nile virus in St John's County, Florida, USA. Parasites Vectors. 2016;9:371.
16. Medley KA. Niche shifts during the global invasion of the Asian tiger mosquito, Aedes albopictus Skuse (Culicidae), revealed by reciprocal distribution models. Glob Ecol Biogeogr. 2009;19:122–33.
17. Senay SD, Worner SP, Ikeda T. Novel three-step pseudo-absence selection technique for improved species distribution modelling. PLoS ONE. 2013;8:e71218.
18. Barbet-Massin M, Jiguet F, Albert CH, Thuiller W. Selecting pseudo-absences for species distribution models: how, where and how many? Methods Ecol Evol. 2012;3:327–38.
19. Thuiller W, Lafourcade B, Engler R, Araújo MB. BIOMOD—a platform for ensemble forecasting of species distributions. Ecography. 2009;32:369–73.
20. Scharlemann JPW, Benz D, Hay SI, Purse BV, Tatem AJ, Wint GRW, Rogers DJ. Global data for ecology and epidemiology: a novel algorithm for temporal fourier processing MODIS data. PLoS ONE. 2008;3:e1408.
21. Breiman L. Random forests. Mach Learn. 2001;45:261–77.
22. Cutler DR, Edwards TC, Beard KH, Cutler A, Hess KT, Gibson J, Lawler JJ. Random forests for classification in ecology. Ecology. 2007;88:2783–92.
23. Landis RJ, Koch GG. The measurement of observer agreement for categorical data. Biometrics. 1977;33:159–74.
24. Brady OJ, Johansson MA, Guerra CA, Bhatt S, Golding N, Pigott DM, Delatte H, Grech MG, Leisnham PT, Maciel-de-Freitas R, et al. Modelling adult Aedes aegypti and Aedes albopictus survival at different temperatures in laboratory and field settings. Parasites Vectors. 2013;6:351.
25. Brown JE, Evans BR, Zheng W, Obas V, Barrera-Martinez L, Egizi A, Zhao H, Caccone A, Powell JR. Human impacts have shaped historical and recent evolution in Aedes aegypti, the dengue and yellow fever mosquito. Evolution. 2013;68:514–25.
26. Mellander C, Lobo J, Stolarick K, Matheson Z. Night-time light data: a good proxy measure for economic activity? PLoS ONE. 2015;10:e0139779.
27. Delatte H, Desvars A, Bouétard A, Bord S, Gimonneau G, Vourc'h G, Fontenille D. Blood-feeding behavior of Aedes albopictus, a vector of chikungunya on La Réunion. Vector Borne Zoonotic Dis. 2010;10:249–58.
28. Cunze S, Kochmann J, Koch LK, Klimpel S. Aedes albopictus and its environmental limits in Europe. PLoS ONE. 2016;11:e0162116.
29. Rochlin I, Ninivaggi DV, Hutchinson ML, Farajollahi A. Climate change and range expansion of the Asian tiger mosquito (Aedes albopictus) in Northeastern USA: implications for public health practitioners. PLoS ONE. 2013;8:e60874.
30. Holstein M. Dynamics of Aedes aegypti distribution, density and seasonal preference in the Mediterranean area. Le Bulletin de l'Organisation Mondiale de la Santé. 1967;36:541–3.

Where do people purchase food? A novel approach to investigating food purchasing locations

Lukar E. Thornton*[iD], David A. Crawford, Karen E. Lamb and Kylie Ball

Abstract

Background: Studies exploring associations between food environments and food purchasing behaviours have been limited by the absence of data on where food purchases occur. Determining where food purchases occur relative to home and how these locations differ by individual, neighbourhood and trip characteristics is an important step to better understanding the association between food environments and food behaviours.

Methods: Conducted in Melbourne, Australia, this study recruited participants within sixteen neighbourhoods that were selected based on their socioeconomic characteristics and proximity to supermarkets. The survey material contained a short questionnaire on individual and household characteristics and a food purchasing diary. Participants were asked to record details related to all food purchases made over a 2-week period including food store address. Fifty-six participants recorded a total of 952 food purchases of which 893 were considered valid for analysis. Households and food purchase locations were geocoded and the network distance between these calculated. Linear mixed models were used to determine associations between individual, neighbourhood, and trip characteristics and distance to each food purchase location from home. Additional analysis was conducted limiting the outcome to: (a) purchase made when home was the prior origin (n. 484); and (b) purchases made within supermarkets (n. 317).

Results: Food purchases occurred a median distance of 3.6 km (IQR 1.8, 7.2) from participants' homes. This distance was similar when home was reported as the origin (median 3.4 km; IQR 1.6, 6.4) whilst it was shorter for purchases made within supermarkets (median 2.8 km; IQR 1.6, 5.6). For all purchases, the reported food purchase location was further from home amongst the youngest age group (compared to the oldest age group), when workplace was the origin of the food purchase trip (compared to home), and on weekends (compared to weekdays). Differences were also observed by neighbourhood characteristics.

Conclusions: This study has demonstrated that many food purchases occur outside what is traditionally considered the residential neighbourhood food environment. To better understand the role of food environments on food purchasing behaviours, further work is needed to develop more appropriate food environment exposure measures.

Keywords: Food environment, Food purchasing, Neighbourhood, Built environment, Geographic information system (GIS)

Background

The potential influence of neighbourhood factors on food purchasing and consumption has received growing attention, however empirical evidence remains inconclusive [1–3]. One of the reasons for this is that research has employed a range of different measures of food store access [4–6]. Two measures are commonly used: proximity to the nearest store, and the count of stores within a neighbourhood [1, 3, 7, 8]. Proximity measures typically ignore other store options nearby, whilst count measures are often limited to specific store types and apply a dichotomous categorisation to stores as being either

*Correspondence: lukar.thornton@deakin.edu.au
Institute for Physical Activity and Nutrition Research, School of Exercise and Nutrition Sciences, Deakin University, Geelong, VIC, Australia

accessible (within buffer) or not accessible (outside the buffer). Furthermore, when buffers are used there is little consensus on an appropriate buffer size, which is important as associations with food behaviours have been shown to be dependent on this [4].

Two additional limitations are common in many studies. First, exposure measures have been limited to a single context, most often within the residential neighbourhood. This ignores the multiple places people visit on a daily basis such as work, schools, and recreational settings. Second, existing measures also assume that all individuals within a particular neighbourhood have an equal ability to access facilities [9] and do not factor in other individual (e.g. cultural, socioeconomic, demographic and mobility) and environmental (e.g. public transport) factors which may influence food store choice [10]. As it stands, there are limited solutions to these problems as appropriate data on where people typically purchase foods to inform such measures are scarce.

A small but growing number of studies internationally have attempted to establish the spatial locations of habitual food purchasing patterns, both among adolescents [11, 12] and adults [13–19]. These studies have broadly concluded that many food purchasing behaviours occur beyond the boundaries of the residential neighbourhood or in stores that are not considered the most proximate to home. For example, Kerr et al. extracted food shopping trips from travel diary data in the US and found return trips between home, the food store, and home again were 5.37 mile (~8.64 km) in length and that trips to grocery stores were on average a distance of 4.67 mile (~7.52 km) from the trip origin, which may have been home, work, or some other location [19]. Whilst this body of work suggest that the access measures commonly applied may be too restrictive, further details related to food purchasing behaviours are required to help understand potential influences.

This paper presents findings from a novel data collection methodology which captured data on food purchasing locations and characteristics associated with food purchasing behaviours over a 2-week period. Data were mapped and distances calculated between the household address and food purchase locations. This study sought to explore purchase location relative to household address. Additional analysis examined whether purchase locations varied by characteristics of the individual, their neighbourhood and the food purchase trip. All food purchases, food purchases made when home was the trip origin, and supermarket purchases were examined separately. Those purchases made when home was the prior location may reflect habitual purchase behaviours that are less likely to be influenced by incidental travel (e.g. to social outings outside of their neighbourhood) and may be more likely

to be influenced by neighbourhood food resources. Purchases made at supermarkets were also examined separately as supermarkets are the predominant location for food expenditure in Australia [20] and therefore have major influence on overall eating behaviours.

Methods
Study sites
This study was conducted within four local governments areas (LGAs) located to the east of the Melbourne CBD (Australia's second largest city). Four Statistical Area Level 1 (SA1) administrative units were chosen within each LGA [average SA1 size within the four selected LGAs: 401 people (SD = 127), 0.215 km^2 (SD = 0.35)]. The SA1s were sampled based on: (1) area-level socioeconomic disadvantage defined by the Australian Bureau of Statistics (ABS) Socio-Economic Indexes for Areas (SEIFA) Index of Relative Socio-Economic Disadvantage (IRSD) [two SA1s in the lowest quartile (low disadvantage termed "high socioeconomic status" (SES)) and two in the highest quartile (high disadvantage termed "low SES")]; and (2) by access to supermarkets (high access: neighbourhoods with two or more Coles or Woolworths (two largest chains (~70% supermarket market share [21]) supermarkets within 2 km; and low access: neighbourhoods with no Coles/Woolworths supermarkets within 2 km). In each LGA, a SA1 was drawn from each quadrant of: low SES-low access; low SES-high access; high SES-low access; high SES-high access. This approach was employed to seek greater heterogeneity amongst participants in terms of socioeconomic and food environment characteristics. Whilst other supermarket chains (e.g. Aldi, IGA) and food store types (e.g. greengrocers) were present in the study region, the access measure was limited to the two dominant chains. However, even when limiting to these two chains, within one of the LGAs, no low SES-low access SA1s could be identified using the criteria above. In this instance the low SES SA1 located furthest (1.4 km) from the nearest (Coles/Woolworths) supermarket was used to represent low SES-low access in this LGA.

Data collection
In October 2014, data collection material including a food purchasing diary and short survey was hand delivered to households within randomly selected streets in the sixteen selected SA1s (data collection tool available in Additional file 1). Supplementary targeted recruitment which involved additional survey deliveries occurred in quadrants of area-disadvantage/supermarket access until a minimum of ten valid food purchasing diaries in each quadrant were received. Fridge magnets were included in the package and were designed as a reminder to record

food purchases. The delivered material was addressed to the main household food purchaser and this person was also required to complete a short questionnaire on their personal and household characteristics (e.g. age, sex, household composition, income). As a gesture of thanks, those who returned valid food purchasing diaries received a $20 gift voucher for a leading retailer and were entered into a prize draw for one of two $100 vouchers.

Food purchasing diary and survey

Within the food purchasing diary, participants were required to record details of all food purchases made over a 2-week period. This included foods made for immediate consumption, restaurant meals, and foods bought to be consumed later including packaged foods. Details to be reported included the date, name and address of store, where they were prior to making the purchase (home, work, other), primary mode of transport to the store (car, public transport, walk/cycle, other, or was home delivered), and what foods they purchased. The diary allowed for multiple purchases to be recorded on any given day and participants were to report if no food was purchased on a particular day.

The specific food items purchased could be recorded in one of two ways. First, participants could record what was purchased by ticking boxes against the categories listed in Additional file 2: Table S1. Second, participants had the option of attaching receipt data. Receipts were later coded against the same categories. Instructions noted that the purchase of multiple items from the same store should be recorded (e.g. hot fast food/takeaway and soft drink). Participants were asked to specify what the "other" item was when this box was checked. Many of these items were able to be recoded into one of the existing categories and therefore the "other" category was not examined further in analysis. Bottled water was also not examined due to the low number of purchases of this item.

Sample and food purchase records

Fifty-six participants returned valid food purchasing diaries [quadrant break-down: low SES-low access ($n = 11$ participants); low SES-high access ($n = 11$); high SES-low access ($n = 19$); high SES-high access ($n = 15$)]. The majority of respondents were female (80%) with fewer participants in the youngest age bracket [18–34 years (20%); 35–54 years (36%); 55 years or over (41%)] (two participants did not report their sex or age).

The 56 participants recorded a total of 952 food purchases. The within-participant average total number of purchases made across the 2 weeks was 16.1 (SD = 7.6) at an average of 10.6 (SD = 5.2) different stores. Out of the 14 days, participants recorded purchases on an average of 9.0 (SD = 2.6) days. Whilst a slightly higher percentage of

all purchases were recorded on Day 1 (11.8%) of the data collection period, purchases were generally spread evenly across the remaining days ranging from 5.3% of all purchases on Day 10 to 9.1% of purchases on Day 3. On Day 14, 6.9% of all purchases were recorded. This indicates that participants continued to report food purchases across the entire study period.

Distance to food purchase location

Each participant's household address (recorded in the consent form and stored separately to the survey) and where they made their food purchases were geocoded in ArcGIS 10.2 [22]. Store name and addresses recorded by participants were verified against online resources to supplement address information where required or to verify the full address. Of the 952 food purchases recorded, 916 were able to be geocoded (96.2%) with those not geocoded due to insufficient store details provided ($n = 28$) or because the purchase occurred interstate and was not considered a regular purchase location ($n = 8$). The shortest network path [8] between household address and food purchase location was calculated using the Network Analyst extension in ArcGIS. Pedestrian network paths were used for when the mode of travel was recorded as walking/cycling whilst street networks were used for all other modes.

Statistical analysis

Data were examined for outliers and distances greater than 35 km (~21.7 mile) were excluded from analysis as these were considered locations that were less likely to be part of a regular routine ($n = 24$; 2.6% of geocoded purchases; distance range 47.3–248 km). This left a final sample of 893 food purchases. The distance between home and food purchase location was examined for all purchases and for two additional dependent variables: (1) distance between home and food purchase location for purchases made when home was reported as the prior location; and (2) distance between home and food purchase location for purchases within supermarkets. Supermarket purchases were defined as purchases within the four largest supermarket chains in Australia which have over 91% of the market share (Coles (market share 32.5%), Woolworths (37.3%), Aldi (12.1%), and IGA (9.7%) [21]). These stores were determined by the store name recorded by participants.

Descriptive statistics for the three different types of food purchase distances by individual and neighbourhood characteristics were generated along with a box-plot of distance from home by food item purchased. The descriptive statistics do not account for within-person clustering. A plot was also created of purchase distance from home for each purchase grouped by individual to visualise the distribution of distance from home.

To visualise the dispersion of purchase locations amongst individuals within the same neighbourhood (SA1), ArcGIS 10.2 was used to create a map with all purchase locations for a single SA1. Added to this were individual-specific standard deviation ellipses which represent the dispersion of purchase locations around the mean centre of these for each of the seven individuals who returned food purchasing diaries from this SA1. Standard deviation ellipses are a common way to represent dispersion of locations and are increasingly applied to studies exploring health behaviours or access to health services [14, 23, 24]. A one standard deviation ellipse was used which captures 68% of all food purchase locations for each individual. In the example SA1, the minimum number of unique purchase locations for an individual was five meaning a sufficient number of unique points were available to generate the ellipses. Household locations were not considered in the generation of these ellipses as the ellipses were created to visualise the dispersion of regular purchase locations which may or may not be near the household location. Food purchase locations are counted each time a purchase is made at that location. This essentially weights a location based on the frequency of trips to that location to purchase food.

Prior to inferential statistical analysis, all distance outcomes were log transformed to account for the skewness in the data and results are presented on these log transformed values. Linear mixed models were used to determine associations between individual, neighbourhoods, and trip characteristics and distance to each food purchase in Stata 14.0 [25] (Table 2). This three-level multilevel analysis examined each purchase accounting for the nesting of purchases within-individuals and within-areas (SA1s). Both the fixed effects and the level of clustering within-individuals and within-SA1s are reported. The clustering [intraclass correlation (ICC)] of purchase distance from home within-individuals and within-SA1s were estimated as part of the mixed effect models. The two ICC values presented are the proportion of the total variance in distance from home that is accounted for by the clustering within-individuals and within-SA1s. Essentially the ICC represents the correlation in the outcome within each cluster. One limitation when interpreting these is that the outcome assessed is distance from home and therefore it is not estimating if the same stores were visited but rather whether the stores visited were a similar distance from home. Two models were fitted for each of the three outcomes (Model 1: Null; Model 2: inclusive of individual characteristics (age, sex), neighbourhood characteristics (combined area-level disadvantage and supermarket access), and trip characteristics (location prior to purchasing (for all purchases and supermarket purchases only), mode of travel (for purchases made

from home only), day of week). Mode of travel was only considered for purchases made when home was the prior location as this was a sensible trip origin to assess this variable. As the outcome assessed is distance from the home and not distance from the origin, results would have been biased if we included, for example, trips made from work during a lunch break where the mode of travel was walking but the actual purchase location is several kilometres from home. Both models were run on all non-missing values for each of the characteristics in Model 2 for comparability (all purchase $n = 845$; purchases made when home was the origin $n = 460$; purchases made within supermarkets $n = 300$). These two models allowed level of clustering within individuals and SA1s to be assessed prior to and after the addition of the individual, neighbourhood and trip characteristics.

Results
Descriptive results
A total of 893 food purchases were considered in the descriptive analysis; 484 (54.2%) of these were made when home was reported as the prior location and 317 (35.5%) were made within supermarkets. Mapped household and food purchase locations are presented in Fig. 1.

Across all purchases, food purchases were found to take place a median distance of 3.6 km (IQR 1.8, 7.2) from participants' homes, with the within-person median ranging from 0.3 to 16.8 km (Table 1). The median distance for purchases made when home was the prior location was only slightly lower than that for all purchases [3.4 km (IQR 1.6, 6.4)] whilst supermarket purchases were generally closer to home [2.8 km (IQR 1.6, 5.6)].

Over 60% of all food purchases occurred beyond 3 km of participant's homes (Table 1). This is demonstrated in Fig. 2 with the 3 km distance (a commonly used buffer size in studies of food environment exposure) marked on this graph to highlight the food purchases taking place beyond this distance. Two participants made all purchases during the 2 weeks within 3 km of their home, whilst six participants made all of their purchases more than 3 km from their home.

Differences in distance between home and purchase location by individual, neighbourhood and trip characteristics are also detailed in Table 1 and are further explored in the multilevel analysis accounting for within-person and within-neighbourhood clustering. Variation in distance to food purchase location from home was also observed by different food items purchased (Fig. 3). The median distance between home and food purchase location was shortest for grocery items (3.2 km; IQR 1.6, 5.7); however, this distance was similar for other fresh and packaged food items (fruit, vegetables, snack food, and soft drink) which reflects the fact many of these items were purchased

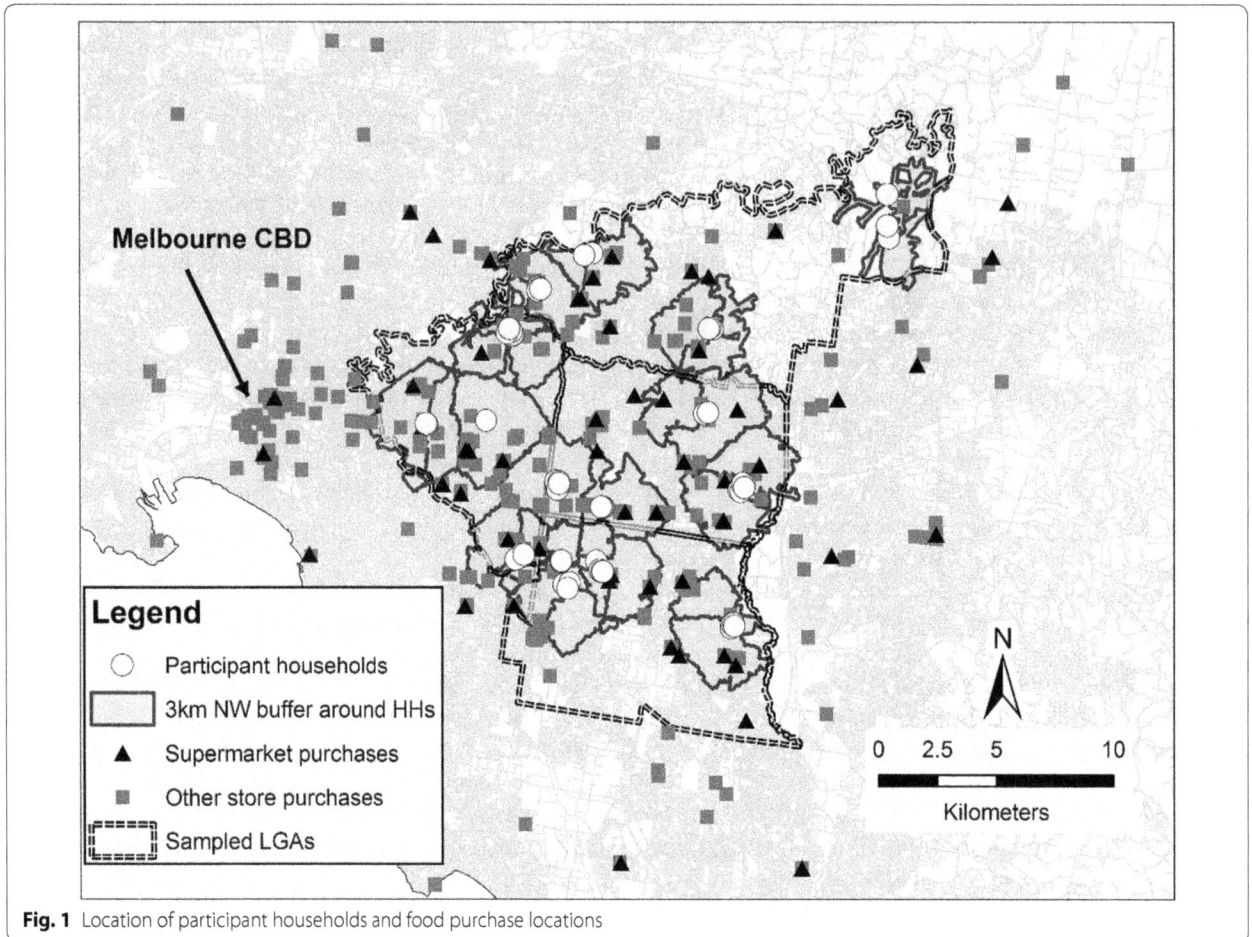

Fig. 1 Location of participant households and food purchase locations

concurrently in supermarkets. Median distances were greater when the item purchased was hot takeaway (4.6 km; IQR 2.6, 13.0), cold takeaway (6.7 km; IQR 2.3, 12.6), and meals in restaurants (6.8 km; IQR 3.4, 15.2).

Figure 4 presents the food purchase locations for all seven individuals living within a single high SES-low access SA1. The standard deviation ellipses presented in this figure highlight the dispersion of purchases locations within individuals but also the similarities and differences in regular purchase locations between individuals who live within close proximity of each other.

Multilevel analysis

For all purchases and for purchases made when home was the prior location, there was evidence to suggest that the distance between home and the food purchase location was greater amongst the youngest age group compared to those aged 55 years and over (Table 2). For the purchases made at supermarkets, age was not associated with distance from home, however supermarket purchases made by men were closer to home than supermarket purchases by women.

Compared to those in low SES-low access SA1s, purchases made by those in high SES-low access SA1s were a further distance from home for all purchases and purchases made when home was the prior location. Purchases were further from home for all three outcomes for those in high SES-low access SA1s compared to low SES-high access SA1s (Additional file 2: Table S2). Conversely, amongst SA1s deemed high SES-high access, purchases were nearer to the home when compared to purchases made by those in high SES-low access SA1s for all outcomes. Amongst those in low SES SA1s, there was no difference in purchase distance from home between those in high access compared to low access neighbourhoods.

When the workplace was the prior location compared to when home was the prior location, all purchases and supermarket purchases were further from home. For purchases made when home was the origin, mode of travel was examined with trips made by walking found to be significantly shorter than trips made by car. For all purchases and purchases made when home was the prior location, purchases made on the weekend were further from the home compared to purchases on the weekday.

Table 1 Descriptive statistics for distance between home and food purchase locations by individual, neighbourhood, and trip characteristics

	All food purchases		Food purchases when origin of trip was home		Food purchases within supermarkets	
	n.	Median (IQR)	n.	Median (IQR)	n.	Median (IQR)
Distance from home (km) (if ≤ 35 km)	893	3.64 (1.82, 7.19)	484	3.40 (1.60, 6.37)	317	2.79 (1.61, 5.59)
Within-person median distance from home (range)	56	min: 0.35 max: 16.81	55	min: 0.33 max: 22.96	56	min: 0.29 max: 15.33
	n.	% of purchases	n.	% of purchases	n.	% of purchases
Distance from home categories (km)						
≤1	93	10.1	60	12.3	54	16.5
>1–2	160	17.5	97	19.9	57	17.4
>2–3	93	10.1	54	11.1	49	15.0
>3–5	196	21.4	100	20.5	67	20.5
>5–10	184	20.1	113	23.2	77	23.5
>10–20	151	16.5	51	10.5	13	4.0
>20–35	16	1.8	9	1.9	0	0
>35 (excluded from analysis)	23	2.5	3	0.6	10	3.1
	n.	Median distance from home (IQR)	n.	Median distance from home (IQR)	n.	Median distance from home (IQR)
Age[a]						
18–34 years	173	4.35 (1.61, 14.35)	85	3.71 (1.48, 7.82)	44	2.16 (0.33, 4.03)
35–54 years	373	3.54 (1.70, 5.98)	164	2.67 (1.61, 5.67)	118	2.62 (1.70, 5.27)
≥55 years	318	3.49 (1.93, 6.74)	219	3.53 (1.96, 6.74)	146	3.38 (1.85, 5.59)
Missing	29	6.61 (1.32, 9.60)	16	6.58 (1.30, 12.57)	9	6.61 (1.27, 9.09)
Sex[b]						
Female	743	3.54 (1.87, 6.56)	401	3.44 (1.70, 5.98)	261	3.29 (1.82, 5.60)
Male	121	5.09 (1.70, 12.43)	67	2.28 (0.63, 8.66)	47	1.70 (0.63, 2.18)
Missing	29	6.61 (1.32, 9.60)	16	6.58 (1.30, 12.57)	9	6.61 (1.27, 9.09)
Neighbourhood characteristics						
Low SES-Low access	200	2.78 (1.31, 4.71)	82	2.09 (1.29, 3.74)	50	2.08 (1.22, 2.85)
Low SES-High access	181	4.03 (0.87, 12.43)	92	2.63 (0.71, 4.35)	58	0.71 (0.63, 2.79)
High SES-Low access	309	5.60 (3.40, 8.43)	192	5.59 (3.38, 7.19)	122	5.59 (3.47, 6.56)
High SES-High access	203	3.17 (1.82, 5.22)	118	2.45 (1.65, 5.03)	87	2.23 (1.56, 3.29)
Origin prior to making purchase						
Home	484	3.40 (1.60, 6.37)	–	–	202	2.62 (1.56, 5.59)
Work	164	5.13 (3.13, 14.83)	–	–	33	2.85 (1.52, 5.13)
Other	226	3.62 (1.96, 7.38)	–	–	74	3.38 (1.90, 4.55)
Missing	19	2.64 (0.85, 6.56)	–		8	2.36 (0.67, 6.12)
Travel mode when origin was home[c]						
Car	–	–	386	3.74 (2.08, 6.65)	–	–
Public transport	–	–	16	4.35 (4.35, 4.62)	–	–
Walk/cycle	–	–	73	0.74 (0.63, 1.58)	–	–
Missing			7	2.09 (1.82, 11.41)		
Day of week						
Weekday	629	3.54 (1.82, 6.74)	307	3.37 (1.58, 5.88)	223	2.62 (1.47, 5.13)
Weekend	264	4.33 (1.82, 8.59)	177	3.74 (1.65, 8.66)	94	3.46 (1.82, 5.75)

[a] Number of participants by age group: 18–34 years *n* = 11 (19.6%); 35–54 years *n* = 20 (35.7%); ≥ 55 years *n* = 23 (41.1%); missing *n* = 2 (3.6%)

[b] Number of participants by sex: female *n* = 45 (80.3%); male *n* = 9 (16.1%); missing *n* = 2 (3.6%)

[c] Results not shown for response categories where fewer than 10 purchases by travel mode (other *n* = 0; home delivery *n* = 2 [4.56 (IQR 3.61, 5.51)]

Nb. reference line at 3km indicates a common buffer size used in neighbourhood food environment studies

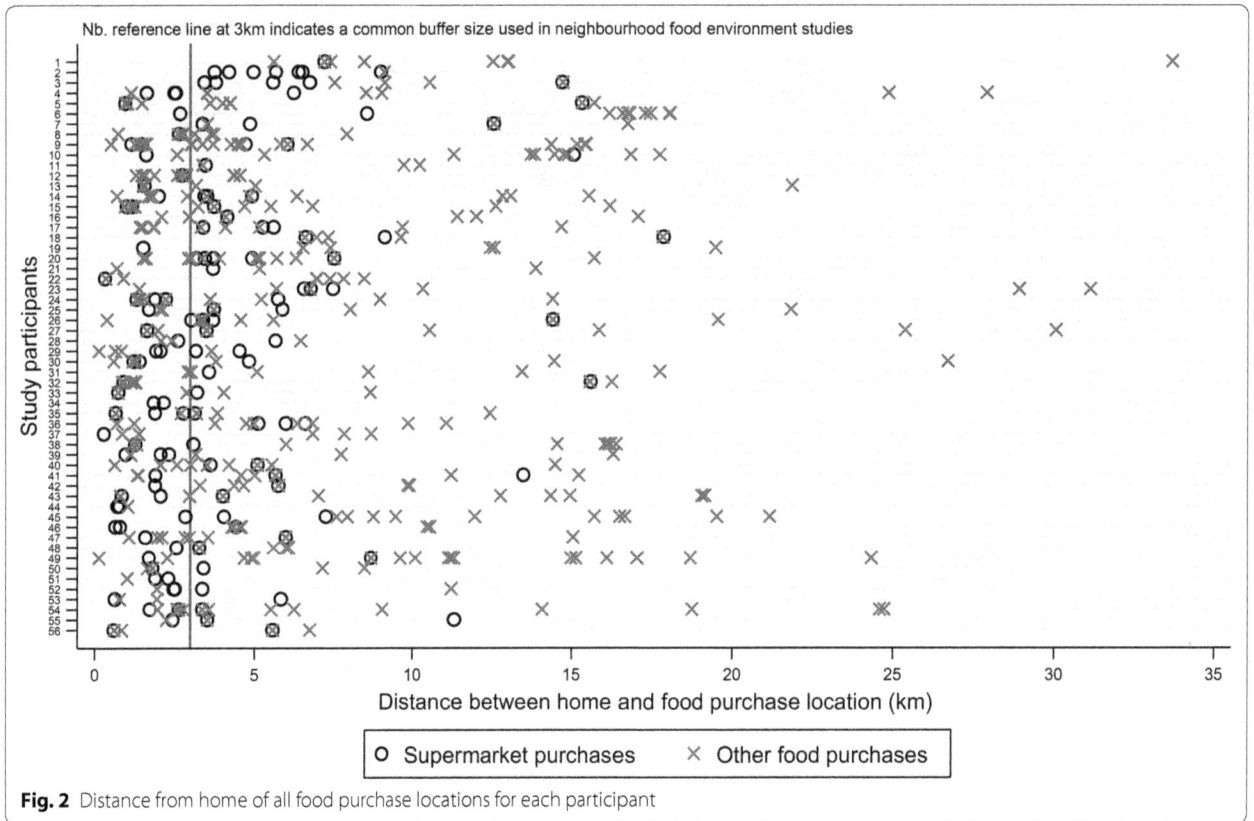

Fig. 2 Distance from home of all food purchase locations for each participant

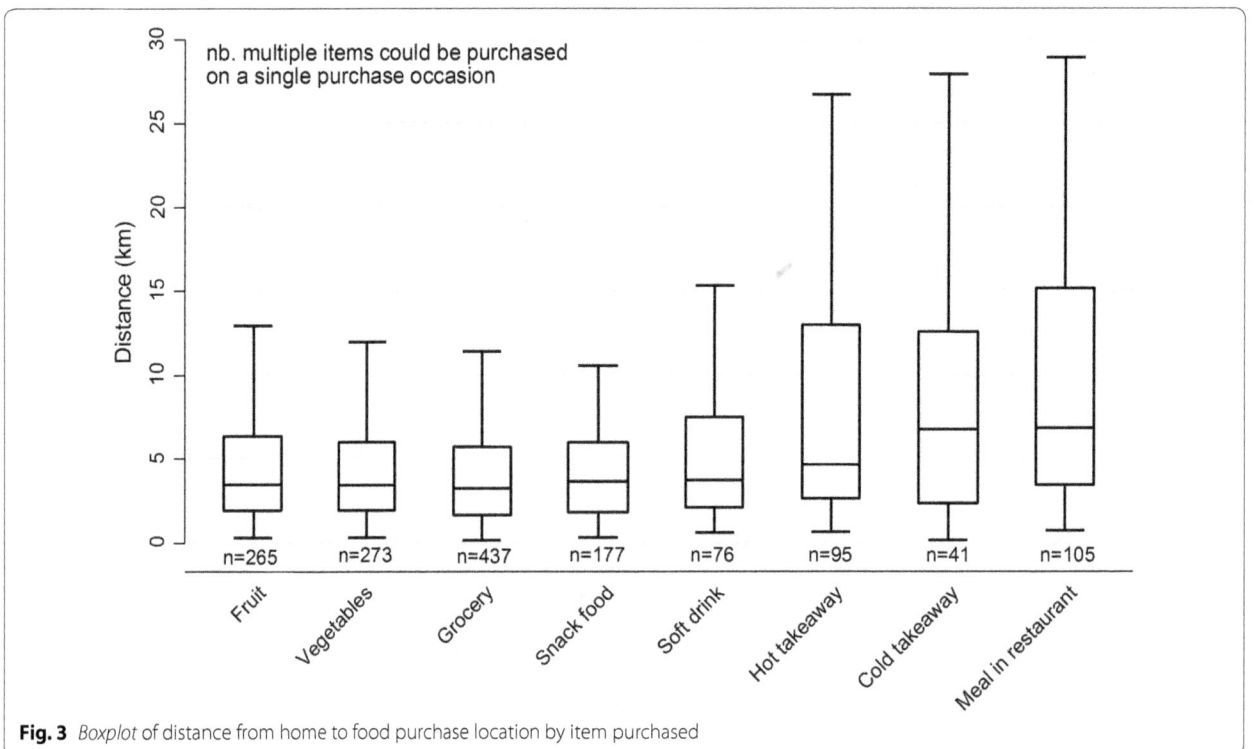

Fig. 3 *Boxplot* of distance from home to food purchase location by item purchased

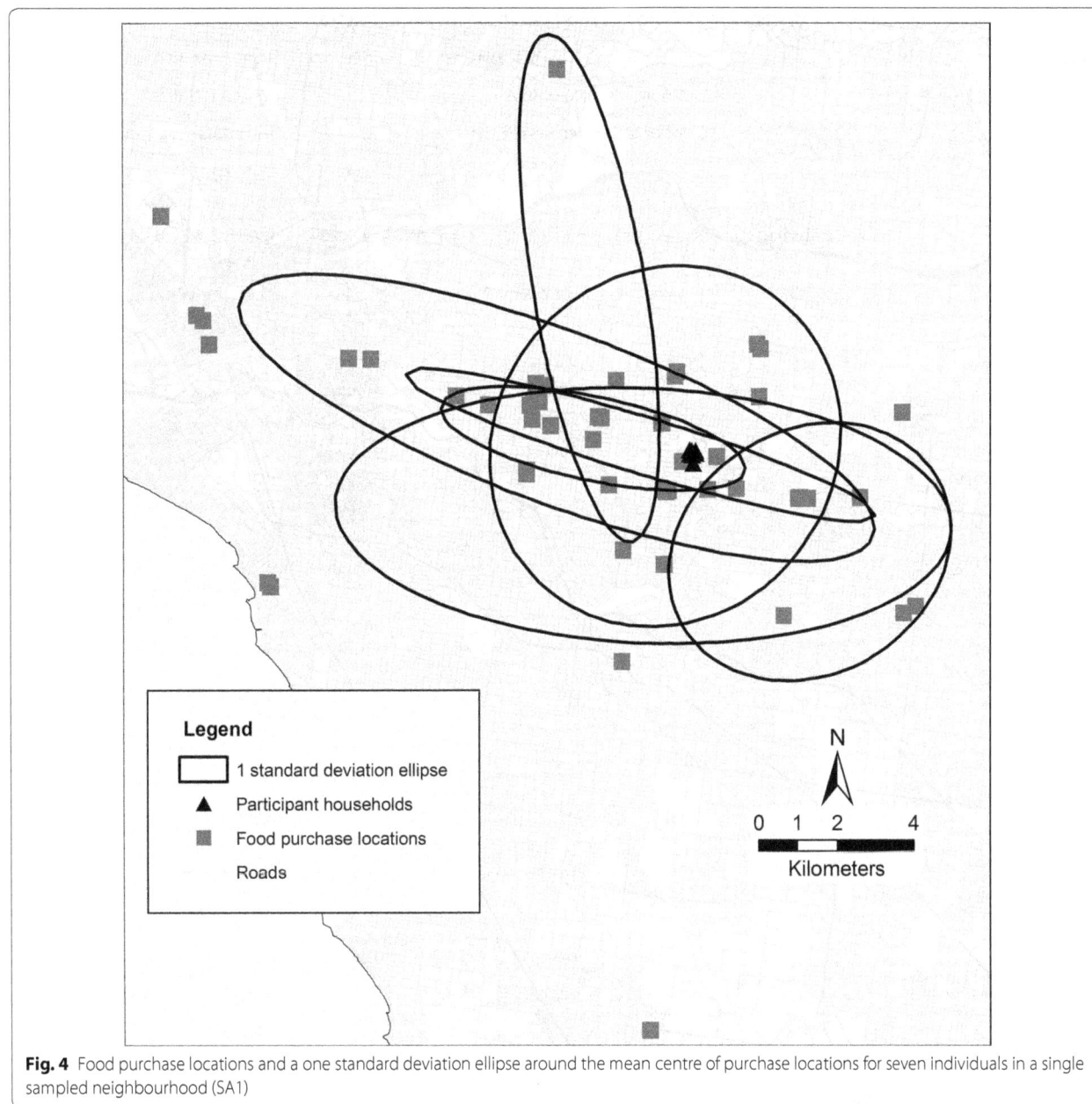

Fig. 4 Food purchase locations and a one standard deviation ellipse around the mean centre of purchase locations for seven individuals in a single sampled neighbourhood (SA1)

No difference in weekend compared to weekday was found for supermarket purchases.

Intraclass correlations

The within-person and within-neighbourhood (SA1) correlations were assessed for both models across the three outcomes. For all purchases in Model 1, the ICC for individuals (18.4%) and for SA1s (20.6%) were similar. The inclusion of individual, neighbourhood, and trip characteristics in Model 2 accounted for some of this ICC with individual ICC reducing to 14.5% and

this ICC with individual ICC reducing to 14.5% and SA1 ICC to 16.8%. For purchases made from home and supermarket purchases, the amount of clustering was higher within SA1s than within individual in the null models. For purchase made from home, the individual and SA1 ICC were more similar when accounting for individual, neighbourhood and trip characteristics (individual ICC: 9.5%, SA1 ICC: 11.6%). For purchases made in supermarkets, the SA1 ICC reduced from 60.6% in Model 1 to 52.8% in Model 2 but still suggested a much higher degree of clustering than within-individuals (6.1%).

Table 2 Linear mixed models for distance from home to food purchase location (log transformed)

All purchases			Purchases made when home was the origin			Purchases made at supermarkets		
Model 1: Null ($n = 845$)			Model 1: Null ($n = 460$)			Model 1: Null ($n = 300$)		
Intraclass correlation (%)			Intraclass correlation (%)			Intraclass correlation (%)		
Individual	18.4		Individual	13.3		Individual	7.4	
SA1	20.6		SA1	28.9		SA1	60.6	
	Model 2: All characteristics ($n = 845$)		Model 2: All characteristics ($n = 460$)			Model 2: All characteristics ($n = 300$)		
	Coef. (95% CI)	p. value	Coef. (95% CI)	p. value		Coef. (95% CI)	p. value	
Age (years)								
18–34	0.56 (0.13, 0.99)	0.011	0.40 (0.02, 0.79)	0.041		0.14 (−0.21, 0.49)	0.437	
35–54	0.21 (−0.12, 0.54)	0.219	−0.16 (−0.45, 0.14)	0.292		0.01 (−0.25, 0.27)	0.938	
55+	Ref.		Ref.			Ref.		
Sex								
Female	Ref.		Ref.			Ref.		
Male	0.10 (−0.25, 0.45)	0.572	−0.06 (−0.37, 0.24)	0.684		−0.34 (−0.60, −0.08)	0.010	
Neighbourhood								
Low SES-Low access	Ref.		Ref.			Ref.		
Low SES-High access	−0.25 (−0.94, 0.44)	0.477	−0.26 (−0.85, 0.32)	0.376		−0.46 (−1.33, 0.40)	0.293	
High SES-Low access	0.70 (0.04, 1.36)	0.037	0.57 (0.07, 1.08)	0.025		0.75 (−0.08, 1.58)	0.077	
High SES-High access	−0.09 (−0.76, 0.59)	0.800	−0.19 (−0.72, 0.34)	0.477		−0.13 (−0.96, 0.71)	0.767	
Location prior to food purchase								
Home	Ref.		n/a			Ref.		
Work	0.59 (0.42, 0.76)	<0.001	–			0.36 (0.15, 0.58)	0.001	
Other	0.13 (−0.01, 0.27)	0.075	–			0.12 (−0.03, 0.27)	0.124	
Mode of travel from home								
Car	n/a		Ref.			n/a		
Public transport	–		0.18 (−0.29, 0.65)	0.445		–		
Walk/cycle	–		−1.15 (−1.38, −0.92)	<0.001		–		
Day								
Weekday	Ref.		Ref.			Ref.		
Weekend	0.17 (0.05, 0.30)	0.008	0.14 (−0.01, 0.29)	0.06		0.10 (−0.04, 0.27)	0.153	
Intraclass correlation (%)			Intraclass correlation (%)			Intraclass correlation (%)		
Individual	14.5		Individual	9.5		Individual	6.1	
SA1	16.8		SA1	11.6		SA1	52.8	

Nb. n. for both Model 1 and Model 2 based on non-missing values in Model 2 for comparability

Discussion

The study builds upon a developing evidence base that demonstrates that the neighbourhood food environment, as traditionally defined, is inadequate for capturing important locations where individuals are exposed to and purchase food. Further, it has shown that distance from home to purchase location varies by the type of food being purchased and also by individual, neighbourhood and trip characteristics. This study's results are supported by prior work from the US. Kerr et al. report the average travel distance (from any origin) to a grocery store to be 4.67 mile (~7.52 km) [19]. They also reported that trips made from home, to a food store, and back home again were an average distance of 5.37 mile [19], or a one way trip of approximately 2.69 mile (~4.32 km). In this present study median distance is reported rather than average due to skewed distribution of the data. The median distance found in the study was 3.40 km but the average distance was 5.03 km.

The sampled neighbourhoods were a mix of those defined as having access to the two major chain supermarkets (Coles and Woolworths) nearby and those without. However, when considering all four major chains (Coles, Woolworth, Aldi and IGA) only three of the 56 participants lived further than 3 km of any supermarket and it is plausible that the presence of a supermarket may be a proxy for the presence of other food retailers. It is therefore unlikely that the lack of nearby food retailers was the key reason that over 60% of all food purchase and over 50% of supermarket purchases occurred more than 3 km from the home.

Distances from home were greatest when the food being purchased was hot takeaway food, cold takeaway food, or meals within sit down restaurants. The location of both the workplace and social activities are likely to be key contributors to this as would an individual's preference for a particular cuisine which may require them to travel a greater distance. US studies have also reported a higher distance to sit down restaurants compared to other store types [17, 19].

In the present study greater distance to food purchase locations was observed among younger age groups which perhaps indicates higher levels of daily mobility. Compared to trips made when home was the origin, distance between home and the purchase location was unsurprisingly greater when workplace was reported as the origin. It is likely this was largely dictated by workplace location. Whilst prior work by this study's authors did not find evidence that the relationship between food stores near home and eating behaviours differed by work status [26], Zenk et al. [14] have previously shown that those employed have larger activity spaces than those not in the labour force suggesting that use of stores further away is more likely. Although that study took place in the US, the clustering of employment opportunities outside of suburban residential areas across Melbourne means this is also likely to be the case in this sample.

Purchases on the weekend were also a greater distance from home than purchases on weekdays (though not to the same extent as the origin of trip differential). Non-work day purchases were also a greater distance from home in Kerr et al.'s study [19]. Purchase locations on the weekend, where more free time is expected, may be more heavily influenced by store preferences and the location of social outings whereas weekday purchase may be determined by time scarcity and convenience.

When home was the prior location, food purchase locations reached by walking or cycling were a median distance of 3 km closer to home than purchase made using a car. This indicates that those engaging in active forms of transport more often used local food stores than those who travelled by car. However, it is not possible to determine whether specific purchases made by active travel were due to personal preference or because of lack of access to a motor vehicle at the time of purchase. Whilst the benefits of active transport are well

established, if purchase location was restricted because of limited vehicle access then this has the potential to result in less healthy food purchases [27].

The linear mixed model results show the neighbourhood of residence (combined area SES and supermarket access) was associated with food purchase distance from home. Participants from high SES-low access SA1s purchased food further from home than participants from each of the other three sampling quadrants. This indicates that whilst nearby supermarkets (and potentially other food stores) may have been located further away, the high SES status of these neighbourhoods could mean that higher levels of employment or greater personal means (e.g. access to a motor vehicle) facilitated the ability and willingness to travel further for food purchases.

Differences in food purchase locations presented in Figs. 3 and 4 highlight that the utilisation of standard food environment exposure measures within a set boundary from household locations may not result in the generation of new and important advances in the field. Whilst the purchase locations and standard deviation ellipses presented in Fig. 4 indicate the home is an important 'anchor point' [9, 28, 29] around which purchases take place, individual variations were apparent. Given differences in individual characteristics, it should not be expected that residents utilise their neighbourhood in the same way. Further, a number of often unmeasured environment differences would also impact on the use of neighbourhoods for food purchasing purposes. For example, neighbourhoods with two supermarkets may differ with regards to a number of other important environmental characteristics (e.g. crime, public transport, walkability) meaning individual use of local supermarkets between these neighbourhoods would likely differ. For this reason, there needs to be a greater emphasis on both individual- and environmental-level moderators.

Kwan has previously described the need to give further consideration to individuals when considering contextual effects [30, 31]. Sharkey and Faber have previously called on researchers investigating residential contextual effects to be more flexible in their approach and answer the questions of where, when, why, and for whom do residential contexts matter [32]. There is an increasing body of food environment research adapting such an approach to investigate where and, in some cases, when food environments matter [12, 33–38]. However, future research needs to continue to evolve to ensure the equally important questions of why and for whom are also answered.

Strengths

The novel data collection method used highlights the potential opportunities provided by studies that collect data on behaviour location. This study was strengthened by the collection of food purchasing data over a 2-week period which allowed for the capture of regular and occasional purchase behaviours. Food purchasing data provides an insight into how individuals interact with the environment and removes assumptions associated with studies that link neighbourhood exposure measures to consumption or health outcomes. Whilst it is not possible to verify missing purchases, the fact participants continued recording data across all fourteen days and that multiple purchases on each day were often recorded indicates good compliance. There were very few problems with the food store data provided (name/address) meaning that over 96% of purchase locations were able to be identified.

Limitations and considerations for future research

This study was limited to a single region of Melbourne, Australia. Whilst an attempt was made to diversify the sample through choosing sample locations that differed by levels of socioeconomic disadvantage and access to major supermarket chains, future work would benefit from being undertaken across a more expansive and diverse area with regards to both population characteristics and the local environments.

A larger study involving more participants would allow for a deeper investigation into the role of individual- and household-level modifiers. Individual and household factors such as age, motor vehicle ownership, disability, family composition (e.g. presence of young children in the household), hours worked per week, workplace location and food preferences are all likely to influence which food stores are visited. Greater consideration of these and other environmental factors (e.g. walkability of neighbourhoods, provision of public transport, and in-store factors such as product range, quality and price) would allow us to understand why two people living in the same neighbourhood access different food stores.

This study objective was to capture the food purchasing locations of the main household food purchaser and consequently the study material was addressed to this person. Whilst this approach potentially captured a large portion of food purchased for consumption by other household members, independent purchases by other household members were not recorded. The completion of the diary by all members of the household would allow for both individual and household purchasing patterns to be assessed.

Future studies should also consider collecting further (precise) address information of the origin of trips (e.g. workplaces). Whilst the addition of GPS data would help

to capture this information, the simple reporting of additional address information on other key origins would provide more context into why purchases are occurring where they do. Whilst this study collected data on work postcode, the large size of these areal units did not provide a meaningful location to be able to calculate purchase distance between work and purchase location when work was the origin. Prior studies suggest food stores outside of the residential context for example, near workplaces, may be important to food behaviours [26, 39]. Therefore it is important that precise address data on workplaces and other frequently visited locations are collected in future studies.

The food categories collected could be further refined (e.g. any vegetables instead of fresh vegetables only which excluded frozen options). This would potentially allow a more detailed analysis on the impact of the food purchase location on the healthiness of food purchases.

Finally, it is acknowledged that the definition of supermarket was different for access (Coles and Woolworths) and purchases (Coles, Woolworths, Aldi and IGA). However, our access measure was based on the two most dominant chains which have ~70% market share and it is unlikely a sufficient neighbourhoods that did not have supermarket access would have been identified if additional supermarket chains were included. Whilst the dominant supermarket chains were used as a proxy for food store access in this study, it is by no means a perfect measure. Future work should pay particular attention to the development of access measures prior to sampling to ensure even greater heterogeneity in neighbourhood food environment measure. This will require access to detailed food retail datasets with accurate and complete data and a range of food store categorisations. Other environmental heterogeneity could also be introduced through the inclusion of other metrics such as walkability.

Conclusions

Through the collection of food purchasing locations this study has been able to demonstrate that many food purchases occur beyond what is commonly defined as the residential neighbourhood food environment. Further, results highlight the potential role of individual and neighbourhood characteristics as an influence on food purchase locations. This study's methods and results can inform our thinking on the appropriateness of using narrowly-focussed neighbourhood exposure measures when trying to understand the associations between food environments and food purchasing behaviours.

Authors' contributions
LT led the conceptualisation and design of the study with input from DC and KB. LT led the analysis and write up of this study. KL advised on the analysis used in this study. DC, KL, and KB provided critical feedback on the drafts of this study. All authors read and approved the final manuscript.

Acknowledgements
The authors would like to acknowledge Ralf-Dieter Schroers, Jennifer McCann, and Kate Parker for their assistance with data collection and data processing.

Competing interests
The authors declare that they have no competing interests.

Funding
Internal funding was used to support project costs.

References

1. Caspi CE, Sorensen G, Subramanian SV, Kawachi I. The local food environment and diet: a systematic review. Health Place. 2012;18:1172–87.
2. Giskes K, van Lenthe F, Avendano-Pabon M, Brug J. A systematic review of environmental factors and obesogenic dietary intakes among adults: are we getting closer to understanding obesogenic environments? Obes Rev. 2011;12(5):e95–106.
3. Ni Mhurchu C, Vandevijvere S, Waterlander W, Thornton LE, Kelly B, Cameron AJ, Snowdon W, Swinburn B. Informas: monitoring the availability of healthy and unhealthy foods and non-alcoholic beverages in community and consumer retail food environments globally. Obes Rev. 2013;14(Suppl 1):108–19.
4. Thornton LE, Pearce JR, Macdonald L, Lamb KE, Ellaway A. Does the choice of neighbourhood supermarket access measure influence associations with individual-level fruit and vegetable consumption? A case study from Glasgow. Int J Health Geogr. 2012;11:29.
5. Ball K, Timperio AF, Crawford DA. Understanding environmental influences on nutrition and physical activity behaviors: where should we look and what should we count? Int J Behav Nutr Phys Act. 2006;3:33.
6. Lytle LA. Measuring the food environment: state of the science. Am J Prev Med. 2009;36(4 Suppl):S134–44.
7. Charreire H, Casey R, Salze P, Simon C, Chaix B, Banos A, Badariotti D, Weber C, Oppert JM. Measuring the food environment using geographical information systems: a methodological review. Public Health Nutr. 2010;13(11):1773–85.
8. Thornton LE, Pearce JR, Kavanagh AM. Using geographic information systems (GIS) to assess the role of the built environment in influencing obesity: a glossary. Int J Behav Nutr Phys Act. 2011;8:71.
9. Perchoux C, Chaix B, Cummins S, Kestens Y. Conceptualization and measurement of environmental exposure in epidemiology: accounting for activity space related to daily mobility. Health Place. 2013;21:86–93.
10. Cummins S. Neighbourhood food environment and diet: time for improved conceptual models? Prev Med. 2007;44(3):196–7.
11. Sadler RC, Clark AF, Wilk P, O'Connor C, Gilliland JA. Using GPS and activity tracking to reveal the influence of adolescents' food environment exposure on junk food purchasing. Can J Public Health-Revue Canadienne De Sante Publique. 2016;107:Es14–20.
12. Shearer C, Rainham D, Blanchard C, Dummer T, Lyons R, Kirk S. Measuring food availability and accessibility among adolescents: moving beyond the neighbourhood boundary. Soc Sci Med. 2015;133:322–30.
13. Chaix B, Bean K, Daniel M, Zenk SN, Kestens Y, Charreire H, Leal C, Thomas F, Karusisi N, Weber C, et al. Associations of supermarket characteristics with weight status and body fat: a multilevel analysis of individuals within supermarkets (RECORD study). PLoS ONE. 2012;7(4):e32908.
14. Zenk SN, Schulz AJ, Matthews SA, Odoms-Young A, Wilbur J, Wegrzyn L, Gibbs K, Braunschweig C, Stokes C. Activity space environment and dietary and physical activity behaviors: a pilot study. Health Place. 2011;17(5):1150–61.
15. Christian WJ. Using geospatial technologies to explore activity-based retail food environments. Spat Spatio-temporal Epidemiol. 2012;3(4):287–95.
16. Hillier A, Cannuscio CC, Karpyn A, McLaughlin J, Chilton M, Glanz K. How far do low-income parents travel to shop for food? Empirical evidence from two urban neighborhoods. Urban Geogr. 2011;32(5):712–29.
17. Liu JL, Han B, Cohen DA. Beyond neighborhood food environments: distance traveled to food establishments in 5 US cities, 2009–2011. Prev Chronic Dis. 2015;12:E126.
18. Cannuscio CC, Tappe K, Hillier A, Buttenheim A, Karpyn A, Glanz K. Urban food environments and residents' shopping behaviors. Am J Prev Med. 2013;45(5):606–14.
19. Kerr J, Frank L, Sallis JF, Saelens B, Glanz K, Chapman J. Predictors of trips to food destinations. Int J Behav Nutr Phys Act. 2012;9:58.
20. Spencer S, Kneebone M. FOODmap: an analysis of the Australian food supply chain. Canberra: Department of Agriculture, Fisheries and Forestry; 2012.
21. Roy Morgan Research. Supermarket sweep: ALDI's share of the Aussie market still rising. http://www.roymorgan.com/findings/6762-supermarket-sweep-aldis-share-of-aussie-market-still-rising-201604142258. Accessed Sept 2016.
22. Environmental Systems Research Institute (ESRI). ArcGIS 10.2 for Desktop. Redland, CA: ESRI; 2013.
23. Sherman JE, Spencer J, Preisser JS, Gesler WM, Arcury TA. A suite of methods for representing activity space in a healthcare accessibility study. Int J Health Geogr. 2005;4:24.
24. Rainham D, McDowell I, Krewski D, Sawada M. Conceptualizing the healthscape: contributions of time geography, location technologies and spatial ecology to place and health research. Soc Sci Med. 2010;70(5):668–76.
25. StataCorp. Stata Statistical Software: Release 14. College Station, TX: StataCorp LP; 2015.
26. Thornton LE, Lamb KE, Ball K. Employment status, residential and workplace food environments: associations with women's eating behaviours. Health Place. 2013;24:80–9.
27. Burns C, Bentley R, Thornton L, Kavanagh A. Associations between the purchase of healthy and fast foods and restrictions to food access: a cross-sectional study in Melbourne, Australia. Public Health Nutr. 2015;18(1):143–50.
28. Chaix B, Meline J, Duncan S, Jardinier L, Perchoux C, Vallee J, Merrien C, Karusisi N, Lewin A, Brondeel R, et al. Neighborhood environments, mobility, and health: towards a new generation of studies in environmental health research. Revue D Epidemiologie Et De Sante Publique. 2013;61:S139–45.
29. Chaix B, Meline J, Duncan S, Merrien C, Karusisi N, Perchoux C, Lewin A, Labadi K, Kestens Y. GPS tracking in neighborhood and health studies: a step forward for environmental exposure assessment, a step backward for causal inference? Health Place. 2013;21:46–51.
30. Kwan MP. From place-based to people-based exposure measures. Soc Sci Med. 2009;69(9):1311–3.
31. Kwan M-P. The uncertain geographic context problem. Ann Assoc Am Geogr. 2012;102(5):958–68.
32. Sharkey P, Faber JW. Where, when, why, and for whom do residential contexts matter? Moving away from the dichotomous understanding of neighborhood effects. Annu Rev Sociol. 2014;40(1):559–79.
33. Crawford TW, Jilcott Pitts SB, McGuirt JT, Keyserling TC, Ammerman AS. Conceptualizing and comparing neighborhood and activity space measures for food environment research. Health Place. 2014;30:215–25.
34. Horner MW, Wood BS. Capturing individuals' food environments using flexible space-time accessibility measures. Appl Geogr. 2014;51:99–107.
35. Kestens Y, Lebel A, Chaix B, Clary C, Daniel M, Pampalon R, Theriault M, Subramanian SVP. Association between activity space exposure

to food establishments and individual risk of overweight. PLoS ONE. 2012;7(8):e41418.

36. Kestens Y, Lebel A, Daniel M, Theriault M, Pampalon R. Using experienced activity spaces to measure foodscape exposure. Health Place. 2010;16(6):1094–103.

37. Widener MJ, Farber S, Neutens T, Horner MW. Using urban commuting data to calculate a spatiotemporal accessibility measure for food environment studies. Health Place. 2013;21:1–9.

38. Widener MJ, Shannon J. When are food deserts? Integrating time into research on food accessibility. Health Place. 2014;30:1–3.

39. Jeffery RW, Baxter J, McGuire M, Linde J. Are fast food restaurants an environmental risk factor for obesity? Int J Behav Nutr Phys Act. 2006;3:2.

Permissions

The contributors of this book come from diverse backgrounds, making this book a truly international effort. This book will bring forth new frontiers with its revolutionizing research information and detailed analysis of the nascent developments around the world.

We would like to thank all the contributing authors for lending their expertise to make the book truly unique. They have played a crucial role in the development of this book. Without their invaluable contributions this book wouldn't have been possible. They have made vital efforts to compile up to date information on the varied aspects of this subject to make this book a valuable addition to the collection of many professionals and students.

This book was conceptualized with the vision of imparting up-to-date information and advanced data in this field. To ensure the same, a matchless editorial board was set up. Every individual on the board went through rigorous rounds of assessment to prove their worth. After which they invested a large part of their time researching and compiling the most relevant data for our readers.

The editorial board has been involved in producing this book since its inception. They have spent rigorous hours researching and exploring the diverse topics which have resulted in the successful publishing of this book. They have passed on their knowledge of decades through this book. To expedite this challenging task, the publisher supported the team at every step. A small team of assistant editors was also appointed to further simplify the editing procedure and attain best results for the readers.

Apart from the editorial board, the designing team has also invested a significant amount of their time in understanding the subject and creating the most relevant covers. They scrutinized every image to scout for the most suitable representation of the subject and create an appropriate cover for the book.

The publishing team has been an ardent support to the editorial, designing and production team. Their endless efforts to recruit the best for this project, has resulted in the accomplishment of this book. They are a veteran in the field of academics and their pool of knowledge is as vast as their experience in printing. Their expertise and guidance has proved useful at every step. Their uncompromising quality standards have made this book an exceptional effort. Their encouragement from time to time has been an inspiration for everyone.

The publisher and the editorial board hope that this book will prove to be a valuable piece of knowledge for researchers, students, practitioners and scholars across the globe.

List of Contributors

Lieze Mertens, Delfien Van Dyck and Ilse De Bourdeaudhuij
Department of Movement and Sport Sciences, Faculty of Medicine and Health Sciences, Ghent University, Watersportlaan 2, 9000 Ghent, Belgium

Delfien Van Dyck, Ariane Ghekiere and Jelle Van Cauwenberg
Research Foundation Flanders (FWO), Egmontstraat 5, 1000 Brussels, Belgium

Ariane Ghekiere, Benedicte Deforche and Jelle Van Cauwenberg
Department of Public Health, Faculty of Medicine and Health Sciences, Ghent University, De Pintelaan 185, 4k3, 9000 Ghent, Belgium
Department of Human Biometry and Biomechanics, Faculty of Physical Education and Physical Therapy, Vrije Universiteit Brussel, Pleinlaan 2, 1050 Brussels, Belgium

Nico Van de Weghe
Department of Geography, Faculty of Sciences, Ghent University, Krijgslaan 281, S8, 9000 Ghent, Belgium

Xiaolu Zhou
Department of Geology and Geography, Georgia Southern University, 68 Georgia Ave, Herty Bldg 0201, Statesboro, GA 30460, USA
Yunnan University of Finance and Economics, Longquan Road 237, Kunming 650221, Yunnan, China

Dongying Li
Department of Landscape Architecture and Urban Planning, Texas A&M University, College Station, TX 77843, USA

Eleonore M. Veldhuizen and Sjoerd de Vos
Department of Human Geography, Planning and International Development Studies, Faculty of Social and Behavioural Sciences, University of Amsterdam, Nieuwe Achtergracht 166, 1018 WV Amsterdam, The Netherlands

Umar Z. Ikram and Anton E. Kunst
Department of Public Health, Academic Medical Centre, University of Amsterdam, Meibergdreef 9, 1105 AZ Amsterdam, The Netherlands

Shaun A. Langley
Urban GIS, 1143 W Rundell Pl Suite 301, Chicago, IL, USA

Joseph P. Messina and Nathan Moore
Center for Global Change and Department of Geography, Environment, and Spatial Sciences, Michigan State University, East Lansing, MI, USA

Linde Van Hecke, Hannah Verhoeven, Benedicte Deforche and Jelle Van Cauwenberg
Department of Public Health, Faculty of Medicine and Health Sciences, Ghent University, Ghent, Belgium

Linde Van Hecke, Hannah Verhoeven and Peter Clarys
Physical Activity, Nutrition and Health Research Unit, Department of Movement and Sport Sciences, Faculty of Physical Education and Physical Therapy, Vrije Universiteit Brussel, Brussels, Belgium

Linde Van Hecke, Hannah Verhoeven, Delfien Van Dyck, Tim Baert and Jelle Van Cauwenberg
Fund for Scientific Research Flanders (FWO), Brussels, Belgium

Delfien Van Dyck
Department of Movement and Sport Sciences, Faculty of Medicine and Health Sciences, Ghent University, Ghent, Belgium

Nico Van de Weghe and Tim Baert
Department of Geography – CartoGIS, Faculty of Sciences, Ghent University, Ghent, Belgium

Sean J. V. Lafontaine
School of Psychology, University of Ottawa, Ottawa, ON K2L 1K9, Canada

M. Sawada
Laboratory for Applied Geomatics and GIS Science (LAGGISS), Department of Geography, Environment and Geomatics, University of Ottawa, Ottawa, ON K1N 6N5, Canada

M. Sawada and Elizabeth Kristjansson
Ottawa Neighbourhood Study (ONS), University of Ottawa, Vanier 5023, 136 Jean Jacques Lussier, Ottawa, ON K1N 6N5, Canada

Elizabeth Kristjansson
School of Psychology and Institute of Population Health, University of Ottawa, Ottawa, ON K2L 1K9, Canada

Tzai-Hung Wen and Ching-Shun Hsu
Department of Geography, National Taiwan University, No. 1, Sec. 4, Roosevelt Road, Taipei City 10617, Taiwan

Ming-Che Hu
Department of Bioenvironmental Systems Engineering, National Taiwan University, No. 1, Sec. 4, Roosevelt Road, Taipei City 10617, Taiwan

Charlene C. Nielsen, Carl G. Amrhein, Alvaro R. Osornio-Vargas a and the DoMiNO Team
Department of Earth and Atmospheric Sciences, University of Alberta, Edmonton, Canada

Charlene C. Nielsen, Alvaro R. Osornio-Vargas and DoMiNO Team
Department of Pediatrics, University of Alberta, 3-591 ECHA, 11,405 87th Avenue, Edmonton, AB T6G 1C9, Canada

Isabel Marzi and Anne Kerstin Reimers
Faculty of Behavioral and Social Sciences, Chemnitz University of Technology, Chemnitz, Germany

Yolanda Demetriou
Department of Sport and Health Sciences, Technical University of Munich, Munich, Germany

Jan van de Kassteele, Laurens Zwakhals, Oscar Breugelmans, Caroline Ameling and Carolien van den Brink
National Institute for Public Health and the Environment - RIVM, 3720BA Bilthoven, The Netherlands

Joseph Gibbons
Department of Sociology Health, San Diego State University, 5500 Campanile Dr., San Diego, CA 92182-4493, USA

Melody K. Schiaffino
Graduate School of Public Health, San Diego State University, 5500 Campanile Dr., San Diego, CA 92182-4493, USA

Naci Dilekli and Kirsten M. de Beurs
Center for Spatial Analysis, University of Oklahoma, 3100 Monitor Ave. Suite 180, Norman, OK, USA

Amanda E. Janitz and Janis E. Campbell
The University of Oklahoma Health Sciences Center, 801 NE 13th Street, Oklahoma City, OK, USA

Naci Dilekli and Kirsten M. de Beurs
Department of Geography and Environmental Sustainability, University of Oklahoma, 100 East Boyd Street, Norman, OK, USA

Daniel Adyro Martínez-Bello and Antonio López-Quílez
Departament d'Estadística i Investigació Operativa, Facultat de Matemátiques, Universitat de València, C/Dr Moliner 50, 46100 Burjassot, Valencia, Spain

Alexander Torres Prieto
Epidemiological Surveillance, Health Office of Department of Santander, Cl. 45 11-52, Bucaramanga 680001, Colombia

Fiona Y. Wong
Faculty of Health and Social Sciences, The Hong Kong Polytechnic University, Kowloon, Hong Kong, China

Els Ducheyne, Ward Bryssinckx, Johannes Charlier, Valérie De Waele and Guy Hendrickx
Avia-GIS, Zoersel, Belgium

Nhu Nguyen Tran Minh, Evans Buliva, Mamunur Rahman Malik and David Roiz
Regional Office for the Eastern Mediterranean, World Health Organisation, Cairo, Egypt

Nabil Haddad
Laboratory of Immunology and Vector-Borne Diseases, Faculty of Public Health, Lebanese University, Fanar, Lebanon

David Roiz, Frédéric Simard and David Roiz
MIVEGEC Lab, IRD/CNRS/UM, Montpellier, France

Osama Mahmoud
Directorate General for Disease Surveillance and Control, Ministry of Health, Muscat, Sultanate of Oman

Muhammad Mukhtar
Directorate of Malaria Control, Islamabad, Pakistan

Ali Bouattour
Institut Pasteur Tunis, Tunis, Tunisia

Abdulhafid Hussain
Vector Control Focal Point, Ministry of Health, Puntland, Somalia

Lukar E. Thornton, David A. Crawford, Karen E. Lamb and Kylie Ball
Institute for Physical Activity and Nutrition Research, School of Exercise and Nutrition Sciences, Deakin University, Geelong, VIC, Australia

Index

A

Accelerometers, 15, 17, 26-27, 50-52, 61-62, 64-65
Active Transport, 1, 12-13, 51, 64, 133, 223
Aedes Aegypti, 93, 95, 175, 201-202, 205, 211-213
Aedes Albopictus, 201-202, 207, 212-213
Aedes-borne Diseases, 201, 210
Aesthetics Index Scores, 66, 69, 71, 73-76
Arboviral Disease, 174
Auditing, 65-67, 77, 79

B

Block Weight, 164
Bmi, 4-6, 51, 66, 73, 75-78, 118, 199
Breast Cancer, 111, 116, 149-150, 152, 155, 157-159
Built Environment, 1-2, 11-13, 15, 26, 40, 64, 66-67, 77, 79-80, 119, 132-133, 214, 225

C

Cancer Screening, 149-150, 152, 155, 157, 159
Ceteris Paribus, 150
Chikungunya, 201-202, 206, 210, 212-213
Children's Independent Mobility (CIM), 117-118
Coarse Resolution, 161-162
Colon Cancer, 189
Comma Separated Value, 55, 63

D

Dengue Fever, 81, 83, 94-95, 175, 187-188
Direct Observation, 65-67, 78
Disease Mapping, 174-175, 177, 187-188
Dna, 97

E

Epidemic Diffusion, 81-82
Ethnic Heterogeneity, 28, 30, 32-34, 36-37

F

Food Environment, 26, 214, 217, 223-225

G

Geographically Weighted Regression, 28, 149-150, 156, 158, 160
Geoimputation Methods, 161, 168
Global Positioning Device, 50

Global Positioning System (GPS), 15, 190
Gtx-3, 54

H

Hazard Mapping, 103, 111
Health-related Indicators, 134-136, 140, 143-144, 146-147
Human Mobility, 26, 81-82, 84, 87-95

I

Individual Activity Tracking, 15
Infectious Disease, 81, 83
Intraclass Correlation, 73-74, 78, 217, 222

K

Kernel Density, 96, 99-100, 105, 116, 153

L

Land Surface Temperature (LST), 174, 176
Leisure Time, 50-52, 60, 62, 197, 200
Lipid Disorders, 189
Liver Cancer, 161
Location-based Step, 15

M

Maximum Imputation Centroid, 161, 167
Melanoma, 161, 172
Mental Health, 26, 30, 36, 38, 66, 115, 225
Mesothelioma, 161
Micro-environment, 1-2, 12
Moderate- to Vigorous- and Vigorous-intensity Physical Activity, 50

N

Neogeography, 39, 48
Normalized Difference Vegetation Index (NDVI), 174

P

P-splines, 135, 137, 144, 146, 148
Polychlorinated Biphenyls (PCBS), 161
Probability Surface, 16, 19, 21-23

S

Satellite Images, 174-176, 185-187

Sedentary Lifestyle, 189

Sedentary Time, 50-52, 54, 56-60, 62-64

Self-reported Health, 28-30, 38, 135

Small for Gestational Age (SGA), 96-97, 102, 105-106

Spatial Epidemiology, 161

Spatial Heterogeneity, 82, 94, 138, 142, 149-151, 154-156

Spatial Regression, 81, 87, 92, 95, 175

Spatially Correlated Random Effects, 134

Spearman's Rank Correlation, 76, 99, 103

Stratified Sampling, 66

Structured Additive Regression, 134, 137, 147-148

T

Timely Mammography Screening, 149, 158

Traffic Density, 1, 3-4, 6-12

V

Vector-borne Infectious Disease, 81

Virtual Environments, 14, 66

Volunteered Geographic Information, 26, 39-40, 46, 48-49, 240

Y

Yellow Fever, 201-202, 206, 212-213

ESSAI HISTORIQUE

SUR LES

PRINCIPAUX INSECTES

Qui ravagent les céréales panifiables et leurs produits

EN TOURAINE.

ENTOMOLOGIE APPLIQUÉE A L'AGRICULTURE

PAR M. G. CHARLOT,

Lauréat de la Société impériale et centrale d'agriculture de Paris, Membre de la Société d'agriculture d'Indre-et-Loire, Correspondant de la Société académique de Blois, des Sociétés d'agriculture de Châteauroux, de la Sarthe, etc., etc.

> L'art ne peut que gagner en aidant
> la nature.　　　M. MOREAU.

TOURS

IMPRIMERIE LADEVÈZE

1861.

ESSAI HISTORIQUE

SUR

L'ALUCITE DES GRAINS

EN TOURAINE.

———

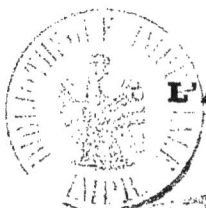

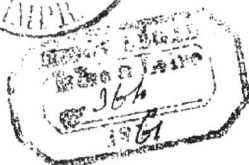

> Il n'y a rien de fait, tant qu'il
> reste quelque chose à faire.

I.

Le grain de nos céréales panifiables **a** quatre ennemis qu'il est bon d'étudier : l'humidité, la chaleur, l'air et les insectes. Parmi ces derniers, la classe des granivores renferme le charançon, la teigne des blés, l'alucite, le trogosite et l'yponomeute, qui sont les plus dangereux ennemis de nos récoltes. Nous ne nous occuperons ici que de l'alucite et de la teigne des blés.

Il y a quelques années, nos recherches nous avaient conduit à constater que la Touraine est, dans sa presque totalité, exempte de ce fléau ; c'est seulement sur les limites sud de notre département que l'alucite se tient depuis plus d'un siècle, et infeste souvent les grains d'une manière fâcheuse. Je demandais, en 1849, si ce fait n'est pas dû à la nature géologique du sol ou à notre climat, et je proposais d'inviter le gouvernement à faire étudier par des hommes compétents les causes de ce phénomène vraiment curieux (1). Il y a peu d'années, M. Doyère a été envoyé en mission par le Ministre

---

(1) *Annales de la Société d'Agriculture d'Indre-et-Loire*, 1849, page 147.

M. Dumas ; en 1850, ce savant a parcouru les quatorze départements infestés d'alucite, et le nôtre est compris dans ce nombre ; quelques remarques faites par M. Doyère sont venues confirmer nos prévisions (1).

Nos cultivateurs n'ont que des idées fausses ou erronées sur tout ce qui est relatif aux mœurs, aux moyens de propagation du papillon des grains et de sa chenille ; c'est pour cela que nous entrerons, à ce sujet, dans quelques détails, et que nous rapporterons succinctement les résultats de quelques-unes de nos observations.

L'alucite semble s'être impatronisée dans les champs et les greniers de certaines contrées ; elle s'y propage à tel point dans certaines circonstances, qu'on a constaté qu'un seul litre de froment avait suffi au développement de plus de quinze mille de ces insectes. Leurs dégâts sont si prompts lorsque la saison, le climat et le sol leur conviennent, qu'on a vu du blé perdre, par leur fait, 25 pour cent de son poids en moins de vingt jours, parce que la chenille, une fois introduite dans le grain, en dévore la substance farineuse sans attaquer l'enveloppe et sans lui faire perdre sa couleur ni sa forme, mais seulement son poids.

Nous avons constaté plusieurs fois que l'ensemencement du grain contenant des larves d'alucite favorise la conservation de l'espèce ; que fort peu de chenilles périssent dans le sol ; que leur métamorphose s'y accomplit aussi régulièrement que dans les granges et les greniers, et que les papillons en sortent à l'époque la plus favorable de l'année, pour aller déposer leurs œufs sur les épis des nouvelles récoltes.

On s'est souvent demandé : que faire du blé infesté d'alucite ? du pain ? mais, comment faire du pain avec du blé dont la farine a été en grande partie dévorée, et dont le peu qui reste se trouve souillé par les ordures qu'y déposent ces myriades d'insectes ? Ce sont ces causes qui font repousser ce pain,

(1) *Recherches sur l'Alucite des céréales*, par M. Doyère, Paris, 1863.

même par les animaux domestiques. Pour semence? C'est le pire des emplois ; nous avons constaté que les grains avaient le germe ou entièrement rongé ou fortement attaqué, et que le peu qui levait périssait l'hiver ou au moment de l'épiage ; mais le plus grand inconvénient d'employer le blé *alucité* comme semence, c'est de jeter des germes d'alucite dans le sol, où ils se conservent pour l'année suivante.

L'immensité des ravages du papillon a éveillé plusieurs fois l'attention du gouvernement et des sociétés savantes ; la Société d'agriculture d'Indre-et-Loire proposa, en 1835, un prix au meilleur moyen pratique de prévenir et d'arrêter les ravages de cet insecte : elle n'obtint aucune réponse.

L'alucite attaque plus particulièrement le blé froment, rarement le seigle, l'orge et l'avoine ; ce n'est que quand elle est pressée par la faim qu'elle se porte sur ces trois derniers.

En 1838, le Ministre du commerce évaluait à 500,000 hectolitres la quantité de blé détruit par l'alucite. MM. Richard et Guérin-Menneville ont posé, sans contestation, les chiffres suivants :

En France, le dégât annuel sur les récoltes, par les insectes, n'est pas moindre d'un dixième; parfois, c'est le quart.

D'après les relevés statistiques du ministère du commerce publiés en 1841, le département d'Indre-et-Loire produit :

En froment, 1,082,097 hectolitres ;

Méteil, 286,544 hectolitres ;

Seigle, 329,384 hectolitres ;

Orge, 310,823 hectolitres.

Et les habitants consomment, en froment seulement, 794,136 hectolitres.

Qu'on fasse à ces chiffres l'application des résultats posés par MM. Guérin-Menneville et Richard, et qu'on en déduise les conséquences !

II.

L'alucite, à l'état parfait, est de l'ordre des lépidoptères, de la famille des séticornes, du genre phalène de Linnée, nommé *alucite* par Fabricius, *œcophore* par Latreille (1). Cette famille comprend la pyrale de la vigne et la teigne qui ronge nos vêtements de laine, tous insectes nuisibles qui se ressemblent beaucoup.

La propagation de ce papillon est rapide et immense, puisqu'une seule femelle pond de 70 à 80 œufs d'un volume presque imperceptible; elle fait souvent deux ou trois pontes par an, ce qui donne d'innombrables générations.

La femelle du papillon dépose au printemps ses œufs par paquets sur le blé encore vert des champs; ils sont huit ou dix jours avant d'éclore. La petite chenille, en sortant de l'œuf, va chercher le meilleur et le plus beau grain encore tendre, et s'y introduit en y faisant une ouverture avec ses mandibules.

Duhamel fixe à cinquante jours le cercle entier de la vie de cet insecte; mais ses métamorphoses subissent l'action des variations atmosphériques. Lorsque les fraîcheurs commencent, les œufs et les chenilles restent stationnaires, et attendent les chaleurs du printemps, qui favorisent leur parfait développement; c'est ce qui explique comment des tas de grains ont pu être entièrement dévorés au printemps, quand on avait à peine remarqué quelques chenilles avant l'hiver.

L'accouplement pour les mâles, et la ponte pour les femelles, sont les derniers actes de la vie chez ces insectes.

Quelquefois on confond l'alucite avec une espèce appelée, par Réaumur, la *fausse-teigne*, qui est la teigne des entomologistes modernes; elle est moins grosse que l'alucite; sa

(1) Ouvrage de Constant Duméril.

chenille a une manière de vivre différente ; c'est seulement au milieu des tas de blé qu'elle vit, et non dans les gerbes; elle file un fourreau auquel elle agglutine quelques grains de blé, et elle attaque le grain à l'intérieur, sans s'y loger ; quelquefois on trouve les teignes avec l'alucite ; mais, je ne sache pas que les teignes se soient tellement multipliées qu'elles puissent être considérées comme un fléau. C'est en unissant leurs dégâts à ceux de l'alucite, que les teignes causent des ravages importants.

III.

Réaumur a décrit l'alucite des entomologistes modernes en 1736 ; on lui avait envoyé cet insecte des campagnes du Poitou, où il causait alors des ravages considérables sur les grains (1).

Ce fut en 1760 que cet insecte reparut en multitudes désastreuses dans le Poitou et l'Angoumois, où Duhamel et Tillet l'étudièrent avec soin et indiquèrent quelques moyens (2) pour le combattre. Ce fléau régna jusqu'en 1763 ; on le revit de 1781 à 1783.

L'alucite ne reparut plus sous forme de fléau, dans nos contrées, qu'au commencement du siècle, de 1800 à 1805, et de 1808 à 1812 : le papillon était alors à Châtillon-sur-Indre, sur les confins de notre département. En 1815, on en constatait la présence dans plusieurs de nos communes, sur les bords de la Creuse et de la Claise ; depuis cette époque, il semble avoir fait peu de progrès sur notre territoire, si ce n'est récemment, pendant les trois années de sécheresse extrême que nous venons de traverser.

En 1827-28-29, on retrouve le papillon dans les départements voisins du nôtre et dans les communes de nos frontières

---

(1) *Mémoires de Réaumur.*
(2) *Histoire d'un insecte qui dévore les grains,* Paris, 1763.

méridionales ; pendant les années 1834-35-36-37, 1846-47-48-49-50-51, on vit l'alucite des grains causant toujours des ravages dans les vallées de la Creuse et de la Claise (1).

En 1857-58-59, années chaudes et sèches, outre les lieux qu'elle habitait depuis plus d'un siècle, nous en avons constaté la présence pour la première fois, en grande quantité, dans les varennes des environs de Tours, et un peu dans la vallée de l'Indre, aux environs de Loches ; mais ce fut particulièrement dans les communes de La Riche, St-Genouph, Berthenay, St-Pierre-des-Corps, la Ville-aux-Dames; fort peu sur les plateaux de Ballan et de Savonnières. L'alucite cessa ses dégâts en Touraine pendant l'été froid et humide de 1860; mais elle reparût, durant l'été chaud et sec de 1861, dans les lieux ci-dessus.

Cet insecte attaquait particulièrement le froment tendre, dit de St-Laud. En cherchant le lieu de provenance de cet ennemi redoutable, nous avons appris qu'une grande quantité de blé *papillonné*, apporté des frontières méridionales du département, avait été vendue à la halle de Tours, et que beaucoup de ces blés avaient été déposés dans des magasins de cette ville.

Une autre cause qui a contribué à répandre l'alucite dans les varennes des environs de Tours, c'est que beaucoup de cultivateurs de cette contrée vont habituellement chercher à St-Laud, près d'Angers, dans les vallées de la Maine et de la Loire, du blé pour renouveler leurs semences, et que l'alucite existe dans ce pays depuis quelques années.

A ces deux causes, joignez la légèreté du sol et la douceur habituelle de la température qui règne dans les vallées du Cher et de la Loire.

(1) Nous avons trouvé ces dates dans les *Annales de la Société d'Agriculture d'Indre-et-Loire*, dans le *Journal d'Indre-et-Loire*, et dans les *Éphémérides de la Société d'Agriculture du département de l'Indre*.

Au nord de la Loire, les terrains argileux de ces plateaux étant généralement plus froids, plus compactes, et les terrains légers, sablonneux de ce pays étant froids et humides, circonstances peu favorables au développement de l'alucite, ce fléau y est inconnu. On y cultive aussi des blés plus durs, le *poulard* et le blé roux.

Nous avons observé, avec l'alucite, la coexistence d'un autre insecte, son ennemi, et qu'on nomme *ichneumon ceraphron destructor*, que nos cultivateurs nomment *mouches*, et qu'ils regardent, à tort, comme un insecte destructeur de leur grain, tandis qu'il en est le protecteur. Ce petit animal dépose un ou deux œufs dans le corps de la chenille vivante de l'alucite ; la larve y croît aux dépens de cette chenille, et finit par la tuer. Réaumur rapporte, dans ses Mémoires, un autre fait digne d'être noté, et que nous avons aussi observé en juillet 1860 : c'est que les jeunes sujets se livrent des combats mortels, ce qui contribue à la décroissance de cet insecte.

On sait que l'alucite est un insecte nocturne, ou plutôt crépusculaire, qu'il ne sort que le soir à la brune. Nous avons vu, en mai et juin 1859, beaucoup de blé fortement endommagé dans plusieurs magasins de Tours ; au mois de juillet de la même année, le soir, au crépuscule, des nuées de papillons sortaient de ces greniers, allant vers la campagne pour y pondre leurs œufs sur les blés encore debout ; des chauves-souris voltigeaient autour de ces greniers pour saisir les papillons au moment de leur sortie, et en détruisaient un grand nombre ; nous nous sommes convaincu de ce fait en faisant l'ouverture d'une de ces chauves-souris (1).

Nous devons encore citer, parmi les causes naturelles défavorables à la propagation de l'alucite, le retour, après une ou plusieurs années chaudes et sèches, d'étés froids et humides : ces saisons lui sont évidemment contraires, et font cesser mo-

(1) Voir à ce sujet nos réflexions sur la destruction des oiseaux entomovores, publiées en 1835.

mentanément le fléau. Les années froides et humides de 1816, 1830 et 1860 en sont des exemples très-remarquables, et dont nous avons été témoins. Malheureusement, la destruction d'une espèce nuisible quelconque ne peut jamais être complète.

Considérée non comme fléau, mais comme espèce entomologique, nous avons trouvé l'alucite, en 1848 et 1849, aux environs de Tours et aux environs d'Amboise, dans la vallée de la Loire. C'est fin de juin et commencement de juillet, le soir, qu'il faut chercher cet insecte. Nous tenons à constater ici que notre province, depuis un siècle environ, est, sur l'extrême limite des régions agricoles du nord et de l'est, celle où l'alucite n'a pas causé de ravages sérieux ; tandis que dans les régions plus chaudes du centre, du midi, en Espagne et en Algérie, l'alucite se propage d'une manière désastreuse. Tout ce qu'on a dit de l'alucite au nord de la Loire doit être, selon nous, attribué à la teigne des blés, avec laquelle on confond souvent l'alucite (1).

IV.

Nous ne pouvons terminer cette notice sans rappeler aux agriculteurs les principaux moyens qui ont été recommandés pour combattre cet ennemi. Parmi ceux qui nous ont paru offrir quelque chance de succès, nous dirons que le blé, une fois égrené, pourra être soumis à la chaleur, au choc mécanique, à l'ensilage, ou réduit en farine, afin d'être préservé du papillon et des autres insectes granivores.

Il nous faudrait faire un volume, s'il nous fallait passer en revue et décrire avec soin tous les moyens qu'on a proposés

(1) M. Herpin, de l'Indre, a eu tort de dire, en 1836, que la Touraine était entièrement envahie par l'alucite ; à la vérité il confond ces deux insectes. Voir sa notice, *Sur l'alucite ou teigne des blés*, Paris, 1860, pages 5-7.

pour la destruction de l'alucite et du charançon ; ils se réduisent à cinq principaux :

1° L'asphyxie ; en privant l'insecte d'air oxygéné, on finit par le détruire ; c'est une expérience de laboratoire, mais difficile à appliquer en grand sur les gerbes et le grain. On a proposé le gaz acide carbonique, le gaz sulfureux et plusieurs autres ; et, dès 1853 (1), nous combattions ces moyens comme impraticables ;

2° La chaleur est, sans contredit, l'un des moyens les plus avantageux qui ait été indiqué jusqu'à ce jour. Depuis les expériences de Duhamel, qui datent d'un siècle, quantité de machines ont été proposées pour détruire l'insecte, sa chenille et sa chrysalide ; mais la difficulté consiste à donner juste le degré de chaleur pour leur destruction sans ôter au blé ses propriétés germinatives et panifiables. Tous les inventeurs de machines sont d'accord sur ce point, qu'il ne faut pas porter la température au-dessus de 55 degrés centigrades. Passé 60 degrés, le germe du blé est altéré ; et au-dessus de 70 degrés la farine, ou plutôt le gluten du blé commence à éprouver une certaine altération ; la pâte et le pain provenant de blés trop chauffés perdent beaucoup de leurs qualités ;

3° La *compression* et le *choc* furent proposés dès 1844 par M. Arnaud. En 1850, M. le docteur Herpin (de l'Indre) proposa une machine pour détruire l'alucite, la teigne et le charançon, basée aussi sur le choc et la compression ; il obtint, à l'exposition de 1855, une médaille de première classe pour son tarare brise-insecte, qui remplace avec économie le pelletage, même pour les blés sains. En 1841, notre honorable collègue M. Derouet-Bruley proposa d'appliquer les greniers Vallery et Salaville, basés, à peu de chose près, sur le même

(1) *Annales de la Société d'Agriculture de Tours,* année 1853, page 50, et voir page 30 de cet opuscule.

(2) Voir une note de M. Charlot sur d'anciens silos, tome IV des *Mémoires de la Société archéologique de Touraine,* année 1850, page 27.

principe ; et plus tard le même membre rappela les savantes recherches de M. Doyère sur l'ensilage des grains ;

4° En 1853, M. Doyère proposa l'ensilage des grains, et rappela l'emploi des silos Grecs et Romains (2) pour conserver longtemps les grains et les préserver des insectes granivores. En novembre 1860, des silos furent établis à la colonie de Mettray, et en février 1861 on en constata les résultats ;

5° En 1859, un cinquième moyen fut proposé par notre honorable collègue et compatriote, M. Emile Pavy, de Girardet ; l'emploi de son grenier améliorateur du grain présente des avantages réels pour conserver longtemps les céréales et les préserver des insectes qui les dévorent.

Tous les remèdes proposés jusqu'à ce jour sont restés infructueux lors des grandes multiplications de la teigne et de l'alucite. Cependant, ne les repoussons pas ; espérons que la science n'a pas dit son dernier mot.

En attendant, ne dédaignons point les auxiliaires que la nature nous envoie ; invoquons le secours des oiseaux entomovores, des ichneumons, des pluies froides et continuelles pendant l'éclosion des chenilles, et n'oublions pas la sage maxime de notre bon La Fontaine : *aide-toi, le ciel t'aidera.*

PRINCIPAUX INSECTES

QUI ATTAQUENT LES CÉRÉALES.

Aux travaux qu'exige la culture des céréales se joignent les soins qu'on doit prendre contre les insectes, dont plusieurs espèces exercent de grands ravages sur les plantes et leurs produits.

Les céréales panifiables ont reçu la grande mission de servir de principale nourriture aux hommes ; aussi, les insectes qui s'y développent et les ravages qu'ils font excitent notre curiosité, notre intérêt, et ils appellent tous nos soins et notre vigilance à les combattre. Au point de vue de la science, il faut aborder sérieusement cette étude, si on veut se rendre compte de bien des mystères de végétations incomplètes ou étiolées.

Pour mettre un peu d'ordre, nous diviserons notre travail en quatre chapitres.

1er Insectes attaquant les céréales sur pied ;

2e Insectes dévastant les grains ;

3e Insectes dévorant la farine des céréales ;

4e Des moyens destructifs et préventifs qu'emploient la nature et l'homme contre les insectes.

CHAPITRE PREMIER.

Insectes attaquant les céréales sur pied.

Le genre *cécidomyie*, de l'ordre des diptères, renferme quantité d'espèces très-nuisibles aux végétaux que l'agriculteur cultive ; quelques-unes font naître sur les plantes des gibbosités et des excroissances où leurs larves vivent et se développent aux dépens des sucs nourriciers.

Nous ne nous occuperons ici que des deux espèces qui attaquent nos céréales en vert :

1° La *cécidomyie du froment*. — Ce diptère, à l'état parfait, a, ainsi que les autres espèces du même genre, deux ailes nues, une bouche sans mâchoire, armée d'un suçoir saillant.

Ce sont de très-petites mouches jaunâtres, qui ont, par leur apparence et leurs formes sveltes et grêles, quelque rapport avec les *cousins* vulgaires, dont elles sont voisines dans la classification naturelle.

Les cécidomyies font leur apparition au commencement de juin ; et leur ponte la plus active, en Touraine, s'effectue de la mi-juin à la mi-juillet ; on les voit, par une belle soirée, quitter leur retraite du bas de la tige du blé, où elles se sont abritées durant la chaleur du jour. Elles viennent déposer leurs œufs sur les épis au moment où le blé sort de son fourreau, commençant à fleurir ; leurs œufs mettent huit ou neuf jours avant de donner naissance à des larves, pour lesquelles est nécessaire une nourriture presque liquide : le grain se formant aussitôt après sa fécondation, il serait trop dur pour nourrir ces larves naissantes ; aussi, ces mouches ne confient-elles jamais leurs œufs à un épi défleuri.

Quand les larves de la cécidomyie ont atteint leur entier développement, elles gagnent la terre en se laissant tomber ; elles s'abritent dans le sol durant l'hiver, passent à l'état de nymphes, et deviennent insectes parfaits au printemps suivant. Quelques-unes restent dans l'épi, s'y transforment en chrysalide dans les granges, et au mois de juin elles prennent leur vol vers les champs de blé.

Les épis et épillets victimes des dégâts de cet insecte jaunissent plus tôt que les autres.

2° *La cécidomyie destructive, cécidomyie trici* de Lat. Ce que nous venons de dire de la cécidomyie du froment pour ses métamorphoses est applicable à la cécidomyie destructive; seulement, celle-ci dépose ses œufs près du collet de la racine, vers le premier nœud de la tige; la larve qui naît de cet œuf vit aux dépens des sucs de la tige et l'étiole, fait avorter l'épi sans nuire beaucoup à son développement extérieur; puis, un peu avant la maturité, on voit les épis rester debout et jaunir avant les autres; les vents un peu forts les renversent. Je crois que cette cécidomyie fait moins de dégâts dans nos contrées que la cécidomyie du froment.

L'ordre des diptères contient en outre quelques autres individus, dont les larves vivent sur plusieurs de nos céréales d'automne; nous noterons :

3° Le *chlorops lineata*. — C'est une petite mouche qui paraît chez nous au milieu de l'automne; elle dépose sur les jeunes plants de blé, de seigle, d'orge et d'avoine d'hiver, un seul œuf sur chaque pied nouvellement levé; peu de temps après, il sort de cet œuf une larve qui ronge la tige jusqu'à sa base : la plante continue à végéter d'une manière languissante, et elle devient informe; c'est ce que nos cultivateurs désignent sous les noms de blé *culoté, bourdé, échaudé,* etc.

Quand on voit un brin de blé rabougri, petit, dont l'épi n'est pas dégagé de la feuille supérieure qui l'enveloppe encore, si l'on détache cette feuille de la tige, souvent de fois on découvre un long sillon, profondément creusé, contenant une poussière, grossière comme du bran de scie, et une larve qui est celle du chlorops à lignes. La paille ainsi attaquée se flétrit ainsi que l'épi, et le grain est desséché par une maturité

précoce. Cette larve produit une mouche noirâtre par tout le
corps, à l'exception des pieds, qui sont fauves. J'ai vu des
individus ayant des lignes jaunes sur le corps : c'est probablement une espèce différente ; mais les larves causent les
mêmes dégâts. Le chlorops nous a paru, en 1812, 1839, 1856 et
1861, plus nombreux sur les plateaux que dans les vallées de
notre département ; cela tient peut-être au sol et aux assolements plus variés.

4° Le *chlorops frit.*, de Linnée. — Les larves de ce diptère
vivent au nombre de huit ou dix dans chaque épi ; elles en rongent la fleur et font avorter le grain. Je n'ai pas eu l'occasion de
constater son existence dans notre département ; peut-être un
jour l'y trouvera-t-on.

5° Une mouche de l'ordre des diptères attaque l'avoine ; elle
est plus petite, ainsi que sa larve, que le chlorops : c'est
l'*agromyze à torses noires.* Elle dépose ses œufs à la base de
cette plante nouvellement levée, dont elle arrête le développement ; il se forme une tumeur, au centre de laquelle se trouve
le ver ou larve.

Nos cultivateurs connaissent cette altération et la carac-
térisent par le nom d'avoine *bourdée*, *culotée.* Quant à la cause,
ils ignorent que ce soit l'effet de la piqûre d'une mouche ; ils
l'attribuent à la *brouissure.*

Dans la partie tuméfiée de l'avoine, en juin, on trouve, en
l'ouvrant, une larve qui s'attache à l'endroit où la hampe de
l'épi se réunit à la feuille ; elle y creuse un sillon en hélice de
manière à intercepter les sucs nourriciers ; elle rabougrit la
plante et empêche la maturité du grain, quelquefois, au printemps, ce ver parvient à détacher la hampe de la tige.

Cette larve se transforme en nymphe dans la terre et à
l'automne elle produit une très-petite mouche noire, à l'exception des pieds qui sont jaunâtres.

Les diptères contiennent encore la *tipule des prés ;* ses larves
rongent les racines de l'avoine et soulèvent la terre, ce
qui dessèche et fait périr cette plante.

6° Le genre *cephus* de Lat., *sirex* de Lin., de l'ordre des hyménoptères, renferme quelques espèces nuisibles aux céréales, notamment le *cephus pygmeus*. Cette espèce renferme plusieurs variétés d'insectes à quatre ailes ; l'abdomen de la femelle est terminé par un aiguillon en forme de scie, avec lequel elle insère au mois de mai un œuf dans une tige ; la larve provenant de cet œuf se nourrit de la moëlle du chaume, perce les cloisons, et parvient, peu de jours avant la moisson, au terme de sa croissance ; arrivée à l'extrémité du chaume, un peu au-dessous du sol, elle s'y transforme en chrysalide, et au mois d'août suivant elle passe à l'état d'insecte parfait. Cette larve produit sur le blé et le seigle un singulier effet : huit ou douze jours avant la moisson, on voit la paille et les épis ne contenant rien, ou renfermant un très-petit nombre de grains racornis. La coupure qu'a faite la larve du cephus à la base du chaume fait que les vents un peu forts le brisent et le font tomber : cette larve a été très-commune en 1861.

En 1829, M. de la Tremblais constatait les dégâts de la larve du cephus dans sa belle propriété, à Clion, près Châtillon-sur-Indre, sur les confins de notre département. Ce ver, dit-il, était assez abondant cette année sur les blés dits *échaudés* ; il trouva des cantons où le dixième, le tiers, et même les quatre cinquièmes des tiges du blé étaient attaqués. M. de la Tremblais voulut étudier cet ennemi, mais il ne vit sortir que des parasites des larves qu'il avait renfermées (1).

7° Le *saperda gracilis* de Guer., est un petit coléoptère, nommé par quelques agriculteurs *aiguillonnier* ; il paraît chez nous dans le courant de juin, quand les blés sont en fleur. La femelle du saperde perce d'un trou la tige du blé près de l'épi, et y introduit un œuf qui donne naissance à une larve, laquelle dévore intérieurement la tige ; ce qui fait dessécher et tomber l'épi ; le cultivateur dit alors que son blé est *aiguillonné*. En 1857, nous avons vu beaucoup de champs où le blé

(1) Procès-verbal de la Société d'agriculture de Loir-et-Cher, de 1829, p. 131.

était ainsi sans épi. La larve continue son ravage jusqu'au bas de la tige, en perçant les nœuds, et va passer l'hiver dans le chaume, très-près de terre; puis l'insecte paraît au printemps.

8° Les coléoptères fournissent encore le *taupin strié,* le *taupin bronzé,* que l'on désigne vulgairement sous le nom de *maréchal*, ainsi que deux petits *hannetons.* Les larves de ces insectes rongent les racines du blé, du seigle, de l'orge et de l'avoine jusqu'au collet, et font périr la plante; c'est en avril et mai que les larves de ces coléoptères font leurs ravages. On voit çà et là les pieds de blé, ainsi attaqués, se faner et périr, et quand on les arrache ils n'ont plus de racines.

9° Le seigle est aussi quelquefois attaqué par la chenille d'une *phalène*, de l'ordre des *lepidoptères crépusculaires.* Elle vit dans l'épi, qu'elle ronge à l'intérieur, et le fait avorter. Le seigle a encore pour ennemi la chenille d'un petit papillon de nuit, *pyralis secalis,* dont la larve se tient dans les tiges, et en ronge l'intérieur; mais ces deux larves ne causent pas, en Touraine, de dégâts notables.

10° La classe des hémiptères donne une espèce de *puceron;* très-petit insecte, qui établit sa résidence à la base de l'épi, détourne une partie des sucs nourriciers de leur cours naturel; conséquemment, il nuit à la formation du grain, et souvent le fait avorter.

On reconnaît les épis qui viennent d'être attaqués par ce puceron à une espèce d'écume blanche, destinée à protéger cet insecte; et quand le blé commence à durcir, le brin semble être plus tôt mûr que les autres.

11° Parmi les lepidoptères nous devons noter la noctuelle du blé, *noctua segetis,* dont la larve attaque le blé et le seigle; elle fait de grands dégâts certaines années, comme en 1861, quand les grains sont encore dans les champs. Cette chenille commence ses ravages chez nous ordinairement dès les premiers jours de juillet, et ne les finit que quand le blé est sec et rentré dans la grange, où elle meurt, ayant besoin d'humidité et de terre pour se transformer en nymphe.

La larve de cette noctuelle est de couleur brune, un peu velue, petite, elle a seize pattes; elle creuse le grain en s'y logeant, comme les larves du charançon et de l'alucite; quelque fois elle le ronge comme celle de la teigne du blé sans s'y loger, elle perce la balle du grain d'un trou rond pour entrer et sortir; elle se métamorphose dans la terre.

L'insecte parfait est un petit papillon de nuit, d'un gris cendré en dessus, les ailes supérieures ont des raies ondulées, les ailes inférieures plus blanches, avec le bord noirâtre.

Nos cultivateurs confondent, sous le nom de *ver du blé*, trois larves appartenant à des espèces différentes : celle du *cephus pygmeus*, qui vit dans l'intérieur de la tige; celle du *chlorops lineata*, qui attaque à l'extérieur la tige abritée par la feuille; enfin, la larve de la *noctuelle segetis*, qui ronge l'intérieur du grain encore sur l'épi. Les causes de cette confusion proviennent de ce qu'on trouve souvent ces trois larves sur le blé du même champ; mais jamais tous les trois sur le même brin.

Ces trois larves se sont montrées en très-grand nombre, en 1861, dans les blés, fort peu dans le seigle et l'orge d'hiver, et quelque peu sur l'avoine de printemps; les dégâts qu'elles ont causés ont encore augmenté le déficit de la récolte, déjà si médiocre, de l'année.

12° Quelquefois les *sauterelles* et les *criquets* font du tort dans les champs de blé placés près des prairies, après la coupe des foins; ces insectes, de la classe des *orthoptères*, que tout le monde connaît (mais on confond en Touraine les *criquets* et les *sauterelles* sous cette dernière dénomination) ne se jettent qu'accidentellement sur les blés de nos grandes vallées du Cher, de la Vienne et de la Loire, ainsi que nous l'avons vu plusieurs fois, notamment durant les étés chauds et secs de 1858 et 1859. Ils étaient très-nombreux dans ces vallées; ils dévastèrent quelques parties de champs de blé, situées à la proximité des prairies; ils détruisirent les feuilles et couchèrent les épis sur terre.

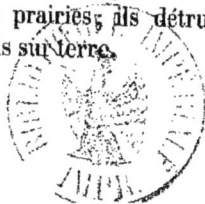

Notre pays est fort heureusement exempt du passage de ces insectes ravageurs, comme en signalent les historiens sacrés et profanes, pour l'Égypte et le midi de la France. Grégoire de Tours en rapporte plusieurs exemples; mais je ne sache pas qu'il ait parlé d'émigrations de sauterelles ayant causé de grands ravages en Touraine. Cependant, Shaw rapporte qu'en 1748 les criquets pénétrèrent de la Barbarie en Allemagne, en Hollande, en Angleterre, en Suède, et jusqu'à l'extrémité occidentale de notre hémisphère; pour parvenir de la Barbarie et se rendre en Angleterre, ils passèrent par la France, où ils causèrent de grands désastres; ce qui nous porte à croire que la Touraine a dû se ressentir de ce passage, ou de quelques émigrations semblables.

Les criquets sont plus abondants et plus communs en Touraine que les sauterelles, où ils se reproduisent. Les criquets qu'on trouve le plus communément en notre pays sont le criquet *stridulé, l'azuré, le bleuâtre, le germanique, le gros à cuisse rouge, le bimoucheté et le verdâtre*. Ces deux derniers sont communs dans les prés, les luzernes, les lieux ombragés et frais.

Les sauterelles les plus communes, et qui se reproduisent dans nos prairies à terrains sablonneux, sont la sauterelle *émigrante,* la sauterelle *ronge-verrue,* la *verte*, etc. On les trouve dans les mêmes stations que les criquets; on voit aussi dans nos chaumes et les blés la sauterelle à demi-étui, de couleur grisâtre; mais les dégâts qu'elle cause aux blés sont peu de chose et passent inaperçus.

13° Nous ne devons pas quitter le chapitre des insectes nuisibles aux céréales sans signaler un fait dont nous avons été plusieurs fois témoin. Nous voulons parler de la larve d'un insecte qui cause certains dégâts dans les cultures du millet *panicum miliacum*, et sur le sorgho, *holcus sorgho*. La semence de ces deux plantes contribue aussi à la nourriture de l'homme, et entre fort souvent dans les assolements de nos varennes du val de la Loire, à l'ouest de Tours. Les mœurs de cette larve nous portent à croire que c'est une espèce de *cephus*, car nous n'avons pu encore voir l'insecte parfait. Cette larve s'insinue dans l'intérieur du chaume de ces deux graminées, pour se repaître de la substance médullaire. Ces plantes ne peuvent plus arriver à la maturité, ou ne donnent que de faibles produits ; cet insecte descend jusqu'au collet de la racine, et probablement il y passe l'hiver, s'y transforme en nymphe et en insecte parfait, et au printemps suivant il recommence la même série de métamorphoses.

Le maïs est attaqué par les larves de deux lépidoptères nocturnes :

La chenille du *leucania zea* attaque l'épi et pénètre entre les enveloppes qui le recouvrent.

Le *Botys silacealis*, sa larve pénètre dans la moëlle du maïs, la dévore, fait jaunir et mourir cette plante.

Nous aurions pu parler dans ce chapitre de beaucoup d'autres insectes vivant au dépens des céréales sur pied ; nous les passons sous silence, afin de ne point étendre démesurément cette notice. Il en est quelques-uns visibles à l'œil nu ; il y en a beaucoup d'autres qui sont microscopiques ; mais la plupart vivent sur certaines céréales cultivées hors de notre département ou qui n'y sont cultivées qu'en fort petite quantité; puis, ces insectes sont généralement mal connus ; enfin, ils ne sont jamais en assez grand nombre pour compromettre l'avenir de nos indispensables récoltes et déterminer d'affreuses disettes.

CHAPITRE II.

Insectes dévastant le grain des céréales.

Dans ce chapitre sont compris l'*alucite* et la *teigne des blés*. Nous avons parlé assez longuement de ces deux insectes dans la première partie, à laquelle nous renvoyons le lecteur.

Nous ne parlerons ici que des mœurs de trois autres insectes qui attaquent le blé en grain : ce sont deux coléoptères et un lépidoptère.

1° Le *trogosite mauritanique* de Lat., ou *trogosite caraboide* de Fabri, de la classe des coléoptères. Sa larve a été bien décrite par l'immortel Parmentier, qui lui donna le nom de *cadelle*. Elle est blanchâtre, longue d'environ dix millimètres ; elle attaque le grain indifféremment par tous les côtés ; il est rare de voir cette chenille à l'extérieur des tas de blé, si ce n'est quand elle gravit contre les murs du grenier pour chercher un lieu propice à sa métamorphose. On a remarqué que cette larve a besoin de l'anfractuosité des murs et des planches pour se changer en nymphe ; et, quand elle n'en trouve pas, elle périt, vu qu'elle ne peut monter sur les corps polis, tels que le marbre, et les murs très-unis, surtout quand ils sont inclinés et en forme de voûte ; aussi, est-ce un moyen que nous avons conseillé d'employer dans les greniers pour s'en débarrasser.

Le trogosite mauritanique a été connu des agronomes sous la forme de larve, avant qu'on ne connût l'insecte parfait ; actuellement, on sait que c'est un petit coléoptère ayant environ cinq millimètres de long, noirâtre, le corps allongé, l'abdomen séparé du corselet par un petit pédoncule ; il est très-fécond ; il pond sur le grain beaucoup d'œufs, ayant besoin d'un climat chaud pour se propager en grande quantité ; aussi ne se propage-t-il chez nous que médiocrement, si ce n'est dans les années très-chaudes, comme 1822-1858-1859. Nous ne l'avons observé que dans le Berry.

2° Le *charançon du blé*, connu aussi sous le nom de *calandre becmare*, est malheureusement trop connu des cultivateurs de nos contrées, ce qui nous dispensera de le décrire. Sa larve, souvent en peu de jours, détruit d'immenses quantités de grain : comme celle de l'alucite, elle en ronge tout l'intérieur ; elle se métamorphose sans révéler sa présence au dehors. On a calculé qu'un couple de charançons peut, dans l'espace de cinq mois, donner naissance à plus de six mille petits.

Quelquefois nous avons trouvé dans le même tas de blé des charançons, des fausses teignes et des alucites, causant en peu de jours des dégâts énormes, surtout dès les premières chaleurs du printemps. Il y a longtemps que ce fléau préoccupe nos agriculteurs. Les premières Annales de la Société d'agriculture d'Indre-et-Loire contiennent plusieurs mémoires et recettes sur la manière de détruire le charançon.

3° L'*yponomeute*, l'*innéelle* de Lat., est un petit lépidoptère nocturne, dont la larve est nuisible au blé en grain, et que l'on confond souvent avec celle de l'alucite, de la fausse-teigne et du trogosite, sous le nom commun de *ver* du blé ; mais ces larves, une fois transformées, sont facilement reconnaissables.

Les larves ou chenilles de l'yponomeute sont grises, blanchâtres ; elles s'insinuent une seule en chaque grain de blé, elles en dévorent la farine, puis elles lient plusieurs de ces grains ensemble, et forment des tuyaux d'une soie blanche pour se convertir en nymphes et se transformer. Le papillon ressemble beaucoup à la teigne du blé. Les saisons chaudes favorisent la multiplication de cet insecte. Comme les larves de l'alucite, de la teigne, du blé, et celle du *charançon*, elles fuient le grand jour, le mouvement ; aussi emploie-t-on les mêmes moyens pour s'en débarrasser.

CHAPITRE III.

Insectes dévorant la farine.

La farine des céréales est souvent ravagée par plusieurs petits insectes à peine visibles à l'œil nu ; ils s'y multiplient à l'infini ; tant qu'ils trouvent des vieilles farines confectionnées, ainsi que leurs issues, et surtout dès qu'elles commencent à fermenter; ils leur communiquent une odeur et un goût désagréables, qui se transmettent au pain. On trouve ces insectes dans les moulins, chez les boulangers et dans les magasins de farine ; ils font perdre en peu de temps beaucoup de poids aux farines.

1° La *blatte* des cuisines est de l'ordre des *orthoptères*, appelée vulgairement *bête noire*, qu'on trouve dans les boulangeries, les cuisines; elle se sert rarement de ses ailes, mais elle court vite; son odeur nauséabonde se communique au moindre contact; elle butine, pendant la nuit, la plupart des substances qui servent à la nourriture de l'homme, la farine, le pain, la viande cuite; mais elle en gâte bien plus qu'elle n'en mange. Notre climat tempéré n'est pas très-favorable à sa propagation ; aussi ne la trouve-t-on que dans les lieux chauds et obscurs; la blatte disparaît pendant l'hiver, elle fuit les habitations froides ; les grands froids la font mourir.

Les orthoptères renferment aussi *le grillon domestique,* que tout le monde connaît; il se nourrit de farine, de pain, et attaque tous nos comestibles.

2° Le *ténébrion de la farine, tenebrio molitor,* de la classe des coléoptères, est commun en Touraine, chez les boulangers, dans les magasins de farine ; ses larves vivent dans la farine, le pain, le sucre et les substances sucrées ; il est connu sous le nom de *vers* de farine. Il fait quelquefois assez de tort pour mériter qu'on cherche les moyens de le détruire.

3° Le *ptine larron, ptinus fur. lat.,* très-petit coléoptère qui, à l'état de larve et d'insecte parfait, attaque la farine des céréales, d'après les observations de l'académicien Audouin.

4° Les *acarus* ou *cirons,* qu'on nomme vulgairement *mites,* genre d'insecte aptères, renfermant un très-grand nombre d'espèces, toutes nuisibles à nos provisions de bouche et aux collections d'histoire naturelle. La plus commune est la mite domestique, qui détruit la farine et le vieux pain. La farine non blutée contenant le son est bien plus sujette à être ravagée des mites et à fermenter que les fleurs, surtout quand elle provient de grain récolté pendant une année humide comme 1860 ; les farines détériorées par ces insectes se reconnaissent aisément à l'odeur qu'elles exhalent, à l'aspect qu'elles présentent : elles sont quelquefois d'un blanc terne ou rougeâtre, et laissent dans la bouche une impression âcre, piquante ; ces farines sont tout à fait impropres à la fabrication du pain, le gluten ayant été altéré par les insectes.

5° Il y a aussi la pyrale de la farine, *pyralis farinalis*, de l'ordre des lépidoptères nocturnes, dont les larves dévorent la farine et le pain.

CHAPITRE IV.

Des moyens destructifs et préservatifs qu'emploient la nature et les hommes.

Nous diviserons ce chapitre en deux sections :

1° Les auxiliaires employés par la nature ;

2° Les moyens que l'homme emploie.

DES AUXILIAIRES DE LA NATURE.

La nature, toujours prévoyante et habile conservatrice de ses œuvres, n'a pas accordé aux insectes le pouvoir de se propager outre mesure, de manière à détruire ce qu'elle a créé, et à troubler l'harmonie qu'elle a établi ; elle a donné aux espèces opprimées des armes diverses, afin de résister à la rapacité de leurs nombreux ennemis et de ne pas disparaître entièrement. La force a été chez elles remplacée par une variété de moyens, de ruses, de stratagèmes qui attestent, là comme partout, la fécondité de ses ressources et sa divine prévoyance.

Les moyens employés par la nature sont nombreux et variés ; ils peuvent se diviser en deux catégories :

1° Les parasites ;

2° L'intempérie des saisons.

1° Les Parasites.

C'est particulièrement dans la classe des hyménoptères que se rencontrent les principaux parasites, qu'on pourrait appeler *insectirodes,* rongeurs d'insectes, parce qu'ils déposent leurs œufs dans les larves des insectes dévastateurs ; ils sont généralement du genre ichneumon. C'est pour aider à les distinguer les uns des autres, que nous avons fait dessiner les principaux.

Il nous semble que chaque insecte a son parasite attaché à son existence ; le plus ordinairement il ne se développe que dans l'intérieur de la chrysalide, dont il sort à l'état parfait.

A la vue des ravages que causent certains insectes, les agriculteurs, rapportant tout à leur intérêt personnel, frappent indistinctement de proscription tous ceux qu'ils trouvent dans leurs cultures et sur leurs produits, quoiqu'il en soit parmi eux qui leur sont de puissants auxiliaires contre les espèces nuisibles.

Ils sont inappréciables, les services que nous rendent ces parasites ; trop souvent ignorés des cultivateurs, qui les prennent à tort pour les ennemis de leurs récoltes, dont ils sont au contraire les protecteurs.

Les ichneumons de Linné sont des insectes de la classe des hyménoptères, ayant les antennes soyeuses, vibratiles, fort longues, l'abdomen cylindrique, avec une tarière longue,

garnie de trois filets. Dans les femelles, ils sout particulière-
meut les parasites des *cephus,* des *cécidomyies* et du *ceraphron
destructeur :* ces petites mouches n'arrêtent pas immédiate-
ment le ravage des insectes, puisqu'elles ne les frappent pas
de suite de mort ; mais elles sont d'un bon augure pour l'année
snivante, quand on les voit en grande quantité, puisqu'elles
arrêtent souvent la grande propagation des ravageurs.

On a remarqué qu'au bout de deux ou trois ans de ravages
des cécidomyies, souvent les parasites prenaient le dessus, et
les récoltes revenaient à leur cours ordinaire.

L'alucite a pour parasite une petite mouche noire, que l'on
croit être la même que celle de la cécidomyie. C'est pour aider
à la distinguer, que nous avons fait dessiner l'une et l'autre,
car il y a fort peu de différence.

Ici se présente une question : Doit-on détruire les insectes
ravageurs à l'état parfait ou à l'état d'œufs, de larve ou de
chrysalide ? Les avis sont partagés. Quelques praticiens font
incinérer les chaumes après la récolte pour détruire les larves
des cécidomyies et celles des cephus.

D'autres battent de suite leurs gerbes, nettoient le grain et
font brûler les criblures. De cette manière, ils détruisent
beaucoup d'œufs, de larves et de chrysalides. Quelques per-
sonnes pensent qu'agir ainsi c'est se priver du chaume et des
criblures qui peuvent rendre quelques services. C'est se
priver aussi du secours des parasites qui sont dans les larves.
Elles préfèrent qu'on détruise l'insecte ailé ; nous pensons
qu'en théorie ces derniers ont raison ; car, en détruisant l'insecte non parfait, c'est se priver du concours des parasites,
qui, par la ponte de leurs œufs, détruiraient des centaines de
cécidomyies ou d'alucites, puisqu'ils ne déposent qu'un œuf
dans chaque larve. Nous pensons aussi que la difficulté gît
dans la possibilité d'atteindre l'insecte parfait en assez grande
quantité. Puis beaucoup ont une existence éphémère et ne
revêtent la dernière forme que pour pondre et mourir peu

après. Pourrait-on saisir le moment opportun ? Le cultivateur doit, selon nous, être continuellement sur la défensive, et saisir toutes les occasions pour combattre l'ennemi de ses récoltes. Il doit le détruire, sous toutes les formes que l'ennemi revêt.

Outre les parasites, les insectes ont encore une infinité d'ennemis dans la classe des oiseaux insectivores, tels que les mésanges, les bergeronnettes, les fauvettes, les hirondelles, les moineaux francs, etc., ainsi que les chauves-souris, qui sont d'un autre ordre. Les gallinacées de nos basses-cours sont aussi très-avides des sauterelles et des criquets.

Nous avons vu avec peine quelques cultivateurs détruire les fauvettes, les rouge-gorges, les verdiers, etc. Nous croyons qu'ils commettent un acte inintelligent en tuant ces oiseaux occupés à chercher dans les épis les larves des cécidomyies et celles des phalènes du seigle; ils croient à tort que ces charmants petits oiseaux mangent le grain quand il est à peine à demi-mûr; qu'ils sachent donc que ces oiseaux sont des auxiliaires inappréciables qui détruisent les ennemis de leurs céréales, et qu'il faut les respecter, l'homme n'ayant encore que de très-faibles moyens de destruction à sa disposition (1).

Les cécidomyies et l'alucite ont aussi pour ennemie une petite araignée qui tend ses toiles sur les tiges du blé; nous avons vu plusieurs de ces insectes y trouver la mort.

Si la nature est la conservatrice par excellence de ses œuvres, elle en est aussi, dans bien des circonstances, la plus grande destructrice, afin de maintenir l'ordre, l'harmonie qu'elle établit. En effet, combien d'insectes qui périssent par milliers, par millions, lors des inondations, à la suite des longues pluies d'orages, des neiges durables, etc. Enfin, le

(1) Voir nos réflexions sur les oiseaux entomovores, de 1836.

manque de nourriture les fait mourir d'inanition, ou les force
à se dévorer eux-mêmes... O éternelle Providence ! !

2° De l'intempérie des saisons.

L'intempérie des saisons est un des grands moyens qu'emploie la nature pour arrêter la trop grande propagation des insectes destructeurs des céréales ; mais il est des conditions vec lesquelles ces intempéries doivent coïncider, pour être salutaires. Ainsi, les cultivateurs comptent beaucoup trop sur es hivers rigoureux, les fortes gelées, pour détruire les œufs les larves et les chrysalides.

Depuis les belles expériences de Réaumur, les entomologistes savent, et ils se sont convaincus que les insectes, à l'état dormant, passent et bravent impunément les hivers rigou-ux, surtout dans les terrains secs.

Il n'en est pas de même des chaleurs ; rien n'est plus funeste aux chrysalides, aux larves et aux œufs, qu'un soleil desséchant ; les étés secs sont contraires au développement des noctuelles, des cephus, des cécidomyies, etc. ; c'est pour cela qu'on a conseillé des labours, des hersages aussitôt après la récolte, soit pour enterrer outre mesure les œufs et les larves, soit pour les exposer aux dernières chaleurs de l'été et à celles de l'automne.

Un puissant moyen de destruction, ce sont les pluies froides au moment de l'éclosion des chenilles et de la transformation de celles-ci en papillons, ainsi que les pluies venues au moment de la ponte. Il est rare que les lépidoptères résistent aux pluies froides survenues à ces époques ; la Touraine en a vu des exemples très-frappants en 1816-1830, et récemment en 1860. Les intempéries de l'été dernier causèrent assurément beaucoup de tort aux agriculteurs ; nous devons dire, pour être justes, qu'elles les débarrassèrent de plusieurs insectes redoutablés pour leurs récoltes, comme la teigne-padelle, qui dévastait les pommiers depuis trois ans (1), l'alucite et la teigne des blés, qui infestaient les grains ; ces trois lépidoptères disparurent comme par enchantement ; ce qui fut une légère compensation aux dégâts que ces pluies causèrent à nos récoltes.

DES MOYENS QUE L'HOMME EMPLOIE.

Les moyens que l'homme emploie pour combattre les insectes qui attaquent les grains sont fort nombreux assurément. Nous ne rappellerons pas ici les moyens que nous avons indiqués dans la première partie pour les teignes et les alucites ; nous y renvoyons le lecteur. Ceux que nous indiquerons se divisent naturellement en deux catégories :

1° Ceux qu'on peut employer dans les champs ;

2° Ceux qu'on peut pratiquer sur le grain et la farine dans les habitations.

Première catégorie — Parmi les premiers, nous devons compter les labours, les défrichements ; la charrue est le grand ennemi des sauterelles, des criquets, des cephus. etc. ; elle enterre profondément les œufs, ou les expose aux ardeurs du soleil.

Nous devons signaler aussi les assolements perfectionnés, alternes et variés : ainsi nos varennes, malgré la douceur de leur climat, la légèreté de leurs terrains sablonneux, sont, proportion gardée, moins sujettes aux ravages des insectes que les champs de nos plateaux ; ils y trouvent d'autres plantes moins

(1) La chenille qu'on a remarquée sur les pommiers en mai, juin et juillet 1861, était la *pyrale oporante* de Bosc, et non la teigne padelle de 1860 ; elles ne font pas leurs métamorphoses à la même époque, puis leurs dégâts ne sont pas de même nature.

convenables à leur nourriture ; puis, les fréquents labours et les sarclages souvent renouvelés sont sans doute contraires à leurs habitudes et à leurs moyens de propagation.

Nous devons aussi comprendre parmi les moyens destructeurs l'excellente méthode de couper les céréales très-près de terre et d'enlever le chaume de suite après la récolte ; par ces moyens, on enlève les larves de quantité d'insectes qui ont déposé leurs œufs dans la tige, et on les empêche de se métamorphoser ; elles finissent par périr et dessécher, faute d'humidité ; on voit que toutes les bonnes méthodes agricoles concourent à préserver nos cultures de céréales du fléau des insectes.

On a aussi conseillé l'emploi de certains engrais mis en couverture au printemps, comme les tourteaux de colza, de navette, la chaux, le plâtre en poudre : ce sont souvent pour beaucoup d'insectes des poisons très-énergiques, ou ces substances contrarient leur goût, leurs mœurs.

Nous avons conseillé d'allumer des feux le soir auprès des pièces de blés menacées d'alucite, de cécidomyie et de phalènes ; ces insectes viennent s'y brûler en assez grand nombre. En juillet 1859, nous vimes dans la varenne de La Riche, au moment où l'on brûlait des chiendents, des alucites, des noctuelles, et autres lépidoptères venir y brûler leurs ailes.

On a recommandé de semer tard ou de semer tôt, afin, disait-on, par ce moyen, de changer l'époque de la floraison ; on pensait échapper à la ponte des cécidomyies et à celle des alucites. C'est une erreur, car il n'appartient pas à l'homme de retarder ni d'avancer la floraison ; d'ailleurs l'insecte, par instinct, prolonge son existence jusqu'à ce qu'il ait rempli l'acte de la reproduction, qui est le but de la nature.

Enfin, que le laboureur sache bien que ce n'est qu'aux dépens de ses intérêts qu'il intervertit l'ordre naturel de ses récoltes.

DEUXIÈME CATÉGORIE. — Les moyens que l'on peut pratiquer sur le grain et la farine, dans les réserves, pour combattre les insectes, sont encore plus nombreux que ceux employés dans les champs ; on pourrait plutôt dire qu'il n'y en a
pas, puisqu'aucun n'est entré dans la pratique, et qu'on en
cherche et propose de nouveaux chaque jour.

C'est à prévenir l'invasion des insectes que doit s'appliquer
le cultivateur ; les moyens les plus usités sont l'aération, la
ventilation, l'éclairage des magasins et greniers à blé, puis le
pelletage, le criblage et le vannage des grains. On sait que
les insectes qui attaquent le grain aiment la tranquillité,
qu'ils fuient le bruit et la lumière. Aussi le cultivateur intelli-
gent met à profit ces mœurs.

La transformation des greniers à blés infestés en greniers à
fourrages, pendant deux ou trois ans, suffit ordinairement
pour les chasser. Les greniers très-éclairés, bien ventilés,
ayant des murs inclinés et très-polis, ne présentant aucune
anfractuosité ni crevasses, sont aussi d'une grande ressource
pour préserver le grain des cadelles, des charançons, des
yponomeutes, etc. L'emploi du grenier conservateur de notre
honorable collègue, M. Pavy, de Girardet, remplace avec
succès tous les moyens ci-dessus indiqués.

Les moyens de détruire les insectes qui attaquent les farines sont assez restreints. On ne peut utilement proposer de
moyen direct pour détruire les *blattes* et les *ténébrions*, car ils
ne sortent que la nuit, et ils se sauvent dès qu'ils voient la
lumière ; on ne peut en tuer qu'un petit nombre en leur faisant la chasse ; l'empoisonnement avec les substances corro-
sives serait un moyen assez sûr, s'il n'entraînait pas de graves
inconvénients.

Le bluttage, le tamisage des farines plusieurs fois par an
est un bon moyen pour les débarrasser des larves. La pro-
preté, l'aération dans les boulangeries, dans les magasins de

farine, leur éclairage, et le recrépissage exact des murs sont les moyens préservatifs les plus certains.

Nous tenons à consigner ici le résultat d'expériences que nous avons faites en 1836, et qui nous ont prouvé que le charançon est extrêmement vivace et très-difficile à tuer, et qu'il est habitué à vivre dans des lieux presque privés d'air oxygéné. Nous avons vu des centaines de charançons vivre des mois entiers dans un bocal bien fermé contenant du blé, et de l'acide carbonique en telle quantité, que la lumière d'une bougie s'y éteignait; au bout de deux mois de séjour dans ce bocal; ils paraissaient morts; étant exposés à l'air pur et chaud, ils reprirent peu à peu la vie et le mouvement; ils n'étaient donc qu'engourdis.

M. le docteur Herpin (de l'Indre) rapporte un fait curieux qui vient à l'appui de nos observations : « J'ai vu, dit-il, des « charançons que j'avais noyés et conservés dans de l'alcool « pendant plusieurs jours, reprendre la vie et s'enfuir après « que l'alcool fut évaporé spontanément (1). » M. Doyère dit qu'il a trouvé des charançons vivant fort bien dans les silos remplis de blés; on sait que le grain fermente toujours et dégage de l'acide carbonique à cause de sa composition complexe (2). Le charançon peut donc vivre dans un air très-pauvre en oxygène.

Nous pourrions rapporter, à l'appui de notre assertion, les belles expériences que l'académicien Biot fit sur les insectes pour combattre les idées émises par plusieurs théoriciens, qui posent en principe, « que tout ce qui vit et respire a besoin « d'air oxygéné pour vivre. »

Dès 1853, je combattais les idées d'un de mes honorables collègues, M. Brame, qui, partant du même principe, proposait de détruire les charançons par l'emploi de gaz délétères,

---

(1) *Notice sur l'alucite*, Paris, 1860.
(2) *De l'alucite des céréales*, Paris, 1853, page 350.

et notamment par le dégagement d'acide carbonique dans les tas de blé des greniers et des magasins. Après avoir allégué les grands inconvénients que ces dégagements présentent, je lui répondis « qu'il y avait longtemps que j'avais fait des expé-
« riences avec divers gaz délétères sur les charançons ; que
« ces gaz, loin d'atteindre le but que je m'étais proposé, ne
« font qu'engourdir ces coléoptères, qui sont rappelés à la vie
« dès qu'ils sont exposés à l'air pur ; et j'ajoutais que tous les
« moyens de ce genre, préconisés jusqu'à ce jour, sont tout à
« fait impuissants ; que la science, malgré toutes les décou-
« vertes faites, n'a encore rien trouvé qui puisse combattre ce
« fléau avec succès (1). »

L'asphyxie par les gaz délétères est une expérience de labo-ratoire, mais difficile à appliquer en grand sur les gerbes et les tas de grains. Il faut, en agriculture, des moyens géné-raux peu coûteux, facilement praticables, et qui surgissent, pour ainsi dire, des actes mêmes de la vie et des mœurs des insectes.

Aussi, M. Delamarre, peu satisfait de tous les moyens connus, proposait en 1852 au gouvernement de décerner un prix très-élevé, « un million, à celui qui trouvera le moyen
« certain de détruire l'alucite, l'aiguillonnier et le charan-
« çon, etc. (2). »

La science et l'étude des insectes sont presque complètes. Ce qu'il s'agit de faire aujourd'hui, c'est d'étudier leurs mœurs, leurs habitudes ; car nous pensons que c'est de là que doivent sortir les moyens pratiques pour les détruire, ou du moins amoindrir leurs ravages.

Plus on étudie les insectes, plus on est porté à admirer la sage prévoyance de la nature pour conserver ce qu'elle a

(1) *Annales de la Société d'agriculture d'Indre-et-Loire*, tome XXXIIIe, page 50.

(2) *De l'alimentation des peuples et des réserves de grain*, Paris, 1852, page 138.

créé ; on voit que chaque individu satisfait instinctivement, et concourt, à son insu, à l'harmonie générale.

Nous pourrions être effrayés à la vue de tant d'ennemis qui sont d'une grande fécondité : mais, indépendamment des moyens qui sont en notre pouvoir, une loi bienfaisante de la nature a établi un équilibre qui s'oppose à l'accroissement d'une race aux dépens des autres.

Nous ne terminerons pas sans dire quelles agréables distractions, quelles douces jouissances nous ont procurées les études auxquelles nous nous sommes livrés sur les insectes, et les observations utiles et curieuses qu'elles nous ont amené à faire. Ici encore, nous avons retrouvé la trace de ces admirables lois de la nature qui nous montrent, jusque dans les infiniments petits, la prévoyance constante, la sollicitude merveilleuse qui préside à tous les phénomènes du monde physique. Notre but a été de populariser l'entomologie, et de chercher à tirer parti de cette science dans l'intérêt de l'agriculture. Puissions-nous avoir atteint ce but.

C'est à MM. les curés, à MM. les instituteurs, et aux hommes de bon sens vivant à la campagne, que nous recommandons l'étude de l'entomologie appliquée à l'agriculture. Tout en s'amusant agréablement, ils pourront faire quelques observations utiles aux cultivateurs, intéressantes pour la science, importantes pour tout le monde.

Tours, imp. Ladevèze.

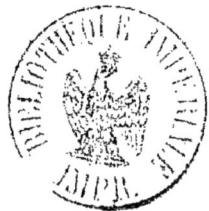

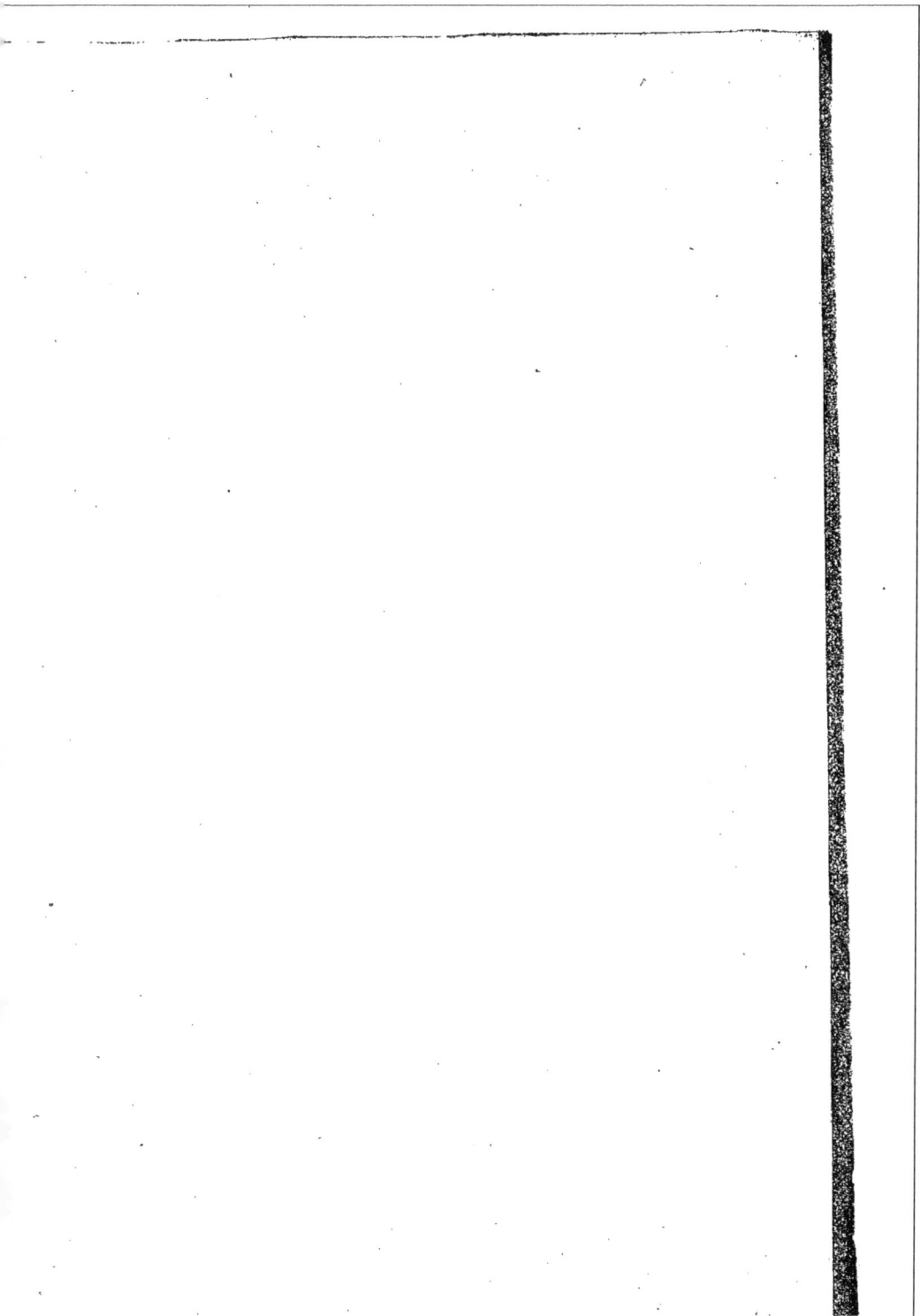

OUVRAGES DU MÊME AUTEUR.

Réflexions sur la destruction des oiseaux entomovores, 1835.

De l'état de l'agriculture en Touraine, 1851.

Notice sur la conservation des bois d'ouvrage, 1854.

Essai historique sur la meunerie et la boulangerie
en Touraine, 1855.

Notice sur les pucerons et autres insectes nuisibles
aux végétaux, 1856.

Essai historique sur la sériciculture de Chenon-
ceaux, 1860.

En collaboration avec M. Alonzo Péan :

Notice sur le canton de St-Aignan (Loir-et-
Cher), 1837.

Excursions archéologiques sur les bords du Cher,
avec carte, trois gravures et fac-similé, 1845.

En collaboration avec M. l'abbé Chevalier :

Études sur la Touraine, hydrographie, géologie,
agronomie, statistique, 1 volume de 400 pages avec
cartes et tableaux, à Tours, Guilland-Verger, libraire-
éditeur, 1858.

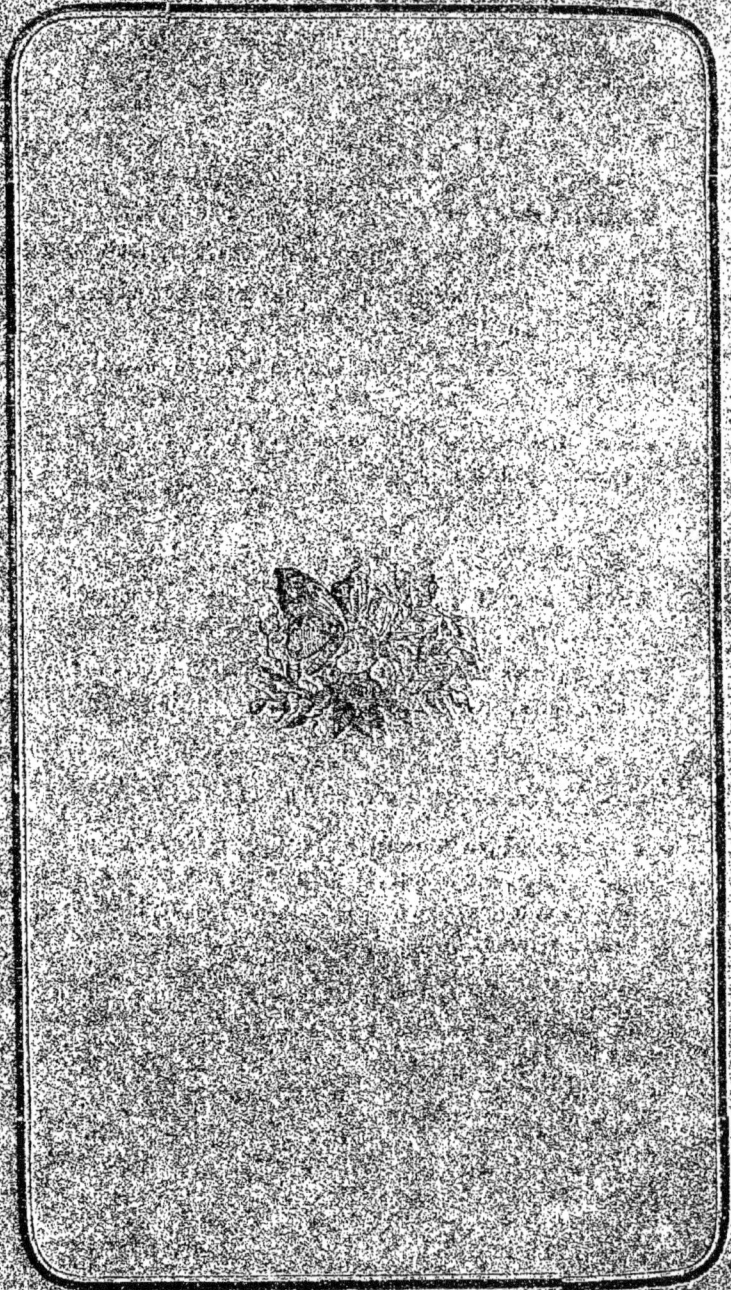

www.ingramcontent.com/pod-product-compliance
Lightning Source LLC
Chambersburg PA
CBHW060455210326
41520CB00015B/3954